Clinical Chemistry

Clinical Chemistry

Ninth Edition

William J. Marshall
MA PhD MSc MB BS FRCP FRCPath FRCPEdin FRSB FRSC

Emeritus Reader in Clinical Biochemistry, King's College London;
formerly Consultant Clinical Biochemist and Director of Pathology,
The London Clinic, London, UK

Marta Lapsley
MB BCh BAO MD FRCPath

Formerly Consultant Chemical Pathologist,
Epsom and St Helier University Hospitals NHS Trust, Epsom, Surrey, UK

Andrew Day
MA MSc MB BS FRCPath

Consultant in Clinical Biochemistry and Metabolic Medicine,
University Hospitals Bristol NHS Foundation Trust, Bristol, UK

Kate Shipman
MA BMBCh MRCP FRCPath

Consultant Chemical Pathologist, Western Sussex NHS Foundation Trust, Chichester, UK

ELSEVIER

Elsevier
3251 Riverport Lane
St. Louis, Missouri 63043

CLINICAL CHEMISTRY, NINTH EDITION
INTERNATIONAL EDITION
Copyright © 2021 by Elsevier Inc. All rights reserved.

ISBN: 978-0-702-0-7936-8
ISBN: 978-0-702-0-7930-6

Previous editions copyrighted 2017, 2012, 2008, 2004, 2000, 1995, 1992, and 1988.

Library of Congress Control Number: 2020936207

Content Strategist: Jeremy Bowes
Content Development Specialist: Dominque McPherson
Publishing Services Manager: Deepthi Unni
Project Manager: Srividhya Vidhyashankar
Design Direction: Bridget Hoette

Printed in Scotland

Last digit is the print number: 9 8 7 6 5 4 3 2

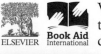

Preface

The information resources currently available to students are varied and numerous. However, despite the widespread availability of electronic materials, the appeal of a book has not lessened. This tangible tool remains popular, and with the ninth edition of this text and online extras, we hope to fulfil all the requirements of those seeking an introduction to clinical chemistry. Please do look at the electronic version for interactive diagrams and multiple-choice questions at varying levels of complexity.

This book was originally written primarily for medical students. However, the utility of a succinct review of the topic has been recognized by many disciplines, both clinical and scientific, and at all stages of training. With the help of comments received from readers around the world, we hope that we fulfil such varied requirements. Please do continue to provide us with your invaluable feedback so that we can further improve the book in future editions.

Each chapter includes a summary of the basic biochemistry and physiology upon which understanding clinical biochemistry depends. The nature, choice, use and limitations of laboratory investigations naturally comprise the bulk of each chapter, but clinical biochemistry is only one part of laboratory medicine, and laboratory tests comprise only one group among the many types of investigation available to support diagnosis and management. Other investigations—for example imaging—are mentioned and overviews of management options are provided; however, we stress that this book is not, and is not intended to be, a textbook of metabolic medicine.

Maybe we should not be surprised by the considerable number and rate of developments since the previous edition, but progress never ceases to amaze. In preparing this edition, there has been significant movement of material between chapters as well as an update and deletion of obsolete material, we hope in a logical manner. Throughout the text, there are new 'red flag sections' indicated by an exclamation mark heading in their respective boxes to emphasise biochemical findings that almost always indicate serious pathology.

We are fortunate enough to have a global readership, but when referring to best practice, UK guidelines are primarily used. Such 'local' guidance is clearly highlighted, but it should be borne in mind that population and service setup variations throughout the world may result in differences between what is considered gold standard and what is practical to provide.

At Elsevier, we have been ably supported by Jeremy Bowes and his fantastic team whose patience and professionalism have made the process a joy. Their cheerful encouragement and expertise have been much appreciated. We are indebted to the designers, copyeditor and indexer whose work has been essential to the production of the book.

At home, once again, Wendy (Marshall), Michèle (Day), Michael (Lapsley) and Alexa (Shipman) have been unstinting in their support and encouragement. We thank them for their significant, albeit indirect, contribution to this book.

William J. Marshall
Andrew Day
Marta Lapsley
Kate Shipman

Further Reading

To seek the most up-to-date information on a topic, readers are recommended to use one of the bibliographic databases that specialize in medical and scientific journals, for example Medline (the database of the National Library of Medicine in the USA, which encompasses references to reviews and papers published in more than 5000 journals and can be accessed via PubMed, www.ncbi.nlm.nih.gov/pubmed/).

Journals that publish articles and reviews relating to clinical chemistry include *Annals of Clinical Biochemistry* and *Clinical Chemistry*. Each issue of *Endocrine and Metabolism Clinics of North America* comprises sets of reviews on related topics, most of which are of direct relevance to clinical chemistry. General medical journals, such as the *British Medical Journal, Lancet* and *New England Journal of Medicine*, carry editorials and reviews of topics related to clinical chemistry from time to time. The monthly issues of *Medicine* together comprise a textbook of medicine, which is updated on a 3-year cycle and is highly recommended.

Many organizations produce guidelines for the investigation and treatment of various disorders, which are usually available online. In the UK, these include the National Institute for Health and Care Excellence (NICE, www.nice.org.uk) and the Scottish Intercollegiate Guidelines Network (SIGN, www.sign.ac.uk). A number of specialist societies produce and regularly update guidelines that are of relevance to the material discussed in this book. Some of these are listed below, and readers are encouraged to visit their websites for further information. Information about individual laboratory tests is available from Lab Tests Online-UK (http://labtestsonline.org.uk), a non-commercial website organized by the Association for Clinical Biochemistry and Laboratory Medicine.

And we would particularly draw attention to the American Association for Clinical Chemistry that hosts the Clinical Chemistry Trainee Council (https://www.aacc.org/clinical-chemistry-trainee-council). This fantastic and free resource is a repository for cases, questions, podcasts, lectures and guidance provided in several languages for trainees in clinical chemistry throughout the world.

Some specialist organizations that produce clinical guidelines

American Association of Clinical Endocrinologists	www.aace.com
Association for Clinical Biochemistry and Laboratory Medicine	www.acb.org.uk
British Association for Enteral and Parenteral Nutrition	www.bapen.org.uk
British Cardiovascular Society	www.bcs.com
British Endocrine Society	www.endocrinology.org
British Inherited Metabolic Diseases Group	www.bimdg.org.uk
British Society of Gastroenterology	www.bsg.org.uk
British Society for Haematology	www.b-s-h.org.uk
British Society for Rheumatology	www.rheumatology.org.uk
British Thyroid Association	www.british-thyroid-association.org

Diabetes UK	www.diabetes.org.uk
European Atherosclerosis Society	www.eas-society.org
Endocrine Society	www.endocrine.org
European Porphyria Network	www.porphyria.eu
European Renal Best Practice Group	www.european-renal-best-practice.org
European Society of Cardiology	www.escardio.org
Imperial Centre for Endocrinology (Endocrine Bible)	www.imperialendo.com/for-doctors/endocrine-bible
National Metabolic Biochemistry Network	www.metbio.net
Renal Association	www.renal.org

Content

Clinical Chemistry

Chapter | 1 |

An introduction to biochemistry and cell biology

Units and Measurements

The data generated by clinical biochemistry (chemical pathology) laboratories are primarily numerical and are mainly expressed as concentrations or units themselves based on concentrations or, in the case of enzymes, activities. Concentrations comprise two variables: the amount of the substance being measured and the amount of substance in which it is distributed. The Système Internationale (SI) paradigm for measurement expresses concentrations in molar terms – typically, in the case of substances measured in a fluid, as most of the substances of interest in clinical biochemistry are, in mmol/L (10^{-3} mol/L) or μmol/L (10^{-6} mol/L), nmol/L (10^{-9}/L) or pmol/L (10^{-12} mol/L). A mole is the amount of a substance equal to the molecular mass expressed in grams – thus, a mole of glucose ($C_6H_{12}O_6$) is $(6 \times 12) + (12 \times 1) + (6 \times 16) = 180$ g, where the second value in each set of parentheses is the atomic mass of the component elements. For substances for which the molecular mass is not known, concentrations may be expressed in units per litre (U/L), where a unit is usually traceable to a single preparation of known purity, or in mass units (g, mg or μg/L). Whereas the SI nomenclature is the standard in the UK and in many countries, mass units are still widely used in the USA and some other countries and, confusingly, are used even in the UK for some drugs.

In this book, in accord with UK practice, we use SI units except where mass units are still preferred, but readers should be aware that typical values and reference intervals will be different between the two systems.

Although an SI unit for enzyme activity exists (the katal (abbreviated as kat), defined as the amount of enzyme that will catalyse the reaction of 1 mol of substrate under specified conditions), even in the UK, enzyme activities are usually expressed as U/L, where a unit is traceable to a preparation with known activity.

Using SI units, the partial pressures of gases (i.e. the component of overall gas pressure exerted by an individual component of a gas mixture) are expressed in kilopascals (kPa), but the former nomenclature (millimetres of mercury [mmHg]) is still widely used. By way of example, the percentage of oxygen in the atmosphere is approximately 21%; the atmospheric pressure at sea level is approximately 101 kPa, so the partial pressure of oxygen (Po_2) is: $0.21 \times 101 = 21$ kPa.

Readers should also be aware that all numerical measurements are subject to imprecision (the inherent variability of any measurement), and effective appreciation of the significance of biochemical data depends on an understanding of the concept of precision. Precision is discussed further in Chapter 2.

Analytical Techniques

It is beyond the scope of this book to discuss the techniques used in the laboratory to generate biochemical data, which include photometric techniques (in which the presence of an analyte generates a change in the intensity of emitted visible or ultraviolet radiation), ion-selective electrodes and separation techniques (e.g. chromatography in its many formats). Although the exact procedure used in different laboratories may vary (largely because the manufacturers of analytical equipment adopt slight variations in their methods), the results generated will typically be relatively independent of the precise method and are comparable between different instruments and, thus, different laboratories.

In brief, **photometric techniques** involve the reaction of the analyte in either a chemical or enzyme-catalysed reaction to cause a change in the concentration of a substance that in turn causes a change in the absorption or emission of radiation at a specific wavelength. Many enzyme-based methods ultimately depend on the conversion of NAD^+ to NADH (or vice versa) and consequent change in the absorption of radiation at 360 nm. (Note that in this context, enzymes are being used as reagents: it is not the enzyme activity that is being measured, although many enzymes are measured using such techniques so that the reaction mixture contains both the enzyme being measured and the enzyme[s] used to generate the signal that is detected by the analytical instrument.)

Ion-selective electrodes are used for measuring ions such as Na^+, K^+ and H^+. These work on the principle that the analyte generates a potential difference (voltage) across a selective membrane (i.e. one that is permeable only to the ion in question), which can be measured using a sensitive voltameter. Measurement of the partial pressure of carbon dioxide (P_{CO_2}) also uses an ion-selective electrode, and that of oxygen (P_{O_2}) uses a related technique.

Atomic emission spectroscopy—the detection of the radiation emitted by a substance when it is heated in a flame (the bright red colour produced in strontium-containing fireworks is a familiar example)—was previously widely used to measure sodium, potassium and lithium, but it has been largely superseded by the use of ion-selective electrodes. **Atomic absorption spectroscopy**, where the absorption of radiation of a specific wavelength by a substance is quantified, is still widely used for measuring the concentration of metals such as copper, although more accurate and reliable techniques are now available and are typically used in laboratories that specialize in such investigations.

Separation techniques are widely used in clinical biochemistry either alone (as with capillary zone **electrophoresis** to detect paraproteins; see Chapter 16) or as a preliminary to measurement by one of many techniques depending on the nature of the analyte. The introduction of **chromatography coupled to detection by mass spectrometry** has been of particular importance in measuring metabolites of interest in relation to inherited metabolic diseases, drugs and hormones, and it allows accurate measurements at very low concentrations.

To be of value, analytical methods must be both specific (measuring only the substance of interest) and sensitive (able to measure biologically relevant concentrations with precision [i.e. reproducibly] and accurately [i.e. correctly]). Note that the terms 'sensitivity' and 'specificity' are used in other contexts in clinical biochemistry, as discussed in Chapter 2.

Whereas some substances measured in clinical biochemistry laboratories are present in serum or urine (the most frequent fluids in which measurements are made) at relatively high concentrations (e.g. sodium ~140 mmol/L, albumin 40 g/L), others, particularly some hormones, are present at only very low concentrations (e.g. picomolar, that is, 10^{-12} mol/L). This poses huge technical challenges. In general, assays become less precise at low concentrations, and in some cases, it may (at least at present) be impossible to measure accurately such concentrations even if they are biologically relevant. For this reason, some reference intervals (the range of values typical of a defined population, see Chapter 2) may not have a defined lower limit. It is then usual to give the lower limit as zero, but it is more informative to quote the lower limit of detection – that is, the lowest measurable concentration that can be reliably distinguished from zero. These limitations can be classified as chemical or physical. This is an important consideration in attempting to measure reduced concentrations of substances, where the limitations of the method may prevent a distinction being made between a normal and a reduced value.

Laboratory measurements are made to detect and monitor pathological changes, but it is important to be aware that **many measurements are affected by a range of physiological and environmental factors** (e.g. time of day, relation to meals), and these must be borne in mind when interpreting the result of laboratory tests. This topic is discussed further in Chapter 2. Finally, drugs are a frequent cause of assay interference, either through a direct effect on the assay itself (i.e. behaving like the analyte of interest, an example being prednisolone, which reacts in many assays for cortisol) or through a pharmacological effect (certain diuretics that cause hypokalaemia, for example). Further instances are discussed where relevant in the ensuing chapters of this book.

Particular problems are posed by **immunoassays**, widely used for measuring hormones (both peptide and steroid hormones), other peptides, proteins (including most tumour markers) and some drugs. Immunoassays are based on antibodies that are chosen to react specifically with individual molecular species. Two major problems arise from this: first, antibodies may (and often do) lack specificity (i.e. they may bind to structurally closely related molecules to that of interest – e.g. 11-deoxycortisol is detected by many cortisol assays); and second, the antibodies developed and used by different suppliers of analytical instruments may react with different epitopes on the surface of the target molecule. Assay interference and variability between different manufacturers' methods is a potential problem with all immunoassays but is particularly so with tumour markers.

Ions and Molecules of Biological Importance

A considerable range of substances are of biological importance. **Ions** are atoms or molecules that carry an electric charge, either overall positive or negative (or sometimes carrying charges that cancel each other out, e.g. one positive and one negative charge: these are termed 'zwitterions'). Important chemical groups that can readily ionize include amino ($-NH_2$) and carboxyl ($-COOH$) groups: amino groups readily gain a proton (i.e. a hydrogen ion, H^+) to become $-NH_3^+$, whereas carboxyl groups readily lose a proton to become $-COO^-$. **Groups that can release a proton are termed 'acidic'; those that can gain a proton are called 'basic'.** Whether a molecule forms an ion depends on the prevailing hydrogen ion concentration. Hydroxyl ($-OH$) groups do not ionize but can interact with other hydroxyl groups (including those in water) in a process called 'hydrogen bonding'. Substances that are capable of becoming charged are termed 'polar'. Water is a strongly polar molecule (capable of dissociation into positively charged hydrogen ions (H^+) and negatively charged hydroxyl ions (OH^-). Because of this, polar entities are typically soluble in aqueous media such as plasma but can only cross cell and intracellular membranes through special channels, access through which is often subject to control. This is because the outward-facing surfaces of such membranes are non-polar. On the other hand, non-polar entities are insoluble in aqueous media, and in the plasma circulate bound to soluble proteins, for example, albumin. However, they can typically cross cell and intracellular membranes unaided. Many molecules have both polar and non-polar regions. In proteins, for example, the non-polar (also termed 'lipophilic' or 'hydrophobic') regions tend to be in the interior of the molecule, whereas the polar (lipophobic, hydrophilic) regions face outwards. The same is true of molecular aggregates, for example, lipoproteins (see Chapter 17).

Small ions of biological importance include sodium and potassium, which carry single positive charges, and calcium and magnesium, which carry two positive charges. Positively charged ions are termed **cations**. Hydrogen ions (single positive charge) are particularly important cations. their concentration in a fluid determines the extent of ionization of all polar entities. Negatively charged ions include chloride and bicarbonate (one charge) and phosphate (one, two or three charges, according to the prevailing hydrogen ion concentration). These are collectively known as **anions**.

Several groups of small molecules are of major biological importance. Simple **carbohydrates** (sugars, Fig. 1.1), such as glucose, fructose, ribose and deoxyribose, consist of carbon, hydrogen and oxygen. These are readily soluble in water because of the interaction of their hydroxyl groups with water molecules ($H-O-H$). Carbohydrates are important energy sources and, in the case of ribose and deoxyribose, are components of nucleic acids (deoxyribonucleic acid [DNA], the repository of genetic information, and ribonucleic acid [RNA], important in the translation of genetic information into the synthesis of functional proteins, respectively). Nucleic acids are polymers of **nucleotides** (comprising ribose or deoxyribose linked to

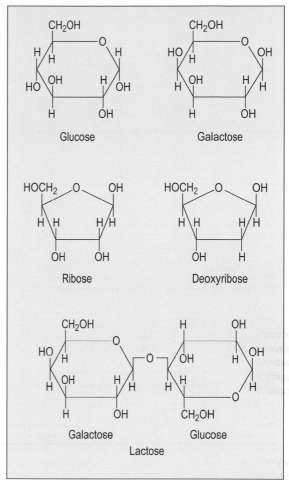

Fig. 1.1 Examples of single carbohydrates (monosaccharides) and a disaccharide (lactose, comprising one molecule of glucose and one of galactose). Glucose and galactose are hexoses (six carbon atoms); ribose and deoxyribose are pentoses (five carbon atoms).

a phosphate residue and a purine or pyrimidine, Fig. 1.2). Individual nucleotides (e.g. adenosine triphosphate [ATP]) play a major role in providing energy to power chemical reactions in cells. Simple sugars can bind to other sugars to form disaccharides, trisaccharides and polysaccharides. The latter include glycogen, an important energy store in the body, starch and dietary fibre (Fig. 1.3).

Fatty acids also comprise carbon, hydrogen and oxygen, and they consist of a chain of hydrogenated carbon atoms of variable length (an alkyl chain) with a terminal carboxyl group (Fig. 1.4). Short-chain fatty acids are soluble in water, but solubility decreases with increasing length of the carbon chain. Fatty acids can be either **saturated** or **unsaturated**. In saturated fatty acids, each carbon atom in the

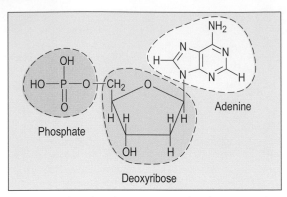

Fig. 1.2 A nucleotide, adenosine monophosphate, comprising a phosphorylated pentose linked to a nitrogenous base, in this case, adenine. DNA and RNA consist of linear chains of nucleotides. In DNA, the pentose is deoxyribose, in RNA, it is ribose. The base can be a purine, either adenine or guanine, or a pyrimidine (thymine or cytosine in DNA, cytosine or uracil in RNA). The double-stranded structure of DNA is maintained through hydrogen bonding between pairs of bases.

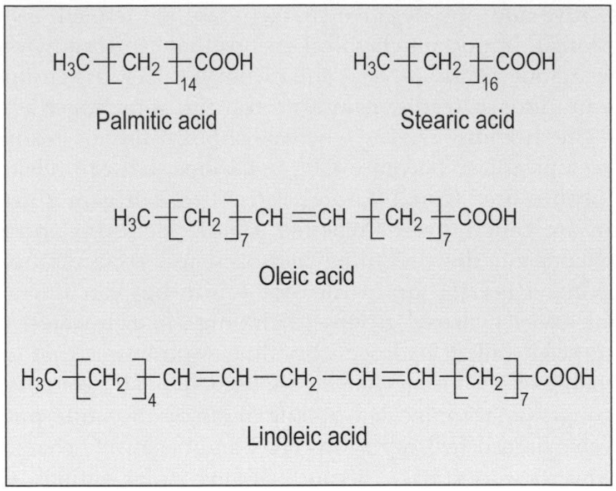

Fig. 1.4 Long-chain fatty acids. The most commonly occurring in the human body are palmitic and stearic acids. Oleic acid is a monounsaturated fatty acid; linoleic acid is a polyunsaturated fatty acid.

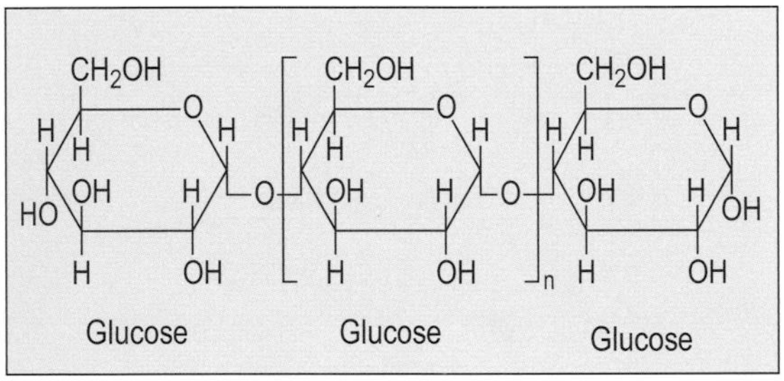

Fig. 1.3 Amylose, a polysaccharide, is a linear polymer of glucose and a component of starch. Glycogen is also a polymer of glucose but has a branched structure.

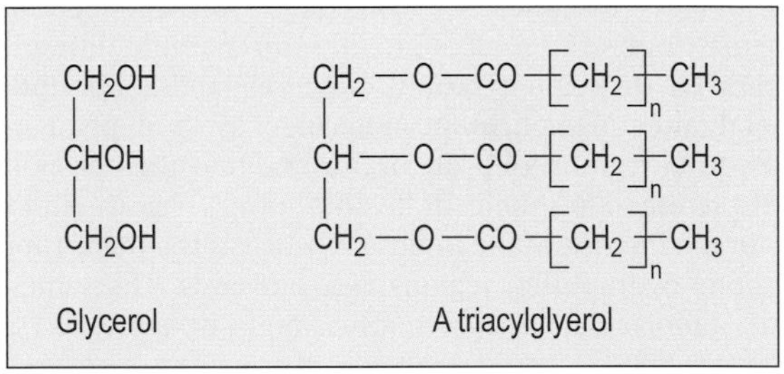

Fig. 1.5 Glycerol and triacylglycerols (triglycerides). In tripalmityl glycerol, n = 14. In any one molecule, the fatty acids are always the same.

chain carries two hydrogen atoms—that is, is a methylene group—except for the first, which carries three (a methyl group): the carbon atoms in the chain are linked by single covalent bonds. In unsaturated fatty acids, an even number of adjacent carbon atoms carry only one hydrogen, and these carbons are linked by double bonds.

Alcohols are substances that carry one or more hydroxyl groups. The simplest is methanol, CH_3OH. The most important in mammalian biochemistry is glycerol (Fig. 1.5), a trihydric (three –OH groups) alcohol, which can combine with fatty acids (esterification) to form **triacylglycerols** (often referred to as **triglycerides**, see Fig. 1.5). These substances are all discussed in detail in Chapter 17. They are important for energy storage. Entities in which two of the hydroxyls of glycerol are combined with fatty acids and the third with a phosphate- or nitrogen-containing substance are important structurally, particularly in cell and intracellular membranes (Fig. 1.6).

Amino acids contain at least one carboxyl and one amino group (Fig. 1.7). When there is one of each, an amino acid is said to be neutral: those with two carboxyl and one amino group are acidic, and those with one carboxyl and two amino groups are basic. With the exception of glycine, all amino acids contain a carbon atom with four different substituents (i.e. covalently bound to four different groups). These groups can be arranged spatially in two different ways; these are termed **stereoisomers**. They have the same chemical composition, but their physical structure is different. Stereoisomers are termed either D- or L-. All amino acids that occur in humans (and other mammals) are L-isomers. Some amino acids can be synthesized in the body; others cannot and must be provided in the diet. The former amino acids are termed 'non-essential' and the latter are termed 'essential'. Amino acids can combine together to form **peptides** (Fig. 1.8). These can comprise small or large numbers of amino acids (oligopeptides and polypeptides, respectively). The former peptides include many hormones, growth factors and other signalling molecules, particularly cytokines (chemokines, lymphokines, interferons, tumour necrosis factor and interleukins). Polypeptides are also termed proteins (see later).

Steroids are complex molecules that share a four-ringed cyclopentaphenanthrene basic structure (Fig. 1.9), usually with methyl groups attached to positions C-10 and C-13 and a substituent or alkyl side chain at C-17. **Sterols** (see Fig. 1.9) are steroid alcohols, with an hydroxyl group at C-3. Biologically important steroids include cholesterol, bile acids and the steroid hormones (sex hormones, glucocorticoids, mineralocorticoids and bile acids all being derived from cholesterol).

These entities are discussed in more detail in later chapters in this book. Steroids are also important components of cell and intracellular membranes (see later).

Proteins are linear polymers of amino acids, linked by peptide bonds, often (arbitrarily) with molecular weights >5 kDa. **Their structure can be described at four levels: primary**—that is, the amino acid sequence; **secondary**—the arrangement of various parts of the sequence into elements with three-dimensional structure; **tertiary**—the folding of these various elements into the functional protein; and **quaternary** (seen only with some proteins)—when these units associate together to form aggregates, for example, haemoglobin, which consists of four globin molecules. Such aggregates may comprise the same molecules or different ones. Haemoglobin, for example, comprises two molecules of α globin and two of β globin.

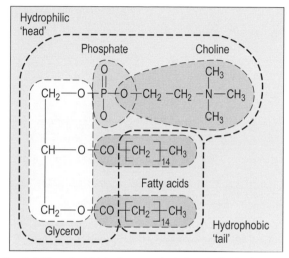

Fig. 1.6 Phosphatidylcholine, a typical phospholipid. These molecules comprise a hydrophobic (non-polar) 'tail' and a hydrophilic (polar) 'head', the former being the fatty acid residues and the latter encompassing the glycerol, phosphate and nitrogenous base residues.

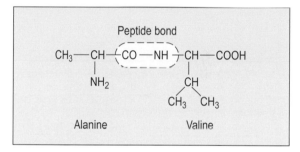

Fig. 1.8 Alanylvaline, a dipeptide. The peptide bond is formed by the elimination of water from the carboxyl group of one amino acid and the amino group of another.

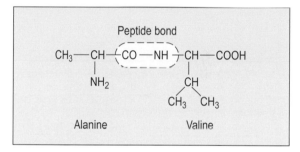

Fig. 1.7 Examples of amino acids. Glycine is the simplest. Phenylalanine is an aromatic amino acid; cysteine contains sulphur; lysine, with two amino groups, is a basic amino acid, and glutamic acid, with two carboxyl groups, is acidic.

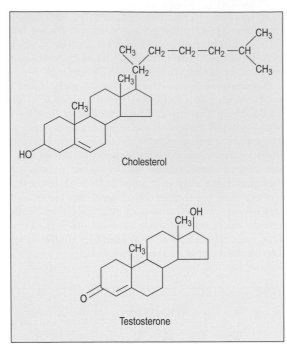

Fig. 1.9 Cholesterol, the precursor molecule of all steroids (e.g. steroid hormones and bile acids), and testosterone, a steroid hormone. These molecules all have a similar basic four-ring structure.

Table 1.1 **Functions of proteins**	
Function	**Example**
buffering	albumin (although all proteins can act as buffers to some extent)
enzymic	alkaline phosphatase (involved in bone mineralization)
	renin (conversion of angiotensinogen to angiotensin)
	complement proteins (complement activation)
humoral immunity	immunoglobulins
maintenance of oncotic pressure	albumin
receptors	low-density lipoprotein receptor
structural	collagen (in bone, connective tissue etc.) spectrin (in red cell membranes)
transport: specific	haemoglobin (oxygen)
	hormone-binding proteins, e.g. thyroid-binding globulin
	glucose transporters
	apolipoproteins
	transferrin (iron)
transport: non-specific	albumin (calcium, fatty acids, bilirubin, drugs)

In the case of enzymes (see later), normal function may depend on the presence of a **prosthetic group** (an entity bound to the protein, e.g. haem in haemoglobin) or one or more **coenzymes** (small molecules that participate in the reaction). Coenzymes and prosthetic groups are often derived from **vitamins**, entities that are essential for life and normal function that must be present in the diet because they are not synthesized in the body (vitamin D, see p. 141, is an exception to this).

Haemoglobin is an example of a protein involved in transport (in this case, of oxygen). There are many other transport proteins, including a number in plasma such as albumin, various hormone-binding proteins and proteins involved in lipid transport (apolipoproteins; see Chapter 17). These proteins are discussed elsewhere in this book. Proteins are also important in facilitating transport across cell membranes (e.g. aquaporins in the kidney collecting ducts, see Chapter 3). Structural proteins include collagen. The immunoglobulins are a group of proteins that comprise an important element of the humoral immune system (see Chapter 16). **Enzymes** are proteins with catalytic activity and are involved in virtually all of the many chemical transformations, both synthetic and catabolic, that occur in

the body. Cell membrane and nuclear receptors (which mediate the interaction of signalling molecules such as hormones with cells) are also proteins. Proteins are synthesized using an RNA template (messenger RNA [mRNA]) derived from genomic DNA, in the rough endoplasmic reticulum of cells, but may undergo post-translational modification involving the addition of carbohydrate and other side chains. Receptors can bind both agonists (resulting in activation) and antagonists (having the opposite effect, often by blocking the binding of an agonist). Although many receptors are highly specific, some are not. For example, cortisol can bind to (and activate) the receptor for aldosterone. Many drugs exert their effects by binding to receptors. The functions of proteins are summarized in Table 1.1.

Elements of Cell Biology

The **cell** (Fig. 1.10) is the basic functional unit of the body. **Tissues** (e.g. adipose tissue) comprise cells of different types (although often with one predominating), and **organs** (e.g. the brain) and organ systems (e.g. the central nervous system) are formed from tissues of various types (e.g. in the case of the brain, nervous tissue, fibrous tissue and vascular tissue). Despite the multiplicity of functions of different cell types in the body, all have some elements in common.

All cells in the body are bounded by a **cell membrane**. These comprise a lipid bilayer (Fig. 1.11) with polar elements exposed to the exterior and interior of the cell, and non-polar elements 'sandwiched' between them. Cell membranes are selectively impermeable. Although some substances can diffuse freely through the membranes, others involve transport proteins, controllable channels (activated by binding of specific ligands) and invagination by the cell membrane to form a vesicle (Fig. 1.12).

Cells contain a fluid called **cytosol**, which surrounds the various intracellular **organelles**. All cells in the body (with the exception of erythrocytes [red blood cells]) contain a **nucleus**. This contains the genetic blueprint in the form of DNA. Apart from germ cells (precursors of ova and sperm), all cells contain a complete set of DNA, although in each cell, only a fraction of this is expressed and used to direct the synthesis of proteins. DNA is complexed with proteins into discrete elements called **chromosomes**, of which there are 46 in each somatic cell. The nucleus is the site of synthesis of mRNA, a process called **transcription**; this is exported from the nucleus to direct the synthesis of proteins (**translation**). The chromosomes are surrounded by a nuclear membrane, similar in composition and structure to the cell membrane. Cell nuclei also contain **nucleoli**, aggregates of RNA and proteins responsible for the assembly of ribosomes (see later).

Mitochondria are the intracellular organelles responsible for the generation of energy (typically in the form of ATP). This process depends on the generation of hydrogen ion gradients across the mitochondrial membrane. Mitochondria also contain small amounts of DNA which, in mammalian cells, is entirely maternally derived.

The **endoplasmic reticulum** consists of a network of membranes. The rough endoplasmic reticulum is studded with ribosomes and is the site of protein synthesis, both of intracellular proteins and proteins destined for export from the cell. The export itself depends on the activity of the membranous **Golgi apparatus**. The smooth endoplasmic reticulum subserves numerous functions, including the synthesis of lipids, phospholipids and steroids, and the inactivation (detoxication) of many drugs and other xenobiotics.

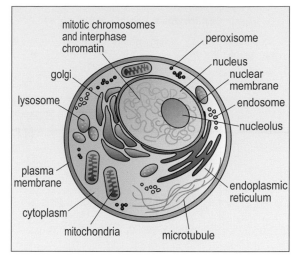

Fig. 1.10 Components of a mammalian cell.

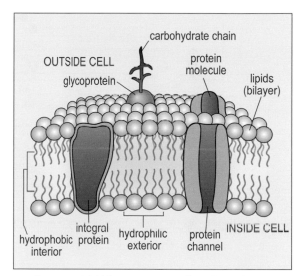

Fig. 1.11 Lipid bilayer structure of a cell membrane.

Vesicles are fluid-filled organelles bound by a bilayer membrane. They are formed during endocytosis (when something external to the cell is surrounded by the cell membrane, which fuses around it and becomes internalized) and exocytosis (the reverse, a mechanism for exporting matter from the cell; see Fig. 1.12). **Lysosomes** are specialized vesicles that contain fluid with a high hydrogen ion concentration relative to the rest of the cell and various lytic enzymes. They can fuse with endocytic vesicles and hydrolyse their contents. In certain inherited metabolic disorders, one of these enzymes is defective and internalized material is not degraded, causing what are termed 'storage disorders'.

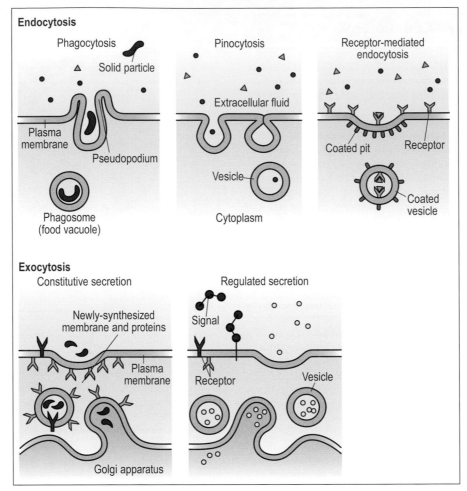

Fig. 1.12 Exocytosis and endocytosis. These processes allow cells to exclude or take up material that is too big to pass directly through the cell membrane. Endocytosis can be receptor mediated or not involve a receptor (the latter process being called 'pinocytosis'). In receptor-mediated endocytosis, the receptors are typically recycled to the cell surface.

Throughout the cytosol, the cellular **cytoskeleton** supports the structure of the cell. It comprises microtubules, microfilaments and intermediate filaments, themselves composed of various proteins including actin and tubulin. The cytoskeleton is particularly well- developed in muscle cells, where it provides the apparatus for muscle contraction.

Transport Mechanisms

Many cells and molecules are mobile in the body, and a variety of transport mechanisms exist that facilitates this. The blood is **pumped** through the vasculature, carrying red and white blood cells and platelets, as well as a huge range of soluble molecules. Substances with limited solubility (e.g. fatty acids) circulate bound to proteins, and many small molecules, for example, hormones, circulate bound to specific transport proteins. Molecules may **diffuse down their concentration gradients** through junctions between cells (e.g. between capillary endothelial cells). Inflammation may increase vascular permeability and increase the passage of larger molecules such as albumin and allow movement of cells such as white blood cells from the vascular to the extravascular compartment.

Several processes permit the transport of molecules into and out of cells. These include **simple diffusion** and **facilitated diffusion** (assisted by a carrier protein), neither of which is energy dependent; **active transport** (energy dependent, with or without the assistance of a transport protein and capable of moving substances against their concentration gradients); and **exocytosis and endocytosis**, involving interaction with the cell membrane and the formation of a vesicle that either is transported into or out of the cell. Transport across cell membranes is ubiquitous: it provides the mechanism for supplying nutrients to cells and removing unwanted substances, but some tissues have highly specialized transport functions. These include the enterocytes of the gut and the cells lining the nephrons in the kidneys, as well as all excitable cells (neurons and myocytes) where the selective transport of ions across cell membranes in response to a signal (e.g. the binding of a neurotransmitter to a receptor) stimulates a rapid, selective change in permeability, leading to the propagation of a nerve impulse or muscle contraction, respectively.

Water is not actively transported in the body (except mechanically in the vasculature and lymphatic system) but (except in parts of the nephrons of the kidneys, see p. 26) moves freely across most cell membranes and between cellular junctions in response to differences in osmolality, that is, the total molar concentration of all the constituent solutes present on either side of the cell membrane or cell junction. The importance of osmolality in determining the movement of water and the maintenance of water homoeostasis is discussed in detail in Chapter 3.

Cell Signalling

The need for cellular controls

Throughout the body, individual cells express selected genes from their identical genomes that allow them to perform their respective functions, e.g. the synthesis of hormones for export in the case of pancreatic beta cells and the detoxification of drugs in hepatocytes. In order to function to fulfil the needs of the body at any time, these processes must be controlled. Thus insulin is secreted in response to an increase in blood glucose concentration, and chronic exposure to some drugs can lead to an increased ability of hepatocytes to detoxify them.

Control is achieved by coordinated **signalling processes**. These fall into two basic categories: **chemical**, involving chemical mediators that are transported in the blood or directly between cells; and **neural**, involving electrical impulses transmitted along specialised cells called neurons.

Types of signalling

Chemical signalling comprises the **endocrine** system (the mediators are released from endocrine glands and are transported throughout the body by the bloodstream, typically to tissues remote from the secreting cells) and **paracrine**

signalling, where the mediators reach their (nearby) target cells by diffusion. In some cases, mediators also act on the cells secreting them (**autocrine** signalling). These mediators, called **hormones**, are typically polypeptides or steroids (the iodine-containing thyroid hormones are an exception). Neurons provide direct connections between the central nervous system and individual cells (which can themselves be neurons), but their effects are mediated through chemicals released from the nerve endings.

Chemical mediators and neural signals must gain access, directly or indirectly, to the interior of their target cells in order to exert their effects. This typically occurs through interaction of the mediators with specific cell-surface **receptors** that transduce the signal from the plasma or through gap junctions that allow direct access of the mediators to the cell cytoplasm. It is beyond the scope of this book to discuss most of the aspects of cell signalling in any detail, but some features are of particular relevance to clinical biochemistry.

The action of chemical mediators

Chemical mediators exert their effects through interaction with specific receptors that recognise and respond to that mediator in particular (i.e. they are **agonists**), although similar chemical entities may also interact with the receptor but have lower affinity and so unless present at high concentrations have a lesser effect (**partial agonists**). Mediators may also bind to a receptor and render it inactive (**antagonists**). The **receptors for polypeptide hormones** are located on cell surfaces. The **receptors for steroid and thyroid hormones** are located on cells' nuclear membranes: these hormones are small enough to be able to diffuse through the plasma membrane of the cell (Fig. 1.13). Binding of mediator to receptor can affect intracellular activity in various ways:

- by direct effects on gene transcription
- by opening an ion channel
- by activating a protein-bound kinase
- by activating a 'G-protein' that in turn initiates a chain of intracellular events involving other messenger molecules (**second messengers**) that themselves mediate the changes in cellular activity typical of the response of the cell to the hormone.

The relevance of signalling systems to clinical biochemistry

It follows that endocrine disorders can arise because of oversecretion or undersecretion of one or more hormones, secretion of a mutant hormone (typically having lower activity) or because of abnormal function of a receptor or one of the events occurring following binding to the receptor. Measurement of the concentrations of hormones

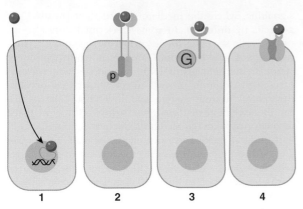

Fig. 1.13 Chemicals can signal cellular response through a variety of mechanisms the commonest of which are seen in this figure. 1. Nuclear receptor; 2. enzyme-linked receptor e.g. kinase; 3. G-protein-coupled receptor; 4. ion channel. G-proteins can then go on and activate other proteins including ion channels and enzymes.

in plasma, a major function of clinical biochemistry laboratories, is of huge importance in the investigation of endocrine diseases, but the intracellular processes are not amenable to biochemical investigation except in specialised laboratories.

Neurotransmitters are typically found at only very low concentrations systemically, and are not routinely measured. Indeed, most neurological disorders are not susceptible to biochemical investigation (see Chapter 18). Exceptions include the individually rare (but hugely important to patients and their families) lysosomal storage disorders. However, molecular genetic analysis is of increasing importance with genetically determined neurological disorders such as Huntington chorea, and measurement of acetylcholine antibodies (which may be performed in either biochemistry or immunology laboratories) is of importance in the diagnosis of myasthenia gravis. The measurement of the neurotransmitter noradrenaline (norepinephrine) is of importance in the diagnosis of tumours of the adrenal medulla and related tissues.

Chapter 2

Biochemical investigations in clinical medicine

Introduction

A central function of the chemical pathology or clinical biochemistry laboratory is to provide biochemical information for the management of patients. Such information will be of value only if it is accurate and relevant, and if its significance is appreciated by the clinician so that it can be used appropriately to guide clinical decision making. This chapter examines how biochemical data are acquired and how they should be used.

Use of Biochemical Investigations

Biochemical investigations are used extensively in medicine, both in relation to diseases that have an obvious metabolic basis (e.g. diabetes mellitus, hypothyroidism) and those in which biochemical changes are a consequence of a disease (e.g. kidney failure, malabsorption) or a treatment. The principal uses of biochemical investigations are for diagnosis, prognosis, monitoring and screening (Fig. 2.1).

The use of biochemistry results within a legal setting, e.g. for investigation of a crime or cause of suspicious death, is termed forensics. This is a specialized subfield due to the additional laboratory requirements to ensure that data are admissible in court. Though forensic work is rare, awareness of protocols, in both those taking and those processing the samples, on how to maintain the evidentiary chain of custody is necessary.

Diagnosis

Medical diagnosis is based on the patient's history, if available, the clinical signs found on examination, the results of investigations and sometimes, retrospectively, on the response to treatment. Frequently, a confident diagnosis can be made on the basis of the history combined with the findings on examination. Failing this, it is usually possible to formulate a differential diagnosis, in effect a short list of possible diagnoses. Selective biochemical and other investigations can then be used to distinguish between them.

It is important that the clinician appreciates how useful the chosen investigations are to help either confirm or refute a diagnosis. Detecting a metabolic abnormality, such as hypoglycaemia, even without a diagnosis of its cause, may allow treatment to be initiated.

Prognosis

Investigations used primarily for diagnosis may also provide prognostic information, while others are used specifically for this purpose. For example, serial measurements of plasma creatinine concentration in progressive kidney disease are used to indicate when dialysis may be required. Investigations can also indicate the risk of development of a particular condition. For example, the risk of coronary artery disease increases with increasing plasma cholesterol concentration. However, such risks are calculated from epidemiological data and cannot give a precise prediction for a particular individual.

Monitoring

A major use of biochemical investigations is to follow the course of an illness and to monitor the effects of treatment. A common example is the use of glycated haemoglobin to monitor the control of blood glucose in patients with diabetes mellitus. Biochemical investigations can also be used to detect complications of treatment, such as hypokalaemia during treatment with diuretics, and possible drug toxicity, such as the hepatotoxicity that may be caused by methotrexate.

11

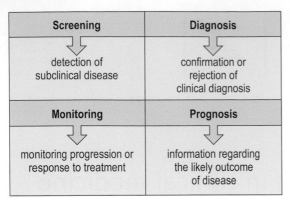

Screening	Diagnosis
⇩	⇩
detection of subclinical disease	confirmation or rejection of clinical diagnosis
Monitoring	Prognosis
⇩	⇩
monitoring progression or response to treatment	information regarding the likely outcome of disease

Fig. 2.1 Principal functions of biochemical tests.

Screening

Biochemical investigations are widely used to determine whether a condition is present subclinically. The best-known example is the mass screening of all newborns for phenylketonuria (PKU), congenital hypothyroidism and some other conditions that is carried out in many countries, including the UK and the USA. This is an example of **population screening**: other types include **selective screening** (e.g. of older people for carcinoma of the colon using the detection of faecal occult blood), **individual screening** (e.g. as part of a health checkup) and **opportunistic screening** (e.g. for hypercholesterolaemia in people found to have hypertension). Factors to consider when designing a screening programme are numerous and summarized in Box 2.1.

Specimen Collection

The test request

The specimen for analysis must be collected and transported to the laboratory according to a specified procedure if the data are to be of clinical value. This procedure begins with the clinician generating a test request, either on paper or electronically. Increasingly, computer systems are becoming more sophisticated, allowing use of 'intelligent' test requesting, where the clinician is presented with relevant information to help with the appropriate choice of test(s). This can inform the user and promote correct test selection as well as provide information on patient preparation, but it can lengthen the time taken to generate the request and is limited by the tests, information and algorithms included in the system. Prompting to provide clinical information can also enable more relevant interpretation of test results.

Box 2.1 Criteria to consider before implementation of a screening programme

The condition is an important health problem, there is a need for case identification
The natural history of the condition is understood
There is an early or latent phase
Treatment is more effective if started early
The treatment is acceptable to patients
That informed consent, confidentiality and autonomy are supported in the programme
The test is acceptable to the population and feasible to administer
The test has appropriate/acceptable characteristics such as sensitivity and specificity
There is a defined population with equity of access to the programme
The facilities to provide the testing and treatment are available
The test and treatment are cost-effective, and benefits outweigh the harm
There is a clear procedure, including education, treatment, quality assurance and evaluation, from the outset
That case-finding should be a continuous process
There is evidence to support effectiveness of a screening programme

The completed request should include:
- patient's name, sex and date of birth
- hospital or other patient identification number
- ward/clinic/address
- name of requesting doctor (telephone/pager number for urgent requests)
- clinical diagnosis/problem
- test(s) requested
- type of specimen
- date and time of sampling
- relevant treatment (e.g. drugs).

It is obviously necessary to provide sufficient information to identify the patient reliably, but the omission of any of the items in this list may either cause delay in analysis and reporting or make it impossible to interpret the results. Many laboratories publish a minimum data set without which they will refuse to analyse samples.

Relevant clinical information and details of treatment, especially with drugs, are necessary to allow laboratory staff to assess the results in their clinical context. Drugs may interfere with analytical methods *in vitro* or may cause changes *in vivo* that suggest a pathological process; for instance, some psychotropic drugs increase plasma prolactin concentration.

Table 2.1 Examples of important factors that influence biochemical variables

Factor	Example of variable affected
age	alkaline phosphatase, urate, cholesterol
sex	gonadal steroids, creatine kinase, HDL-cholesterol
ethnicity	creatine kinase, estimated glomerular filtration rate
pregnancy	urea, alkaline phosphatase, bicarbonate
posture	proteins
exercise	creatine kinase
stress	prolactin
nutritional intake	glucose, triglyceride, testosterone
time of day	cortisol, testosterone
drugs	γ-glutamyl transferase (phenytoin), prolactin (fluoxetine, risperidone)

All laboratories should publish user guides, preferably available online. These should provide information including the test repertoire, specimen requirements (see later), turnaround time, protocols for dynamic function testing and, preferably, local or national guidelines for the investigation or monitoring of particular conditions, together with contact details for making enquiries to the laboratory.

The patient

Some analytes are affected by variables such as posture, fasting status, time of day, etc., and it may be necessary to standardize the conditions under which the specimen is obtained. Factors of importance in this respect are listed in Table 2.1 and are discussed further in subsequent chapters.

Even when standardized conditions are used for sampling, the results of repeated tests (e.g. daily measurements of fasting blood glucose concentration) will show a Gaussian distribution, clustering about the 'usual' value for the individual. Typically, the scatter, which can be assessed by determining the standard deviation (SD), is less for analytes subject to strict regulation (e.g. plasma calcium and fasting glucose concentrations) than for others (e.g. plasma enzyme activities). This **biological variation** can be expressed as the coefficient of variation (CV) for repeated tests, where CV(%) = SD/mean value × 100.

The specimen

The specimen provided must be appropriate for the test requested. Most biochemical analyses are made on serum or plasma (see lightbulb section p. 22), but occasionally whole blood is required (e.g. for blood gases), and analyses of urine, cerebrospinal fluid, pleural fluid, etc. can also be valuable. For most analyses on serum or plasma, either fluid is acceptable, but in some instances it is of critical importance which of these is used; for example, serum is required for protein electrophoresis and plasma for measurement of renin activity. **Haemolysis** must be avoided when blood is drawn and, if the patient is receiving intravenous therapy, blood must be drawn from a remote site (e.g. the opposite arm) to avoid contamination. Haemolysis causes increases in plasma potassium and phosphate concentrations and aspartate aminotransferase activity, because of leakage from red blood cells. Results of other tests may also be affected by haemolysis because of interference in some analytical methods. If there is a delay in centrifugation to separate blood cells from plasma, glucose is metabolized and the concentration will fall, which also prevents the sodium pump from actively maintaining cellular gradients. Leakage from cells *in vitro* can therefore cause increases in plasma potassium and phosphate concentrations even in the absence of obvious haemolysis, particularly in patients with high white blood cell or platelet counts. The laboratory should always draw attention to potentially spurious results.

All specimens must be correctly labelled and transported to the laboratory without delay. There should be a written protocol for discarding incorrectly collected or labelled specimens. For tests on serum or plasma, the fluid is separated from blood cells by centrifugation and then analysed. Specimens must be stored appropriately to prevent degradation of analytes until the analysis is complete. Most laboratories will then refrigerate samples to store them for a short period after analysis and freeze for longer term storage for specific analytes or clinical indications.

Equal care is needed with the collection and transportation of other specimens, such as urine and cerebrospinal fluid. All specimens should be regarded as potentially infectious and handled using appropriate precautions.

Urgent requests

Laboratories should endeavour to generate results within a timescale appropriate to clinical requirements. Some requests will be urgent in that their results may have an immediate bearing on the management of the patient, e.g. the measurement of plasma paracetamol concentration in a patient who has taken a drug overdose. Special provision must be made for such samples to be 'fast-tracked' through the analytical process, albeit in full accordance with

Case history 2.1

The laboratory system flagged up a blood result on a request generated from the diabetes clinic for a pre-appointment check, with the following results:

Results (see Appendix for reference ranges)

Serum:		
	sodium	140 mmol/L
	potassium	12.2 mmol/L
	creatinine	84 µmol/L
	calcium	0.34 mmol/L
	phosphate	1.22 mmol/L

Summary
Severe hyperkalaemia and hypocalcaemia but normal phosphate concentration.

Interpretation
These results must be spurious; hyperkalaemia and hypocalcaemia are unlikely to be compatible with life, and are in keeping with contamination on venesection. Investigation disclosed that the original specimen was collected into the glucose tube, which contained potassium fluoride and oxalate, and then transferred to a plain tube.

Discussion
The degree of contamination and the range of tests requested will affect the ease of its detection. It is worth noting that although extremes of potassium and calcium concentration can occur, more subtle shifts, including of sodium concentrations and enzyme activities, can occur when specimens are introduced into tubes containing incorrect additives. This makes all such preanalytical errors impossible for the laboratory to detect. If users detect potentially spurious results the laboratory should be notified so that, if possible, contamination can be confirmed and the results appropriately flagged or removed from the patient's record.

procedures to ensure quality, and the results reported to the requesting clinician as soon as they have been validated.

Repeat requesting

When biochemical investigations are being used to monitor the progress of a patient's condition, serial analyses will be required, and the question arises of how frequently these should be performed. This will depend on both physiological and pathological factors. For example, in patients being treated with thyroxine for hypothyroidism, it takes several weeks for the plasma concentration of thyroid-stimulating hormone (TSH) to stabilize at a new value after a change in the dose of thyroxine: repeating thyroid function tests in a patient whose dosage of thyroxine has been changed at an interval of <2 months may therefore provide misleading information and could prompt a premature further change of dosage. In contrast, plasma glucose and potassium concentrations can change very rapidly in patients being treated for diabetic ketoacidosis, and it may be appropriate to make measurements as frequently as every 1–2 h. Laboratory user guides may include guidance on repeat testing and minimum repeat intervals, based on locally or nationally agreed protocols. However, it is worth noting that specific patient circumstances may require a departure from generally recommended practice, e.g. more frequent measurement in pregnancy.

Sample Analysis and Reporting of Results

Analysis

The ideal analytical method is **accurate, precise, sensitive** and **specific.** Accurate means that the method gives

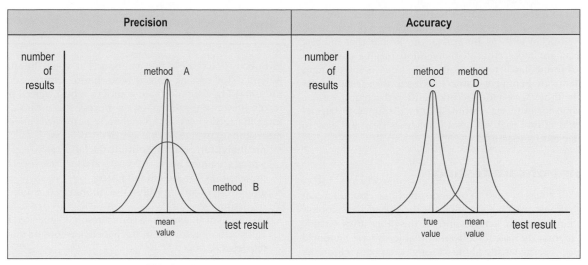

Precision	Accuracy

Fig. 2.2 Precision and accuracy of biochemical tests. Both graphs show the distribution of results for repeated analysis of the same sample by different methods. *Precision:* the mean value is the same in each case, but the scatter about the mean is less in method A than in method B. Method A is, therefore, more precise. *Accuracy:* both are equally precise, but in method D, the mean value differs from the true value. The mean for method C is equal to the true value. Both methods are equally precise, but method C is more accurate.

results that are correct (when compared with an agreed standard: Fig. 2.2) and precise that the result is the same if repeated (see Fig. 2.2). A method is sensitive if able to measure low concentrations of the analyte and specific if not subject to interference by other substances. Note that this should not be confused with the statistical terms of sensitivity and specificity (see p. 19). In addition, it should preferably be cheap, simple and quick to perform. In practice no test is ideal, but laboratory staff make considerable efforts to ensure that the results are sufficiently reliable to be clinically useful. Analytical methods are subject to rigorous quality-control and quality-assurance procedures.

Nevertheless, there will always be a potential for some degree of imprecision or **analytical variation** in a result. The extent of this can be assessed by making repeated analyses (using exactly the same method) on the same sample (to calculate mean and SD) and the imprecision expressed as the analytical CV (cf. biological variation, see earlier). As will be discussed later in this chapter, an understanding of the concepts of both analytical and biological variation is essential to allow informed interpretation of laboratory data.

It is important to appreciate that results obtained using different methods may not be interchangeable. This is particularly relevant when monitoring a single individual over time. Ideally the same analytical method should be used on each occasion; therefore comparison of results from different laboratories or point-of-care testing devices may be misleading.

It is often appropriate to perform a group of related tests on a specimen. For example, plasma calcium and phosphate concentrations and alkaline phosphatase activity all provide information that may be useful in the diagnosis of bone disease; several liver 'function' tests may usefully be grouped together. Such groupings are sometimes referred to as 'biochemical profiles'. Many currently available analysers can perform numerous assays simultaneously on a single specimen. However, although it may be tempting to perform all the assays on every specimen, this approach is costly and generates an enormous amount of information, some of which may be unwanted, ignored or misinterpreted (e.g. an elevated prolactin concentration in someone who is taking psychotropic medication being construed as evidence of a prolactinoma). Worst of all, it may actually divert the clinician's attention from important results. Discrete analysis— that is, performing only the necessary tests required to answer a question (e.g. 'Is the jaundice cholestatic or hepatocellular?')— is the most clinically useful and cost-effective approach.

Reporting results

Once analysis has been completed and the necessary quality-control checks made and found to be satisfactory, a report can be issued. Electronic reporting allows results to be displayed to the clinician in several ways, including as a graph showing the trend for repeated measurements of an analyte, as well as being transmitted directly into the integrated electronic patient record. It may be appropriate for the laboratory to add a comment to a report to assist the clinician with its interpretation. Results that indicate a need for rapid clinical intervention may be communicated immediately to the requesting clinician. Increasingly, patients are being given direct access to their results, especially if they have a long-term condition that requires monitoring, for example, chronic kidney disease. Laboratories should ensure that reports are made as clear and easy to understand as possible.

Point-of-care testing

Not all analyses need to be performed in a central laboratory. Reagent sticks for testing for the presence of glucose, protein, bilirubin, ketones and nitrites in the urine outside the laboratory have long been available, as have handheld devices for the testing of blood for glucose both within the healthcare setting and by patients in the community. Continuing developments have broadened the scope of point-of-care testing including desktop analysers that provide, for example, measurements of hydrogen ion concentration, sodium, potassium and creatinine. The technology continues to develop expanding both the repertoire and locations where testing can be accessed, for example, cholesterol home test kits in pharmacies.

In recent years, manufacturers have developed instruments that can perform a wide range of tests suitable for use at the point of care, but such testing is generally considerably more expensive than laboratory analysis. These instruments allow the more rapid provision of analytical results for patients in whom they are required urgently (e.g. in intensive therapy units) but may also be used for convenience (e.g. in doctors' offices [surgeries]). It is clearly desirable that such instruments are capable of providing results that are as accurate and precise as those provided by the main laboratory. The instruments are designed to be very simple to operate, but it is nevertheless essential that individuals using them, who will usually not be laboratory staff, are properly trained in their use. They should adhere to protocols designed to ensure the quality of results and to provide a robust audit trail so that, for example, should a manufacturer report a problem with a particular test, patients whose results may have been affected can be identified. Both the training and quality issues should be supervised from the laboratory or by similarly qualified professionals.

Some analyses can be performed outside traditional healthcare settings and the results given directly to patients, for example, the measurement of plasma cholesterol concentration in retail pharmacies. Such analyses should be subject to appropriate quality-assurance procedures, and trained personnel should be available to advise patients on the significance of the results.

Sources of Error

Erroneous results are at best a nuisance; at worst, they have potential for causing considerable harm. Errors can be minimized by scrupulous adherence to robust, agreed protocols at every stage of the testing process: this means a lot more than ensuring that the analysis is performed correctly. Errors can occur at various stages in the process:

- **preanalytical,** occurring outside the laboratory (e.g. the wrong specimen being collected, mislabelling, incorrect preservation, the patient not fasted)
- **analytical,** occurring within the laboratory (e.g. human or instrument error)
- **postanalytical,** whereby a correct result is generated but is incorrectly recorded in the patient's record or misinterpreted.

Analytical errors can be *systematic* (also known as bias: different analytical methods may produce results that are higher or lower than the definitive or reference method) or *random*. Many of the few errors that do occur even in good laboratories are detected by quality control procedures, including data-handling software or personal scrutiny of reports by laboratory staff. Some are so bizarre that they are easily recognized for what they are. More subtle ones are more likely to go undetected. Unfortunately, the risk of errors occurring can never entirely be eliminated.

Interpretation of Results

When the result of a biochemical test is obtained, the following points must be taken into consideration:
- Is it normal?
- Is it significantly different from any previous results?
- Is it consistent with the clinical findings?

Is it normal?

The use of the word 'normal' is fraught with difficulty. Statistically, it refers to a distribution of values from repeated measurement of the same quantity and is described by the bell-shaped Gaussian curve (Fig. 2.3). Many biological variables show a Gaussian distribution: the majority of individuals within a population will have a value approximating to the mean for the whole, and the frequency with which any value occurs decreases with increasing distance from the mean. If the variable being measured has a normal (Gaussian) distribution in a population, statistical theory predicts that approximately 95% of the values in the population will lie within the range given by the mean ±2 SDs

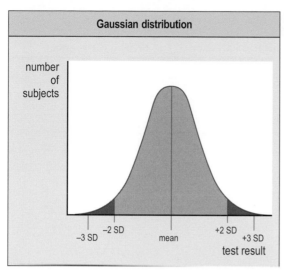

Fig. 2.3 Gaussian distribution. The range of the mean ±2 standard deviations (SDs) encompasses 95.45% of the total number of test results. The range of the mean ±3 SDs encompasses 99.73% of the total number.

(see Fig. 2.3); of the remaining 5%, half the values will be higher and half will be lower than the limits of this range.

For some analytes, the distribution of values is skewed (usually to the right); an example is plasma bilirubin concentration. Such data can often be converted to a normal distribution by logarithmic transformation.

When establishing the range of values for a particular variable in healthy people, it is conventional first to examine a representative sample of sufficient size to determine whether the values fall in a Gaussian distribution. If so, the range (mean ±2 SDs) can then be calculated; this, in statistical terms, is the 'normal range'. Several important points arise from this:

- although it is assumed that the population is healthy, values from 5% of individuals by definition lie outside the normal range. By implication, if the measurements were to be made in a group of comparable individuals, 1 in 20 would have a value outside this range, yet be healthy.

- the specialized statistical use of the word 'normal' does not equate with what is generally meant by the word, that is, 'habitual' or 'usually encountered' or in medical sense 'not diseased'.

- the statistical 'normal' may not be related to another common use of the word, which is to imply freedom from risk. For example, there is an association between increased risk of coronary heart disease and plasma cholesterol concentrations even within the normal range.

Thus, the normal range for an analyte, defined and calculated as described, has considerable limitations. It identifies only the range of values that can be expected to occur most

often in individuals who are comparable with those in the population for whom the range was derived. It is not necessarily normal in terms of being 'ideal', nor is it associated with no risk of having or developing disease. Furthermore, by definition it will exclude values from some healthy individuals.

In all cases, like must be compared with like. When physiological factors affect the concentration of an analyte (see Table 2.1), an individual's result must be assessed by comparing it with the value expected for comparable healthy people. It may, therefore, be necessary to establish normal ranges for subsets of the population, such as various age groups, or male or female individuals only.

To alleviate the problems associated with the use of the word 'normal', the term **reference interval** (RI) (often called the 'reference range') has been widely adopted in clinical biochemistry, using numerical values (reference limits) generally based on the mean ±2 SDs or 95% of the population. Results can be compared with the RI without assumptions being made about the meaning of 'normal'. In practice, however, the term 'normal range' is still in general clinical use. It is used synonymously with RI in this book. Typical RIs for some common analytes are given in the Appendix: these are appropriate for the case histories, but they may not apply to all laboratories because of differences in analytical methods and in the characteristics of the population. Differences between RIs are a particular problem with immunoassays, because different antibodies may vary in their specificity for the analyte and the extent to which they exhibit cross-reactivity with other, similar molecular species. Nevertheless, efforts are being made in the UK to introduce common standards in various areas of pathology, including uniform reference ranges.

In using RIs to assess the significance of a particular result, the individual is being compared with a population. Some analytes show considerable biological variation, but the combined analytical and biological variations will usually be less for an individual than for a population. For example, although the RI for plasma creatinine concentration is 60–110 µmol/L in men, the day-to-day variation in an individual is much less than this. Thus, it is possible for a test result to be abnormal for an individual yet still be within the accepted 'normal range'.

An abnormal result does not always indicate the presence of a pathological process, nor a normal result its absence. However, the more abnormal a result, that is, the greater its difference from the limits of the RI, the greater is the probability that it is related to a pathological process. For some analytes or conditions, a decision threshold may be more appropriate to report than a RI, e.g. the diagnostic threshold of HbA_{1c} for diabetes or a value of prostate specific antigen in a man of the relevant age that should trigger further investigation for possible prostate cancer.

In practice, there is rarely an absolute demarcation between normal values and those seen in disease: equivocal

Table 2.2 Analytical and biological variation

Analyte	Analytical variation	Biological variation	Critical difference
sodium	1.1 mmol/L	2.0 mmol/L	6 mmol/L
potassium	0.1 mmol/L	0.19 mmol/L	0.6 mmol/L
bicarbonate	0.5 mmol/L	1.3 mmol/L	4 mmol/L
urea	0.4 mmol/L	0.85 mmol/L	2.6 mmol/L
creatinine	5.0 µmol/L	4.1 µmol/L	18 µmol/L
calcium	0.04 mmol/L	0.04 mmol/L	0.16 mmol/L
phosphate	0.04 mmol/L	0.11 mmol/L	0.3 mmol/L
total protein	2.0 g/L	1.66 g/L	7 g/L
albumin	1.0 g/L	1.44 g/L	5 g/L
alanine aminotransferase	2 U/L	4 U/L	12 U/L
alkaline phosphatase	5 U/L	4 U/L	18 U/L

Analytical variation: typical standard deviations for repeated measurements made using an automated analyser on a single quality control serum with concentrations within the reference range. *Biological variation:* typical standard deviations for repeated measurements made at weekly intervals in a group of healthy subjects over a period of 10 weeks, corrected for analytical variation. *Critical difference:* 2.8 × total standard deviation for the analyte, which takes into account both the analytical and the biological variation. These are calculated for healthy subjects with values within typical reference ranges.

results must be investigated further. If an important decision in the management of a patient is to be based on a single result, it is vital that the cutoff point, or 'decision level', is chosen to ensure that the test functions efficiently. In screening for PKU, for example, the blood concentration of phenylalanine selected to indicate a positive result must include all infants with the condition; in other words, there must be no false negatives (FNs). Because there is some overlap in the values seen in the presence and absence of PKU, this inevitably means that some healthy children will test positive (false positives [FPs]) and will be subjected to further investigation. Generally, it is unusual to have to determine a patient's management on the basis of one result alone.

It has been explained that 5% of healthy people will, by definition, have a value for a given variable that is outside the RI. If a second and independent variable is measured, the probability that this result will be 'abnormal' is also 0.05 (5%). It follows that the more tests that are performed on an individual, the greater the probability that the result of one of them will be abnormal: for 10 independent variables, the probability is 0.4; in other words, at least one abnormal result would be expected in 40% of healthy people. For 20 variables, the probability is 0.64.

Is it different?

If the result of a previous test is available, the difference can be compared and the significance assessed depending on

the precision of the assay itself (a measure of its reproducibility) and the natural biological variation. Some examples of variation in common analytes are given in Table 2.2.

The probability that the difference between two results is **analytically significant** at a level of $p < 0.05$ is 2.8 times the analytical SD. Thus, for plasma calcium concentration, with an analytical SD of 0.04 mmol/L, an apparent increase in calcium concentration from 2.54 to 2.62 mmol/L ($2 \times$ SD) is within the limits of expected analytical variation, whereas an increase from 2.54 to 2.70 ($4 \times$ SD) is not. However, to decide whether an analytical change is **clinically significant**, it is also necessary to consider the extent of natural **biological variation**. The effects of analytical and biological variation can be assessed by calculating the overall SD of the test, given by:

$$SD = \sqrt{SD_A^2 + SD_B^2}$$

where SD_A and SD_B are the SDs for the analytical and biological variation, respectively. If the difference between two test results exceeds 2.8 times the SD of the test ('critical difference', see Table 2.2), the difference can be regarded as a potential clinical significance: the probability of this difference being a result of analytical and biological variation is <0.05 (Case History 2.2). It should be appreciated, however, that setting the level of significance at a probability of <0.05 is arbitrary (albeit conventional). It does not mean that a difference of less

Case history 2.2

History

A 41-year-old man had been diagnosed as having diabetes mellitus and hypertension six months ago. On review by his general practitioner, the conditions appeared to be well controlled.

Results

Serum creatinine 118 µmol/L. Six months earlier it was 105 µmol/L.

Summary

Increase in creatinine concentration over 6 months in a man with risk factors for kidney disease.

Discussion

The analytical variation for creatinine is 5.0 µmol/L, the biological variation is 4.1 µmol/L (see Table 2.2). The critical difference is:

$$2.8 \times \sqrt{5.0^2 + 4.1^2}$$

that is, 18 µmol/L. Thus, the apparent increase in creatinine is not significant at a level of $p = 0.05$.

than that equating to this probability cannot be of significance, nor that a greater difference necessarily is significant. Before undertaking a major intervention based on a result, the likelihood that it is truly of clinical significance should always be considered. Is it consistent with clinical findings?

If the result is consistent with clinical findings, it is evidence in favour of the clinical diagnosis. If it is not consistent, the explanation must be sought. There may have been a mistake in the collection, labelling or analysis of the sample, or in the reporting of the result. In practice, it may be simplest to request a further sample and to repeat the test. If the result is confirmed, the utility of the test in the clinical context should be considered and the clinical diagnosis itself may have to be reviewed.

The Clinical Utility of Laboratory Investigations

In using the result of a test, it is important to know how reliable the test is and how suitable it is for its intended purpose. Thus, laboratory personnel must ensure, as far as is practicable, that data are accurate and precise, and the clinician should appreciate how useful the test is in the context in which it is used. Various properties of a test can be calculated to provide this information.

Specificity and sensitivity

Earlier in the chapter, the terms 'sensitivity' and 'specificity' were used to describe characteristics of analytical methods. The terms are also widely used in the context of the utility of laboratory tests. The specificity of a test is a measure of the incidence of negative results in persons known to be free of a disease, that is, 'true negative' (TN). Sensitivity is a measure of the incidence of positive results in patients known to have a condition, that is, 'true positive' (TP). A specificity of 90% implies that 10% of disease-free people would be classified as having the disease on the basis of the test result: they would have an FP result. A sensitivity of 90% implies that only 90% of people known to have the disease would be diagnosed as having it on the basis of that test alone: 10% would be FNs.

Specificity and sensitivity are calculated as follows:

$$\text{Specificity} = \frac{\text{TN}}{\text{all without disease (FP + TN)}} \times 100$$

$$\text{Sensitivity} = \frac{\text{TP}}{\text{all with disease (TP + FN)}} \times 100$$

An ideal diagnostic test would be 100% sensitive, giving positive results in all subjects with a particular disease, and also 100% specific, giving negative results in all subjects free of the disease. Because the ranges of results in quantitative tests that can occur in health and in disease almost always show some overlap, individual tests do not achieve such high standards. Factors that increase the specificity of a test tend to decrease the sensitivity, and *vice versa*. To take an extreme example, if it were decided to diagnose hyperthyroidism only if the plasma free thyroxine concentration were at least 28 pmol/L (the upper limit of the reference range is 22 pmol/L), the test would have effectively 100% specificity: positive results (>28 pmol/L) would only be seen in thyrotoxicosis (an exception is a rare condition in which patients are resistant to thyroid hormones). On the other hand, the test would have a low sensitivity in that many patients with mild hyperthyroidism would be not be diagnosed. If a concentration of 18 pmol/L were used, the test would be very sensitive (all those with hyperthyroidism would be correctly assigned) but have low specificity, because many normal people would also be diagnosed as having the condition. These concepts are illustrated in Fig. 2.4.

Whether it is desirable to maximize specificity or sensitivity depends on the nature of the condition that the test is used to diagnose and the consequences of making an incorrect diagnosis. For example, sensitivity is paramount in a screening test for a harmful condition, but the inevitable FP results mean that all positive results will have to be investigated further. However, in selecting patients for a trial of a new treatment, a highly specific test is more appropriate to ensure that the treatment is being given only to

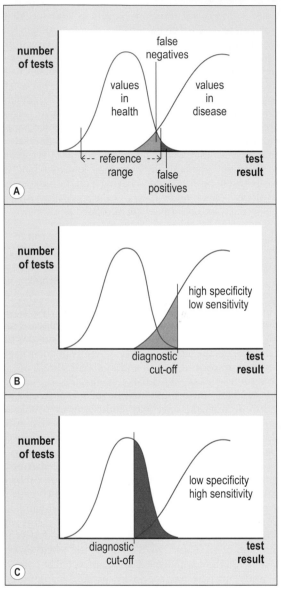

Fig. 2.4 Ranges of values for a test result in health and disease overlap (A), therefore some individuals with disease will have results within the reference range (false negatives), whereas others, free of disease, will have results outside this range (false positives). If the diagnostic cutoff value for a test is set too high (B), there will be no false positives, but there will be many false negatives; specificity is increased, but sensitivity decreases. If the diagnostic cutoff value is set too low (C), the number of false positives, and sensitivity, increases at the expense of a decrease in specificity.

patients who have a particular condition. In some cases, this decision may not be straightforward, for example, in the context of chest pain and suspected acute myocardial infarction, where the possible options are to identify all those who have had a myocardial infarction ('rule in') or to identify all those who have definitely not ('rule out'). The preferred option should depend on the relative outcomes of treatment and non-treatment for patients in the two groups.

One way of comparing the sensitivity and specificity of different tests is to construct **receiver operating characteristic (ROC) curves**. Each test is performed in each of a series of appropriate individuals. The specificity and sensitivity are calculated using different cutoff values to determine whether a given result is positive or negative (Fig. 2.5). The curves can then be assessed to determine which test performs best in the specific circumstances for which it is required. If the line goes through the top left corner (0,1) then the test has perfect diagnostic efficiency, which can also be described as having an area under the ROC curve (AUROC) of 1. An AUROC of 0.5 is a test that is no better than a coin toss, therefore all tests should have an AUROC between 0.5 and 1.0.

Efficiency

The efficiency of a test is the number of correct results divided by the total number of tests. Thus, efficiency is given by:

$$\frac{TP + TN}{\text{total number of tests}} \times 100$$

When sensitivity and specificity are equally important, the test with the greatest efficiency should be used.

Predictive values

Even a highly specific and sensitive test may not necessarily perform well in a clinical context. This is because the ability of a test to diagnose disease depends on the prevalence of the condition in the population being studied (prevalence is the number of people with the condition in relation to the population). This ability is given by the 'predictive value' (PV). The **positive predictive value (PPV) is the percentage of all positive results that are TPs,** that is:

$$PPV = \frac{TP}{TP + FP} \times 100$$

If a condition has a low prevalence and the test is <100% specific, many FPs will result and the PPV will be low.

A high predictive value for a positive test is important if an action based on an FP result could potentially be dangerous. However, when a test is used for **screening** (i.e. the detection of a condition in asymptomatic individuals), the appropriate management is to perform further (diagnostic)

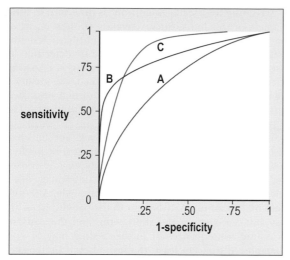

Fig. 2.5 Receiver operating characteristic curves for three hypothetical tests, A, B and C. Examination of the curves shows that test A performs less well in terms of both sensitivity and specificity than tests B and C. Test B has better specificity than C, but C has better sensitivity.

tests; although these may cause inconvenience for subjects with FP results, they are unlikely to be harmful.

In order not to miss cases, a screening test should have a very high **negative predictive value (NPV); this is the percentage of all negative results that are TNs,** that is:

$$NPV = \frac{TN}{TN + FN} \times 100$$

This conclusion follows directly from the fact that the test must be highly sensitive.

For clarity, this discussion has centred on the use of single tests for diagnostic purposes, but in practice, the clinician will combine clinical information and, often, the results of several investigations to make a diagnosis. If the tests are used rationally, the PV of positive results will be higher, as the tests will be used only in patients who have other features suggesting a particular diagnosis (the prevalence of the disease in question would be higher in a group of such people than in the general population). For example, although Cushing disease is rare, making the PV of a positive test for the condition in the general population low, in practice one would only investigate patients suspected on clinical grounds of having the condition and in whom the prevalence will therefore be higher. Therefore, targeted testing is essential to avoid unhelpful, or even misleading, results.

Likelihood ratios

The concept of predictive values is an unfamiliar one for many people: it has no obvious parallel in our everyday

lives. The concept of odds is a more familiar one. **Likelihood ratios (LRs)** express the odds that a given finding (e.g. a particular result) **would occur in a person with, as opposed to without, a particular condition.** The LR for a positive result is given by:

$$LR_{+ve} = sensitivity/(1 - specificity)$$

The LR_{-ve} (the odds that a negative test result would occur in a person with, as opposed to without, a particular condition) is given by:

$$LR_{-ve} = (1 - sensitivity)/specificity$$

LRs can be used to convert the probability of a condition being present before the test was done (in the case of a screening test, this is the prevalence) to the post test probability of its being present. The greater the value of the LR, the more useful the test will have been.

Evidence-based clinical biochemistry

Most clinicians interpret large quantities of clinical and laboratory data intuitively. Ideally, tests should be selected on the basis of their known utility, and their results used on the basis of validated outcome measures as part of an evidence-based approach. The test characteristics, discussed earlier, facilitate this. However, it remains the case that many well-established tests have been introduced into clinical practice without being properly evaluated, and few systematic reviews of existing tests have been performed. Furthermore, new tests are often introduced into laboratories' repertoires without a systematic assessment of their utility having been made, and their value and limitations may only become apparent in the light of experience of their day-to-day use. International groups working to improve the evidence base promote the use of the Standards for Reporting of Diagnostic Accuracy Studies (STARD) reporting guideline for diagnostic accuracy studies.

Clinical Audit

Clinical audit is part of the process of ensuring quality—in this context, of ensuring the provision of a high quality laboratory service. In this respect, it is complementary to the other techniques of quality assurance, which in the main concentrate on the analytical aspects of the service, that is the provision of precise and accurate results. Clinical audit is the process of systematically examining practice to ensure that it is efficient and beneficial to patients. It involves identifying an area of practice, identifying the standards or guidelines (e.g. a protocol for investigation of patients suspected of having a particular condition), measuring performance against these standards, implementing changes designed to achieve these and then examining compliance with them and the effects on patient care. It should be followed by reaudit after an appropriate interval as part of continuing quality improvement. Whether undertaken in the context of formal audit or not, ongoing liaison between the providers and users of laboratory services is essential to ensure that the service meets the latter's clinical needs. It also provides a forum for laboratory staff to educate users about changes in practice designed to improve the service.

The term 'audit' is also applied to procedures used by some laboratory accreditation bodies to examine the internal functioning of laboratories. It is beyond the scope of this book to describe such procedures.

Screening

Screening tests are used to detect disease in groups of apparently healthy individuals or to refine case identification in specific groups. As previously discussed, high sensitivity is particularly desirable for screening tests; to avoid unnecessary further tests in healthy people, high specificity is also an important consideration. Screening tests for PKU are designed to maximize sensitivity but are also highly specific. However, PKU has a low incidence, so that even with a sensitivity of 100% and specificity of 99.9%, the predictive value of a positive test is only 9%, that is, 10 of 11 positive tests will be shown on further investigation to be FPs. On the other hand, the predictive value of a negative test will be 100%, confirming that no cases will be missed using the screening test. These calculations are made as follows:

1. incidence of PKU = 1 in 10 000 live births
2. sensitivity = 100%, that is, all with PKU will test positive (1 TP and 0 FN in 10 000 infants)
3. number of infants without PKU = 9999
4. specificity = 99.9%, that is, 99.9% of those without PKU will test negative (9989 TN) and 0.1% will test positive (10 FP)
5. predictive value of a positive test

$$\left(\frac{TP}{TP + FP} \times 100 \right) = \frac{1}{11} \times 100 = 9\,\%$$

6. predictive value of a negative test

$$\left(\frac{TN}{TN + FN} \times 100 \right) = \frac{9989}{9989 + 0} \times 100 = 100\,\%$$

Screening for specific conditions is discussed in other chapters of this book. Such screening is often based on the use of considerably less specific but highly sensitive tests, and therefore has a low efficiency for detecting disease. Indiscriminate biochemical profiling is also inefficient. The more tests that are performed, the greater is the probability that an apparently abnormal result will arise that is not the result of a pathological process (see p. 18).

When multiple analyses are performed and an unexpected abnormality is found, a decision must be made as to what action to take. The abnormality may be considered insignificant in some clinical circumstances, but if it is not, further investigations must be made. Although these may be of ultimate benefit to the patient, he or she may suffer anxiety in the short term, and the cost and economic consequences of further testing may be considerable. At the very least, the tests should be repeated to ensure that the abnormality was not due to analytical error.

The ready availability of an investigation often leads to it being used unnecessarily or inappropriately. Healthcare professionals should be encouraged to be selective in making test requests. Before requesting a test, one should know how the result will influence the management of the patient: if it will not have an influence, it should not be requested.

Plasma and serum

Plasma is the aqueous phase of blood, preserved *in vitro* by the inclusion of an anticoagulant in the collection tube; note that it therefore contains clotting factors, which is why 'fresh frozen plasma' can be given to patients with bleeding crises. Serum is the aqueous phase of blood that has been allowed to clot, therefore for urgent analysis, plasma may be the preferred sample type, as up to 30 min is required for the clotting process to complete. Both are obtained by centrifugation which deposits the cells to the bottom of the tube leaving the aqueous phase on top. For technical reasons, many biochemical measurements are more conveniently made on serum, but the concentrations of most analytes are effectively the same in both fluids. In this book, the term 'plasma' is used to describe the concentrations of substances in blood, and the term 'serum' refers to actual measurements made in serum (e.g. in the case histories) and in the few instances where serum must be used for analysis.

SUMMARY

- Biochemical investigations are used for diagnosis, monitoring, screening and assessing prognosis.
- **Specimens for analysis** must be collected and transported to the laboratory under appropriate conditions.
- Analytical results are affected by both **analytical** and **biological variation.**
- Results can be compared either with **reference intervals**, decision thresholds or with the results of previous tests.

- **The utility of test results** depends on many factors: an 'abnormal' result should not be assumed to indicate a pathological process, nor a 'normal' one to exclude disease or potential disease.
- The utility of tests can be measured and described mathematically: applying this information can considerably enhance the value of laboratory test results in clinical practice.

Chapter | 3 |

Water, sodium and potassium

Introduction

Water distribution

Water accounts for approximately 60% of body weight in men and 55% in women, the difference reflecting the typically greater body fat content in women. Approximately 66% of this water is in the intracellular fluid (ICF) and 33% is in the extracellular fluid (ECF); only 8% of body water is in the plasma (Fig. 3.1). Water is not actively transported in the body. It is, in general, freely permeable through the ICF and ECF, and its distribution is determined by the osmotic contents of these compartments. Except in the kidneys, the osmotic concentrations, or osmolalities, of these compartments are always equal: they are isotonic. Any change in the solute content of a compartment engenders a shift of water, which restores isotonicity.

The major contributors to the osmolality of the ECF are sodium (a cation, see p.2) and its associated anions, mainly chloride and bicarbonate; in the ICF, the predominant cation is potassium. Other determinants of ECF osmolality include glucose and urea, although urea diffuses freely across the plasma membranes, so changes in ECF urea concentration do not affect water distribution. Protein makes a numerically small contribution of approximately 0.5%. This is because osmolality is dependent on the molar concentrations of solutes: although the total concentration of plasma proteins is approximately 70 g/L, their high molecular mass results in their combined molar concentrations being <1 mmol/L. However, because the capillary endothelium is relatively impermeable to protein and the protein concentration of interstitial fluid is much less than that of plasma, **the osmotic effect of proteins is an important factor in determining water distribution between these two compartments**. The contribution of proteins to the osmotic pressure of plasma is known as the 'colloid osmotic pressure' or 'oncotic pressure' (see Chapter 16).

Under normal circumstances, the amounts of water taken into the body and lost from it are equal over a period of time. Water is obtained from the diet and oxidative metabolism, and it is lost through the kidneys, skin, lungs and gut (Box 3.1). About 170 L water is filtered by the kidneys every 24 h, and almost all of this is reabsorbed. In adults, the minimum volume of urine necessary for normal excretion of waste products is about 500 mL/24 h, but as a result of obligatory losses by other routes, the minimum daily water intake necessary for the maintenance of water balance is approximately 1100 mL. This increases if losses are abnormally large, for example, with excessive sweating or diarrhoea. Water intake is usually considerably greater than this minimum requirement, but the excess is easily excreted through the kidneys.

Sodium distribution

The body of an adult man contains approximately 4000 mmol sodium, 70% of which is freely exchangeable, the remainder being complexed in bone. The majority of the exchangeable **sodium is extracellular**: normal ECF sodium concentration is 133–146 mmol/L, whereas that of the ICF is only 4–10 mmol/L. Most cell membranes are relatively impermeable to sodium, but some leakage into cells occurs and the gradient is maintained by active pumping of sodium from the ICF to the ECF by Na^+,K^+-ATPase (the sodium–potassium pump).

As with water, sodium input and output normally are balanced. The normal intake of sodium in the developed world is 100–200 mmol/24 h, but the obligatory sodium loss, via the kidneys, skin and gut, is <20 mmol/24 h. Thus, the sodium intake necessary to maintain sodium balance is much less than the normal intake; excess sodium is excreted in the urine. Despite this, excessive sodium intake may be harmful: there is evidence that it is a contributory factor in hypertension.

It is important to appreciate that there is a massive internal turnover of sodium. Sodium is secreted into the gut at

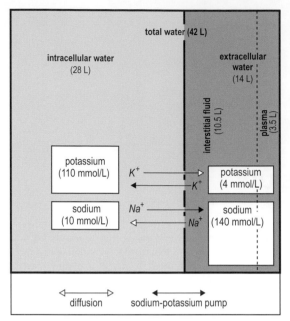

Fig. 3.1 Distribution of water, sodium and potassium in the body of a 70-kg man. In women, the distribution is similar but water accounts for a lower percentage of body weight (50–55%). In children and infants, the proportion of interstitial fluid water is higher and water makes up a higher percentage of body weight (75–80%). Note that although plasma volume is approximately 3.5 L, blood volume in a 70-kg man is approximately 5.5 L.

a rate of approximately 1000 mmol/24 h and is filtered by the kidneys at a rate of 25 000 mmol/24 h, the vast majority being regained by reabsorption in the gut and renal tubules, respectively. If there is even a partial failure of this reabsorption, sodium homoeostasis will be compromised.

Potassium distribution

Potassium is the predominant intracellular cation. Some 90% of the total body potassium is free and therefore exchangeable, whereas the remainder is bound in red blood cells, bone and brain tissue. However, only approximately 2% (50–60 mmol) of the total is located in the extracellular compartment (see Fig. 3.1), where it is readily accessible for measurement. Plasma potassium concentration is not, therefore, a reliable index of total body potassium status, but because of the effect of potassium on membrane excitability, it is important in its own right. The potassium concentration of serum is 0.2–0.3 mmol/L higher than that of plasma (see p.22), because of the release of potassium from platelets during clot formation, but this difference is not usually of practical significance.

Box 3.1 **Daily water balance in an adult**

Obligatory losses	mL	Sources	mL
skin	500	water from oxidative metabolism	400
lungs	400	minimum in diet	1100
gut	100		
kidneys	500		
total	**1500**	**total**	**1500**

The minimum intake necessary to maintain balance is approximately 1100 mL. Actual water intake in food and drink is usually greater than this: the excess over requirements is excreted in the urine.

There is a constant tendency for potassium to diffuse down its concentration gradient from the ICF to the ECF, opposed by the action of Na^+,K^+-ATPase, which transports potassium into cells. Potassium homoeostasis and its disorders are described later in this chapter.

Water and Sodium Homoeostasis

Water and extracellular fluid osmolality

Changes in body water content independent of the amount of solute will alter the osmolality (Fig. 3.2). The **osmolality of the ECF** is normally maintained in the range 275–295 mmol/kg water. Any loss of water from the ECF, such as occurs with water deprivation, will increase its osmolality and result in movement of water from the ICF to the ECF. However, a slight **increase in ECF osmolality** will still occur, stimulating the hypothalamic thirst centre, causing thirst and thus promoting a desire to drink, and stimulating the hypothalamic osmoreceptors, which causes the release of **vasopressin** (antidiuretic hormone [ADH]).

Vasopressin renders the renal collecting ducts permeable to water (its combination with V2 receptors results in the insertion of aquaporins [water channels] into the normally impermeable apical membrane of the cells of the collecting tubules), permitting water reabsorption and concentration of the urine. The maximum urine concentration that can be achieved in humans is about 1200 mmol/kg. The osmoreceptors are highly sensitive to osmolality, responding to a change of as little as 1%. Plasma vasopressin concentration declines to very low values at an osmolality of 284 mmol/kg, but it increases sharply if osmolality increases above this level (Fig. 3.3A). However, if an

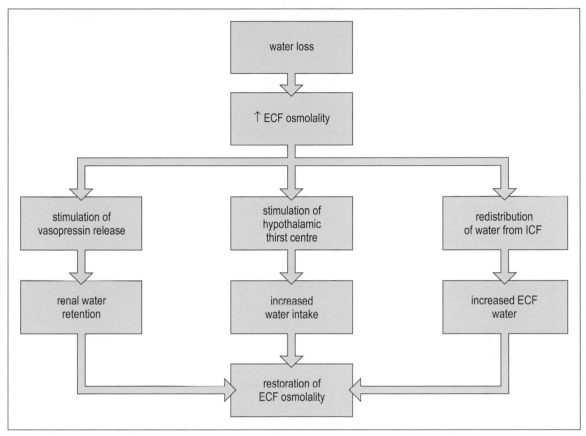

Fig. 3.2 Physiological responses to water loss. ECF, extracellular fluid; ICF, intracellular fluid.

increase in ECF osmolality occurs as a result of the presence of a solute such as urea that diffuses readily across cell membranes, ICF osmolality also increases and osmoreceptors are not stimulated.

If **ECF osmolality declines**, there is no sensation of thirst and vasopressin secretion is inhibited. Dilute urine is produced, allowing water excretion and restoration of ECF osmolality to normal. The vasopressin responses to changes in osmolality occur rapidly. In health, the ingestion of water surplus to requirements leads to a rapid diuresis, and water depletion leads to a rapid increase in the concentration of the urine.

Other stimuli that affect vasopressin secretion include arterial and venous baroreceptors and angiotensin II (in response to reduced effective blood volume), stress, pain, nausea and a range of drugs (Box 3.2). Hypovolaemia and hypotension increase the slope of the vasopressin response to an increase in osmolality (see Fig. 3.3A) and lower the threshold osmolality for vasopressin secretion. The vasopressin response to a decline in plasma volume is exponential: it is relatively small with small decreases in plasma

volume, but greater declines cause a massive increase in vasopressin secretion (see Fig. 3.3B). Also, osmolar controls are overridden, so that ECF volume is defended (by stimulating water retention) at the expense of a decrease in osmolality.

Sodium and extracellular fluid volume

The volume of the ECF is directly dependent on the total body sodium content: sodium is very largely confined to the ECF, and water intake and loss are regulated to maintain a constant ECF osmolality, and hence sodium concentration.

Dietary **sodium intake** is highly variable. Sodium balance is maintained by regulation of its excretion by the kidneys. **Sodium excretion** requires glomerular filtration, but the glomerular filtration rate (GFR) appears to become an important limiting factor in sodium excretion only at extremely low rates of filtration (sodium retention is a late feature of chronic kidney disease). Normally, approximately 70% of filtered sodium is

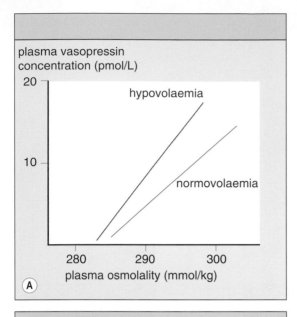

A, plasma vasopressin concentration (pmol/L)

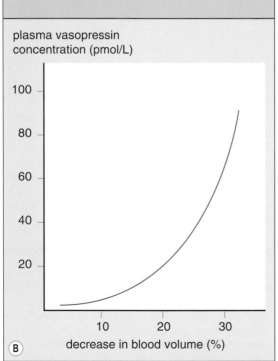

B, plasma vasopressin concentration (pmol/L)

Fig. 3.3 A, Vasopressin secretion is stimulated by an increase in extracellular fluid osmolality above a threshold of approximately 284 mmol/kg; in hypovolaemia (blue line), this threshold is reduced and the response is greater. **B,** Vasopressin secretion is stimulated exponentially by hypovolaemia. Note the difference in the scales of the vertical axes.

Box 3.2 Control of vasopressin secretion

Stimulating factors	Inhibiting factors
increased ECF osmolality	decreased ECF osmolality
severe hypovolaemia (via angiotensin II and arterial and venous receptors)	hypervolaemia
stress, including pain	alcohol
nausea	
exercise	
drugs	
amiodarone	
analgesics, e.g. NSAIDs, opiates	
antidepressants, e.g. SSRIs	
anticonvulsants, e.g. carbamazepine, sodium valproate, lamotrigine	
antipsychotics, e.g. phenothiazines, butyrophenones	
anticancer drugs, e.g. vinca alkaloids, platinum compounds, melphalan, cyclophosphamide, methotrexate	
MDMA ('ecstasy')	
proton pump inhibitors	

ECF, extracellular fluid; MDMA, 3,4-methylenedioxymethamphetamine; NSAID, non-steroidal anti-inflammatory drug; SSRI, selective serotonin reuptake inhibitor.

actively reabsorbed in the proximal tubules, with further reabsorption in the loops of Henle. Sodium reabsorption is reduced in the proximal tubules if blood volume increases (because this is associated with a decline in the oncotic pressure in peritubular capillary blood) and if sympathetic activity decreases (such as also tends to occur with an increase in blood volume). Only <5% of filtered sodium reaches the distal tubules and collecting ducts, but these comprise the major site for the fine control of sodium excretion.

Aldosterone, released from the adrenal cortex in response to activation of the renin–angiotensin system, stimulates sodium reabsorption in the distal parts of the distal tubules and collecting ducts, and it is the major factor controlling renal sodium excretion. The control of renin

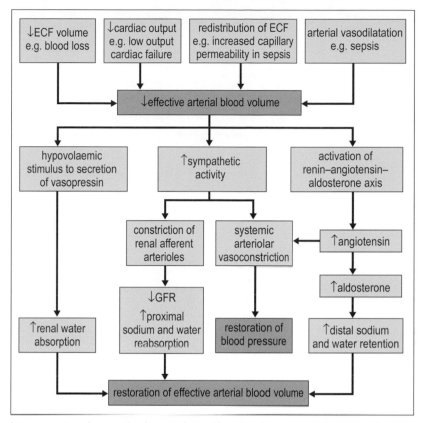

Fig. 3.4 Physiological responses to a decrease in plasma volume. These involve responses to restore plasma volume and to maintain blood pressure. ECF, extracellular fluid; GFR, glomerular filtration rate.

secretion is discussed in detail in Chapter 10, but in essence, renin secretion is stimulated primarily by a decrease in renal perfusion secondary to a decrease in blood volume—specifically a fall in arterial blood volume (effective blood volume, see later).

Natriuretic peptide hormones also have a role in controlling sodium excretion. Atrial natriuretic peptide (ANP) is a 28–amino acid peptide, one of a family of similar peptides, secreted by the cardiac atria in response to atrial stretch after a rise in atrial pressure (e.g. caused by ECF volume expansion). ANP acts both directly by inhibiting distal tubular sodium reabsorption and through decreasing renin (and hence aldosterone) secretion. It also antagonizes the pressor effects of noradrenaline (norepinephrine) and angiotensin II (and thus tends to increase GFR) and has a systemic vasodilatory effect. It appears to provide 'fine-tuning' of sodium homoeostasis but is probably more important in pathological states than physiologically. Two other structurally similar peptides have been identified. One (B-type natriuretic peptide [BNP],

originally discovered in brain) is secreted by the cardiac ventricles in response to ventricular stretching and has similar properties to ANP; the other (C-type natriuretic peptide [CNP]) is present in high concentrations in vascular endothelium and is a vasodilator. Measurement of BNP is of value in the management of patients with suspected cardiac failure (see Chapter 17). Increased secretion of natriuretic peptides has been postulated to be, at least in part, responsible for the natriuresis seen in cerebral salt wasting (see p.39).

In summary, the initial response to a decrease in ECF volume is activation of the renin–aldosterone axis, causing an increase in the secretion of aldosterone and leading to sodium retention. Water reabsorption follows along the resulting osmotic gradient. Maintenance of osmolality takes precedence unless there is a very large decline in plasma volume, which stimulates a massive increase in vasopressin (see Fig. 3.3B) and free water retention. In addition to the changes in sodium and water excretion, there are also changes in the tone of

Box 3.3 **Causes and clinical features of predominant water depletion**

Causes		Clinical features
Decreased intake		**Symptoms**
infancy		thirst
old age		dryness of mouth
unconsciousness		difficulty in swallowing
dysphagia		weakness
restriction of oral intake		confusion
Increased loss		**Signs**
from kidneys	from skin	weight loss
renal tubular disorders	sweating	dryness of mucous membranes
diabetes insipidus	from lungs	decreased saliva secretion
increased osmotic load caused	hyperventilation	decreased urine volume (early)[a]
by diabetes mellitus, osmotic	from gut	
diuretics or high protein	diarrhoea (in infants)	
intake		

[a]Unless caused by renal water loss.

arteriolar smooth muscle, peripheral vascular resistance, renal blood flow and blood pressure. The physiological responses to a decrease in ECF volume are illustrated in Fig. 3.4.

Water and Sodium Depletion

Water depletion, or combined water and sodium depletion, will occur if losses are greater than intake. Depletion of water alone is seen much less frequently than depletion of both water and sodium. Because sodium cannot be excreted from the body without water, sodium loss never occurs alone but is always accompanied by some loss of water. The fluid lost may be isotonic or hypotonic with respect to ECF.

The clinical and biochemical features of water depletion and of isotonic sodium and water loss are quite different, as are the physiological responses, and it is helpful to consider them separately. In clinical practice, however, states of fluid depletion encompass the whole spectrum between these two extremes, and the clinical and biochemical features will reflect this. Furthermore, it should be appreciated that they may have been modified by previous treatment.

Water depletion

Water depletion will occur if water intake is inadequate or if losses are excessive. Excessive loss of water without any sodium loss is unusual, except in diabetes insipidus, but even if there is loss of sodium as well, provided that this is small, the clinical consequences will be related primarily to the water depletion (Box 3.3).

Loss of water from the ECF causes an **increase** in **osmolality**, which, in turn, causes movement of water from the ICF to the ECF, thus lessening the increase. Nevertheless, the increase in ECF osmolality will be sufficient to stimulate the thirst centre and vasopressin secretion. Plasma sodium concentration increases; plasma protein concentration and the haematocrit are usually only slightly elevated. Unless water depletion is due to uncontrolled loss through the kidneys, the urine becomes highly concentrated and there is a rapid decrease in its volume. Because water loss is borne by the total body water pool, and not just the ECF (Fig. 3.5), **signs of a reduced ECF volume are not usually present.** Furthermore, the increased colloid osmotic pressure of the plasma tends to hold extracellular water in the vascular compartment. Circulatory failure is a very late feature of water depletion: it is much more likely to occur if sodium depletion is also present.

Severe water depletion induces cerebral dehydration, which may cause cerebral bleeding through damage to

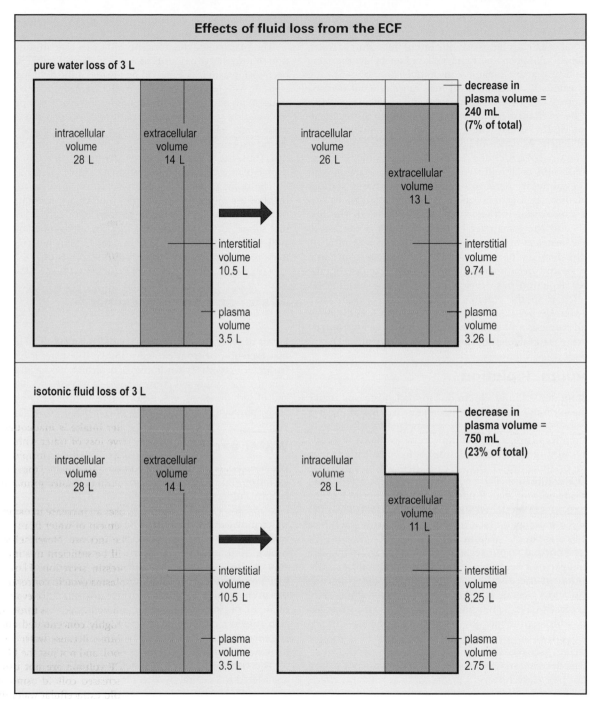

Effects of fluid loss from the ECF

pure water loss of 3 L

intracellular volume 28 L
extracellular volume 14 L

intracellular volume 26 L
extracellular volume 13 L

decrease in plasma volume = 240 mL (7% of total)

interstitial volume 10.5 L
plasma volume 3.5 L

interstitial volume 9.74 L
plasma volume 3.26 L

isotonic fluid loss of 3 L

intracellular volume 28 L
extracellular volume 14 L

intracellular volume 28 L
extracellular volume 11 L

decrease in plasma volume = 750 mL (23% of total)

interstitial volume 10.5 L
plasma volume 3.5 L

interstitial volume 8.25 L
plasma volume 2.75 L

Fig. 3.5 Comparison of the effects of water loss and isotonic fluid loss from the extracellular compartment. When only water is lost from the extracellular fluid (ECF), the increase in osmolality causes water to move from the intracellular fluid (ICF), which minimizes the decrease in plasma volume. When isotonic fluid is lost from the ECF, no osmotic imbalance is produced, there is no movement of water from the ICF and the effect on plasma volume is, therefore, much greater.

blood vessels. In the short term, cerebral shrinkage is mitigated somewhat by movement of extracellular ions into cerebral cells, causing an osmotic intracellular shift of water. If dehydration persists, brain cells adapt by synthesizing osmotically active organic compounds ('osmolytes'), and overzealous fluid replacement may cause cerebral oedema because of rapid intracellular movement of water (Fig. 3.6B).

The **management** of water depletion requires treatment of the underlying cause and replacement of the fluid deficit. Water should preferably be given either orally or via a nasogastric tube. If this is not possible, 5% dextrose should be administered intravenously, together with 0.9% saline if there has been accompanying sodium depletion. As a general guide, the aim should be to correct approximately two- thirds of the deficit in the first 24 h and the remainder in the next 24 h while avoiding a decrease in sodium concentration of >10 mmol/L in the first 24 h. How rapidly the sodium concentration should be normalized depends on how quickly the water depletion has developed. If it is long-standing (as it often is in the elderly), a decrease of no more than 0.5 mmol/L per hour is recommended, but initially more rapid correction (1 mmol/L per hour) may be appropriate in acute water depletion (more common in children).

Sodium depletion

Sodium depletion is seldom due to inadequate oral intake alone, although sometimes inadequate parenteral input is responsible. More often, it is a consequence of excessive sodium loss (Box 3.4). Sodium can be lost from the body either isotonically (e.g. in plasma) or hypotonically (e.g. in sweat or dilute urine). In each case, there will be a **decrease in ECF volume** (see Fig. 3.5), but this will be less if the fluid lost is hypotonic than if it is isotonic, because some of the water loss will be shared with the ICF. The clinical features of sodium depletion (see Box 3.4) are primarily a result of the decrease in ECF volume.

The **normal responses to hypovolaemia** are an increase in aldosterone secretion, stimulating renal sodium reabsorption in the distal convoluted tubules and collecting ducts, and a decline in urine volume as a consequence of a decreased GFR. Significantly increased vasopressin secretion, which stimulates the production of highly concentrated urine, occurs only with more severe ECF volume depletion (see Fig. 3.3).

The decrease in GFR may lead to pre-renal acute kidney injury (see Case history 5.1). In contrast with the effects of pure water depletion, plasma protein concentration and the haematocrit are usually clearly increased in sodium depletion, unless this is a result of the loss of plasma or blood. Furthermore, because the fluid loss is borne mainly by the ECF, signs of a reduced ECF volume are usually present, and there is a greater risk of peripheral circulatory

failure than in water depletion. The features of sodium and water depletion are compared in Table 3.1.

The plasma sodium concentration can give an indication of the relative amounts of water and sodium that have been lost: plasma sodium will be normal if the fluid lost is isotonic with respect to the ECF and increased if it is hypotonic. With severe sodium depletion, increased vasopressin secretion secondary to the resulting hypovolaemia may cause water retention; plasma volume is then maintained at the expense of osmolality and hyponatraemia develops. Thus, the plasma sodium concentration in a sodium-depleted patient may be high, normal or low (Table 3.2).

The **management** of sodium depletion involves treatment of the underlying cause and, if necessary, restoration of the intravascular volume by giving isotonic fluid ('normal saline' [0.9% sodium chloride]) by intravenous infusion. This can usually be done rapidly, but any associated free water deficit requires more cautious correction.

Water and Sodium Excess

Excess of water and sodium can result from a failure of normal excretion or from excessive intake. The latter is often iatrogenic. As with the syndromes of depletion, it is helpful to consider the causes and consequences of excess water alone and of sodium excess with isotonic retention of water separately, although in practice there is often a degree of overlap.

Water excess

Water excess is usually related to an impairment of water excretion (Box 3.5). However, the limit to the ability of the healthy kidneys to excrete water is about 20 mL/min, and occasionally, excessive intake is alone sufficient to cause water intoxication. This can sometimes occur in patients with psychiatric disorders. It has also been described in people drinking large amounts of beer with a low solute content, because this results in a low osmotic load for excretion and there is a minimum osmolality below which the urine cannot be diluted further. Increased thirst can occur in organic brain disease (particularly trauma and after surgery), although decreased thirst is more common. Hyponatraemia is invariably present in water overload. The increased water load is shared by the ICF and ECF.

The **clinical features** of water overload (see Box 3.5) are related to cerebral overhydration; their incidence and severity depend on the extent of the water excess and its time course. Thus, a patient with a plasma sodium concentration of 120 mmol/L, in whom water retention has occurred gradually over several days, may be asymptomatic, whereas one in whom this is an acute phenomenon may show signs of severe water intoxication. In the short

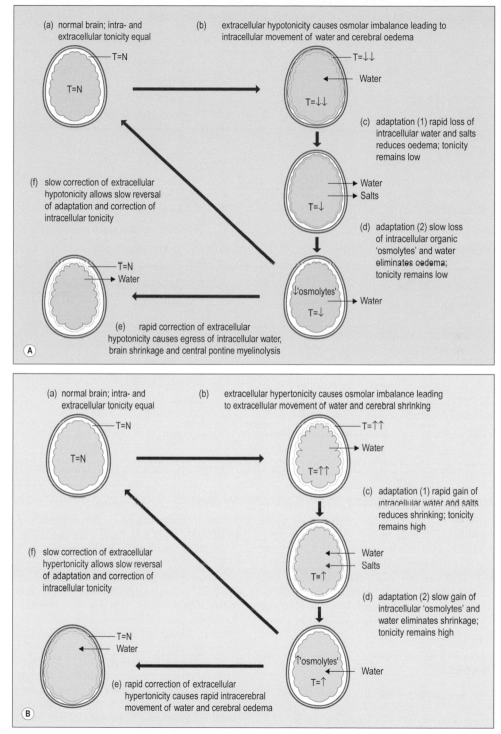

Fig. 3.6 Effects of hyponatraemia **(A)** and hypernatraemia **(B)** on the brain, adaptive changes and the effects of rapid correction. T, tonicity; N, normal.

Box 3.4 **Causes and clinical features of predominant sodium depletion**

Causes	Clinical features
Excessive loss	**Symptoms**
from kidneys	weakness
diuretic phase of acute kidney injury	apathy
diuretic therapy	postural dizziness
mineralocorticoid deficiency	syncope
cerebral salt wasting	confusion, coma (late)
other salt-losing states	
from skin	**Signs**
massively increased sweating	weight loss
cystic fibrosis	related to decreased plasma volume
widespread dermatitis	tachycardia
burns	hypotension (initially postural)
from gut	peripheral circulatory failure
vomiting, diarrhoea	oliguria
fistulae	related to decreased interstitial fluid
ileus	decreased intraocular pressure
intestinal obstruction	decreased skin turgor
Inadequate intake	
sodium deletion will occur whenever intake is inadequate to	
balance excessive losses; inadequate intake alone is rarely	
a cause of depletion	

term, the effects of hypotonicity are mitigated to some extent by a movement of ions out of cerebral glial cells; more chronically (days), a decrease in intracellular organic 'osmolytes' further reduces intracellular water content (see Fig. 3.6A). As is the case with water depletion, this adaptation necessitates a cautious approach to treatment, particularly in chronic water overload. The **management** of water overload is discussed together with that of hyponatraemia on p. 38.

Sodium excess

Sodium excess can result from increased intake or decreased excretion. The **clinical features** are related primarily to **expansion of ECF volume** (Box 3.6). When related to excessive intake (e.g. the inappropriate use of hypertonic saline), a rapid shift of water from the intracellular compartment may also cause cerebral dehydration. When sodium overload is due to excessive intake, hypernatraemia is common (see Case history 3.5).

Sodium overload is more often due to impaired excretion than to excessive intake. The most frequent cause is secondary aldosteronism. This is seen in patients who, despite clinical evidence of increased ECF volume (e.g. peripheral oedema), appear to have a decreased effective arterial blood volume, for example, caused by venous pooling or a disturbance in the normal distribution of ECF between the vascular and extravascular compartments. This phenomenon is particularly associated with cardiac failure, hypoalbuminaemia and hepatic cirrhosis. Many such patients with sodium excess are, paradoxically, hyponatraemic, implying the coexistence of a defect in free water excretion. This is probably in part due to an increase in vasopressin secretion as a result of

Table 3.1 Clinical and laboratory findings in sodium and water depletion

	Sodium depletion	Water depletion
plasma [Na[a]]	normal or ↓	↑
haematocrit	↑↑↑[a]	normal or slightly ↑
ECF volume	↓↓↓	usually normal
plasma [urea]	↑	high normal
urine volume	↓	↓↓↓
urine concentration	↑	↑↑↑
thirst	late	early
tachycardia, hypotension	early	late

[a]Unless caused by loss of blood.

Table 3.2 Plasma sodium concentration with various causes of sodium depletion

Mechanism of sodium depletion	Plasma sodium concentration
sodium and water loss, waterloss predominating, e.g.excessive sweating	increased
isotonic sodium and waterloss, e.g. burns, haemorrhage	normal
Sodium loss with water retention, e.g. treatment of isotonic sodium depletion with low sodium fluids	decreased

Box 3.5 Causes and clinical features of excess body water

Causes	Clinical features
Increased intake	behavioural disturbances
compulsive water drinking	confusion
excessive parenteral fluid administration	headache
water absorption during bladder irrigation	convulsions
	coma
	muscle twitching
Decreased excretion	extensor plantar responses
chronic kidney disease (severe)	
cortisol deficiency	
inappropriate or ectopic secretion of vasopressin	
drugs:	
stimulating vasopressin release (see Box 3.2)	
potentiating the action of vasopressin, e.g. chlorpropamide	
vasopressin (V2) agonists, e.g. oxytocin	
interfering with renal diluting capacity, e.g. thiazide diuretics	

leads to sodium retention and modest expansion of the ECF volume (but to an insufficient extent to cause oedema), but sodium balance is then restored and a new steady state is achieved. It is thought that the increased arterial filling leads to a decrease in sympathetic activity and secretion of angiotensin II, with a consequent increase in renal perfusion and GFR, together with the increased secretion of ANP. The net result is an increase in the delivery of sodium to the distal nephrons, which, together with ANP, counters the sodium-retaining action of aldosterone. In oedematous states, relative arterial underfilling leads to a decline in GFR, increased proximal tubular sodium reabsorption, and decreased delivery of sodium to the distal nephrons. Even though there is increased secretion of ANP, its ability to cause natriuresis is limited by this decreased sodium delivery.

The **management** of sodium excess should be directed towards the cause, where possible. In addition, diuretics (including spironolactone if secondary aldosteronism is a contributory factor) can be used to promote sodium excretion. Sodium intake must be controlled. Dialysis or

the decreased effective blood volume. Also, the decrease in GFR and consequent increase in proximal tubular sodium reabsorption decreases the delivery of sodium and chloride to the loops of Henle and distal tubules. This reduces the diluting capacity of the kidneys, thereby compromising water excretion. Kidney disease is a relatively uncommon cause of sodium excess, as is increased mineralocorticoid secretion caused by primary adrenal disease (Conn syndrome, see p. 184).

It is noteworthy, however, that oedema is not a feature of Conn syndrome: furthermore, in healthy individuals, the administration of high doses of mineralocorticoids initially

Box 3.6 Causes and clinical features of predominant sodium excess

Causes	Clinical features
Increased intake	peripheral oedema
excessive parenteral administration	dyspnoea
absorption from saline emetics	pulmonary oedema
	venous congestion
Decreased excretion	hypertension
decreased glomerular filtration:	effusions
acute and chronic kidney disease	weight gain
increased tubular reabsorption:	
primary mineralocorticoid excess:	
Cushing syndrome	
Conn syndrome	
secondary mineralocorticoid excess:	
congestive cardiac failure	
nephrotic syndrome	
hepatic cirrhosis with ascites	
renal artery stenosis	

The 'U&E' profile

U&E, standing for urea and electrolytes, is the term given to a long-established profile aimed at testing kidney function and fluid and electrolyte status. In most circumstances, however, creatinine is a better first-line test of kidney (or more precisely glomerular) function. Some laboratories automatically include creatinine in the 'U&E' profile, but creatinine alone should be requested if only a screening test for kidney function is required. An electrolyte is any substance that dissociates into free ions when it dissolves in water, and can therefore conduct electricity and move along an electrochemical gradient. Positively charged electrolytes are cations and negatively charged ones are anions. Conventionally, the two electrolytes included in the U&E profile are sodium and potassium, which are measured by near-identical methods in the laboratory and almost invariably requested and reported as a pair. There are, however, a large number of atomic and molecular ions in plasma, all of which are electrolytes.

Laboratory Assessment of Water and Sodium Status

Plasma **sodium concentration is dependent on the relative amounts of sodium and water** in the plasma. In isolation, therefore, plasma sodium concentration provides no information about the sodium content of the ECF. It may be high, normal or low in states of sodium excess or depletion, according to the amount of water in the ECF.

The plasma sodium concentration is one of the most frequent measurements made in clinical chemistry laboratories (largely for historical reasons), but definite indications for its measurement are few and results are often misinterpreted. Plasma sodium concentration should be measured in the following situations:

- patients with dehydration or excessive fluid loss, as a guide to appropriate replacement
- patients on parenteral fluid replacement
- patients with unexplained confusion, abnormal behaviour or signs of central nervous system (CNS) irritability.

In the assessment of a patient's water and sodium status, **clinical observations**, such as assessment of central venous pressure, fluid balance and body weight, may all provide

haemofiltration may be necessary if kidney function is poor, and it is occasionally necessary in acute sodium overload associated with the use of hypertonic fluids.

vital information, although each is open to inaccuracy or misinterpretation. In the intensive care setting, indicators of cardiac output such as transoesophageal echocardiography provide more precise measures of intravascular volume. An increase in the concentration of plasma proteins or in the haematocrit suggests haemoconcentration. Other abnormal results may suggest specific conditions; for example, hyperkalaemia in a patient with hyponatraemia with clinical evidence of sodium depletion would suggest adrenal failure.

Measurement of urine osmolality and sodium can provide valuable information, although the results may be misleading (e.g. in patients on steroids or diuretics). A urine osmolality of >100 mmol/kg in a patient with hyponatraemia indicates water retention, which may be inappropriate (e.g. in **syndrome of inappropriate antidiuresis (SIAD**, see p. 40), and failure to produce a concentrated urine in hypernatraemia may point to diabetes insipidus. Urine sodium concentration is a useful marker of arterial blood volume because it reflects the renal response to aldosterone: a value ≤30 mmol/L usually indicates intravascular volume depletion, although total ECF volume could be high if there is

abnormal fluid distribution between compartments. However, natriuresis in a patient with sodium depletion could imply either a failure of aldosterone secretion or a failure of the kidneys to respond to the hormone (Case history 3.1).

Sodium measurement

Sodium concentration is usually measured by ion-selective electrodes which, strictly speaking, determine the activity of sodium rather than its concentration, that is, the number of atoms that act as true ions in a defined volume of water. Plasma normally comprises around 93% water by volume (the remaining 7% comprises proteins and lipoproteins): ion-selective electrodes are calibrated to allow for this, and they produce results that are a close estimate of plasma sodium concentration.

Laboratory analyzers dilute the plasma before analysis (indirect analysis), whereas most point-of-care testing instruments measure sodium concentration directly in undiluted plasma (direct analysis). Under most circumstances, the two techniques give results that are very similar.

Case history 3.1

History

A 50-year-old woman with a long history of rheumatoid disease complained of fainting episodes after an attack of gastroenteritis.

Examination

Blood pressure 102/72 mmHg when lying down, 78/56 when standing.

Results (see Appendix for reference ranges)

Serum:	sodium	118 mmol/L
	potassium	3.9 mmol/L
	urea	9.1 mmol/L
	creatinine	74 μmol/L
	eGFR	77 mL/min/1.73 m²

ACTH (tetracosactide [Synacthen]) test: normal cortisol response to ACTH

Plasma: aldosterone (recumbent)	1420 pmol/L (100–450)
Plasma: renin activity (recumbent)	15.6 nmol/L per hour (1.1–2.7)
24-h urinary sodium excretion	118 mmol

Summary

Severe hyponatraemia with slightly raised urea. High renin and aldosterone and natriuresis.

Interpretation

The hyponatraemia with a slightly raised urea is consistent with sodium depletion producing hypovolaemia. The result of the ACTH stimulation test is normal, excluding adrenal failure, and renin and aldosterone are appropriately raised. The patient's urinary sodium excretion is excessive: although the input was not assessed, the expected response in a volume-depleted patient is sodium retention by the kidneys.

Discussion

Postural hypotension may be caused by hypovolaemia, autonomic neuropathy or hypotensive drugs. This patient was not taking such medication and there was no other evidence of neuropathy. It was important to rule out adrenal insufficiency, and she was shown to have a normal renin and aldosterone response to volume depletion. The normal renal response to volume depletion is to conserve sodium, with a urine sodium concentration of <30 mmol/L.

It was concluded that the patient had a renal salt-losing state such that the kidneys could not respond to the normal physiological stimuli to retain sodium. She became symptomatic only when diarrhoea and vomiting caused further fluid loss. This was later confirmed by sodium balance studies and the patient was found to have renal papillary necrosis, an occasional complication of the use of certain analgesic drugs, which principally affects renal tubular function.

However, if the fractional plasma water content is decreased, as it is in severe hyperlipidaemia or hyperproteinaemia, the sodium concentration, measured (after dilution) by an indirect ion-selective electrode, will be an underestimate of true sodium activity because the dilution is of total plasma volume, not just water volume. Direct ion-selective electrodes give a more accurate estimate of the concentration of sodium in plasma under these circumstances.

This effect, known as **pseudohyponatraemia**, is only seen with severe hyperlipidaemia (when the plasma will usually appear turbid to the naked eye) and with large increases in total protein concentration caused by paraproteinaemia (see p. 292). If it is suspected, plasma osmolality should be measured because it is a direct measure of solute activity in plasma water. Plasma osmolality should be normal in a patient with pseudohyponatraemia.

Measurement of osmolality

Given that it is osmolality, rather than sodium concentration, that is controlled by the hypothalamus, it might appear logical to measure plasma osmolality rather than sodium concentration. The measurement of osmolality is, however, less precise than that of sodium and is not easily automated. It is nevertheless useful under certain circumstances.

Measurement of osmolality can help in the interpretation of a low plasma sodium concentration and is necessary in water deprivation tests for possible diabetes insipidus (see Chapter 9). It can also be useful in the investigation of patients suspected of having ingested substances such as ethanol or ethylene glycol (see Case history 21.5) because, if present, these increase the plasma osmolality. This can be revealed by comparing the measured osmolality with the approximate expected value using a formula that adds together the main osmolar plasma constituents to calculate osmolarity (see the following).

Measured osmolality (in mmol/kg of water) and calculated osmolarity (in mmol/L of solution) are normally numerically very similar. Significant discrepancies (an **osmolar gap**) occur when abnormal osmotically active species are present in plasma (as may occur in poisoning, and perhaps in some cases of the sick cell syndrome) and when the fractional water content of plasma is reduced, as in severe hyperlipidaemia or hyperproteinaemia (**pseudohyponatraemia**).

Measurement of anions (bicarbonate and chloride)

A change in plasma sodium concentration must be matched by a change in anion concentration. The major anions of the ECF are chloride and bicarbonate. Bicarbonate (strictly, total carbon dioxide, but this mostly comprises bicarbonate ions, see p. 58) is frequently measured because it reflects the extracellular buffering capacity (note that the measurement must be made on a fresh sample to obtain an accurate result, because of the loss of carbon dioxide to the atmosphere on standing). The measurement of plasma chloride rarely adds useful information in the diagnosis of disorders of sodium and water homoeostasis. However, it may have a role in the detection of harmful hyperchloraemia in patients receiving large volumes of chloride-rich intravenous fluids (see p. 63), and it may occasionally be helpful in the diagnosis of patients with non-respiratory acidoses or rare chloride-losing states (as it is used in the calculation of the anion gap, see p. 59).

Osmolality and osmolarity

Plasma **osmolality** is a measure of the number of osmotically active particles per kilogram of plasma water (expressed as **mmol/kg**). It is a true physicochemical entity that determines the colligative properties of a solution, including osmotic pressure. **Osmolarity** is an estimate of osmolality that is derived by adding together the concentrations, in **mmol/L** of the solutes that are present at highest concentration in plasma, but doubling that of sodium to allow for the anions that inevitably accompany cations. The most commonly used formula is:

$$osmolarity = 2 \times [Na^+] + [urea] + [glucose]$$

where all concentrations are measured in mmol/L. The factor 2 is to allow for the major anions (chloride and bicarbonate); other formulae include potassium and a slightly smaller multiplier, to allow for the fact that some anions and cations act as ion pairs rather than as individual moieties

---

Hyponatraemia

A slightly low plasma sodium concentration is a frequent finding. The median plasma sodium concentration of hospital inpatients is ~5 mmol/L lower than in healthy control subjects. Mild hyponatraemia is seen with a wide variety of illnesses and may be multifactorial in origin (see the 'Sick cell syndrome' section, p. 42). It is essentially a secondary phenomenon that reflects the presence of disease; treatment should be directed at the underlying cause and not at the hyponatraemia. Hyponatraemia itself may warrant primary treatment, but usually only when it is severe or is associated with clinical features of water intoxication (see Box 3.5).

Causes

It has been emphasized that plasma sodium concentration depends on the amounts of both sodium and water in the plasma, so a low sodium concentration does not necessarily imply sodium depletion. Indeed, hyponatraemia is more frequently a result of a defect in water homoeostasis that causes water retention and hence dilution of plasma sodium. One of three mechanisms is usually primarily responsible for the development and maintenance of hyponatraemia, although in individual patients more than one factor may be involved. These mechanisms are:

- **sodium depletion** (hypovolaemic hyponatraemia)
- **water excess** (euvolaemic hyponatraemia)
- **water and sodium excess** (hypervolaemic hyponatraemia).

For an explanation of the connection between sodium status and plasma volume, see p. 27

Sodium depletion

Sodium cannot be lost without water, and isotonic or hypotonic loss would not be expected to cause a decline in plasma sodium concentration. However, hyponatraemia can occur in patients with sodium depletion, and it is due either to inappropriate replacement of fluid (e.g. containing insufficient sodium) or, in severe sodium depletion, to the hypovolaemic stimulus to vasopressin secretion, which overrides the osmotic control and permits water retention at the expense of a decrease in osmolality. A patient with adrenal failure with hyponatraemia as a result of sodium depletion is presented in Case history 10.1.

Clinical signs of hypovolaemia (see Box 3.4) may be present in patients with hyponatraemia caused by sodium depletion. Unless the sodium loss is occurring through the kidneys, increased aldosterone secretion should cause maximal renal sodium retention and the urinary sodium concentration will be low (<30 mmol/L). This finding is a valuable aid to the diagnosis of extra-renal sodium depletion as a cause of hyponatraemia. In contrast, in hypovolaemia caused by renal sodium losses, urine sodium concentration is often much greater than 30 mmol/L.

The **management** of hyponatraemia associated with sodium depletion involves correction of the underlying cause and appropriate fluid replacement (e.g. physiological [0.9%] saline). It is important to monitor plasma sodium concentration: restoration of plasma volume will suppress any hypovolaemic stimulus to vasopressin secretion, causing a relative water diuresis.

Plasma sodium concentration is usually normal in patients treated with diuretics, but these drugs have complex effects on sodium and water homoeostasis. Although primarily tending to cause sodium depletion, the blocking of sodium reabsorption in the cortical diluting segment of the nephrons may impair free water excretion. This, perhaps exacerbated by the effect of vasopressin secretion secondary to hypovolaemia and an increase in water intake because of thirst, can result in hyponatraemia. This is usually mild, but it can be more severe, particularly in patients receiving treatment with thiazides. Treatment with diuretics is the most frequent cause of hypovolaemic hyponatraemia in ambulant patients.

Cerebral (or central) salt wasting describes the combination of hyponatraemia and natriuresis in the presence of cerebral pathology. It is particularly associated with brain injury and cranial surgery. The pathogenesis is uncertain: mechanisms may include release of natriuretic peptides by the brain and increased centrally mediated sympathetic activity, leading to dopamine release and increased renal perfusion pressure. It is sometimes mistaken for SIAD (see later). The critical practical difference between cerebral salt wasting and SIAD is that patients with cerebral salt wasting should have clinical and biochemical features of hypovolaemia: indeed, it should not be diagnosed unless there is evidence of hypovolaemia (patients with SIAD are typically euvolaemic), marked natriuresis (urine sodium >100 mmol/L) and diuresis. The distinction is vital, because the management of the two conditions is quite different: patients with cerebral salt wasting require intravenous isotonic saline, often in large volumes, to replace the sodium that is being lost. SIAD, in which the basic problem is water retention, is usually treated by water restriction or, in severe cases, a vasopressin receptor antagonist (see p. 40).

Water excess

Water excess causes **dilutional hyponatraemia** with reduced plasma osmolality. It can occur acutely purely because of excessive water intake, but this is rare. Normal kidneys are capable of excreting 1 L water per hour: water intoxication and hyponatraemia will thus be seen only when very large quantities of fluid are ingested rapidly, as is seen in some patients with psychoses. It can also occur in people who drink large quantities of weak beer (see p. 32). Far more frequently, however, the acute development of water excess and hyponatraemia is a result of a combination of excessive hypotonic fluid intake and impairment of diuresis. Because osmolality is normally precisely controlled, the persistence of dilutional hyponatraemia implies a failure of diuresis, which must be caused by either continued (and inappropriate) production of vasopressin (or the presence of a drug having a vasopressin-like action) or an impairment of the renal diluting mechanism.

SIAD is essentially a diagnosis of exclusion. It is frequently diagnosed on insufficient evidence without regard

Case history 3.2

History

A man who had undergone major abdominal surgery 36 h earlier and was still receiving intravenous fluid replacement was reviewed by the ward junior doctor.

Examination

He was alert and appeared neither underhydrated nor overhydrated. He had received a total of 3.5 L of dextrose-saline since his operation, and examination of the fluid balance chart showed that he had a positive balance of 2 L.

Results

Serum:
	sodium	127 mmol/L
	urea	4.0 mmol/L
	creatinine	68 µmol/L
	eGFR	>90 mL/min/1.73 m^2

Summary

Moderate hyponatraemia, other results unremarkable.

Interpretation

Hyponatraemia resulting from excessive administration of hypotonic intravenous fluids.

Discussion

Hyponatraemia is a very common finding in postoperative patients on intravenous fluid infusions. It is usually, as in this case, a reflection of excessive administration of hypotonic fluids (5% dextrose or 'dextrose-saline') at a time when the ability of the body to excrete water is depressed as part of the normal metabolic response to trauma, which includes increased release of vasopressin. If, as is usually the case, there are no clinical features of water intoxication, the only action necessary is adjustment of the fluid input.

to other possible causes of hyponatraemia. Both clinical information and laboratory data are important. It is essential to measure urine and plasma osmolalities: plasma osmolality is low and the urine should be less than maximally dilute (i.e. osmolality >100 mmol/kg). The **laboratory criteria for the diagnosis** are:

- hyponatraemia
- decreased plasma osmolality
- inappropriately concentrated urine (it is sometimes stated that the osmolality of the urine should be greater than that of the plasma, but it is sufficient that it is not maximally dilute)
- continued natriuresis (>30 mmol/L)

- no clinical evidence of volume depletion (e.g. due to diuretics) or oedema
- normal renal function
- normal adrenal function
- normal thyroid function (although only profound hypothyroidism causes hyponatraemia)
- clinical and biochemical response to fluid restriction.

Oedema is not a feature of SIAD: the excess of water is distributed throughout both the ICF and the ECF, and the effect on ECF volume is insufficient to cause oedema. Measurement of vasopressin concentration is seldom helpful in differential diagnosis: raised values are present in the majority of patients with hyponatraemia, irrespective of the cause.

There are at least four different types of SIAD:

- tumours may produce the hormone (ectopic production)
- abnormal regulation of vasopressin release, for example, stimulation of thoracic volume receptors during artificial ventilation or resetting of the 'osmostat' so that osmolality is still controlled but at a lower level, perhaps as a result of decreased intracellular organic solute ('osmolyte') content
- incomplete suppression of vasopressin release when osmolality falls (a 'vasopressin leak')
- inappropriate activation of the aquaporin water channel, because of genetic mutations of the vasopressin V2 receptor gene, has been described in a few patients.

Conditions associated with SIAD are listed in Box 3.7. In addition, certain drugs either stimulate vasopressin release (see Box 3.2) or have a vasopressin-like action on the kidneys.

This syndrome was previously called 'syndrome of inappropriate antidiuretic hormone secretion' or SIADH, but because inappropriate secretion of the hormone is not always present in patients satisfying its diagnostic criteria, and vasopressin is now the accepted name for 'antidiuretic hormone', the newer term syndrome of inappropriate antidiuresis is more appropriate.

Severe hyponatraemia has been reported in individuals undertaking endurance athletic events, such as marathon running. This is due to stress-mediated secretion of vasopressin combined with an inappropriately high intake of low-solute fluids.

The **management of dilutional hyponatraemia** (i.e. water overload) depends on its severity and the time course over which it develops. The latter is relevant because of the adaptive responses to water overload (see Fig. 3.6 and p. 32). As a general principle, hyponatraemia should be corrected at a rate that reflects the rate of its development, but in severely symptomatic patients, it is often necessary to effect partial correction rapidly to control symptoms.

Case history 3.3

History

An elderly man was admitted to hospital in an acute confusional state. No history was available.

Examination

He had finger clubbing and tar staining indicating that he was a heavy smoker. There were signs of a right-sided pleural effusion, but no other obvious abnormality was detected. He was neither dehydrated nor oedematous.

Investigations

A chest radiograph confirmed the presence of the effusion and showed a mass in the right lower zone with an appearance typical of a carcinoma.

Results

Serum:	sodium	114 mmol/L
	potassium	3.6 mmol/L
	bicarbonate	22 mmol/L
	urea	2.5 mmol/L
	creatinine	55 μmol/L
	eGFR	>90 mL/min/1.73 m^2
	total protein	48 g/L
	osmolality	236 mmol/kg
Plasma:	glucose	4.0 mmol/L
Urine:	osmolality	350 mmol/kg
	sodium	50 mmol/L

Summary

Severe hyponatraemia with low serum urea and protein concentrations. Relatively high urine osmolality and ongoing natriuresis in the presence of hypo-osmolal plasma.

Interpretation

The patient is not clinically dehydrated, and the low serum protein and urea concentrations suggest that the hyponatraemia is dilutional. The normal response should be for vasopressin secretion to be inhibited, resulting in the production of dilute urine. However, in this case, the urine is inappropriately concentrated in relation to the serum, implying continuing secretion of vasopressin resulting in SIAD. The chest radiograph indicates that the likely source is ectopic secretion of vasopressin by a bronchial carcinoma.

Discussion

In SIAD, there is inappropriate concentration of the urine and continued natriuresis despite the low plasma sodium concentration because plasma volume is maintained by water retention; therefore, there is no hypovolaemic stimulus to renin, and hence aldosterone, secretion. Hyponatraemia with natriuresis can also occur in adrenal failure and in renal disorders, and these must be excluded before a diagnosis of SIAD can be made. Water intoxication should always be considered as a possible cause of a confusional state, especially in the elderly.

Patients with mild acute and chronic hyponatraemia ([Na$^+$] 125–130 mmol/L) are usually asymptomatic, although even they may have an increased incidence of osteoporosis and falls. The underlying cause must be addressed, but if this is not possible, the logical treatment is to restrict the patient's water intake to less than that required to maintain normal water balance, for example, to 500–1000 mL/24 h, until the plasma sodium concentration has become normal. However, water restriction is unpleasant and impractical to sustain long term. Demeclocycline, a drug that antagonizes the action of vasopressin on the renal collecting ducts, has been used for this purpose, but it can cause photosensitivity and is potentially nephrotoxic. V2 vasopressin receptor antagonists (vaptans) are now available for the treatment of SIAD, although they are expensive and patients require careful monitoring of water and electrolyte status during treatment.

If patients are severely symptomatic (e.g. experiencing convulsions; see Box 3.5), as is more likely if the hyponatraemia is severe or has developed rapidly, urgent correction of the hyponatraemia will be necessary. Hypertonic saline (1.8%, 2.7% or 3%) should be infused at a rate sufficient to increase the plasma sodium concentration initially by 1 mmol/L per hour (0.5 mmol/L per hour if onset is more than 48 h previously) but not by >10 mmol/L over 24 h. (Note that hypertonic saline should not be given to patients who are experiencing fluid overload.) Paradoxically, giving a loop diuretic at the same time can be beneficial: this reduces the slight increase in ECF volume that is present, stimulates distal renal tubular sodium retention and increases free water excretion. Regular clinical assessment and measurement of plasma sodium concentration are essential. The infusion should be stopped when patients become asymptomatic, irrespective of sodium concentration, or when plasma sodium concentration reaches 120 mmol/L. In chronic dilutional hyponatraemia, correcting the sodium concentration

Box 3.7 **Conditions associated with the syndrome of inappropriate antidiuresis**

Ectopic secretion

bronchial carcinomas

other tumours, e.g. thymus, prostate

Inappropriate secretion

pulmonary diseases

   pneumonia

   tuberculosis

   positive pressure mechanical ventilation

cerebral diseases

   head injury

   encephalitis

   tumours

   aneurysms

miscellaneous

   pain, e.g. postoperative, acute intermittent

      porphyria, Guillain–Barré syndrome,

         hypothyroidism (profound), drugs (see **Box 3.2**)

---

too rapidly risks causing central pontine myelinolysis (see Fig. 3.6A), a brain syndrome characterized by spastic quadriplegia, pseudobulbar palsy and cognitive changes. Hypoxaemia, a history of alcohol excess or the presence of chronic liver disease may increase this risk. This condition has a poor prognosis.

It is possible to calculate the approximate infusion rate of hypertonic saline required to achieve a given increase in sodium concentration, but doing so must never be used as a substitute for careful clinical and biochemical monitoring.

Combined water and sodium excess

Combined water and sodium excess is a frequent cause of hyponatraemia. It underlies the hyponatraemia of congestive cardiac failure, hypoproteinaemic states and some patients with liver failure. The mechanism is discussed on p. 34. The fact that there is sodium excess is indicated by signs of increased ECF volume (e.g. peripheral oedema or ascites). The logical treatment in these patients involves measures to treat the underlying cause and remove the excess sodium and water (e.g. with diuretics). Despite the

hyponatraemia, saline should not usually be given, because these patients are already experiencing sodium overload.

Other causes of hyponatraemia

Decreased fractional water content of plasma, causing pseudohyponatraemia, can occur with severe hyperproteinaemia and hyperlipidaemia (see p. 38).

Addition of a solute to the plasma that is confined to the ECF will tend to increase ECF osmolality. The most common example is hyperglycaemia (Case history 3.4): a decline in plasma sodium is a normal response to hyperglycaemia, and it is essential to measure plasma glucose concentration in all patients with unexplained hyponatraemia. Acutely, there is a shift of water from the ICF to the ECF, lowering the ECF sodium concentration, and the increase in ECF osmolality stimulates vasopressin secretion, leading to water retention. The resulting increase in ECF volume inhibits aldosterone secretion, leading to natriuresis. Movement of water from the ICF to the ECF does not occur in uraemia because urea equilibrates between the ECF and the ICF, thus preventing an osmotic imbalance.

The 'sick cell syndrome'

Hyponatraemia is frequently observed in patients with either acute or chronic illness, without any obvious cause. The term 'sick cell syndrome' has been used to describe this phenomenon, which previously was attributed to an increase in the permeability of cell membranes to sodium with or without a decrease in the activity of the sodium pump. However, any transmembrane shift of sodium would be expected to be accompanied by an iso-osmotic movement of water, and thus should not affect plasma sodium concentration, although it is possible that sodium could become bound to intracellular macromolecules, thus nullifying its effect on osmolality. A raised osmolar gap (see p. 38), presumed to be due to loss of intracellular organic molecules through leaky cell membranes, has been observed in some patients, and the accompanying iso-osmotic shift of water to the extracellular compartment would dilute its sodium concentration. Depletion of intracellular organic solutes may also reset the hypothalamic osmostat. Many sick patients may have a degree of stress-related increased vasopressin secretion or another cause of SIAD.

In practice, however, the mechanism of the hyponatraemia of the 'sick cell syndrome' is relatively unimportant. The hyponatraemia reflects the presence of the underlying disease, and it is this that should be treated, not the hyponatraemia.

Case history 3.4

History

A patient with insulin-treated diabetes woke up feeling hypoglycaemic and drank two glasses of a sugar-rich drink, which abolished the symptoms. She had a hospital appointment that morning and, worried that she might become hypoglycaemic while driving, decided to omit her usual injection of insulin. She felt quite well on arrival at the hospital. Blood was taken for routine monitoring tests.

Results

Plasma:	glucose	28 mmol/L
Serum:	sodium	126 mmol/L
	osmolality	290 mmol/kg

Serum urea, creatinine, potassium and bicarbonate concentrations were normal.

Summary

Hyponatraemia with hyperglycaemia.

Interpretation

The hyponatraemia is dilutional. It is the result of a movement of water from the ICF to the ECF to maintain isotonicity as the plasma glucose concentration increases. In the short time since onset, there was no significant osmotic diuresis, and thus no dehydration.

Discussion

Lowering of plasma sodium concentration is a normal response to hyperglycaemia. It is observed in patients with diabetes and occasionally when glucose is administered at a rate greater than it can be metabolized during parenteral nutrition. It can also occur after mannitol infusion. Mannitol may be given to patients with cerebral oedema, to reduce intracellular water content, and is also used as an osmotic diuretic.

Acute hypervolaemic hyponatraemia may be fatal as it causes cerebral oedema (see Fig. 3.6). Acute-onset hyponatraemia with **sodium <120 mmol/L** requires urgent assessment and management (see p. 41). Children are at higher risk of cerebral oedema so **sodium <130 mmol/L in patients aged <16 years** should be managed with the same degree of urgency.

A simple algorithm for the diagnosis of hyponatraemia is given in Fig. 3.7. Some of the commoner causes of hyponatraemia are indicated in Table 3.3, and some investigations that may help in elucidating its cause are presented in Box 3.8. It must be emphasized, however, that an appreciation of the underlying physiological principles and their clinical correlates is vital for correct interpretation of their results.

Management of hyponatraemia

Hyponatraemia is essentially a feature of a disorder involving water or sodium homoeostasis, or both. As has been discussed, measures to treat the causative condition may need to be supplemented by direct measures to correct the imbalance of sodium and water. These will vary according to the mechanism of the hyponatraemia, and it is therefore essential both to diagnose the cause and to understand the pathogenesis. If symptoms of water intoxication are present, urgent (though cautious) correction will be required.

Hypernatraemia

Hypernatraemia is less common than hyponatraemia but is much more frequently of clinical significance. The causes include pure water depletion, combined sodium and water depletion with water loss predominating, or sodium excess; of these, excess sodium is the least common. Hypernatraemia is a relatively frequent finding in elderly people, as a result of inadequate water intake; in hospitals, it is often iatrogenic.

In most patients with hypernatraemia, the cause is obvious from the history and clinical observations. Diabetes insipidus is an important cause, and the investigation of patients suspected of having this condition is considered in Chapter 9.

Regardless of its cause, hypernatraemia should be treated by administration of hypotonic fluids such as water (orally) or 5% dextrose (parenterally). In patients with sodium overload, measures to remove excess sodium may have to be considered. As already emphasized, it is important that hypernatraemia caused by water depletion is not corrected too rapidly.

Investigation of hyponatraemia

In many instances, the cause of hyponatraemia can be recognized clinically and additional investigations add little to the management of the patient. Careful clinical evaluation and study of fluid balance charts (if reliable) will often indicate the underlying mechanism or mechanisms, and thus point the way to a diagnosis. Hyponatraemia caused by sodium depletion may be accompanied by physical signs of a decrease in ECF volume, whereas this will be normal in patients with water excess, and in combined water and sodium excess the signs will be those of ECF expansion. Not infrequently, however, clinical assessment of fluid volume status may be difficult, and a systematic process of biochemical investigation is necessary.

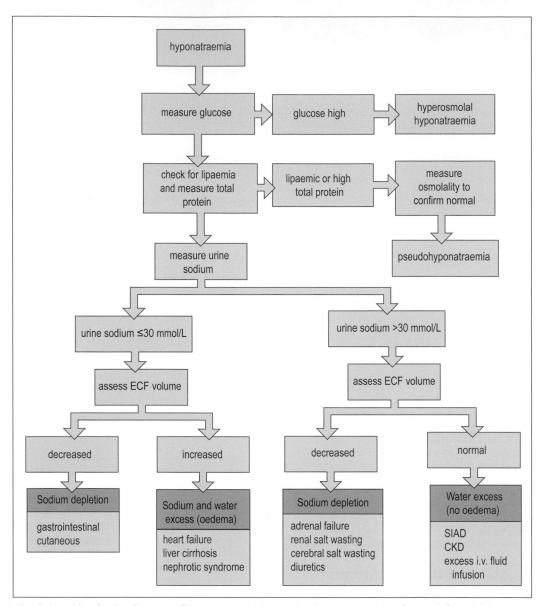

Fig. 3.7 Simple algorithm for the diagnosis of hyponatraemia. In practice, hyponatraemia is often multifactorial, but one cause may predominate and determine the clinical features. ECF, extracellular fluid; i.v., intravenous; SIAD, syndrome of inappropriate antidiuresis; CKD, chronic kidney disease.

Potassium Homoeostasis

Dietary potassium intake is of the order of 75–150 mmol /24 h, values higher in the range being associated with a high intake of fruit and vegetables. Extracellular potassium balance is controlled primarily by the kidneys and, to a lesser extent, by the gastrointestinal tract. In the kidneys, filtered potassium is almost completely reabsorbed in the proximal tubules. Some active potassium secretion takes place in the most distal part of the distal convoluted tubules, but potassium excretion is primarily a passive process. The active reabsorption of sodium generates a membrane potential that is neutralized by the movement of

Table 3.3 Some common causes of hyponatraemia

Cause	Mechanism	ECF volume
syndrome of inappropriate antidiuresis	water excess	normal
increased gastrointestinal output	sodium depletion	decreased
inappropriate i.v. fluids	water excess	normal or increased
congestive cardiac failure and hypoproteinaemic states	sodium and water retention	increased
diuretic therapy	sodium depletion and water retention (see text)	decreased
adrenal insufficiency	sodium and water depletion	decreased
hyperglycaemia	isotonic redistribution	normal
non-specific ('sick cell syndrome')	see text	normal

ECF, extracellular fluid; i.v., intravenous.

Box 3.8 Some laboratory investigations of value in the investigation of hyponatraemia

inspection of serum for limpaemia

serum

    osmolality

    potassium

    urea

    creatinine

    total protein

    TSH and free T4

haematocrit

ACTH (tetracosactide [Synacthen]) stimulation test

urine

    sodium

    osmolality

ACTH, adrenocorticotrophic hormone; TSH, thyroid-stimulaing hormone.

Case history 3.5

History

A male infant aged 15 weeks was admitted to hospital for the investigation of recurrent diarrhoea. He had been well until 8 weeks of age, when the first episode had occurred. Since then, there had been several further attacks.

Examination

There were clinical signs of dehydration and he had lost weight.

Results

Serum:	sodium	167 mmol/L
	potassium	4.9 mmol/L
	urea	2.6 mmol/L
Urine:	sodium	310 mmol/l

Summary

Severe hypernatraemia with high urine sodium concentration.

Interpretation

The combination of high urine sodium excretion with hypernatraemia suggests salt overload. In most patients with chronic diarrhoea, the kidneys conserve sodium in response to dehydration and there is hyponatraemia, because of loss of sodium with inadequate replacement.

Discussion

Stool chromatography revealed the presence of an abnormal sugar, which was identified as lactulose. Lactulose is a non-absorbed osmotic laxative. Careful observation confirmed the suspicion that the child's mother was adding salt and lactulose to his feeds. She was not allowed to stay with him unattended, and the diarrhoea and electrolyte abnormalities resolved rapidly. This was a case of child abuse (fabricated or induced illness, sometimes referred to as 'Munchausen syndrome by proxy').

potassium and hydrogen ions from tubular cells into the lumen. Thus, **urinary potassium excretion** depends on several factors:

- the circulating concentration of aldosterone
- intravascular volume (reduction stimulates aldosterone secretion)
- the relative availability of hydrogen and potassium ions in the cells of the distal tubules and the collecting ducts

- the capacity of these cells to secrete hydrogen ions
- the rate of flow of tubular fluid: a high flow rate (e.g. osmotic diuresis, treatment with diuretics) favours the transfer of potassium into the tubular lumen
- the amount of sodium available for reabsorption in the distal convoluted tubules and the collecting ducts
- dietary potassium intake (the kidneys' capacity to retain potassium is enhanced by low intake, and vice versa): the mechanism for this is uncertain
- magnesium status: magnesium depletion increases potassium secretion from the distal nephron (it also impairs the action of the sodium–potassium pump responsible for the uptake of potassium into the ECF).

In the distal nephrons, potassium is secreted in exchange for either sodium or hydrogen ions: increased delivery of sodium increases the potential secretion of potassium. Aldosterone stimulates potassium excretion both indirectly, by increasing the active reabsorption of sodium in the distal convoluted tubules and the collecting ducts, and directly, by increasing active potassium secretion in the distal part of the distal convoluted tubules. Aldosterone secretion from the adrenal cortex is stimulated indirectly by activation of the renin–angiotensin system in response to hypovolaemia (see p. 28) and directly by hyperkalaemia.

Because both hydrogen and potassium ions can neutralize the nephron membrane potential generated by active sodium reabsorption, there is a **close relationship between potassium and hydrogen ion homoeostasis**. In an acidosis, hydrogen ions will tend to be secreted in preference to potassium; in alkalosis, fewer hydrogen ions will be available for excretion and there will be an increase in potassium excretion. Thus, there is **a tendency towards hyperkalaemia in acidosis** and towards **hypokalaemia in alkalosis**. In addition, the active secretion of hydrogen ions in the distal nephron is partly balanced by a reciprocal reabsorption of potassium. An exception to this tendency is renal tubular acidosis caused by defective renal hydrogen ion excretion (see p. 97). In this condition, because of the decrease in hydrogen ion excretion, potassium secretion must increase to balance sodium reabsorption. The result is the unusual combination of hypokalaemia with acidosis.

The capacity of the distal nephrons to excrete potassium is, in part, determined by intracellular magnesium concentration. Magnesium depletion (e.g. resulting from

---

Case history 3.6

History

After surgery for major abdominal injuries sustained in a knife fight, a young man was fed parenterally with a regimen including 17 g nitrogen as amino acids and 500 g glucose, and artificially ventilated. On day four he become pyrexial, and positive blood cultures were subsequently obtained.

Examination

His fluid balance chart showed that in the previous 24 h his fluid intake had been 3000 mL, urine output had been steady at 90–100 mL/h, and 300 mL fluid had been aspirated via a nasogastric tube. The sodium intake had been 70 mmol. A request for biochemistry testing was made, and the sample was collected the following morning.

Results

Serum:		
	sodium	150 mmol/L
	potassium	4.2 mmol/L
	urea	10.2 mmol/L
	creatinine	102 µmol/L
	eGFR	>90 mL/min/1.73 m^2
	glucose	25 mmol/L

Summary

Hypernatraemia with hyperglycaemia with raised urea and normal creatinine concentrations.

Interpretation

Sodium input is not excessive; water depletion is the more likely cause of the hypernatraemia. His measured net fluid balance is only 400 mL positive. This is insufficient to balance insensible losses, which will have been increased by the pyrexia and possibly by ventilation. The urine output has not decreased; therefore there has also been an excessive renal water loss. This is due to an osmotic diuresis as a result of glycosuria and a high urea output. The high urea concentration relative to that of creatinine is typical of fluid depletion (see Box 5.1).

Discussion

Glucose intolerance may be a problem in patients receiving parenteral nutrition and can be exacerbated by sepsis, which causes insulin resistance. Parenteral administration of excessive nitrogen will result in increased formation of urea, which will also contribute to an osmotic diuresis: this patient was receiving amino acids equivalent to >100 g protein/day, more than his probable requirements. Inadequate humidification of inspired air may also be a causative factor in water depletion in such circumstances.

increased gastrointestinal or renal loss) results in increased tubular potassium secretion.

Healthy kidneys are less efficient at conserving potassium than sodium: even on a potassium-free diet, urinary excretion remains at 10–20 mmol/24 h. Because there is also an obligatory loss from the skin and gut of approximately 15–20 mmol/24 h, the kidneys cannot compensate if intake declines to much less than 40 mmol/24 h.

Potassium is secreted in gastric juice (5–10 mmol/L) and much of this, along with dietary potassium, is reabsorbed in the small intestine. In the colon and rectum, potassium is secreted in exchange for sodium, partly under the control of aldosterone. Stools normally contain some potassium, but considerable amounts (up to 30 mmol/L) can be lost in patients with fistulae or chronic diarrhoea, or in patients who are losing gastric secretions through persistent vomiting or nasogastric aspiration.

Movement of potassium between the intracellular and extracellular compartments can have a profound effect on plasma potassium concentration. Potassium ions move into cells from the ECF in exchange for sodium, via the transmembrane, energy-dependent sodium–potassium pump (Na^+,K^+-ATPase). Hyperkalaemia can result if the activity of this pump is impaired or if there is damage to cell membranes. Potassium uptake into cells is stimulated by insulin and β-adrenergic stimulation; α-adrenergic stimulation has the opposite effect. Potassium uptake is impaired in magnesium depletion, but the concurrent increased loss of potassium through the kidneys results in net potassium depletion and hypokalaemia.

Transcellular shifts of hydrogen ions can cause reciprocal shifts in potassium and vice versa. In a systemic acidosis, intracellular buffering of hydrogen ions results in the displacement of potassium into the ECF. In alkalosis, there is a shift of hydrogen ions from the ICF to the ECF, and a net movement of potassium ions in the opposite direction, which tends to produce hypokalaemia. Similarly, potassium depletion can lead to systemic alkalosis (see Chapter 4).

Potassium Depletion and Hypokalaemia

Potassium depletion occurs when output exceeds intake. Except in patients who are fasting, inadequate intake is rarely the sole cause of potassium depletion. However, **increased loss of potassium, either from the gut or (more often) through the kidneys, is a frequent occurrence**. If renal potassium excretion is <20 mmol/L in a patient with hypokalaemia, excessive renal excretion is unlikely to be the cause. Drug therapy is often implicated in the pathogenesis of potassium depletion. Hypokalaemia, although usually only mild (3.0–3.5 mmol/L), is the most frequently occurring electrolyte abnormality.

The **causes of hypokalaemia** are shown in Box 3.9. By far the most common causes are loss of potassium from the gut and treatment with diuretics. When hypokalaemia is a result of potassium depletion, it usually develops slowly and is only corrected slowly when the cause is effectively treated. In contrast, hypokalaemia as a result of redistribution of potassium from the extracellular to the intracellular compartment usually develops acutely and can normalize rapidly. Bartter, Liddle and Gitelman syndromes are rare

---

Box 3.9 Principal causes of hypokalaemia

Decreased K⁺ intake
oral (rare)
parenteral

Transcellular K⁺ movement
alkalosis
insulin administration
β-adrenergic agonists
refeeding syndrome
rapid cellular proliferation (e.g. anabolic phase after starvation)

Increased K⁺ excretion
renal
  diuretics
  diuretic phase of acute kidney injury
  nephrotoxic drugs (e.g. amphotericin)
  mineralocorticoid excess:
    primary aldosteronism
    secondary aldosteronism
    Cushing syndrome
    carbenoxolone, liquorice (see p. 184)
    renal tubular acidosis (types 1 and 2)
  Bartter, Liddle and Gitelman syndromes (see Table 3.4)
  magnesium depletion
extrarenal
  diarrhoea
  purgative abuse
  villous adenoma of the rectum
  vomiting, gastric aspiration
  enterocutaneous fistulae
  excessive sweating

Table 3.4 Inherited disorders of renal tubular function that are associated with hypokalaemic alkalosis

Syndrome name	Inheritance	Renin and aldosterone	BP	Other features	Cause	Usual age of clinical onset
Liddle	AD	↓	↑	family history of premature stroke	activating mutation in distal tubule sodium channel	infancy to early adulthood
Gitelman	AR	↑	↓/N	salt wasting hypomagnesaemia hypocalciuria	defect in thiazide-sensitive sodium transporter	adulthood
Bartter	AR	↑	↓/N	salt wasting short stature	impaired sodium reabsorption in loop of Henle	infancy to early childhood

AD, autosomal dominant; AR, autosomal recessive; BP, blood pressure.

inherited disorders caused by mutations in renal tubular ion transport proteins. Their biochemical and clinical features are summarized in Table 3.4.

Clinical features

Even severe hypokalaemia may be asymptomatic. Hypokalaemia causes hyperpolarization of excitable membranes, thus decreasing their excitability. When symptoms are present, they are related primarily to disturbances of neuromuscular function (Table 3.5): muscular weakness, constipation and paralytic ileus are common problems. Cardiac dysrhythmias can be fatal: characteristic electrocardiographic (ECG) findings include ST segment depression and a prominent U wave. Hypokalaemia also potentiates digoxin toxicity. This is an important practical consideration, because diuretics and digoxin may be prescribed together, although the latter drug is now used less frequently than in the past. Hypokalaemia results in increased synthesis of prostaglandins, which antagonize the action of vasopressin, leading to polyuria and secondary polydipsia.

Investigation of hypokalaemia

As indicated in Box 3.9, the causes of hypokalaemia can be divided into decreased potassium intake, redistribution of potassium into cells and increased potassium excretion. The first two groups are usually clinically apparent: low potassium intake is usually a chronic problem, whereas abnormal transcellular movement of potassium is more likely to be an acute disorder. Current and recent drug treatment should be reviewed for thiazide or loop diuretics and potentially nephrotoxic drugs such as amphotericin or cisplatin, all of which cause increased urinary potassium loss. Because increased

Table 3.5 Clinical features of hypokalaemia

Disorder	Feature
neuromuscular	weakness
	constipation, ileus
	hypotonia
	depression
	confusion
cardiac	arrhythmias
	potentiation of digoxin toxicity
	ECG changes (ST depression, T wave depression/inversion, prolonged P-R interval prominent U wave)
renal	impaired concentrating ability leading to polyuria and polydipsia
metabolic	alkalosis

Excitable membranes become hyperpolarized in hypokalaemia, decreasing their excitability The effect on the kidneys is due to increased synthesis of prostaglandins, which antagonize the action of vasopressin.

potassium losses may be either via the kidneys or via other routes (usually gastrointestinal), it is often informative to measure urine potassium output. A random urine potassium concentration >20 mmol/L in the presence of hypokalaemia is inappropriately high and usually indicates that the kidneys are the route of potassium loss.

Most patients with hypokalaemia also have a metabolic alkalosis, the presence of which is indicated by a high plasma bicarbonate concentration: measurement of venous or arterial hydrogen ion concentration (pH) is rarely necessary. Important exceptions are renal tubular acidosis and some instances of increased gastrointestinal loss, which may be associated with the low plasma bicarbonate concentrations that characterize metabolic acidosis.

Patients with increased renal or gastrointestinal potassium excretion often also have increased magnesium excretion; magnesium depletion may exacerbate hypokalaemia by impairing the capacity of the kidney tubules appropriately to reabsorb filtered potassium (see p. 46). Plasma magnesium concentration should therefore be measured if the clinical picture indicates that depletion is likely or in any patient with otherwise unexplained hypokalaemia or hypokalaemia that is resistant to replacement.

Management of hypokalaemia

Although the plasma potassium concentration is a poor guide to total body potassium, a plasma concentration of 3.0 mmol/L generally implies a deficit of the order of 300 mmol. The first step in the management of hypokalaemia should be to identify and treat the causative condition, but potassium replacement is frequently required. Oral supplementation may be appropriate in mild, chronic hypokalaemia, but in more severe or acute cases, intravenous administration is necessary. Because any potassium deficit will be almost entirely from the ICF but administered potassium first enters the ECF, replacement must be undertaken with care, particularly when the intravenous route is used.

As a guide, the following potassium dosages should not be exceeded without good reason: a rate of 20 mmol/h, a concentration of 40 mmol/L in intravenous fluid or a total of 240 mmol/24 h. Thorough mixing with the bulk of the fluid to be infused is vital. Plasma concentrations should be monitored during treatment. If unusually large amounts of potassium are necessary, and particularly if there is impaired kidney function, ECG monitoring is essential, because characteristic changes in the waveform occur with changing plasma potassium concentrations.

Potassium Excess and Hyperkalaemia

Potassium excess can be caused by excessive intake or decreased excretion. A normal intake may be excessive if excretion is decreased (e.g. in kidney failure). Excessive intake is otherwise virtually always iatrogenic and the result of parenteral administration. Drugs are frequently implicated as causes of hyperkalaemia: combinations of potassium-sparing diuretics with angiotensin-converting enzyme inhibitors (ACEIs), angiotensin II receptor blockers

Case history 3.7

History

A 67-year-old woman presented with severe muscular weakness. She had been in the habit of taking large amounts of purgatives and recently had been prescribed a thiazide diuretic for mild hypertension.

Results

Serum:	potassium	2.4 mmol/L
	bicarbonate	36 mmol/L

Summary

Severe hypokalaemia with high serum bicarbonate concentration.

Interpretation

Hypokalaemic alkalosis resulting from both increased losses from the gut, owing to purgative abuse and from the kidneys as a result of a thiazide diuretic.

Discussion

Thiazides act by inhibiting sodium–chloride cotransport in the distal part of the ascending limbs of the loops of Henle and in the first part of the distal tubules. As a result, there is an increase in the amount of sodium delivered to, and available for reabsorption from, the distal tubules: this will tend to increase potassium and hydrogen ion excretion from the kidneys. Loop diuretics similarly increase renal potassium excretion, although to a lesser extent. The doses of thiazide diuretics used to treat hypertension rarely cause significant hypokalaemia unless, as in this case, other causes of hypokalaemia are present.

If necessary, potassium supplements may be prescribed at the same time as diuretics; combined preparations are available but typically provide insufficient potassium. Alternatively, a potassium-sparing diuretic such as amiloride may be co-prescribed. Potassium supplements are probably unnecessary unless the plasma concentration is <3.0 mmol/L, and they are potentially dangerous in patients with renal impairment because hyperkalaemia may result.

(ARBs) or non-steroidal anti-inflammatory drugs (NSAIDs) are particularly hazardous. NSAIDs tend to decrease renal potassium excretion through their effect on eicosanoid synthesis.

Hyperkalaemia (Box 3.10) can result from potassium excess but can also be a result of redistribution of potassium from the intracellular to the extracellular compartment. This mechanism can sometimes cause hyperkalaemia even in a patient with potassium depletion (e.g. in diabetic ketoacidosis). As with hypokalaemia, more than one cause of hyperkalaemia may be present. **Pseudohyperkalaemia**,

History

A 60-year-old man underwent total gastrectomy for a carcinoma. He was malnourished before surgery and it was decided to provide parenteral nutrition postoperatively. On the fifth day, his serum potassium concentration was 3.0 mmol/L, despite the provision of 60 mmol potassium/24 h in the intravenous feed.

Interpretation

The patient is hypokalaemic in spite of the provision of sufficient potassium to cover normal obligatory losses.

Discussion

Potassium excretion increases during the metabolic response to trauma but, once a patient becomes anabolic, the body's requirements increase as potassium is taken up into cells. Furthermore, during total parenteral nutrition, glucose is often the predominant energy source, providing a considerable stimulus to insulin release. Potassium requirements may, therefore, be much greater than normal because insulin stimulates its uptake into cells.

This patient had recently undergone abdominal surgery, and an ileus is usual in these circumstances. This will result in decreased reabsorption of any potassium secreted into the gut and can also contribute to the loss of potassium from the ECF.

Severe hypokalaemia is a feature of the refeeding syndrome that may occur when nutrition is started at an inappropriately high rate (see p. 149).

Box 3.10 **Principal causes of hyperkalaemia**

Spurious

haemolysis

delayed separation of serum from blood cells

contamination (e.g. with potassium EDTA anticoagulant)

abnormal blood cells, e.g. leukaemia, thrombocytosis

Excessive K+ intake

oral, e.g. LoSalt (rare except in chronic kidney disease orf with K+-sparing diuretics)

parenteral infusion

Transcellular K+ movement

tissue damage (e.g. trauma, tumour lysis syndrome)

catabolic states

    systematic acidosis

    insulin lack

    vigorous exercise (transient)

Decreased K+ excretion

acute kidney injury

chronic kidney disease

K+-sparing diuretics

angiotensin-converting enzyme inhibitors

angiotensin II receptor antagonists

non-steroidal anti-inflammatory drugs

mineralocorticoid deficiency:

    Addison disease

    adrenalectomy

    hyporeninaemic hypoaldosteronism

---

caused by the leakage of potassium from blood cells *in vitro*, often occurs. Although often caused by frank haemolysis, this is not invariably the case, especially if there has been a delay in separation of the plasma from the blood cells. The normal clotting process releases potassium from white cells and platelets: this normally contributes a negligible amount to serum potassium concentration, but the effect is exaggerated in patients with high white cell or platelet counts (e.g. in leukaemia).

Investigation of hyperkalaemia

Chronic mild hyperkalaemia, with a serum potassium concentration of 5.3–6.0 mmol/L, is a relatively common finding, especially in elderly patients. In some cases, it is clearly attributable to acute or chronic kidney disease, but in others, no such cause is apparent.

It is important to exclude adrenal insufficiency, if necessary, with an adrenocorticotrophic hormone (ACTH;

tetracosactide [Synacthen]) stimulation test (see p. 179). Mineralocorticoid deficiency often, but not always, results in hyponatraemia, an increase in urea and hyperkalaemia.

A careful drug history may elicit use of 'potassium-sparing' diuretics such as spironolactone. ACEIs or ARBs cause hyperkalaemia, especially in patients with renal artery stenosis (which may be unsuspected clinically), and it is essential to check 'urea and electrolytes' one week after starting drugs of this class. NSAIDs are particularly prone to cause hyperkalaemia in patients taking diuretics.

Haemolysis is an obvious cause of pseudohyperkalaemia, and most laboratories screen for, and report this on all samples, but the same effect occurs in the absence of haemolysis if separation of the plasma from the cells is delayed for more than about 4 h, especially at low temperatures. Pseudohyperkalaemia associated with high white cell or platelet counts can be excluded by measuring a full blood count. Some patients have subclinical red cell abnormalities that result in more rapid cell breakdown in vitro: measurement of potassium using a blood tube containing heparin anticoagulant with rapid centrifugation and separation of the plasma may identify this cause. Pseudohyperkalaemia of any cause is not of direct clinical significance, but patients may need to have their blood samples taken in the hospital phlebotomy clinic and processed rapidly to enable accurate measurement of potassium.

If the above causes are excluded, the patient may have hyporeninaemic hypoaldosteronism. This is particularly prevalent in the elderly and often a feature of early (e.g. diabetic) nephropathy, with hyperkalaemia out of proportion to the reduction in GFR. It may be helpful to measure paired serum and urine potassium concentrations and osmolalities to calculate the transtubular potassium gradient (TTKG), a measure of the ability of the nephrons to excrete potassium appropriately. In hyporeninaemic hypoaldosteronism, the TTKG is low.

Clinical features

Hyperkalaemia is less common than hypokalaemia but is more dangerous: through its effect on the heart, it can kill without warning. It lowers the resting membrane potential, shortens the cardiac action potential and increases the speed of repolarization. Cardiac arrest in asystole or slow ventricular fibrillation may be the first sign of hyperkalaemia. The risk increases significantly with potassium concentrations exceeding 6.5 mmol/L (particularly if the increase has occurred rapidly); this should be treated as a medical emergency. It is therefore necessary to be alert for this disorder in appropriate circumstances, for instance, in acute kidney injury, to ensure that effective early management is instituted. Characteristic ECG changes (initially peaking of T waves, followed by loss of P waves and, finally, the development of abnormal QRS complexes) may precede cardiac arrest. Other clinical features of hyperkalaemia include muscle weakness, and in hyperkalaemia associated with acidosis, hyperventilation (Kussmaul respiration, see Case history 13.2) may be present.

Management

In **acute and severe hyperkalaemia,** intravenous calcium gluconate (10 mL of a 10% solution given over 1 min and repeated as necessary) affords some degree of immediate protection to the myocardium by antagonizing the effect of hyperkalaemia on myocardial excitability. Intravenous infusion of glucose and insulin promotes intracellular potassium

---

Case history 3.9

History

A young man was admitted to hospital after sustaining a fractured femur and ruptured spleen in a motorcycle accident. He underwent splenectomy and was put in traction. Some 24 h after admission, he had passed only 300 mL urine.

Results

Serum:		
	urea	21.5 mmol/L
	creatinine	168 μmol/L
	eGFR	49 mL/min/1.73m^2
	potassium	6.5 mmol/L

Summary

Severe hyperkalaemia with high serum urea and creatinine concentrations.

Interpretation

Oliguria with high serum urea and creatinine concentrations indicates that the patient has developed acute kidney injury; this might be reversible (i.e. pre-renal; see p. 85). The hyperkalaemia is due to a combination of decreased renal perfusion (hypovolaemic shock) and the loss of potassium either from cells damaged directly by trauma or from cells whose membrane integrity is impaired by hypoxia.

Discussion

This case illustrates the risk of severe hyperkalaemia in patients who sustain acute kidney injury owing to hypovolaemic shock. Similar results may be seen in patients who have sustained a gastrointestinal haemorrhage, which may itself cause hypovolaemia, affecting renal function, but in addition, there will be absorption of potassium from red blood cells undergoing lysis in the gut and increased synthesis of urea from the amino acids released.

Note that although the estimated glomerular filtration rate (eGFR) is stated to be 49 mL/min/1.73 m^2, eGFR calculations overestimate the true GFR in patients who are developing acute kidney injury, see p. 82.

---

uptake. Salbutamol, which activates Na^+,K^+-ATPase, has a similar effect. If insulin is used, blood glucose must be monitored for the subsequent 6 h because of the risk of hypoglycaemia. In an acidotic patient, hyperkalaemia can be controlled temporarily by bicarbonate infusion (using a 1.26% solution, not 8.4%, which risks causing ECF volume expansion because of the high sodium concentration).

In acute kidney injury and in other circumstances where the hyperkalaemia is uncontrollable, dialysis or haemofiltration will be required. In chronic kidney disease, restriction of potassium intake and the administration of oral ion-exchange resins are often successful in preventing dangerous hyperkalaemia until such time as dialysis becomes necessary for other reasons.

ECG monitoring can be valuable in patients with hyperkalaemia. Changes in the plasma potassium concentration are reflected by changes in the ECG waveform more rapidly than could be determined by biochemical measurement.

Stable chronic hyperkalaemia with potassium concentration <6.5 mmol/L is not a medical emergency, although there is increased risk of cardiac dysrhythmias if the underlying cause worsens or a second contributory factor arises. Treatment is primarily of the underlying cause, with care to avoid use of drugs that promote renal potassium retention and to restrict overconsumption of potassium-rich foods, such as fruits, or high-potassium salt substitutes (e.g. LoSalt).

Patients with hyporeninaemic hypoaldosteronism may need treatment for acute hyperkalaemia should this supervene, but in the longer term, the mineralocorticoid drug fludrocortisone or the potassium-wasting diuretic furosemide may be useful.

Case history 3.10

History

Blood from an outpatient being treated with diuretics was received in the laboratory for biochemical analysis. The serum potassium concentration was 6.7 mmol/L. There was no visible haemolysis, and the blood was freshly drawn. She was recalled and asked to bring all her tablets with her. It transpired that she had initially been prescribed a loop diuretic and potassium supplements for congestive cardiac failure. However, at an outpatient attendance she had been prescribed spironolactone, an antagonist of aldosterone used as a potassium-sparing diuretic, instead of the potassium supplements. She had misunderstood the instructions given to her, and continued to take both the supplements and the diuretic. She was asked to stop taking the potassium supplements, and her serum potassium concentration was normal when checked 1 week later.

Discussion

Therapeutic drugs are a common cause of hyperkalaemia: potassium-sparing diuretics and angiotensin-converting enzyme inhibitors or aldosterone receptor blockers pose a particular risk, especially in the elderly, in whom renal function may be diminished. Salt substitutes (which contain potassium) are also a potential hazard.

Hyperkalaemia is a medical emergency because it causes potentially fatal cardiac dysthymias. Plasma potassium concentrations may increase rapidly, particularly in patients with defective potassium excretion. **Potassium >6.0 mmol/L** requires urgent repeat and if rising rapidly or **potassium >6.5 mmol/L** the patient must be referred for urgent management in hospital.

Intravenous fluid therapy

The safe and effective provision of appropriate intravenous fluids to patients who are unable to maintain adequate sodium, water and potassium balance is learned through supervised clinical practice but must be informed by a thorough understanding of the underlying physiological and pathological principles. Accurate measurement of fluid losses and assessment of insensible losses is important. Biochemical measurements can provide valuable information but are frequently misinterpreted (e.g. that hyponatraemia necessarily indicates sodium depletion).

Initial assessment of an acutely ill patient will include assessment of whether he or she is hypovolaemic and needs fluids as part of **resuscitation**. Blood (or red cell concentrate) may be required if bleeding has occurred. Patients who are unable to meet their ongoing fluid and electrolyte requirements orally or enterally need provision of intravenous fluids. It is helpful to consider separately the amounts of water and electrolytes needed for **routine maintenance** and to **replace abnormal losses** and **redistribution**.

For replacement of gastrointestinal losses, the choice will be determined by the nature of the fluid being lost; for example, gastric aspirates require isovolumetric replacement with 0.9% sodium chloride (sometimes referred to as 'normal' or 'physiological' saline, although it is neither of these).

The most frequent indication for the use of intravenous fluids outside critical care and high-dependency units is in relation to surgery. Before surgery, steps should be taken to ensure that body water, sodium and potassium status are normal. In emergencies, this may require rapid resuscitation with intravenous fluids or blood. Considerable quantities of water can be lost from exposed mucosal surfaces during surgery, in addition to any loss of blood and other continuing insensible losses.

Postoperatively, the requirement is to maintain fluid balance until the patient is able to take fluids orally. In the immediate postoperative period, the metabolic response to trauma causes relative water retention because of increased secretion of vasopressin. Stress also decreases sodium excretion and there is loss of potassium from damaged cells into the ECF. In the first 24 h after surgery, intravenous fluid administration may need to be limited to no more than 1500 mL if overload is to be avoided, and potassium is not usually required. As the metabolic response to trauma resolves, fluid input can be increased to maintain an adequate urine output. A recommended intravenous postoperative fluid regimen after the first 24 h is 25–30 mL/kg per 24 h water and 1 mmol/kg per 24 h sodium and potassium, but account must also be taken of any additional losses (e.g. from fistulae or gastric aspirates) and the results of measurements of plasma concentrations of sodium, potassium, urea and creatinine. Gastrointestinal losses should usually be replaced with 0.9% sodium chloride, but otherwise Hartmann's solution is preferable to replace sodium, because it contains less chloride and reduces the risk of inducing hyperchloraemic acidosis (see p. 63).

The provision of nutrients postoperatively is discussed in Chapter 8.

The composition of some more frequently used intravenous fluids is shown in Table 3.6.

Table 3.6 The composition of some intravenous fluids

Fluid	Composition	Use
0.9% sodium chloride[a]	sodium 154 mmol/L	isotonic fluid replacement
	chloride 154 mmol/L	
dextrose-saline	sodium 31 mmol/L	balanced sodium and water replacement[b,c]
	chloride 31 mmol/L	
	glucose 222 mmol/L	
5% dextrose	glucose 278 mmol/L	water replacement[b]
1.26% sodium bicarbonate	sodium 150 mmol/L	treatment of acidosis
	bicarbonate 150 mmol/L	
Hartmann's solution	sodium 131 mmol/L	isotonic fluid replacement
('Ringer–lactate',	potassium 5.4 mmol/L	
compound sodium	calcium 2.2 mmol/L	
lactate)	chloride 112 mmol/L	
	lactate 29 mmol/L	

[a]Sometimes referred to as physiological or 'normal' saline.
[b]These solutions are isotonic with plasma, but metabolism rapidly removes the glucose so they are effectively hypotonic.
[c]Dextrose–saline contains sodium and water in suitable proportion to provide total daily sodium and water requirement to an adult who has no deficits or abnormal losses, through use of a single infusion fluid: glucose is used to make the solution isotonic. Note that this is often inappropriate in clinical practice, and many patients require both 0.9% saline or Hartmann's solution and 5% dextrose.

SUMMARY

- **Sodium, potassium and water homoeostasis are closely linked.** Sodium is the principal extracellular cation, and the amount of sodium in the body is the major determinant of ECF volume. Potassium is the major intracellular cation.
- **Sodium and potassium are transported actively** in the body; **water moves passively** in response to changes in the solute contents of the body's fluid compartments.
- **Sodium excretion** is primarily controlled by **aldosterone**, a hormone secreted in response to a decrease in ECF volume that causes sodium retention and loss of potassium.
- **Water excretion** is controlled by **vasopressin** (ADH). This promotes water retention and is secreted in response to an increase in ECF osmolality and a decrease in ECF volume.
- **Potassium excretion** is regulated in part by aldosterone but also depends on extracellular hydrogen ion concentration and sodium and water excretion.
- Disturbances of either water or sodium homoeostasis can produce characteristic clinical and biochemical features, but combined disturbances are common and the features may then be less clear-cut.
- Changes in plasma sodium concentration can be caused by changes in the amounts of extracellular sodium or water, or both. **Hyponatraemia is common**; it is sometimes an appropriate physiological response to disease. **Hypernatraemia is less common** than hyponatraemia and usually is related to a decrease in body water.
- **Plasma potassium concentration** is a poor guide to the body's overall potassium status. Depletion is not always associated with hypokalaemia, nor is hypokalaemia always due to potassium depletion; similar considerations apply to potassium excess and hyperkalaemia.
- **Hypokalaemia** is most frequently a result of excessive gastrointestinal or renal loss of potassium and may be exacerbated by poor intake. It can also be a consequence of increased cellular uptake of potassium from the plasma. It can cause skeletal and smooth muscle weakness, and impairment of myocardial contractility and renal concentrating ability. It also potentiates digoxin toxicity.
- **Hyperkalaemia** is most frequently due to decreased renal excretion or loss of potassium from cells; hyperkalaemia is often iatrogenic, occurring as a result of drug treatment or inappropriate potassium administration. Spurious hyperkalaemia, caused by release of potassium from cells *in vitro*, is common. Hyperkalaemia can cause cardiac arrest: this can occur in the absence of any warning clinical symptoms or signs.

Chapter | 4 |

Hydrogen ion homoeostasis and blood gases

Introduction

The normal processes of metabolism result in the net formation of 40–80 mmol of hydrogen ions per 24 h, principally from the oxidation of sulfur-containing amino acids. This burden of hydrogen ions is excreted by the kidneys in the urine. In addition, there is a considerable endogenous turnover of hydrogen ions as a result of normal metabolic processes. Incomplete oxidation of energy substrates generates acid (e.g. lactic acid by glycolysis or oxoacids [ketoacids] from triacylglycerols [triglycerides]), whereas further metabolism of these intermediates consumes it (e.g. gluconeogenesis from lactate or the oxidation of ketones). Temporary imbalances between the rates of production and consumption may arise in health (e.g. the accumulation of lactic acid during anaerobic exercise), but overall they are in balance and thus make no contribution to net hydrogen ion excretion.

Potentially far more acid is generated as carbon dioxide during energy-yielding oxidative metabolism. In excess of 15 000 mmol/24 h of carbon dioxide is produced in this way and is normally excreted by the lungs. Although carbon dioxide itself is not an acid, in the presence of water it can undergo hydration to form a weak acid, carbonic acid:

$$CO_2 + H_2O \rightleftharpoons H_2CO_3 \qquad [4.1]$$

Carbon dioxide is removed from the body in expired air. As hydrogen ions can be generated stoichiometrically from carbon dioxide, the normal daily production of carbon dioxide is potentially equivalent to at least 15 000 mmol of hydrogen ions. In health, pulmonary ventilation is controlled so that carbon dioxide excretion exactly matches the rate of formation.

The homoeostatic mechanisms for hydrogen ions and carbon dioxide are very efficient. Temporary imbalances can

be absorbed by buffering, and as a result, the hydrogen ion concentration of the body is maintained within narrow limits (35–45 nmol/L [pH 7.35–7.46] in extracellular fluid [ECF]). The intracellular hydrogen ion concentration is slightly higher but is also rigorously controlled. In disease, however, imbalances between the rates of acid formation and excretion can develop and may persist, resulting in acidosis or alkalosis.

Buffering of hydrogen ions

As hydrogen ions are generated, they are buffered, thus limiting the rise in hydrogen ion concentration that would otherwise occur. A buffer system consists of a weak acid—that is, one that is incompletely dissociated—and its conjugate base. If hydrogen ions are added to a buffer, some will combine with the conjugate base and convert it to the undissociated acid. Thus, the addition of hydrogen ions to the bicarbonate–carbonic acid system (Equation 4.2) drives the reaction to the right, increasing the amount of carbonic acid and consuming bicarbonate ions:

$$H^+ + HCO_3^- \rightleftharpoons H_2CO_3 \qquad [4.2]$$

Conversely, if the hydrogen ion concentration falls, carbonic acid dissociates, thereby generating hydrogen ions.

The efficacy of any buffer is limited by its concentration and by the position of the equilibrium. A buffer operates most efficiently at hydrogen ion concentrations that result in approximately equal concentrations of undissociated acid and conjugate base. The bicarbonate buffer system is the most important in the ECF, yet at normal ECF hydrogen ion concentrations, the concentration of carbonic acid is about 1.2 mmol/L, whereas that of bicarbonate is 20 times greater. However, the capacity of the bicarbonate system is greatly enhanced in the body because carbonic acid can readily be formed from carbon dioxide or disposed of by conversion into carbon dioxide and water (see Equation 4.1).

For every hydrogen ion buffered by bicarbonate, a bicarbonate ion is consumed (see Equation 4.2). The bicarbonate must be regenerated to maintain the capacity of the buffer system. Yet, when bicarbonate is formed from carbonic acid (indirectly from carbon dioxide and water), equimolar amounts of hydrogen ions are formed simultaneously (see Equation 4.2). Bicarbonate formation can continue only if these hydrogen ions are removed. This process occurs in the cells of the renal tubules, where hydrogen ions are secreted into the urine and where bicarbonate is generated and retained in the body.

Proteins, including intracellular proteins, are also involved in buffering. The proteinaceous matrix of bone is an important buffer in chronic acidosis. Phosphate is a minor buffer in the ECF but it is of fundamental importance in the urine. The special role of haemoglobin is considered on p. 57.

Bicarbonate reabsorption and hydrogen ion excretion

The glomerular filtrate contains the same concentration of bicarbonate ions as the plasma. At normal rates of glomerular filtration, ~4300 mmol of bicarbonate is filtered by the renal glomeruli each 24 h. If this bicarbonate were not reabsorbed, copious amounts would be excreted in the urine, depleting the body's buffering capacity and causing an acidosis. In health, at normal plasma bicarbonate concentrations, **virtually all the filtered bicarbonate is reabsorbed**.

The luminal surface of renal tubular cells is impermeable to bicarbonate; therefore, reabsorption must occur indirectly after its combination with hydrogen ions to form carbonic acid, which then dissociates to produce carbon dioxide, which diffuses across the luminal cell membrane. Within the renal tubular cells, carbon dioxide reacts with water to form carbonic acid (Fig. 4.1). This reaction (see Equation 4.1) is catalysed in the kidneys by the enzyme carbonate dehydratase (carbonic anhydrase). The carbonic acid thus formed dissociates into hydrogen and bicarbonate ions. The bicarbonate ions pass across the basolateral borders of the cells into the interstitial fluid and are thereby returned to the blood. The hydrogen ions are secreted across the luminal membrane in exchange for sodium ions, which accompany bicarbonate into the interstitial fluid (see Fig. 4.1). The formation of bicarbonate and hydrogen ions is promoted by their continuous removal and by the presence of carbonate dehydratase. This whole process, which takes place primarily in the proximal tubules, effectively results in the reabsorption of filtered bicarbonate.

Although hydrogen ions are secreted into the tubular fluid during bicarbonate reabsorption, this does not represent net acid excretion. The formation of these hydrogen ions merely provides the means for the reabsorption of bicarbonate. **Net acid excretion** depends on the same reactions occurring in the renal tubular cells but, in addition,

requires the presence of a suitable buffer system in the urine. This is because the minimum urinary pH that can be generated, 4.6, is equivalent to a hydrogen ion concentration of only 25 μmol/L. Given a normal urine volume of 1.5 L/24 h, free hydrogen ion excretion can account for less than a thousandth of the total amount that has to be excreted. **The principal urinary buffer is phosphate.** This is present in the glomerular filtrate, ~80% being in the form of the divalent anion, HPO_4^{2-}. This combines with hydrogen ions and is converted to $H_2PO_4^-$:

$$HPO_4^{2-} + H^+ \rightleftharpoons H_2PO_4^- \qquad [4.3]$$

At the minimum urinary pH, virtually all the phosphate is in the $H_2PO_4^-$ form. About 30–40 mmol of hydrogen ions is normally excreted in this way every 24 h.

Ammonia, produced by the deamination of glutamine in renal tubular cells, is also an important urinary buffer. The enzyme that catalyses this reaction, glutaminase, is induced in states of chronic acidosis, allowing increased ammonia production and hence increased hydrogen ion excretion via ammonium ions. Ammonia can readily diffuse across cell membranes, but ammonium ions, formed when ammonia buffers hydrogen ions (Equation 4.4), cannot. Passive reabsorption of ammonium ions is therefore prevented.

$$NH_3 + H^+ \rightleftharpoons NH_4^+ \qquad [4.4]$$

At normal intracellular hydrogen ion concentrations, most ammonia is present as ammonium ions, but diffusion of ammonia out of the cell disturbs the equilibrium, causing more ammonia to be formed.

The simultaneous production of hydrogen ions would seem to negate the role of ammonia as a buffer. However, these hydrogen ions are used up in gluconeogenesis, when they combine with glutamate formed by the deamination of glutamine. There may also be some shift of hepatic urea synthesis (a process that generates hydrogen ions) to glutamine synthesis (which consumes them). Urinary hydrogen ion excretion is summarized in Fig. 4.2. Acidification of the urine takes place primarily in the distal parts of the distal tubules and in the collecting ducts, where an ATP-dependent H^+ pump in the α-intercalated cells secretes hydrogen ions. Electrochemical neutrality is maintained by concurrent secretion of chloride. The activity of this pump is determined largely by intracellular hydrogen ion concentration.

It will be apparent that hydrogen and bicarbonate ions are generated in equimolar amounts in renal tubular cells. This is essential for the reabsorption of filtered bicarbonate, but it also means that when a hydrogen ion is excreted in the urine, a bicarbonate ion is produced and retained. **This process effectively regenerates the bicarbonate ions consumed when hydrogen ions are buffered.**

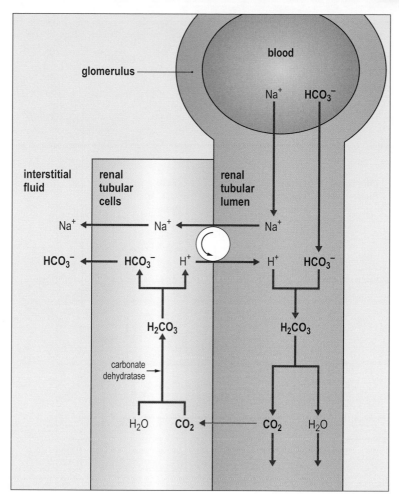

Fig. 4.1 Reabsorption of filtered bicarbonate by renal tubular cells. Bicarbonate cannot be reabsorbed directly. Hydrogen and bicarbonate ions are generated in renal tubular cells and the hydrogen ions are secreted in exchange for sodium into the tubular lumen where they combine with filtered bicarbonate to form carbon dioxide and water. Bicarbonate ions diffuse with sodium from the tubular cells into the interstitial fluid and then into the plasma.

There is considerable secretion of both acid (by the stomach) and bicarbonate (by the pancreas and small intestine) into the gut, but these processes are normally in balance and in health do not contribute to net hydrogen ion excretion.

Transport of carbon dioxide

Carbon dioxide, produced by aerobic metabolism, diffuses out of cells and into the ECF. A small amount combines with water to form carbonic acid, thereby increasing the hydrogen ion concentration of the ECF.

In red blood cells, metabolism is anaerobic and little carbon dioxide is produced. **Carbon dioxide thus diffuses into red cells** down a concentration gradient and carbonic acid is formed, facilitated by carbonate dehydratase (Fig. 4.3).

Haemoglobin buffers the hydrogen ions formed when the carbonic acid dissociates. Haemoglobin is a more powerful buffer when in the deoxygenated state, and the proportion in this state increases during the passage of blood through capillary beds, because oxygen is lost to the tissues.

The overall effect of this process is that carbon dioxide is converted to bicarbonate in red blood cells. This bicarbonate diffuses out of the red blood cells through a specific ion exchange channel because a concentration gradient develops: electrochemical neutrality is maintained by inward diffusion of chloride ions (the chloride shift). **In the lungs**, the reverse process occurs: the oxygenation of haemoglobin reduces its buffering capacity, liberating hydrogen ions; these combine with bicarbonate to form carbon dioxide, which diffuses into the alveoli to be excreted in the expired air while bicarbonate diffuses into the cells from the plasma.

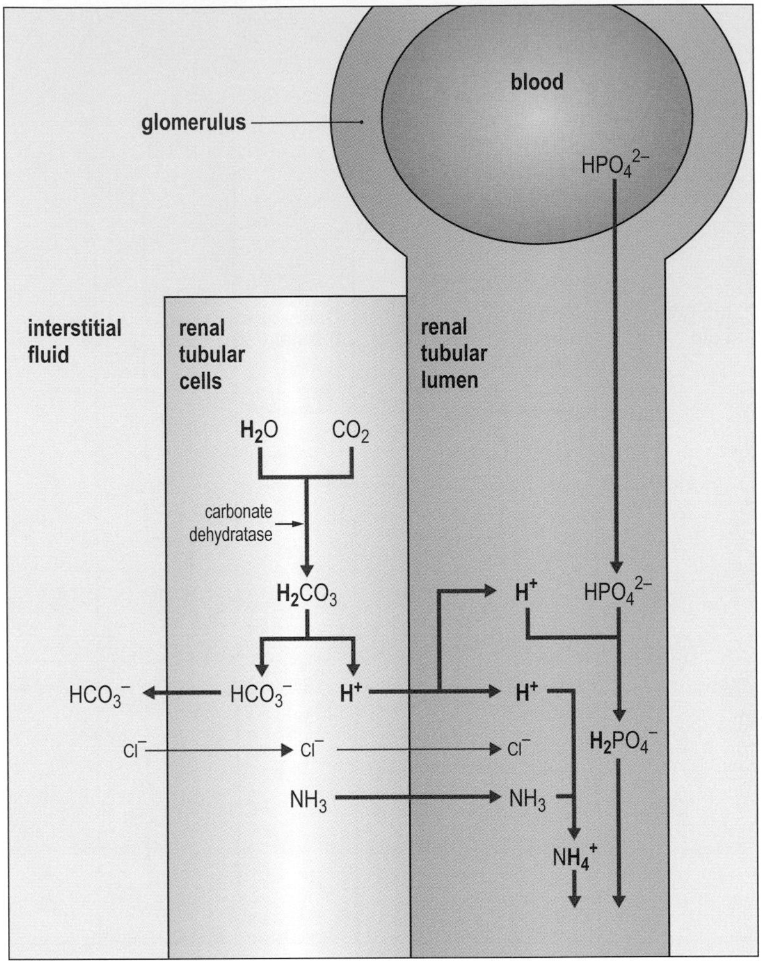

Fig. 4.2 Renal hydrogen ion excretion. Hydrogen and bicarbonate ions are generated in renal tubular cells from carbon dioxide and water by the reversal of the buffering reaction. The hydrogen ions are excreted in the urine buffered by phosphate and ammonia, while the bicarbonate enters the extracellular fluid, replacing that which was consumed in buffering.

Most of the carbon dioxide in the blood is present in the form of bicarbonate. Dissolved carbon dioxide, carbonic acid and carbamino compounds (compounds of carbon dioxide and protein) account for <2.0 mmol/L in a total carbon dioxide concentration of approximately 26 mmol/L. The terms 'bicarbonate' and 'total carbon dioxide' are frequently used synonymously. They are not strictly the same but may be considered to be so for most practical clinical purposes. It is technically difficult to measure bicarbonate concentration alone: most analytical techniques for bicarbonate actually measure total carbon dioxide.

The concentration of carbon dioxide (and of oxygen) in blood is expressed as **partial pressure** (P), which is the pressure that an amount of gas would exert if it occupied the same volume alone (see p. 1). The physicochemical properties of a gas in solution are determined by its partial pressure rather than by molar concentration. Using the Système Internationale (SI), partial pressure is measured in kilopascals (kPa), but the alternative conventional unit millimetres of mercury (mmHg) is also in use: for any gas, mmHg = kPa × 7.5.

Clinical and Laboratory Assessment of Hydrogen Ion Status

As discussed in this chapter, many conditions are associated with abnormalities of blood hydrogen ion concentration and partial pressure of carbon dioxide ($P\text{co}_2$). The clinical features associated with both of these abnormalities and with an altered partial pressure of oxygen ($P\text{o}_2$) are shown in Table 4.1.

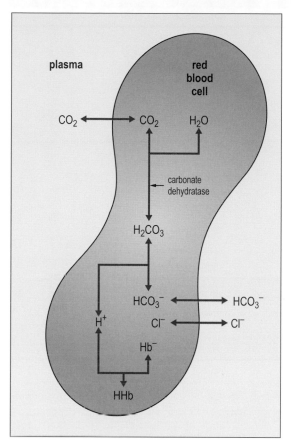

Fig. 4.3 Transport of carbon dioxide in the blood. In capillary beds, carbon dioxide diffuses into red blood cells and combines with water to form carbonic acid; the reaction is catalysed by carbonate dehydratase. The carbonic acid dissociates to form hydrogen ions (which are buffered by haemoglobin) and bicarbonate, which diffuses out of the cell; chloride diffuses in to maintain electrochemical neutrality. In the alveoli, the process reverses; carbon dioxide is produced from bicarbonate and is excreted in the expired air.

It is usual to measure hydrogen ion concentration [H+] in arterial blood anticoagulated with heparin. The arteriovenous difference for [H+] is small (<2 nmol/L), but the difference is significant for P_{CO_2} (~1 kPa higher in venous blood) and P_{O_2} (~8 kPa lower in venous blood).

By the law of mass action, it follows from the equations describing the dissociation of carbonic acid (Equations 4.1 and 4.2) that [H+] is directly proportional to P_{CO_2} and inversely proportional to bicarbonate concentration; that is, it is determined by the ratio of P_{CO_2} to bicarbonate:

$$[\mathrm{H^+}] = K\frac{P_{CO_2}}{\left[\mathrm{HCO_3^-}\right]} \qquad [4.5]$$

The constant, K, embraces the dissociation constants for Equations 4.1 and 4.2 and the solubility coefficient of carbon dioxide, which governs the concentration of the gas in solution at a given partial pressure. When [H+] is measured in nmol/L, bicarbonate in mmol/L and P_{CO_2} in kPa, the value of K is approximately 180 at 37°C; if P_{CO_2} is measured in mmHg, the value of K is 24.

Blood gas analyzers derive bicarbonate concentration using this formula. It is not the same as the bicarbonate (strictly, total carbon dioxide) measured by most laboratory analyzers. There has been considerable argument over whether this approach is valid, given that the values of the constants involved are based on observations in supposedly ideal solutions, which biological fluids are not. However, for most practical purposes the derivation is an acceptable one. Confusingly, this derived parameter is sometimes described as 'actual bicarbonate', and it is important to be aware that it is different from 'standard bicarbonate' (see later and also p. 69).

An appreciation of the relationship between [H+], bicarbonate concentration and P_{CO_2} is of fundamental importance to an understanding of the pathophysiology of hydrogen ion homoeostasis. It will be apparent from Equation 4.5 that the relationships between [H+] and P_{CO_2} and between bicarbonate concentration and P_{CO_2} are linear. These relationships have been quantified by measurements made *in vivo*; therefore, it is possible to predict the effect of a change in one variable on another, for example, the effect of an acute rise in P_{CO_2} on [H+]. This information is an important aid in the interpretation of acid–base data. Many blood gas analyzers convert [H+] to pH:

$$\mathrm{pH} = \log_{10}\frac{1}{[\mathrm{H^+}]} \qquad [4.6]$$

However, this transformation is unhelpful because it obscures the linear relationships.

The relationships between [H+], P_{CO_2} and bicarbonate concentration are plotted in Fig. 4.4. This diagram may be useful as an *aide-mémoire* to the interpretation of acid–base data but should not be used as a substitute for a full understanding of the underlying principles.

Many instruments for blood gas analysis generate other data such as standard bicarbonate and base excess. The definitions, uses and misuses of these terms are described later.

Disorders of Hydrogen Ion Homoeostasis

Four components can be identified in the pathophysiology of hydrogen ion disorders (acid–base disorders):

- generation
- buffering

Table 4.1 Effects of change in partial pressure of carbon dioxide and oxygen and concentration of hydrogen ion in the blood

	Increase	Decrease
P_{CO_2}	peripheral vasodilatation	paraesthesiae
	headache	dizziness
	bounding pulse	muscle cramps
	papilloedema	headache
	flapping tremor } late signs	tetany
	drowsiness, coma	
P_{O_2}	pulmonary and retinal fibrosis (only with prolonged use of high inspiratory P_{O_2}, particularly in infants)	breathlessness
		cyanosis
		drowsiness, confusion and coma
		pulmonary hypertension (in chronic hypoxaemia)
[H⁺]	hypoventilation	hyperventilation
	increased catecholamine release	
	hyperkalaemia	paraesthesiae
	decreased myocardial contractility	muscle cramps
	} severe	dizziness headache
	CNS depression } acidosis only	
		tetany
		drowsiness, confusion and coma

Paraesthesiae, dizziness, muscle cramps and tetany are related to a decrease in ionized calcium.
CNS, central nervous system; PCO_2, partial pressure of carbon dioxide; PO_2, partial pressure of oxygen; [H⁺], hydrogen ion concentration.

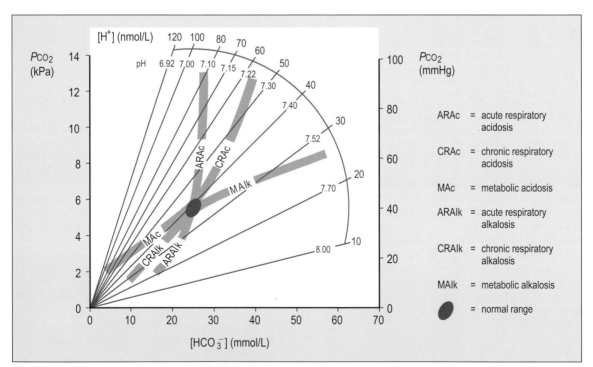

Fig. 4.4 Relationship between partial pressure of carbon dioxide (PCO_2), hydrogen ion concentration and bicarbonate concentration. Shaded areas represent the ranges of values found in simple disturbances of acid–base homoeostasis. Data falling outside these areas indicate mixed disturbances.

- compensation
- correction.

It is helpful to consider these separately, although in reality they may occur concurrently, albeit with different time courses.

Acid–base disorders are classified as either **respiratory** or **metabolic** (or **non-respiratory**) according to whether there is a primary (causative) change in P_{CO_2}. The term **acidosis** signifies a tendency for the [H$^+$] to be above normal, and **alkalosis** for it to be below normal.

Metabolic (non-respiratory) acidosis

The primary abnormality in metabolic acidosis is **either increased production or decreased excretion of hydrogen ions** other than from carbon dioxide. In some cases, both may contribute. **Loss of bicarbonate** from the body can also, indirectly, cause acidosis. Causes of metabolic acidosis are given in Box 4.1. Excess hydrogen ions are buffered by bicarbonate (Equation 4.2) and other buffers. The carbonic acid thus formed dissociates (Equation 4.1), and the carbon dioxide is lost in the expired air. This buffering limits the potential rise in hydrogen ion concentration, but at the expense of a reduction in bicarbonate concentration, which is a constant feature of metabolic acidosis.

Compensation is affected by hyperventilation, which increases the removal of carbon dioxide and decreases the P_{CO_2}. The P_{CO_2}/[HCO$_3^-$] ratio falls, thus tending to reduce the [H$^+$] (Equation 4.5). Hyperventilation is a direct result of the increased [H$^+$] stimulating the respiratory centre. Respiratory compensation cannot completely normalize the [H$^+$], because it is the high concentration itself that stimulates the compensatory hyperventilation. Furthermore, the increased work of the respiratory muscles produces carbon dioxide, thereby limiting the extent to which the P_{CO_2} can be lowered.

If the cause of the acidosis is not corrected, a new steady state may be attained, with a raised [H$^+$], low bicarbonate and low P_{CO_2}. In the steady state, the decrease in P_{CO_2} attributable to respiratory compensation is approximately 0.17 kPa for each 1 mmol/L decrement in bicarbonate concentration. The extent to which compensation can take place will be limited if respiratory function is compromised. Even with normal respiratory function, it is exceptional for a P_{CO_2} <1.5 kPa to be recorded, no matter how severe the metabolic acidosis.

In a healthy person, hyperventilation would produce a respiratory alkalosis. In general, the compensatory mechanism for any acid–base disturbance involves the generation of a second, opposing disturbance. In the case of a metabolic acidosis, compensation is through the generation of a respiratory alkalosis (although this

> **Box 4.1 Principal causes of metabolic (non-respiratory) acidosis**
>
> ### Increased H$^+$ formation
> ketoacidosis (usually diabetic, also alcoholic)
> lactic acidosis
> poisoning, e.g. ethanol, methanol, ethylene glycol and salicylate
> inherited organic acidosis
>
> ### Acid ingestion
> acid poisoning
> excessive parenteral administration of amino acids, e.g. arginine, lysine and histidine[a]
>
> ### Decreased H$^+$ excretion
> renal tubular acidoses (types 1 and 4)[a]
> generalized established kidney failure[a]
> carbonate dehydratase inhibitors[a]
>
> ### Loss of bicarbonate
> diarrhoea[a]
> ileostomy[a]
> pancreatic, intestinal and biliary fistulae or drainage[a]
> renal tubular acidosis (type 2)[a]
>
> ---
> [a]Acidosis with normal anion gap.

only limits the severity of the acidosis: the patient does not become alkalotic). In a respiratory acidosis, compensation is through the generation of a metabolic alkalosis (see later).

If renal function is normal in a patient with metabolic acidosis, excess hydrogen ions can be excreted by the kidneys. However, in many cases there is impairment of renal function, although this may not be the primary cause of the acidosis.

The complete **correction** of a metabolic acidosis requires reversal of the underlying cause; for example, rehydration and insulin for diabetic ketoacidosis (see Case history 13.2) and treatment of sepsis if this is the cause of a lactic acidosis. It is important to maintain adequate renal perfusion to maximize renal hydrogen ion excretion. The use of exogenous bicarbonate to buffer hydrogen ions is discussed later in this chapter and on p. 241.

Increased production of hydrogen ions

Increased production of hydrogen ions is the cause of the acidosis in ketoacidosis (diabetic or alcoholic), lactic acidosis and acidosis seen in poisoning, for example, with salicylate or ethylene glycol.

Decreased excretion of hydrogen ions

Acidosis occurs in kidney failure (see Case history 5.2), when the decreased glomerular filtration causes a reduction in the amount of sodium that is filtered and, therefore, available for exchange with hydrogen ions. The amount of phosphate filtered and available for buffering also decreases. Renal tubular acidoses are discussed in Chapter 5.

Loss of bicarbonate

Loss of bicarbonate and retention of hydrogen ions can result in acidosis in patients losing alkaline secretions from the small intestine (e.g. through fistulae). In the stomach, bicarbonate generated in the parietal cells from carbon dioxide and water diffuses into the blood and hydrogen ions are secreted into the lumen (Fig. 4.5). In the pancreas and small intestine, the movements of bicarbonate and hydrogen ions occur in the opposite directions (see Fig. 4.5); thus, hydrogen ions that are secreted into the stomach lumen are neutralized by bicarbonate in the small intestine.

Under normal circumstances, as most of the fluid and ions secreted into the gut are reabsorbed, the gut is effectively a closed system with regard to acid–base balance. If, however, alkaline secretions are lost, the patient is at risk of becoming acidotic. Increased renal hydrogen ion excretion (with generation and retention of bicarbonate) may prevent this, but excessive fluid loss from the gut may deplete the ECF to such an extent that the glomerular filtration rate falls and the kidneys are no longer able to compensate.

Excessive infusion of 'normal' (0.9%) saline

Infusion of 0.9% saline can cause acidosis because it contains chloride at a considerably higher concentration than that in normal plasma, and the resultant hyperchloraemia generates acidosis. Expansion of ECF volume also reduces renal bicarbonate reabsorption because of inhibition of aldosterone-driven sodium reabsorption.

The anion gap

When bicarbonate concentration falls in a metabolic acidosis, electrochemical neutrality must be maintained by other anions. In many cases, anions are produced simultaneously and equally with hydrogen ions, for example, acetoacetate and β-hydroxybutyrate in diabetic ketoacidosis and lactate in lactic acidosis. When this does not occur (e.g. in renal tubular acidoses and acidosis secondary to loss of bicarbonate from the gut), the deficit is met by chloride ions.

Case history 4.1

History

A 60-year-old man was admitted to hospital with severe abdominal pain that had begun 2.5 h earlier. He was not taking any drugs.

Examination

He was shocked (blood pressure 92/55 mmHg) and had a distended, rigid abdomen; neither femoral pulse was palpable.

Results (see Appendix for reference ranges)

Arterial blood:		
	hydrogen ion	90 nmol/L (pH 7.05)
	$P\text{CO}_2$	3.5 kPa
	$P\text{O}_2$	12 kPa
	bicarbonate	7 mmol/L

Summary

High [H+] with low $P\text{CO}_2$.

Interpretation

The high [H+] indicates that he is acidotic, and this must be metabolic in origin because the $P\text{CO}_2$ is not raised. Indeed, $P\text{CO}_2$ is decreased, reflecting compensatory hyperventilation.

Discussion

Compensatory hyperventilation may be clinically obvious (Kussmaul respiration, see Case history 13.2). An even lower $P\text{CO}_2$ might have been expected in someone with metabolic acidosis of this severity, but splinting of the abdominal muscles (the abdomen is rigid) will have restricted respiratory movements. The low bicarbonate concentration reflects the primary abnormality: bicarbonate is consumed as hydrogen ions are buffered. If there is no respiratory component to an acidosis, the plasma bicarbonate concentration is a good guide to its severity.

The clinical diagnosis (which was confirmed at laparotomy) was a ruptured abdominal aortic aneurysm. The patient was in severe shock after extravasation of blood from the aneurysm. Impaired tissue perfusion had led to inadequate oxygenation, despite the normal arterial $P\text{O}_2$, with consequently increased anaerobic metabolism of glucose to lactic acid.

Lactic acid is a normal metabolite of muscle and is converted back to glucose in the liver (the Cori cycle). However, with greatly increased production and possible impairment of hepatic metabolism because of poor perfusion, lactic acid accumulates. If renal function is compromised, for instance, by hypoperfusion, the ability of the kidneys to excrete excess hydrogen ions may also be impaired.

Other causes of lactic acidosis are given in Box 4.2.

Box 4.2 Causes of lactic acidosis

Tissue hypoxia

decreased perfusion
reduced Pao_2

Drugs, etc.

ethanol, methanol
metformin (rarely)
fructose, sorbitol

Congenital

glucose 6-phosphatase deficiency
other inherited diseases with defective gluconeogenesis
    or pyruvate oxidation

Lactic acidosis is sometimes classified as type A (tissue hypoxia) and type B (all other causes), with further division of type B into B1 (with lactic acid generated as a result of endogenous factors, e.g. ketoacidosis); B2, where toxins are implicated; and B3 as a result of inherited metabolic disorders.

Pao_2, arterial partial pressure of oxygen.

The difference between the sums of the concentrations of the principal cations (sodium and potassium) and of the principal anions (chloride and bicarbonate) is known as the 'anion gap':

$$\text{Anion gap} = \left([Na^+] + [K^+]\right) - \left([Cl^-] + [HCO_3^-]\right) \quad [4.7]$$

In health, the anion gap has a value of 14–18 mmol/L and mainly represents the unmeasured net negative charge on plasma proteins.

In an acidosis in which anions other than chloride are increased, the anion gap is increased. In contrast, in an acidosis caused by loss of bicarbonate—for example, renal tubular acidosis—plasma chloride concentration is increased and the anion gap is normal.

In the majority of cases of acidosis, the cause is obvious clinically and can be confirmed by the results of simple tests. The anion gap may, however, be useful in the analysis of complex acid–base disorders, as shown by Case history 4.7. Many laboratories do not routinely measure chloride as part of an 'electrolyte profile', but it should be requested if calculation of the anion gap is necessary.

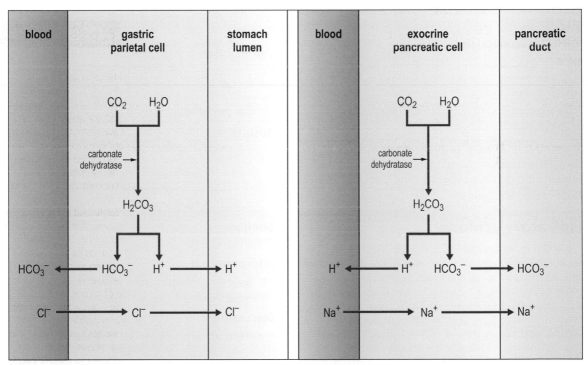

Fig. 4.5 Generation of acidic gastric and alkaline pancreatic secretions. Hydrogen and bicarbonate ions are generated from carbon dioxide and water, catalysed by carbonate dehydratase. In the stomach, the hydrogen ions are secreted whereas bicarbonate is retained. The reverse process occurs in the pancreas.

Management

The management of metabolic acidosis should be directed at reversing the underlying cause. When this is not immediately possible, bicarbonate is sometimes given to buffer hydrogen ions, although except for certain specific indications (renal tubular acidoses and the acidosis of acute kidney injury, especially if hyperkalaemia is present), there is no general agreement as to when it should be used and little evidence of benefit. However, many would consider it prudent to give bicarbonate when the arterial [H⁺] is >100 nmol/L (pH < 7.0) and there is no immediate prospect of lowering it by other means, particularly in a patient whose clinical condition is generally poor. If bicarbonate is used, it should usually be given in small quantities, using an isotonic (1.26%, 150 mmol/L) solution, and the effect on the arterial [H⁺] should be measured regularly. Large amounts of bicarbonate, given rapidly in an attempt to correct an acidosis, can be harmful. Overprovision may produce an alkalosis. Also, the reaction of bicarbonate with hydrogen ions produces carbon dioxide, adding to the load that must be excreted by the lungs, and its rapid diffusion into cells may increase intracellular acidosis. The use of hypertonic (8.4%, 1.0 mol/L) bicarbonate risks causing expansion of the ECF volume, as it is given as the sodium salt.

The characteristic biochemical changes seen in the blood in metabolic acidosis can be summarized as follows:

Metabolic acidosis

$[H^+]$	↑
pH	↓
P_{CO_2}	↓
$[HCO_3^-]$	↓↓

Changes caused by the underlying condition will also be present. Hyperkalaemia is common in patients with acidosis, except in bicarbonate-wasting conditions, for reasons discussed in Chapter 3.

Respiratory acidosis

Some of the many conditions associated with the development of respiratory acidosis are shown in Box 4.3. They are all characterized by an increase in P_{CO_2}. For every hydrogen ion that is produced, a bicarbonate ion is also generated. With an acute rise in P_{CO_2}, every 1 kPa increase is associated with a concomitant increase in bicarbonate concentration of 0.5–1 mmol/L, but in [H⁺] of only 5.5 nmol/L: this seeming discrepancy occurs because the majority of the hydrogen ions are buffered by intracellular buffers, particularly haemoglobin (see Fig. 4.3). In chronic carbon dioxide retention, when renal compensation is maximal, the [H⁺] is increased by only 2.5 nmol/L for each 1 kPa rise in P_{CO_2}, whereas bicarbonate concentration increases by 2–3 mmol/L.

A respiratory acidosis can only be corrected by means that restore the P_{CO_2} to normal, but if a high P_{CO_2} persists, compensation occurs through increased renal hydrogen ion excretion.

In acute respiratory acidosis, unless very severe, the bicarbonate concentration, although increased, is usually within the reference range. If the bicarbonate concentration is clearly elevated in a respiratory acidosis, either a more chronic course with renal compensation (Case history 4.3) or a coexisting metabolic alkalosis is suggested. A low bicarbonate would suggest a coexisting metabolic acidosis.

Management

The aim when treating respiratory acidosis is to **improve alveolar ventilation** and lower the P_{CO_2}. In acute alveolar hypoventilation, however, it is usually hypoxaemia rather than hypercapnia that poses the main threat to life, unless the P_{O_2} is being maintained by the supply of

---

Case history 4.2

History

A young man sustained injury to the chest in a road traffic accident.

Examination

Part of his ribcage moved inwards during inspiration, in a manner typical of a flail segment resulting from multiple rib fractures. This was sufficiently severe to compromise effective ventilation.

Results

Arterial blood:	P_{O_2}	8 kPa
	P_{CO_2}	8 kPa
	hydrogen ion	58 nmol/L (pH 7.24)
	bicarbonate	25 mmol/L

Summary

High [H⁺] with raised P_{CO_2}.

Interpretation

The raised P_{CO_2} indicates that his acidosis (high [H⁺]) is respiratory in origin.

Discussion

The magnitude of the increase in [H⁺] and the within reference range bicarbonate suggest that no renal compensation has occurred. Such compensation can take several days to become fully effective, in contrast with the rapid respiratory compensation in metabolic disorders.

Box 4.3 **Principal causes of respiratory acidosis**

Airway obstruction

chronic obstructive pulmonary disease, e.g. bronchitis, emphysema
bronchospasm, e.g. in asthma
aspiration

Depression of respiratory centre

anaesthetics
sedatives
cerebral trauma
tumours

Neuromuscular disease

poliomyelitis
Guillain–Barré syndrome
motor neurone disease
tetanus, botulism
neurotoxins, curare

Pulmonary disease

pulmonary fibrosis
severe pneumonia
respiratory distress syndrome

Extrapulmonary thoracic disease

flail chest
severe kyphoscoliosis

additional oxygen. If ventilation were to cease abruptly, death from hypoxaemia would occur in approximately 4 min; the $P\text{CO}_2$ by comparison rises at a rate such that it would take more than 10 min for it to reach a lethal level.

In chronic respiratory acidosis, it is seldom possible to correct the underlying cause: treatment is directed at maximizing alveolar ventilation by, for example, utilizing physiotherapy, bronchodilators and antibiotics. If artificial ventilation becomes necessary, it is vital to monitor the patient's arterial blood gases and hydrogen ion concentration to avoid overcorrection of the respiratory acidosis. Artificial ventilation is discussed in more detail on p. 74.

Oxygen may safely be used at high concentrations in patients with acute respiratory failure. In many patients with chronic carbon dioxide retention, however, the respiratory centre becomes insensitive to carbon dioxide and hypoxaemia provides the main stimulus to respiration. It is usual to control oxygen administration (e.g. 24% or 28% of the inspired gas) in such patients to prevent abolition of this stimulus, although the importance of doing this is considered to be less now than formerly.

It is important to appreciate that, from the data alone, it would not be possible to determine whether results in sample C in Case history 4.3 represent a state of either compensated chronic carbon dioxide retention or acute carbon dioxide retention developing in a patient with a pre-existing metabolic alkalosis. The management of these two states would not be the same. The clinical context is of crucial importance in distinguishing between them.

The characteristic biochemical changes in arterial blood in acute and chronic respiratory acidosis can be summarized as follows:

	Respiratory acidosis	
	Acute	**Chronic**
$[\text{H}^+]$	↑	Slight ↑ or high–normal
pH	↓	Slight ↓ or low–normal
$P\text{CO}_2$	↑	↑
$[\text{HCO}_3^-]$	Slight ↑	↑

Metabolic (non-respiratory) alkalosis

Metabolic alkalosis is characterized by a primary increase in the ECF bicarbonate concentration, with a consequent reduction in $[\text{H}^+]$ (see Equation 4.5). In healthy subjects, the consequent increased glomerular filtration of bicarbonate exceeds its tubular reabsorption rate; therefore, there is excretion of bicarbonate in the urine. Massive quantities of bicarbonate must be ingested to produce a sustained alkalosis.

Because the body is a net producer of acid, it might be supposed that metabolic alkalosis would be corrected by normal acid production. In practice however, and in contrast with metabolic acidosis and respiratory disorders of acid–base balance, a metabolic alkalosis may persist even after the primary cause has been corrected. It is thus necessary to consider both the mechanisms that can cause metabolic alkalosis and those that can perpetuate it.

Causes of metabolic alkalosis are shown in Box 4.4. They can be divided into those associated with chloride or ECF volume depletion (sometimes termed 'saline responsive') and those in which there is potassium depletion; in some instances, both are present. Alkali loading causes only a transient alkalosis unless there are additional factors operating to sustain it. The **maintenance** of a metabolic alkalosis requires inappropriately high (as far as hydrogen ion homoeostasis is concerned) renal bicarbonate reabsorption and hydrogen ion excretion. Factors that may be responsible for this include a decrease in ECF volume, mineralocorticoid excess and potassium depletion.

Loss of gastric acid is an important cause: as discussed earlier, the generation of gastric acid (effectively hydrochloric acid) results in the formation of bicarbonate ions, which are

Case history 4.3

History

A 70-year-old man, known to suffer from chronic obstructive pulmonary disease, was admitted to hospital with an acute exacerbation of his illness. Arterial blood analysis was carried out on admission (results sample A). In spite of vigorous physiotherapy and medical treatment, his condition deteriorated (results sample B), and it was decided to start artificial ventilation. Analysis was repeated after 6 h (results sample C). After 12 h he had a generalized fit (results sample D).

Results

Arterial blood	A	B	C	D
P_{CO_2} (kPa)	9.5	11.0	7.7	5.7
hydrogen ion (nmol/L)	50	58	40	29
pH	7.30	7.24	7.40	7.54
bicarbonate (mmol/L)	35	35	34	35

Sample A

The results on admission indicate an acidosis. This is of respiratory origin, because the P_{CO_2} is raised. However, the [H+] is only slightly elevated, indicating that renal compensation is occurring, as would be expected in a patient with chronic carbon dioxide retention. The raised bicarbonate, which suggests a metabolic alkalosis, is the result of the compensatory increase in renal hydrogen ion excretion. Indeed, the commonest causes of raised plasma bicarbonate concentration in the elderly are chronic carbon

dioxide retention and diuretic-induced potassium depletion (see p. 47).

Sample B

A more severe acidosis subsequently develops, commensurate with the rise in P_{CO_2}. This is a result of further carbon dioxide retention with no corresponding increase in renal hydrogen ion excretion.

Sample C

Artificial ventilation lowers the P_{CO_2} rapidly; the [H+] is now normal, although the P_{CO_2} is still elevated. This represents this patient's normal steady state, in which there is an almost complete renal compensation of the acidosis.

Sample D

Continued ventilation reduces the P_{CO_2} to within the normal range for a healthy subject, but to less than this patient's normal. He has become alkalotic and suffers a fit as a consequence. The alkalosis is due to the continued high rate of renal hydrogen ion excretion in response to the chronically raised P_{CO_2}. Adaptation of renal hydrogen ion excretion in response to a change in P_{CO_2} takes several days. Thus, rapid reduction of the P_{CO_2} exposes the compensatory, secondary response, which then appears to be the sole acid–base abnormality. The compensatory mechanism in respiratory acidosis involves the generation of a metabolic alkalosis.

retained. Loss of chloride can also occur from lower in the gut. In both cases, there is also loss of sodium and water, tending to reduce ECF volume, stimulating renal sodium retention via renin and aldosterone, and the simultaneous excretion of potassium and hydrogen ions (the latter always being accompanied by retention of bicarbonate). Note that, paradoxically, as a result of the increased renal hydrogen ion excretion, the urine may be acidic in patients with a metabolic alkalosis—exactly the opposite of what is required to correct the disturbance. It would appear that the mechanisms that protect ECF volume take precedence over those that regulate acid–base status. A metabolic alkalosis caused by loss of gastric acid may occur in patients undergoing nasogastric aspiration, but it is not usually a feature of vomiting if the pylorus is patent, as the additional loss of alkaline secretions from the upper small intestine counteracts the effect of the retention of bicarbonate ions generated by gastric parietal cells. Vomiting with **pyloric stenosis** is an unusual cause of metabolic alkalosis, but the disturbance can be severe; other causes rarely result in such a severe disturbance.

Loop and thiazide diuretics also cause loss of chloride, sodium and water, and increase delivery of sodium to the distal parts of the nephron, thus increasing the amount that is available for reabsorption in exchange for potassium and hydrogen ions. A mild alkalosis may develop during the treatment of oedema with diuretics ('contraction alkalosis'): the loss of chloride-rich fluid causes a decrease in the volume of the ECF in which bicarbonate is distributed, thus increasing its concentration, while renal bicarbonate reabsorption is stimulated.

In **potassium depletion** ('saline-unresponsive alkalosis'), loss of intracellular potassium leads to an intracellular shift of hydrogen ions, tending to cause an extracellular alkalosis. In addition, potassium depletion results in there being less potassium available to exchange for hydrogen ions when sodium reabsorption occurs in the distal nephron. This effect will be exacerbated if there is increased aldosterone secretion (which may be the primary cause of potassium depletion or result from a decrease in effective arterial blood volume). A third factor relating potassium depletion and alkalosis is that potassium depletion

Box 4.4 Principal causes of metabolic alkalosis

Primarily related to volume depletion/hypochloraemia

gastrointestinal
    gastric aspiration
    vomiting with pyloric stenosis
    congenital chloride-losing diarrhoea
renal
    diuretic therapy (not K^+-sparing)

Primarily related to potassium depletion

inadequate intake
increased excretion
mineralocorticoid excess
    Conn syndrome (primary aldosteronism)
    Cushing syndrome
    Bartter syndrome and related conditions (see Table 3.4)
secondary aldosteronism
drugs increasing mineralocorticoid activity
    carbenoxolone

Administration of alkali

inappropriate treatment of acidotic states
chronic alkali ingestion

Potassium-sparing diuretics tend to be weak diuretics, having a lesser chloriuretic effect than loop and thiazide diuretics, and not causing potassium depletion. In some instances (e.g. secondary aldosteronism), there is both an effective decrease in circulating volume and potassium depletion.

---

stimulates the formation of ammonia, increasing the capacity of the kidneys to excrete acid. In metabolic alkalosis caused by potassium depletion, urine chloride concentration is typically >20 mmol/L; in saline-responsive alkalosis, it is usually <20 mmol/L.

The **correction** of a metabolic alkalosis requires reversal both of the primary cause and of the mechanism responsible for its perpetuation. The expected **compensatory change** would be an increase in P_{CO_2}, which would increase the ratio $P_{CO_2}/[HCO_3^-]$ and thus $[H^+]$ (see Equation 4.5). Low arterial $[H^+]$ inhibits the respiratory centre, causing hypoventilation, and thus an increase in P_{CO_2}. However, as an increase in P_{CO_2} is itself a powerful stimulus to respiration, this compensation is self-limiting, particularly in acute metabolic alkalosis. In more chronic disorders, significant compensation may occur, presumably because the respiratory centre becomes less sensitive to carbon dioxide. Should hypoventilation lead to significant hypoxaemia, however, this will provide a powerful stimulus to respiration and prevent further compensation.

Management

The management of a metabolic alkalosis depends on the severity of the condition and on the cause. When hypovolaemia and hypochloraemia are present, they can be corrected simultaneously by an infusion of isotonic sodium chloride solution ('normal saline'), which will also improve renal perfusion and allow excretion of the bicarbonate load. It is only very rarely necessary to attempt rapid correction of metabolic alkalosis by infusion of hydrochloric acid or its precursor, ammonium chloride.

The treatment of metabolic alkalosis associated with potassium depletion should be directed at the underlying cause. Potassium replacement should be given to correct the hypokalaemia and may be sufficient on its own to correct the alkalosis, particularly if this is only mild. The management of primary aldosteronism is considered in Chapter 10.

The biochemical features of metabolic alkalosis can be summarized as follows:

Metabolic alkalosis

$[H^+]$	↓
pH	↑
P_{CO_2}	↑
$[HCO_3^-]$	↑↑

Respiratory alkalosis

The main **causes** of respiratory alkalosis are shown in Box 4.5. The common feature and cause of the alkalosis is a fall in P_{CO_2}, which reduces the ratio of P_{CO_2} to bicarbonate concentration (see Equation 4.5). In acute respiratory alkalosis, the $[H^+]$ falls by approximately 5.5 nmol/L for each 1.0 kPa fall in P_{CO_2}.

The fall in P_{CO_2} causes a small decrease in bicarbonate concentration. **Compensation** occurs through a reduction in renal hydrogen ion excretion, which further decreases plasma bicarbonate concentration. Renal compensation in a respiratory alkalosis develops slowly, as it does in a respiratory acidosis. If a steady P_{CO_2} is maintained, maximal compensation with a new steady state develops within 36–72 h.

Management

As with other disturbances of acid–base homoeostasis, the management of patients with respiratory alkalosis should be directed towards the underlying cause, although this is frequently not possible. Fortunately, a chronic compensated respiratory alkalosis is not, in itself, dangerous. Increasing the inspired P_{CO_2} by making

67

Case history 4.4

History

A 45-year-old man was admitted to hospital with persistent vomiting. He had a long history of dyspepsia but had never sought advice for this, preferring to treat himself with proprietary remedies.

Examination

He was dehydrated and his respiration was shallow.

Results

Arterial blood:	hydrogen ion	28 nmol/L (pH 7.56)
	P_{CO_2}	7.2 kPa
	bicarbonate	45 mmol/L
Serum:	sodium	146 mmol/L
	potassium	2.8 mmol/L
	urea	34.2 mmol/L

Gastroscopy, performed after this metabolic imbalance had been corrected, showed pyloric stenosis, thought to be due to scarring caused by peptic ulceration.

Summary

Low [H⁺] with high P_{CO_2}. Raised urea and hypokalaemia.

Interpretation

The patient is alkalotic and, because the P_{CO_2} is high, this must be metabolic (non-respiratory) in origin. The raised urea is consistent with the clinical signs of dehydration, but the presence of hypokalaemia is unusual in this state (see discussion).

Discussion

The increase in P_{CO_2} is a result of compensatory hypoventilation leading to carbon dioxide retention. In chronic metabolic alkalosis, as in this case, each increment of 1 mmol/L in bicarbonate concentration typically causes an increase in P_{CO_2} of approximately 0.1 kPa.

The alkalosis is a result of loss of unbuffered hydrogen ions in gastric juice with concomitant retention of bicarbonate. The dehydration is caused by gastric fluid loss. (When dehydration is caused by conditions other than gastric fluid loss, a raised plasma urea concentration is more likely to be accompanied by a low plasma bicarbonate concentration and high plasma potassium concentration, as a consequence of impaired renal perfusion). Fluid loss stimulates renal sodium reabsorption, but sodium can only be reabsorbed either with chloride or in exchange for hydrogen and potassium ions. Gastric juice has a high concentration of chloride, and patients losing gastric secretions become hypochloraemic. This means that less sodium than usual can be reabsorbed with chloride. However, it appears that the defence of ECF volume takes precedence over acid–base and electrolyte homoeostasis, and further sodium reabsorption occurs in exchange for hydrogen ions (perpetuating the alkalosis) and potassium ions (leading, together with potassium loss in the gastric juice, to potassium depletion). This explains the apparently paradoxical finding of acidic urine and a high urine potassium concentration in patients with severe metabolic alkalosis.

Box 4.5 Principal causes of respiratory alkalosis

Increased respiratory drive secondary to hypoxia

high altitude
severe anaemia
  pulmonary disease, e.g. pulmonary embolism,
  pulmonary oedema, acute asthma

Other causes of increased respiratory drive

cerebral disturbances, e.g. trauma, infection, tumours
respiratory stimulants, e.g. salicylates
liver failure
gram-negative septicaemia
hyperventilation syndrome
voluntary hyperventilation

Mechanical overventilation

the patient rebreathe into a paper bag may abort the clinical features of acute hypocapnia in acute hyperventilation, but this is only a temporary measure and risks causing hypoxia.

The biochemical features of respiratory alkalosis can be summarized as follows:

	Respiratory alkalosis	
	Acute	Chronic
[H⁺]	↓	Slight ↓ or low–normal
pH	↑	Slight ↑ or high–normal
P_{CO_2}	↓	↓
[HCO₃⁻]	Slight ↓	↓

Interpretation of Acid–Base Data

A thorough understanding of the pathophysiology of acid–base homoeostasis is essential for the correct interpretation of laboratory data, but these data should always be considered in the clinical context.

The starting point in any evaluation should be the hydrogen ion concentration or pH. This will indicate whether the predominant disturbance is an acidosis or an alkalosis. However, a normal value does not exclude an acid–base disorder. There may be either a fully compensated disturbance or two primary disturbances whose effects on hydrogen ion concentration cancel each other out.

If the P_{CO_2} is abnormal, there must be a respiratory component to the disturbance. If the P_{CO_2} is raised in an acidosis, the acidosis is respiratory and comparison of the hydrogen ion concentration with that predicted for an acute change in P_{CO_2} (bearing in mind that an increase [decrease] in P_{CO_2} of 1 kPa typically causes an increase [decrease] in [H$^+$] of 5.5 nmol/L) will indicate whether there is an additional metabolic component, although it is important to appreciate that this may be a compensatory change. If the P_{CO_2} is low in an acidosis, the acidosis is metabolic and there is an additional respiratory component, which will often reflect compensation. A similar rationale applies to alkalotic states. An algorithm for the analysis of acid–base data is given in Fig. 4.6.

Because the bicarbonate is calculated by the blood gas analyzer from the P_{CO_2} and [H$^+$], it does not provide any more information than these two measurements alone. However, knowing the bicarbonate concentration may simplify the interpretation of acid–base data. Its concentration is always decreased in metabolic acidosis and increased in metabolic alkalosis, regardless of whether there is compensation.

Mixed acid–base disturbances occur frequently and appear complex. Correct diagnosis requires a logical approach and a clear understanding both of the relevant pathophysiology and of the quantitative relationships between [H$^+$] and P_{CO_2}. The biochemical changes that are characteristic of the various acid–base disturbances are shown in Table 4.2. With this physiological approach, calculated parameters such as 'standard bicarbonate' and 'base excess' are redundant.

The standard bicarbonate is a calculated estimate of the bicarbonate concentration that would be present if the P_{CO_2} were normal, and thus reflects only the metabolic influences on bicarbonate. The base excess is a calculated estimate of the metabolic influences on total buffering capacity. These parameters were introduced with a view to distinguishing between the respiratory and metabolic components in acid–base disorders, but they take no account of normal physiological responses. An abnormal standard bicarbonate or base excess indicates the presence of a metabolic acidosis or alkalosis. It does not, however, indicate whether this is either part of a mixed disturbance of

---

Case history 4.5

History

A 19-year-old student was brought by her friends to the emergency department with an acute asthma attack. An arterial blood sample was taken, but before oxygen could be administered she began to experience tingling in her fingers and toes.

Examination

She was highly anxious and agitated, with tachypnoea (respiratory rate 26 breaths/min).

Results

Arterial blood:	hydrogen ion	30 nmol/L (pH 7.52)
	P_{O_2}	9.2 kPa
	P_{CO_2}	3.5 kPa
	bicarbonate	21 mmol/L

Summary

Low [H$^+$], with a reduced P_{CO_2}. Low P_{O_2} consistent with hypoxia.

Interpretation

The low P_{CO_2} indicates respiratory alkalosis, a result of her tachypnoea. The extent of the decrease in [H$^+$] indicates that there is neither compensation nor an additional acid–base disturbance.

Discussion

No metabolic compensation would be expected to have occurred during this acute episode. The tingling symptoms are a result of a decrease in the plasma concentration of ionized calcium, caused by increased binding of calcium to albumin owing to the alkalosis (see p. 255). These symptoms, and the alkalosis, improve rapidly after administration of oxygen, which increases the P_{O_2} and reduces the hypoxia-driven respiratory drive, thus allowing the P_{CO_2} to rise. The presence of a high P_{CO_2} at presentation and before administration of oxygen in patients with acute asthma, in contrast, indicates critical, potentially life-threatening hypoventilation.

Case history 4.6

History

A young woman was admitted to hospital unconscious, following a head injury. A skull fracture was demonstrated on radiography, and a computed tomography (CT) scan revealed extensive cerebral contusions. The respiratory rate was increased, at 38 breaths/min. Three days after admission, the patient's condition was unchanged.

Results

Arterial blood:	hydrogen ion	36 nmol/L (pH 7.44)
	P_{CO_2}	3.6 kPa
	bicarbonate	19 mmol/L

Summary

[H+] at the lower limit of normal, with low P_{CO_2} and reduced bicarbonate.

Interpretation

Compensated respiratory alkalosis. The P_{CO_2} is reduced as a result of hyperventilation but the [H+] is being maintained in the low-normal range as a result of a compensatory increase in renal bicarbonate excretion.

Discussion

Abnormalities of respiration (hypoventilation and hyperventilation) are common in patients with head injuries. Hyperventilation can occur with injuries involving the brainstem and as a result of raised intracranial pressure. Even though a low P_{CO_2} is also characteristic of the respiratory compensation in metabolic acidosis, the history and normal [H+] preclude this diagnosis. Also, a much lower bicarbonate concentration would be expected in a metabolic acidosis.

Case history 4.7

History

A young woman was admitted to hospital 8 h after she had taken an overdose of aspirin.

Results

Arterial blood:	hydrogen ion	30 nmol/L (pH 7.53)
	P_{CO_2}	2.0 kPa
	bicarbonate	12 mmol/L

Summary

Low P_{CO_2} and bicarbonate with slightly reduced [H+].

Interpretation

The patient is alkalotic, and the low P_{CO_2} indicates a respiratory cause. However, the [H+] is not as low as would have been expected as a result of an acute fall in P_{CO_2}. The data would be appropriate for a chronic, compensated respiratory alkalosis, but such a low P_{CO_2} would be exceptional, and this interpretation is not compatible with the history. The alternative is that there is an acute respiratory alkalosis with a coexistent metabolic acidosis. This combination is characteristic of salicylate poisoning, where initial respiratory stimulation causes a respiratory alkalosis but later the metabolic effects of salicylate tend to predominate, producing an acidosis.

Discussion

This case history illustrates the importance of considering the clinical setting when analyzing acid–base data. Calculation of the anion gap might have been helpful here. It would have been increased by the presence of organic anions, indicating a coexisting metabolic acidosis. Note that, although the low bicarbonate indicates the presence of a metabolic acidosis, it is not necessary to know the bicarbonate concentration to reach this conclusion.

Case history 4.8

History

An elderly man was admitted to hospital in a confused state. He was dyspnoeic and had a cough productive of sputum. He was unable to give a coherent history, but one of the casualty officers knew him to be a patient with insulin-treated diabetes with a long history of chronic bronchitis.

Results

Arterial blood:	hydrogen ion	66 nmol/L (pH 7.18)
	P_{CO_2}	7.4 kPa
	bicarbonate	20 mmol/L

Summary

Very high [H+] with moderately raised P_{CO_2}.

Interpretation

The patient is acidotic, and the raised P_{CO_2} indicates a respiratory component. However, the [H+] is higher than would be expected in an acute respiratory acidosis with a P_{CO_2} at this level. Therefore, there must also be a metabolic component to the acidosis.

Discussion

From these data alone, it is not possible to determine whether the respiratory disturbance is acute or chronic. These results could, for example, represent the results of the concurrent development of a respiratory and a metabolic acidosis. In contrast, they are also compatible with the presence of metabolic acidosis in a patient with chronic carbon dioxide retention. Given that the patient is known to suffer from chronic bronchitis, the second interpretation is more likely.

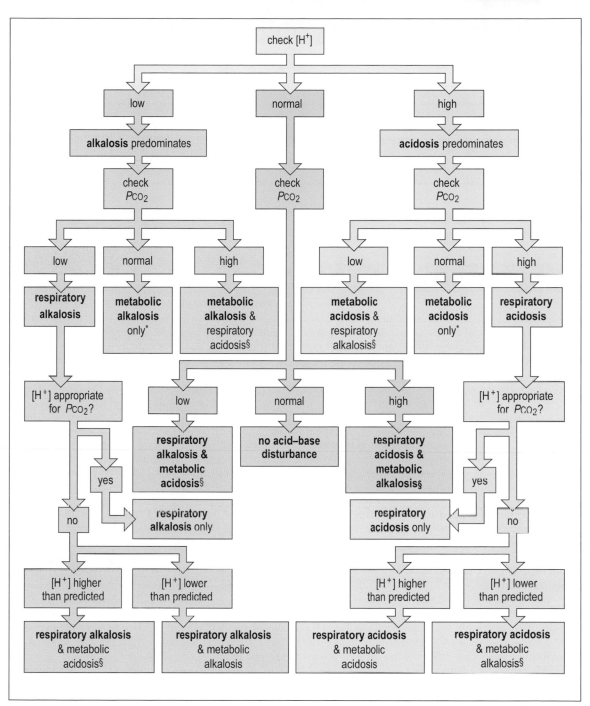

Fig. 4.6 Algorithm for the analysis of acid–base data. Where two disturbances are shown, the predominant one is in bold type. §A disturbance that would be expected to develop as a result of physiological compensation but could be a coexisting pathological process. *Because compensation for metabolic disorders develops so rapidly, 'pure' (i.e. uncompensated) metabolic disorders do not occur unless the normal respiratory response is prevented (e.g. in a ventilated patient). Acutely, compensation for metabolic alkalosis is less efficient than for acidosis.

Table 4.2 Biochemical changes characteristic of disturbances of acid–base homoeostasis

	Acidosis				Alkalosis		
	METABOLIC	RESPIRATORY			METABOLIC	RESPIRATORY	
	Acute	*Chronic*			*Acute*	*Chronic*	
[H*]	↑	↑	slight ↑ or high–normal	↓	↓	slight ↓ or low–normal	
pH	↓	↓	slight ↓ or low–normal	↑	↑	slight ↑ or high–normal	
P_{CO2}	↓	↑	↑	↑	↓	↓	
[HCO$_3$]	↓↓	slight ↑	↑	↑↑	slight ↓	↓	

acid–base homoeostasis or related to normal physiological compensation.

Oxygen Transport and Its Disorders

In patients with respiratory disorders, a disturbance of the arterial partial pressure of oxygen (Pao_2) may be of greater clinical significance than either an abnormal arterial partial pressure of carbon dioxide ($Paco_2$) or abnormal [H$^+$]. Although oxygen and carbon dioxide diffuse in opposite directions between the alveoli and the bloodstream, their respective partial pressures do not necessarily change in a reciprocal fashion. There are two reasons for this: first, carbon dioxide is generally more diffusible than oxygen, with the result that, in pulmonary oedema and interstitial lung disease, hypoxaemia develops but the $Paco_2$ may not increase; and second, very little oxygen is carried in physical solution in the blood, and haemoglobin is normally nearly fully saturated with oxygen. As a result, hyperventilation cannot increase Pao_2 significantly, but can reduce the $Paco_2$. A raised Pao_2 is seen only in patients given supplementary oxygen, which increases the proportion of oxygen in the inspired gas (Fio_2) and results in an increased inspired Po_2. It is essential to know the Fio_2 to interpret Pao_2 correctly.

The **oxyhaemoglobin dissociation curve**, which relates blood Po_2 to the percentage of the maximum saturation of haemoglobin with oxygen, is sigmoid (Fig. 4.7). As a consequence, a considerable drop in Po_2 can occur without a significant effect on the amount of oxygen carried in the blood. Saturation falls below 90% only when Po_2 (reference range 11–15 kPa) falls below about 8 kPa, but if Po_2 decreases further, saturation declines rapidly.

There are many causes of **hypoxaemia** (Table 4.3). The reasons for the hypoxaemia associated with hypoventilation, venous-to-arterial shunting and impaired diffusion are self-evident. However, in many respiratory diseases,

such as lung collapse (atelectasis) and pneumonia, there is an imbalance between ventilation and perfusion of the alveoli. Blood leaving poorly ventilated, well-perfused alveoli will have a low Po_2 and a raised Pco_2. The effect on Pco_2 can be compensated in normally perfused and ventilated alveoli by hyperventilation. This removes additional carbon dioxide but cannot compensate for the low Po_2 in blood from poorly ventilated alveoli because the haemoglobin in blood from well-perfused alveoli will be fully saturated; thus, the amount of oxygen carried cannot be increased significantly, even by increasing the proportion of oxygen in the inspired gas, because this can only increase the (relatively small amount) of oxygen transported in physical solution in the blood. The poorly perfused alveoli are effectively dead space. With moderate degrees of ventilation/perfusion imbalance, Pao_2 is reduced and $Paco_2$ is either normal or even reduced. With severe imbalance, hyperventilation cannot compensate through increased removal of carbon dioxide from normally ventilated and perfused alveoli, and $Paco_2$ becomes elevated.

Although an adequate Pao_2 is essential for normal tissue oxygenation, it is not the only factor involved. The amount of oxygen delivered to tissues depends on arterial oxygen content and their blood supply.

The oxygen content of blood depends on haemoglobin concentration and on its saturation, which is a function of the affinity of haemoglobin for oxygen and the Po_2. Haemoglobin saturation can be measured *in vitro* or, more usually in clinical practice, *in vivo* with an oximeter. Pulse oximeters are lightweight devices designed to be clipped to an earlobe or fingertip. They measure oxygen saturation (SpO_2) (p = peripheral) by monitoring the absorption of light by oxyhaemoglobin and deoxyhaemoglobin in the underlying tissue. Various factors can affect the affinity of haemoglobin for oxygen, and thus the percentage saturation at a given Po_2. 2,3-Diphosphoglycerate (2,3-DPG) is an important physiological regulator. An increase in red cell 2,3-DPG causes a shift in the oxyhaemoglobin dissociation curve to the right,

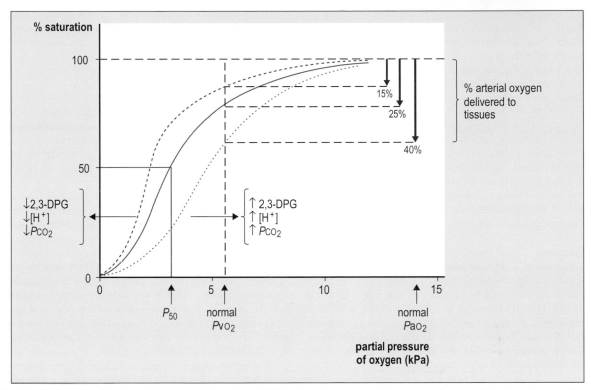

Fig. 4.7 Oxyhaemoglobin dissociation curve. Normal arterial (Pa_{O_2}) and venous partial pressure of oxygen (Pv_{O_2}) are shown. The effect of a right or left shift in the amount of oxygen delivered to tissues is indicated. A right shift causes an increase, a left shift a decrease. P_{50} is the Po_2 at which haemoglobin is 50% saturated with oxygen. 2,3-DPG, 2,3-diphosphoglycerate.

Table 4.3 **Causes and mechanisms of hypoxaemia**	
Cause	**Mechanism**
Low inspired oxygen	
low barometric pressure low % oxygen in inspired air	low alveolar Po_2
Alveolar hypoventilation	
respiratory depression neuromuscular disease	low alveolar Po_2
Venous-to-arterial shunt	
cyanotic congenital heart disease	admixture of arterial blood (high Po_2) with venous blood (low Po_2)
Impaired diffusion	
pulmonary fibrosis	inadequate arterial oxygenation despite normal alveolar Po_2
Ventilation/perfusion imbalance	
chronic obstructive pulmonary disease	blood perfuses non-aerated parts of lung and is not oxygenated
Po_2, partial pressure of oxygen.	

which facilitates oxygen uptake by tissues (see Fig. 4.7). Red cell 2,3-DPG concentrations are increased in chronic hypoxia. Acidosis and an increase in P_{CO_2} also shift the curve to the right.

Knowing SpO_2, the capillary blood P_{O_2} can be calculated from the oxyhaemoglobin dissociation curve. This quantity can be used as a surrogate for Pa_{O_2}, although its value is typically lower (but never higher). In ventilated patients, end-tidal expired carbon dioxide (E_TCO_2) can be used as a surrogate for Pa_{CO_2}, in both cases avoiding the need for arterial blood sampling.

Tissue blood supply depends on the cardiac output and local vascular resistance. Thus, tissue hypoxia can be caused not only by hypoxaemia but also by anaemia, impaired haemoglobin function, decreased cardiac output or vasoconstriction. Even if oxygen delivery to tissues is adequate, utilization may be impaired by poisons such as cyanide.

An **increase in plasma lactate** concentration (as a result of anaerobic metabolism) is often characteristic of tissue hypoxia, but it should be appreciated that it is a relatively late sign. Hyperlactataemia is a marker of the severity of septic shock: accumulation of lactate occurs both as an effect of tissue hypoxia and as a result of the metabolic response to sepsis, which includes increased glycolysis and reduced metabolic lactate consumption.

Respiratory Failure and Respiratory Support

The respiratory apparatus consists of the lungs (where gas exchange takes place) and a ventilatory pump (the respiratory muscles acting on the thorax). Respiratory failure (that is, inadequate oxygenation of or removal of carbon dioxide from the blood) is conventionally divided into type 1 (hypoxaemic, where the primary problem is with gas exchange) and type 2 (hypercapnic, or ventilatory failure). Typically, in type 1 (caused by parenchymal lung damage, e.g. pneumonia, pulmonary oedema), alveolar P_{O_2} (PA_{O_2}) is low and Pa_{CO_2} is normal or low; in type 2 (causes include chronic obstructive pulmonary disease and diseases causing respiratory muscle weakness), Pa_{O_2} is low and Pa_{CO_2} is high. Note, however, that there is often overlap, and patients with some conditions (notably severe asthma) can progress from type 1 to type 2 or develop either type of respiratory failure. Some of the abbreviations most commonly used in the description of respiratory failure and respiratory support are listed in Table 4.4.

The management of type 1 and type 2 respiratory failure is different. If the distinction cannot be made clinically, it is helpful to calculate the PA_{O_2} using the alveolar gas equation, a simplified version of which is:

$$PA_{O_2} = PI_{O_2} - Pa_{CO_2}/RQ$$

where PI_{O_2} is the partial pressure of oxygen in the inspired gas and RQ is the respiratory quotient (typically ~0.8). The normal alveolar–arterial difference in P_{O_2} is <2 kPa in healthy young adults, increasing slightly with age: it is increased in type 1, but not type 2, respiratory failure.

If a patient is unable to maintain an adequate Pa_{O_2} by breathing room air, it may be possible to overcome this by increasing the oxygen supply, for example, by using some form of face mask or nasal cannulae. This increases alveolar P_{O_2} in poorly ventilated areas but is of no value in hypoxaemia caused by shunts. The efficacy can be checked by pulse oximetry and measurement of Pa_{O_2}. High concentrations (40–60%) using a high-flow-rate mask are typically prescribed in acute type 1 respiratory failure (e.g. as a result of pneumonia), but lower concentrations (24% or 28%, achieved using Venturi-type low flow rate) are preferred in type 2 respiratory failure (see p. 65).

If adequate oxygenation (i.e. Pa_{O_2} >8.0 kPa) cannot be achieved using supplementary oxygen alone, even when augmented by, for example, the use of aggressive physiotherapy to remove secretions and bronchodilators to reduce airways resistance, some form of respiratory support will be required. Other factors that are taken into consideration when considering the need for respiratory support are the presence of acidosis, tachypnoea and the use of accessory muscles of respiration.

It is beyond the scope of this book to discuss these techniques in any detail, but their principal features are summarized in Table 4.5. They are divided into negative pressure and positive pressure, the latter being either non-invasive or invasive (i.e. delivered via an endotracheal or tracheostomy tube). Positive pressure is the type most frequently used in hospitals: techniques range from supporting the patient's own breathing to taking over the work of breathing completely. Modern ventilators are capable of operating in multiple modes. The technique used depends on the clinical circumstances.

There are, however, adverse aspects to mechanical ventilation. These include damage to the lungs (e.g. because of the positive pressure of the inspired gas) and decreased venous return to the heart (leading to decreased cardiac output and to sodium and water retention).

Blood samples for blood gases and acid–base analysis

Acquisition of appropriate high-quality blood samples is particularly important in the context of accurate measurement of blood gases and [H+]. Analysis is performed on whole blood, so special syringes that are preloaded with heparin must be used and fully mixed with the blood by gentle rolling so that it is fully anticoagulated and will not block the analyzer.

Arterial blood is necessary to assess **respiratory function** by analysis of Po_2 and Pco_2. Venous blood gas results reflect a mix of central respiratory function and peripheral extraction, which is rarely informative (Po_2 is usually ~8 kPa lower and Pco_2 1 kPa higher in venous blood, but this is very variable). An unexpectedly low Po_2 result may lead to suspicion that a venous sample was taken by mistake. **Venous blood** can be used for measuring **hydrogen ion concentration** (pH) alone, for example, during the monitoring of diabetic ketoacidosis, because the arteriovenous difference in [H+] is small and venous blood samples can be obtained more safely and less painfully than arterial samples.

The most appropriate sample site for arterial blood is the radial artery. Brachial or femoral arteries can be used, but sampling is more difficult and more prone to complications such as damage to neighbouring structures and the hypoxic effects of vasospasm because they have a less extensive collateral circulation. Painful vasospasm may occur and occasionally a vasovagal response causes syncope, so the patient should lie flat and be reassured by the operator. A local anaesthetic may be used; aseptic procedure must be adopted. The syringe needle should be introduced accurately at a 45-degree angle, and blood should be allowed to fill the barrel spontaneously under arterial blood pressure rather than by withdrawing the plunger. The risk of haematoma is higher for arterial than for venous phlebotomy, so prolonged pressure should be applied to the puncture site until bleeding has stopped.

Any air that enters the syringe must be expelled before the syringe is capped before analysis because equilibration between blood gases and ambient air will occur rapidly and affect the blood gas partial pressures. Care must be taken to avoid needlestick injury. Ideally, sample analysis should be performed immediately using a point-of-care testing analyzer; if the sample is to be transported, it must be placed in crushed ice water and taken rapidly to the laboratory or remote analyzer. Some analyzers allow the patient's temperature to be inputted, to enable more accurate derivation of the calculated parameters such as bicarbonate.

All personnel, including junior medical staff, must receive training before attempting to use blood gas analyzers; the results must be fully documented in the patient record in accordance with local policies and current inspired oxygen concentration should also be recorded.

Table 4.4 Abbreviations commonly used in the description of respiratory failure and respiratory support

Term	Abbreviation	Example
partial pressure (general term)	P	Po_2
arterial partial pressure	Pa	Pao_2
alveolar partial pressure	P_A	P_{AO_2}
inspired gas partial pressure	Pi	Pio_2
end-tidal expired partial pressure	E_T	E_Tco_2
proportion of gas in mixture	Fi	Fio_2
gas saturation	Si	Sio_2

Table 4.5 Techniques of ventilatory support

Non-invasive

negative airways pressure (NAP)	negative pressure is applied to thorax • cuirass; whole body ('iron lung') (rarely used)
positive airways pressure (PAP)	applied via a close-fitting mask; suitable for patients who are conscious and able to cooperate and protect their airway • at constant pressure throughout the respiratory cycle (continuous PAP (CPAP)) • at two pressures (higher in inspiration) (bilevel PAP (BiPAP)) • intermittently (non-invasive positive pressure ventilation (NIPPV))

Invasive

partial support	requires intubation augments patient's own breathing • synchronized intermittent mandatory ventilation (SIMV) allows voluntary breaths between mandatory breaths and can be used with or without positive end-expiratory pressure (PEEP), intended to prevent the collapse of alveoli • pressure support ventilation (PSV) (positive pressure augments patients' own breaths)
full support	requires sedation; ventilator controls respiration • controlled mandatory ventilation (CMV): constant rate with control of either volume or pressure, with PEEP (constant positive pressure ventilation) or without; does not allow spontaneous breaths
extracorporeal	does not use mechanical ventilator • extracorporeal gas exchange (ECGE), either membrane oxygenation (ECMO) or carbon dioxide removal (ECCO$_2$R); requires venovenous bypass through 'artificial lung'

SUMMARY

- **Hydrogen ion homoeostasis** depends on buffering in the tissues and bloodstream, acid excretion by the kidneys and excretion of carbon dioxide (hydration of which forms carbonic acid) through the lungs.
- Blood **hydrogen ion concentration is directly proportional to the partial pressure of carbon dioxide (Pco$_2$), and inversely proportional to the concentration of bicarbonate,** the principal extracellular buffer.
- **Acidosis** (increased [H$^+$]) can be caused by retention of carbon dioxide (**respiratory acidosis**) or ingestion/increased production/decreased excretion of acid or loss of bicarbonate (non-respiratory or **metabolic acidosis**). **Alkalosis** can be caused by hyperventilation (**respiratory alkalosis**), leading to a fall in Pco$_2$, or increased loss of acid (non-respiratory or **metabolic alkalosis**).
- Physiological **compensatory mechanisms** operate to oppose the change in [H$^+$]: compensation in effect causes the generation of an opposing disturbance; for example, in respiratory acidosis, compensation is through increased renal acid excretion.

- Ultimate **correction** of an acidosis or alkalosis usually requires correction of the underlying cause.
- **Mixed disturbances**, with respiratory and metabolic components, occur frequently. Even in these cases, a diagnosis can be made based on clinical assessment and logical consideration of the arterial hydrogen ion concentration and Pco$_2$.
- **Maintenance of a normal Pao$_2$** requires an adequate oxygen content in the inspired gas and normal alveolar ventilation and perfusion. The **oxygen content of blood** depends on Po$_2$, red cell haemoglobin content and normal haemoglobin function; **oxygen delivery** to tissues additionally depends on the adequacy of tissue perfusion.
- Various techniques of ventilatory support are available for patients with respiratory failure, ranging from simple augmentation of oxygen supply for a patient able to breathe normally to complete mechanical ventilation or, occasionally, extracorporeal gas exchange.

Chapter | 5 |

The kidneys

Introduction

The kidneys have three major functions:
- excretion of waste
- maintenance of extracellular fluid (ECF) volume and composition, including acid–base balance
- hormone synthesis.

They also contribute to glucose supply in the fasting state through gluconeogenesis. Each kidney comprises approximately 1 million functional units, called 'nephrons'.

The kidneys have a rich blood supply and normally receive about 25% of the cardiac output. Most of this is distributed initially to the capillary tufts of the glomeruli, which act as high-pressure filters. Blood is separated from the lumen of the nephron by three layers: the capillary endothelial cells, the basement membrane and the epithelial cells of the nephron (Fig. 5.1). The endothelial and epithelial cells are in intimate contact with the basement membrane; the endothelial cells are fenestrated, and contact between the epithelial cells and the membrane is discontinuous so that the membrane is exposed to blood on one side and to the lumen of the nephron on the other side.

The glomerular filtrate is an ultrafiltrate of plasma; that is, it has a similar composition to plasma except that it is almost free of large proteins. This is because the endothelium provides a barrier to red and white blood cells, and the basement membrane, although permeable to water and low molecular mass substances, is largely impermeable to macromolecules. This impermeability is related to both molecular size and electrical charge. Proteins with molecular masses lower than that of albumin (68 kDa) are filterable, at least to some extent; negatively charged molecules are less easily filtered than those bearing a positive charge. Almost all the protein in the glomerular filtrate is reabsorbed and catabolized by proximal tubular cells, with the result that normal urinary protein excretion is <150 mg/24 h.

Filtration is a passive process. The total filtration rate of the kidneys is mainly determined by the difference between the blood pressure in the glomerular capillaries and the hydrostatic pressure in the lumen of the nephron, the nature of the glomerular basement membrane and the number of glomeruli. The difference in the osmotic pressures of the plasma and the ultrafiltrate provides a small force that opposes filtration. In adults, the **normal glomerular filtration rate** (GFR) is approximately **120 mL/min**, equivalent to a volume of about 170 L/24 h. However, urine production is only 1–2 L/24 h, depending on fluid intake; the bulk of the filtrate is reabsorbed further along the nephron.

The glomerular filtrate passes into the **proximal tubules**, where much of it is reabsorbed. Under normal circumstances, about 75% of the sodium is reabsorbed isotonically and all the glucose, amino acids, potassium and bicarbonate are reabsorbed here by energy-dependent mechanisms.

Medullary hyperosmolality, which is vital for the further reabsorption of water, is generated by the countercurrent system, summarized in Fig. 5.2. Chloride ions, accompanied by sodium, are pumped out of the ascending limbs of the **loops of Henle** into the surrounding interstitial fluid, and then diffuse into the descending limbs. Because the ascending limbs of the loops of Henle are impermeable to water, the net effect is an exchange of sodium and chloride ions between the ascending and descending limbs. This alters the osmolality of both the fluid within the nephrons and the surrounding interstitial fluid. A gradient of osmolality is set up between the isotonic corticomedullary junction and the extremely hypertonic (~1200 mmol/L) deep medulla. Diffusion of urea from the collecting ducts into the interstitium and then into the loops of Henle also makes an important contribution to medullary hypertonicity. It is noteworthy that urinary concentrating ability is impaired in malnourished children mainly because of decreased availability of urea but can be restored by increasing their dietary protein intake.

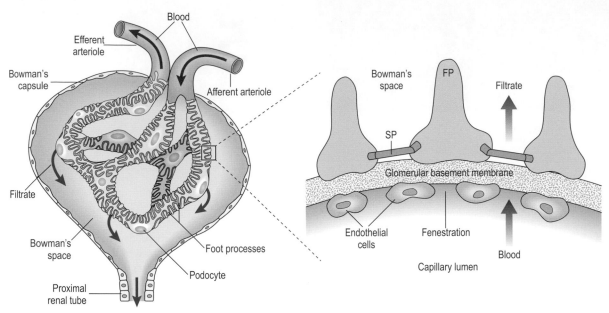

Fig. 5.1 Glomerular capillary, with detail showing fenestrations in endothelial cells, basement membrane and epithelial cells (podocytes) with slit pores or diaphragms (SP) between interdigitating foot processes (FP).

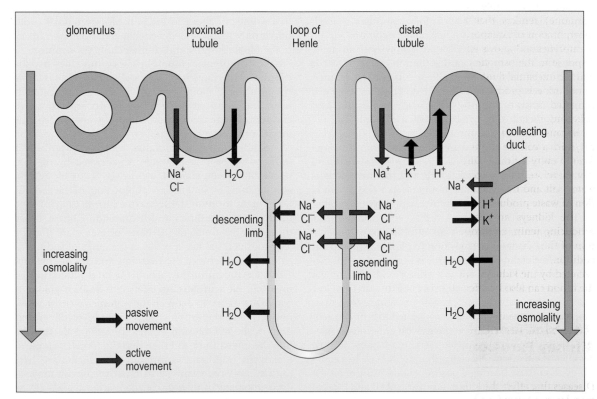

Fig. 5.2 Movements of major ions, passive movement of water and changes in osmolality in the nephron. In the ascending loop of Henle, chloride ions are actively transported and sodium ions accompany them to maintain electrochemical neutrality.

The tubular fluid becomes increasingly dilute as it passes up the ascending limbs of the loops of Henle, as a result of the continued removal of chloride and sodium ions. Fluid entering the **distal tubules** is hypotonic (~150 mmol/kg) with respect to the glomerular filtrate. Further dilution takes place in the early part of the distal tubules.

Approximately 90% of the filtered sodium and 80% of the filtered water has been reabsorbed from the glomerular filtrate by the time it reaches the beginning of the distal tubules. In the distal tubules, further sodium reabsorption takes place, in part controlled by aldosterone; this generates an electrochemical gradient that is balanced by the secretion of potassium and hydrogen ions. Ammonia is also secreted in the distal tubule and buffers hydrogen ions, being excreted as ammonium ions (see p. 56).

Whereas the proximal tubules are responsible for bulk reabsorption of the glomerular filtrate, the distal tubules and the collecting ducts exert fine control over the composition of the tubular fluid, depending on the requirements of the body.

Tubular fluid then passes into the **collecting ducts**, which extend through the hypertonic renal medulla and discharge urine into the renal pelvices and then through the ureters into the bladder. The cells that line the collecting ducts are normally impermeable to water. Vasopressin (antidiuretic hormone) renders them permeable by stimulating the incorporation of aquaporins (water channels) into the cell membranes and allows water to be reabsorbed passively in response to the osmotic gradient between the duct lumen and the interstitial fluid. Thus, in the absence of vasopressin, dilute urine is produced; in its presence, the urine is concentrated. Some reabsorption of sodium also occurs in the collecting ducts under the stimulus of aldosterone.

Because the normal adult GFR is approximately 120 mL/min, a volume of fluid equivalent to the entire ECF is filtered every 2 hours. Disease processes affecting the kidney therefore have a considerable potential for affecting water, salt and hydrogen ion homoeostasis and the excretion of waste products.

The kidneys are also important **endocrine organs**, producing renin, erythropoietin and calcitriol. The secretion of these hormones may be altered in renal disease. In addition, several other hormones are either inactivated or excreted by the kidneys, and hence their concentrations in the blood can also be affected by kidney disease.

The Biochemical Investigation of Kidney Function

Diseases that affect the kidneys can selectively damage glomerular or tubular function, but isolated disorders of tubular function are relatively uncommon. In acute and chronic kidney injury, there is effectively a loss of function of whole nephrons, and because the process of filtration is essential to the formation of urine, **tests of glomerular function are almost invariably required in the investigation and management of any patient with kidney disease**. The principal function of the glomeruli is to filter water and low-molecular-weight components of the blood while retaining cells and high-molecular-weight components. The most frequently used tests are those that assess either the GFR or the integrity of the glomerular filtration barrier.

It should be noted that the GFR declines with age, and this must be taken into account when interpreting results.

Measurement of glomerular filtration rate

Clearance

An estimate of the GFR can be made by measuring the urinary excretion of a substance that is completely filtered from the blood by the glomeruli and is not secreted, reabsorbed or metabolized by the renal tubules. Experimentally, inulin (a plant polysaccharide) has been found to meet these requirements. The volume of blood from which inulin is cleared or completely removed in 1 min is known as the inulin clearance, and it is equal to the GFR.

Measurement of inulin clearance requires the infusion of inulin into the blood and is not suitable for routine clinical use. The most widely used biochemical clearance test is based on measurements of creatinine in plasma and urine. This endogenous substance is derived mainly from the turnover of creatine in muscle, and daily production is relatively constant, being a function of total muscle mass. A small amount of creatinine is derived from meat in the diet. **Creatinine clearance** is calculated using the following formula:

$$\text{Clearance} = \frac{U \times \dot{V}}{P} \; \text{mL/min} \qquad [5.1]$$

U = urine creatinine concentration (µmol/L)
$\dot{V}$ = urine flow rate (mL/min or (L/24 h)/1.44)
P = plasma creatinine concentration (µmol/L)

Creatinine clearance in healthy adults is ~120 mL/min, but a normal GFR for a small person will be lower than for a large person. Results can be corrected to a standard body surface area of 1.73 m² using formulae that incorporate weight and height; this allows easier comparison between individuals. It should be noted that the clearance formula is valid only for a steady state, that is, when kidney function is not changing rapidly.

Creatinine is actively secreted by the renal tubules and, as a result, the creatinine clearance is higher than the true GFR. The difference is of little significance when the GFR is normal, but when the GFR is low (<10 mL/min), tubular secretion makes a major contribution to creatinine excretion and creatinine clearance significantly overestimates the GFR. The effect of creatinine breakdown in the gut also becomes significant when the GFR is very low. Certain drugs, including spironolactone, cimetidine, fenofibrate, trimethoprim and amiloride, decrease creatinine secretion and thus can reduce creatinine clearance. In the calculation of creatinine clearance, two measurements of creatinine concentration and one of urine volume are required. Each of these has an inherent imprecision that can affect the accuracy of the calculation, resulting in a coefficient of variation of up to 30% in hospital patients, mostly related to the difficulty of collecting a timed urine sample (usually 24 hours).

Thus, although previously widely used, measurements of creatinine clearance are potentially unreliable and no longer recommended in routine practice. Alternative methods should be used if a reliable calculation of GFR is required, for example in the assessment of potential kidney donors, investigation of patients with minor abnormalities of kidney function and calculation of the initial doses of potentially toxic drugs that are eliminated from the body by renal excretion.

There are two main alternative approaches to determining the GFR in clinical practice. These are to derive an estimated GFR (eGFR) from the plasma creatinine concentration (see p. 81) or to use exogenous markers of clearance. GFR can be calculated by measuring the disappearance from the blood of a test substance that is completely filtered by the glomeruli and neither secreted nor reabsorbed by the tubules, after a single injection. This approach has the advantage that a urine collection is not required. Suitable substances for this purpose include ^{51}Cr-labelled ethylenediaminetetraacetic acid (EDTA), ^{125}I-iothalamate (for which the decline in plasma radioactivity is monitored) and iohexol, a non-radioactive x-ray contrast medium that can be measured using high-performance liquid chromatography. Typically, blood samples are taken at 2, 3 and 4 hours after injection, although samples taken over a longer period may be required in patients with renal impairment.

Plasma creatinine

Plasma creatinine concentration is the most reliable simple biochemical test of glomerular function. Ingestion of a meat-rich meal can increase plasma creatinine concentration by as much as 20 µmol/L for up to 10 hours afterwards, so ideally blood samples should be collected after an overnight fast. Strenuous exercise also causes a transient, slight increase. Plasma creatinine concentration is related to muscle bulk, and therefore, a value of 100 µmol/L could be normal for an athletic young man but would suggest renal impairment in a thin 70-year-old woman. Although muscle bulk tends to decline with age, so too does the GFR,

and hence plasma creatinine concentrations remain fairly constant.

Some older laboratory methods for the measurement of creatinine can suffer from interference, for example from bilirubin and ketones. The laboratory should be able to advise on whether this may be a problem in individual cases.

The reference range for plasma creatinine in the adult population is around 50–110 µmol/L, but the day-to-day variation in an individual is much less than this range. Equation 5.1 indicates that **plasma creatinine concentration is inversely related to the GFR**. GFR can decrease by 50% before plasma creatinine concentration rises beyond the reference range; plasma creatinine concentration doubles for each further 50% decline in GFR. Consequently, **a normal plasma creatinine concentration does not necessarily imply normal kidney function**, although a raised concentration does usually indicate impaired renal function (Fig. 5.3). Furthermore, a change in creatinine concentration, provided that it is outside the limits of normal biological and analytical variation, does suggest a change in GFR, even if both values are within the population reference range (see Case history 2.2).

Changes in plasma creatinine concentration can occur, independently of kidney function, because of changes in muscle mass. Thus, a decrease can occur as a result of starvation and in wasting diseases, and immediately after surgical amputation of a limb; an increase can occur during refeeding. However, changes in creatinine concentration for these reasons rarely lead to diagnostic confusion.

In pregnancy, creatinine concentrations decrease, partly because of an increase in GFR and partly because of haemodilution from the increase in circulating plasma volume.

Kidney function in the elderly

The glomerular filtration rate (GFR) decreases with age in otherwise healthy people and so does the clearance of creatinine. However, plasma creatinine concentration changes little because creatinine production also falls with age; this reflects a decrease in muscle mass and sometimes also in meat consumption. Despite the decline in the GFR, kidney function remains sufficient for most normal processes, but the decreased reserve capacity may become apparent in even mild disease. A small acute decrease in GFR may result in failure of homoeostasis, and some drugs may not be adequately excreted. Renal responsiveness to vasopressin, thirst sensation and the aldosterone response to renin all decrease with increasing age, putting elderly people at greater risk of disorders of fluid balance and composition. They are also at greater risk of developing acute kidney injury if they become ill for other reasons.

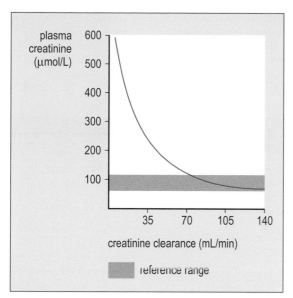

Fig. 5.3 Relationship between creatinine clearance and plasma creatinine concentration.

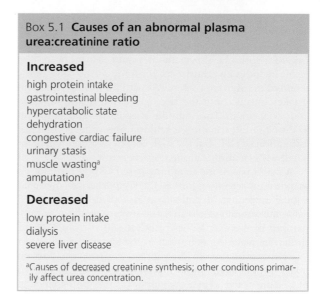

Box 5.1 **Causes of an abnormal plasma urea:creatinine ratio**

Increased

high protein intake
gastrointestinal bleeding
hypercatabolic state
dehydration
congestive cardiac failure
urinary stasis
muscle wasting[a]
amputation[a]

Decreased

low protein intake
dialysis
severe liver disease

[a]Causes of decreased creatinine synthesis; other conditions primarily affect urea concentration.

Plasma urea

Urea is synthesized in the liver, primarily as a by-product of the deamination of amino acids. Its elimination in the urine represents the major route for nitrogen excretion. It is filtered from the blood by the glomeruli, but significant tubular reabsorption occurs through passive diffusion.

Plasma urea concentration is a less reliable indicator of renal glomerular function than creatinine. Urea production is increased by a high protein intake, in catabolic states, and by the absorption of amino acids and peptides after gastrointestinal bleeding. Conversely, production is decreased in patients with a low protein intake and sometimes in patients with liver disease. Tubular reabsorption increases at low rates of urine flow (e.g. in fluid depletion), and this can cause increased plasma urea concentration even when kidney function is normal.

Factors that affect the ratio of plasma urea to creatinine are summarized in Box 5.1. Changes in plasma urea concentration are a feature of renal impairment, but it is important to consider possible extrarenal influences on urea concentrations before ascribing any changes to an alteration in kidney function.

Urea diffuses readily across dialysis membranes and, during renal dialysis, a decline in plasma urea concentration is a poor guide to the efficacy of the process in removing other toxic substances from the blood.

Cystatin C

Cystatin C is low molecular mass peptide (13 kDa) that is produced by all nucleated cells. It is cleared from the plasma by glomerular filtration, and its plasma concentration reflects the GFR more accurately than creatinine. It is not much influenced by sex or muscle mass but may be increased in malignancy, hyperthyroidism and by treatment with corticosteroids. Although not widely available in routine laboratories, measurement may have a role in the detection of early renal impairment in patients in whom creatinine is affected by unusual muscle bulk (e.g. body builders, teenage boys, the frail elderly [especially women] and patients with wasting muscle disorders) or in whom the significance of a mildly reduced eGFR is uncertain. Several formulae for eGFR (see next section) have been devised that are either based on cystatin C concentration alone or include both creatinine and cystatin C values. They are considered to give better estimates of GFR than those based on creatinine alone.

Estimated glomerular filtration rate

An alternative to a formal measurement of creatinine clearance is to calculate an estimate of the clearance from the serum creatinine concentration. Various formulae have been derived for this purpose by comparing serum creatinine concentrations with formal measurements of GFR in large groups of individuals. These formulae take into account factors that predict muscle mass, and therefore, creatinine production rate, such as age, body weight, sex and racial origin.

The recommended formula for routine use in the UK is the **Chronic Kidney Disease Epidemiology Collaboration**

(CKD-EPI). It is based on pooled data from several studies and correlates better with measured GFR than the previously used Modification of Diet in Renal Disease (MDRD) formula, especially at values >60 mL/min. The result includes an adjustment for body surface area and is reported as mL/min/1.73 m^2. As with the MDRD equation, it takes into account the sex, age, serum creatinine value and racial origin. The addition of cystatin C concentration to the CKD-EPI equation is said to improve the accuracy of estimation of GFR, but the high cost of measurement compared with creatinine alone restricts its use.

A major use of the creatinine-based CKD-EPI formula is as a tool for screening for CKD. UK guidelines recommend annual screening of patients at risk of developing CKD, using measurements of eGFR and urinary albumin, as summarized in Box 5.2. Values of eGFR >60 mL/min/1.73 m^2 should be regarded as normal in the absence of clinical or laboratory evidence of kidney disease (e.g. abnormalities on imaging, proteinuria or haematuria). Note that calculations of GFR are not valid in acute kidney disorders, pregnancy, in conditions in which there is severe muscle wasting or oedematous states. Calculations of eGFR in children require specific formulae that take height into account.

Although now less widely used and not validated for use in screening for CKD, the **Cockcroft–Gault formula** also provides an estimate of the creatinine clearance and hence GFR. Many drug dosing regimens, such as some of those used in cancer chemotherapy, are based on this, despite being derived using old creatinine assays that were in use before international standardization. The formula takes into account body weight in addition to sex, age and serum creatinine concentration. It is not adjusted for body surface area, so it gives an absolute value for GFR in mL/min.

A calculator for all of these equations is available at www.kidney.org/professionals.

Box 5.2 Early identification of chronic kidney disease

Offer annual testing using eGFR and urinary protein excretion (preferably albumin) for patients with the following risk factors:

diabetes

hypertension

history of acute kidney injury

cardiovascular disease
   ischaemic heart disease
   chronic heart failure
   peripheral vascular disease
   cerebral vascular disease

structural renal tract disease, recurrent kidney stones or prostatic hypertrophy

systemic disorders known to affect kidneys, e.g. systemic lupus erythematosus

family history of kidney failure or hereditary kidney disease

haematuria detected for other reasons

taking nephrotoxic drugs, e.g. lithium, NSAID (eGFR only)

---

eGFR, estimated glomerular filtration rate (using creatinine CKD-EPI formula); NSAID, non-steroidal anti-inflammatory drug.

Estimated glomerular filtration rate

Although eGFR calculations can be very useful for clinicians and are more helpful than creatinine measurements alone, they are not valid in all clinical circumstances. When renal function is changing rapidly—for instance, in acute kidney injury (AKI)—the eGFR may not reflect the severity of the injury. In patients who are overloaded with fluid or have an abnormal muscle mass, the concentration of creatinine, and therefore the eGFR, will not be a reliable indicator of kidney function.

Several formulae have been devised to estimate the GFR from single measurements of plasma creatinine (e.g. CKD-EPI, see p.81). They all assume that in any individual, the plasma creatinine concentration is not changing rapidly and that the patient has normal muscle mass and a normal total body water content. Most laboratories now automatically report eGFR with every adult creatinine value, regardless of whether the calculation is valid in the clinical scenario. Thus, it is important to realize that reported eGFR values may be misleading in many circumstances including:

• AKI

• increased volume of distribution for creatinine, such as with the oedema of heart failure or nephrotic syndrome
• pregnancy
• decreased muscle mass, such as with paraplegia, amputations or muscle wasting disorders
• increased muscle mass in athletes and body builders
• extremes of age
• ethnic groups in whom the formula has not been validated
• malnutrition and obesity
• after a meat-rich meal
• treatment with drugs that interfere with creatinine secretion by the renal tubules.

eGFR is not reliable enough in situations where a precise knowledge of GFR is required, such as for calculating doses of some toxic drugs that are excreted through the kidneys and for the assessment of potential living kidney donors. In these circumstances, a formal measurement of GFR is recommended.

Assessment of glomerular integrity

Impairment of glomerular integrity results in the filtration of large molecules that are normally retained and is manifest as proteinuria. Proteinuria can, however, occur for other reasons (see p. 94). **Clinical proteinuria** was originally defined as proteinuria that can be reliably detected by dipstick testing (>300 mg/L), but in the UK it is now defined by formal laboratory measurement of protein or albumin:creatinine ratio in a 'spot' urine sample (Table 5.1). The significance of **microalbuminuria** (increased urinary albumin excretion, but not to an extent that can be detected by conventional dipsticks) in patients with diabetes mellitus is considered in Chapter 13.

With severe glomerular damage, red blood cells are detectable in the urine (haematuria). Although haematuria can occur as a result of lesions anywhere in the urinary tract, the red cells often have an abnormal morphology in glomerular disease, because of their passage through the basement membrane. The presence of red cell casts (cells embedded in a proteinaceous matrix) in urinary sediment is strongly suggestive of glomerular dysfunction.

Tests of renal tubular function

Formal tests of renal tubular function are performed less frequently than tests of glomerular function. Many rely on the detection of increased quantities of substances in the urine that are normally reabsorbed by the tubules. The presence of **glycosuria** in a subject with a normal blood glucose concentration implies proximal tubular malfunction that may be either isolated (renal glycosuria) or part of a generalized tubular defect (renal Fanconi syndrome). **Amino aciduria** can occur with tubular defects and may also be generalized or specific to a few amino acids. Tests of proximal tubular **bicarbonate reabsorption** may be required in the assessment of proximal renal tubular acidosis (RTA). The small amount of (principally low molecular weight) protein that is filtered by the glomeruli is normally almost completely reabsorbed by and catabolized in the proximal renal tubular cells. The increased excretion of **low-molecular-weight proteins** in urine can indicate renal tubular damage. β_2-Microglobulin quantitation has been used for this purpose but it is unstable in acidic or infected urine. The measurement of retinol-binding protein or α_1-microglobulin is more reliable but, in practice, specific evidence of tubular damage is rarely required clinically. Notably, albumin is also filtered to a small extent, although it is normally almost entirely reabsorbed, and proximal tubular damage may result in increased urinary excretion in the microalbuminuria range.

The only tests of distal tubular function in widespread use are the **water deprivation test**, to assess renal concentrating ability (see p. 170), and tests of **urinary acidification**, to diagnose distal RTA.

Haematuria

Haematuria can be macroscopic (visible to the naked eye) or microscopic ('invisible haematuria' detected by dipstick testing). If it is invisible and no cause is immediately apparent, a second urine sample should be tested to confirm the finding. Haematuria of 1+ or more always requires further investigation even if the patient is taking anticoagulant medication. The commonest causes are urinary tract infections, kidney stones, urothelial malignancies and glomerulonephritis, many of which are also associated with significant proteinuria. If no cause is found in someone with persistent invisible haematuria without proteinuria, they should be monitored annually to check for deterioration in kidney function and blood pressure control as long as the haematuria persists.

Table 5.1 Approximate relationship of urine total protein and albumin

Albumin: creatinine ratio (mg/ mmol)	Total protein: creatinine ratio (mg/ mmol)	24-h urine protein (mg)	Comments
3.0	15	150	usual upper limit of reference range
30	50	500	referral threshold for people with dipstick-detectable haematuria
70	100	1000	referral threshold without haematuria (in non-diabetic subjects)
>250	>300	>3000	'nephrotic range' proteinuria

In the UK, 24 h urine collections for protein are no longer recommended.

Imaging and Renal Biopsy

It is important to appreciate that biochemical tests of renal function are only one part of the repertoire of investigations available to the renal physician. Ultrasound scanning is recommended to assess kidney size and exclude hydronephrosis in patients with newly diagnosed kidney disease. Other techniques include: Doppler studies to assess blood flow, plain and contrast radiography (e.g. arteriography), computed tomography (CT) and magnetic resonance imaging to provide anatomical information, static and dynamic isotope scanning to provide functional information and percutaneous kidney biopsy to provide a histopathological diagnosis. The measurement of specific antibodies in serum (e.g. antiglomerular basement membrane antibodies, positive in Goodpasture disease, a type of glomerulonephritis, and antineutrophil cytoplasmic antibodies, positive in systemic vasculitis) and other proteins (e.g. complement components, often low in systemic lupus erythematosus) can also provide valuable diagnostic information.

Kidney Disorders

Kidney disease is an increasing global problem with a significant economic impact, especially in the developed world. Several organizations have produced guidelines to improve detection and treatment of kidney disorders using internationally agreed nomenclature for describing the stage and type of disease. The standardization of nomenclature allows better comparison of data between different countries and healthcare organizations. Thus, the older terms 'chronic renal failure' and 'acute renal failure' have largely been replaced with **'chronic kidney disease'** and **'acute kidney injury'** (AKI). Similarly, the term 'end-stage renal failure' has been replaced with **'kidney failure'** (KF) or 'established kidney failure'.

Failure of kidney function may occur rapidly, producing the syndrome of AKI. This is potentially reversible. In contrast, CKD often develops insidiously over many years and is irreversible, leading eventually to KF in some patients. Patients with KF require long-term renal replacement therapy (i.e. dialysis or a successful kidney transplant) to survive. Biochemical tests are essential to the diagnosis and management of KF, but seldom provide information of help in determining its cause.

The term **'glomerulonephritis'** encompasses a group of kidney diseases that are characterized by pathological changes in the glomeruli, often with an immunological basis such as immune complex deposition. Glomerulonephritis may present in many ways, for example as acute nephritis with haematuria, hypertension and oedema, as AKI or CKD, or as proteinuria which may lead to the **nephrotic syndrome** (proteinuria, hypoproteinaemia and oedema, often with accompanying hyperlipidaemia).

Many disorders primarily affect renal tubular function, but most are rare. Their metabolic and clinical consequences range from being trivial (e.g. in isolated renal glycosuria) to being serious (e.g. in cystinuria, see p. 98).

Acute kidney injury

AKI is characterized by **rapid loss of kidney function**, with retention of urea, creatinine, hydrogen ions and other metabolic products and, usually but not always, oliguria (<400 mL urine/24 h). The severity of the injury can be graded according to changes in plasma creatinine concentration and urine output (Table 5.2). Although potentially reversible, the consequences for homoeostasis are so profound that this condition continues to have a high mortality. Furthermore, AKI often develops in patients who already have CKD or are severely ill, with multiple organ involvement. Computerised early warning systems are being used increasingly within hospitals to identify patients who are deteriorating clinically and are at high risk of developing AKI.

Table 5.2 **Staging of acute kidney injury in adults**		
Stage	**Creatinine concentration**	**Urine output**
1	≥26 µmol/L increase within 48 h *or* 1.5- to 1.9-fold increase from baseline within 7 days	<0.5 mL/kg per hour for >6 h
2	2- to 3-fold increase from baseline within 7 days	<0.5 mL/kg per hour for >12 h
3	≥354 µmol/L *or* ≥3-fold increase from baseline within 7 days	<0.3 mL/kg per hour for >24 h or anuria for 12 h

The staging based on level of increase can also be applied to changes occurring within 1 year, using the median value of creatinine concentration during that time as the baseline.

Detection of acute kidney injury

In the UK, laboratories are required to apply an algorithm to all reported creatinine results (apart from results from patients in neonatal units and those on dialysis) to detect potential AKI. These are reported as AKI stages 1–3 depending on both the absolute creatinine value and the change in creatinine concentration over the previous year. The hope is that potential AKI will be detected earlier, allowing intervention to protect the kidneys from further damage.

AKI can be divided into **three categories**, according to whether renal functional impairment is related to a decrease in renal blood flow (**pre-renal**), to intrinsic damage to the kidneys (**intrinsic**), or to urinary tract obstruction (**post-renal**) (Box 5.3). Should any of these occur in a patient whose renal function is already impaired, the consequences are likely to be more serious. Some clues to the presence of chronic disease in a patient with AKI ('acute on chronic' kidney disease) are discussed in Case history 5.3.

The terms 'uraemia' (meaning 'urine in the blood') and 'azotaemia' (increase in concentration of nitrogenous compounds) have been used as synonyms for kidney disease (both AKI and CKD).

Pre-renal acute kidney injury

Pre-renal AKI is caused by circulatory insufficiency, as may occur with severe bleeding, burns, fluid loss, heart failure, systemic sepsis or hypotension that leads to renal

hypoperfusion and a decrease in GFR. This may in part be due directly to a fall in systemic blood pressure to below the level at which autoregulation can preserve the GFR, but it can occur even if blood pressure is maintained, as this is achieved by sympathetic activation, which induces intense renal vasoconstriction. Initially, this results in a decrease in GFR with relative preservation of tubular function (allowing conservation of sodium and water, and hence ECF volume). However, if adequate perfusion is not rapidly restored, **pre-renal AKI may progress to intrinsic kidney damage** ('acute tubular necrosis'). Older patients with CKD, diabetes, liver disease or hypertension, or patients exposed to nephrotoxic drugs (e.g. aminoglycosides) or x-ray contrast agents, are at particular risk of such progression. It may be possible to prevent this if renal perfusion can be restored before structural damage has occurred.

Pre-renal AKI is essentially the result of a normal physiological response to hypovolaemia or a fall in blood pressure. Stimulation of the renin–angiotensin–aldosterone system and vasopressin secretion typically results in the production of a small volume of highly concentrated urine with a low sodium concentration (a fact that may be helpful in distinguishing between pre-renal and intrinsic AKI; Case history 5.1; Table 5.3). Renal tubular function is normal, but the decreased GFR results in the retention of substances normally excreted by filtration, such as urea and creatinine. Decreased excretion of hydrogen and potassium ions results in a tendency towards metabolic acidosis and hyperkalaemia (the latter often being exacerbated by tissue damage).

Intrinsic acute kidney injury

Causes and pathogenesis. A wide variety of conditions can cause intrinsic AKI. Many cases are due to nephrotoxic drugs or renal ischaemia secondary to hypoperfusion, leading to 'acute tubular necrosis'. Causes include sepsis, severe bleeding, burns and heart failure. (See Case history 5.2.) Specific kidney diseases and systemic diseases that affect the kidneys are also important but are less common. The pathogenesis of this condition is complex: in any individual case, several factors may be involved. The term **'acute tubular necrosis'** is widely used as a synonym for intrinsic AKI. However, it is not strictly accurate; biopsy, if performed, may reveal ischaemic damage to nephrons, but not usually frank necrosis. Although not yet widely available, measurement of urine kidney injury molecule-1 or neutrophil gelatinase-associated lipocalin may help to identify patients at high risk of progression to intrinsic kidney injury, because their concentrations rise before that of plasma creatinine.

Although primary glomerular damage is uncommon in AKI, secondary damage occurs if there is persistent glomerular hypoperfusion (itself caused by afferent arteriolar vasoconstriction) and the GFR declines further. Contributory

Case history 5.1

History

A 25-year-old man sustained multiple injuries in a motorcycle accident. He received blood transfusions and underwent surgery.

Examination

He was clinically dehydrated and his blood pressure was 90/50 mmHg. The total urine volume passed during his first 24 h of admission was only 500 mL.

Results (see Appendix and Table 5.3 for reference ranges)

Serum:	potassium	5.6 mmol/L
	urea	21.0 mmol/L
	creatinine	140 µmol/L
	eGFR	57 mL/min/1.73 m²
	osmolality	316 mmol/kg
Urine:	sodium	5 mmol/L
	osmolality	650 mmol/kg

Summary

Serum urea is raised to a much greater degree than creatinine. The urine is concentrated but with low sodium.

Interpretation

The results are consistent with pre-renal AKI. The urine contains little sodium and the urine osmolality is twice that of serum (see Table 5.3). These are normal physiological responses, implying that intrinsic renal function is intact and that the ability of the kidneys to function normally is constrained only by hypoperfusion.

Discussion

The distinguishing features of pre-renal AKI as opposed to intrinsic kidney injury are listed in Table 5.3. These features are not absolutely reliable. They are all invalidated if the patient has been given diuretics, and osmolalities are invalidated by the use of x-ray contrast media. In practice, it is often not possible to distinguish between pre-renal and intrinsic renal injury using biochemical tests; furthermore, if untreated, pre-renal AKI progresses to intrinsic renal injury. Concentrated, sodium-poor urine is a more reliable indicator of pre-renal AKI than a dilute sodium-containing urine is of intrinsic renal injury, because the latter is appropriate for a well-hydrated, healthy person. Oliguria, although usually present, is not a constant feature of AKI.

The increase in serum urea concentration in this patient is greater than the increase in creatinine. This is due both to passive reabsorption of urea in the renal tubules and to increased synthesis from amino acids released as a result of tissue damage.

The patient was given extra fluid intravenously and this resulted in a diuresis. The elicitation of this response may be the only way of distinguishing pre-renal from intrinsic kidney injury. His serum urea and creatinine were normal 48 hours later.

Note that most laboratories report eGFR with every plasma creatinine concentration that is measured in an adult. However, the calculation is very misleading in patients with AKI, because the increase in creatinine concentration may lag several hours to days behind the decline in glomerular filtration rate.

Table 5.3 Biochemical values in oliguria of acute kidney injury		
	Pre-renal	**Intrinsic**
urine sodium concentration	<20 mmol/L	>40 mmol/L
urine : plasma urea concentration	>20:1	<10:1
urine : plasma osmolality	>1.5:1	<1.1:1
Intermediate values occur in incipient intrinsic kidney injury.		

factors include intrarenal release of vasoactive substances, obstruction of the tubular lumen by debris and casts, or by interstitial oedema, back leak of glomerular filtrate through damaged tubular epithelium and reperfusion injury. Failure of the GFR to recover after correction of the circulatory deficit is common.

Metabolic consequences. The characteristic biochemical changes in the plasma in AKI are summarized in Box 5.4. **Hyponatraemia** is common. It is due primarily to an excess of water relative to sodium: contributory factors may include decreased excretion and continued intake of water, injudicious fluid administration and increased water formation from oxidative metabolism. **Hyperkalaemia** occurs as a result of decreased renal excretion of potassium, release into the circulation from tissue breakdown and a transcellular shift (retained hydrogen ions are taken up by cells in exchange for potassium as part of the intracellular buffering mechanism). In severe cases, plasma potassium concentration can increase by 1–2 mmol/L in a few hours, although the rise is usually less rapid. Decreased hydrogen ion excretion causes a **metabolic acidosis**.

Retention of phosphate and leakage of intracellular phosphate into the interstitial fluid leads to **hyperphosphataemia**, which inhibits the 1α-hydroxylation of 25-hydroxycholecalciferol to calcitriol (see p. 259). The resulting decreased plasma concentration of calcitriol causes skeletal resistance to the actions of parathyroid hormone (PTH), causing **hypocalcaemia**. Hypercalcaemia in the oliguric phase of AKI raises the possibility of malignancy (see p. 261). **Hypermagnesaemia** is also often present as a result of decreased magnesium excretion. In established AKI, what urine is produced has a similar osmolality and ionic composition to plasma. Proteinuria is always present, and the urine may be dark because of the presence of haem pigments from the blood.

Natural history. There are typically three phases to the course of acute tubular necrosis: the initial oliguric phase, a diuretic phase and a recovery phase. The **oliguric phase** typically lasts for 8–10 days but sometimes is much shorter or persists for several weeks. In an apparently increasing number of patients, there is no oliguric phase. Non-oliguric AKI is particularly associated with aminoglycoside nephrotoxicity and burns. In general, it has a better prognosis than oliguric AKI. When an oliguric phase does occur, it is followed by a diuretic phase, with increasing urine volume. This is the result of an increase in GFR, and initially there is often little improvement in tubular function. The composition of the urine is similar to that of protein-free plasma. During this phase, urine volume may exceed 5 L/day and, because of its high ionic concentration, there is a considerable risk of both dehydration and depletion of sodium and potassium.

Although the onset of the **diuretic phase** often heralds clinical improvement, plasma concentrations of urea and creatinine do not decline immediately, because the GFR is still much lower than normal and insufficient to allow excretion of the surplus. The persisting high urea concentration in the blood, and hence in the glomerular filtrate, contributes to the diuresis by an osmotic effect. The acidosis also persists until tubular function is restored. Plasma calcium concentration may rise during this phase, particularly after crush injuries, because of the release of calcium from damaged muscle. Temporary persistence of any elevation in the plasma concentration of PTH will stimulate calcitriol synthesis, and this may also contribute to hypercalcaemia.

Gradually, in the **recovery phase**, as the tubular cells regenerate and tubular function is restored, the diuresis subsides and the various abnormalities of kidney function resolve. Patients who survive the acute illness may recover completely. There may be some residual impairment of kidney function, but this may not be apparent from simple tests. Patients remain at increased risk of developing CKD or further episodes of AKI and require long-term monitoring.

In very severe cases of AKI, such as may occur after massive antepartum haemorrhage, the ischaemic insult to the kidneys may exceed their regenerative capacity: there is renal cortical necrosis and no recovery of kidney function. A type of KF occurring in patients with chronic liver disease is discussed in Chapter 6.

Post-renal acute kidney injury

Obstruction to the flow of urine leads to an increase in hydrostatic pressure in the collecting ducts, which opposes glomerular filtration and, if prolonged, leads to secondary renal tubular damage. Obstruction that occurs above the level of the urethral insertion into the bladder must be bilateral to have a major effect on urine flow (see Box 5.3). Complete anuria is rare with AKI from other causes and thus is strongly suggestive of obstruction. More often, obstruction is either intermittent or incomplete, and urine production may even be normal in obstruction with overflow. The degree of reversibility of kidney damage in obstructive injury depends to some extent on how long-standing the obstruction is. It is more likely to be reversible if the obstruction is acute.

Management of acute kidney injury

All patients with suspected AKI should have an urgent medication review to minimize exposure to potentially nephrotoxic drugs. Obstruction should be excluded either clinically or by ultrasound examination. If present, the obstruction should be relieved or, if this is not immediately possible, urinary drainage should be established by another means.

Many cases of intrinsic kidney injury are preventable, and if a patient is judged to be at high risk, it is important to attempt to prevent progression to acute tubular necrosis by **measures to maintain kidney perfusion** (e.g. early administration of intravenous fluids to maintain ECF

Case history 5.2

History

A young man was admitted to hospital with severe abdominal injuries after being knocked down by a car.

Examination

He was severely shocked, with a swollen, tender abdomen.

Progress

He was given intravenous fluids and blood, and was taken to the operating theatre. At laparotomy, his spleen was found to be ruptured: splenectomy was performed. There was also mesenteric damage and a tear in the duodenum: the damaged gut was resected.

Three days later he became hypotensive and pyrexial, and was taken back to theatre. Free fluid was present in the peritoneal cavity and a leak was found in a segment of gangrenous small intestine. Appropriate surgical procedures were performed. Following this, the patient became oliguric, despite adequate hydration.

Results

Serum:		
	sodium	128 mmol/L
	potassium	5.9 mmol/L
	bicarbonate	16 mmol/L
	urea	22.0 mmol/L
	creatinine	225 μmol/L
	eGFR	33 mL/min/1.73 m²
	calcium	1.72 mmol/L
	calcium (adjusted)	1.96 mmol/L
	phosphate	2.96 mmol/L

Urine:		
	albumin	28 g/L
	osmolality	324 mmol/kg
	sodium	80 mmol/L

Summary

Markedly raised serum urea and creatinine, with high potassium and phosphate, low bicarbonate and calcium. High urine sodium.

Interpretation

Serum urea and creatinine are increased proportionately, indicating likely intrinsic AKI. There is acidosis reflecting inability to excrete hydrogen ions. His serum potassium is high, secondary to AKI and acidosis. Phosphate retention results in decreased serum calcium concentration. The urine osmolality is similar to the approximate calculated serum osmolarity (see p. 38) and there is significant sodium loss indicating failure to conserve sodium and concentrate urine.

Discussion

These findings are typical of AKI in a septic, catabolic patient (see Table 5.3 and Box 5.4). As AKI progresses, the kidneys lose their ability to conserve sodium and to produce concentrated urine. The patient was treated with haemofiltration; antibiotics were continued and his pyrexia settled. Six days after the accident, the patient's urine output began to increase, as shown in Fig. 5.4. The biochemical changes that occurred before and after the diuretic phase, until recovery of normal renal function, are also shown in Fig. 5.4. Note that the calculated eGFR may be misleading in this case (see p. 82).

> ! Patients who have had an episode of AKI are at increased risk of developing CKD. Their kidney function should be monitored for at least 2–3 years following such an episode.

---

volume). Volume repletion should be monitored with reference to fluid balance charts and measurements of blood flow if available. Loop diuretics are not recommended routinely but may be helpful in patients who are fluid overloaded. Dopamine should be avoided as it can reduce renal perfusion. Hypoxaemia, if present, must be corrected. In critically ill patients, good, but not excessive, glycaemic control is beneficial. If dipstick testing is positive for blood, the patient should be investigated promptly to exclude rapidly progressive glomerulonephritis.

If oliguria persists and acute tubular necrosis is diagnosed, it becomes necessary to minimize the severe adverse consequences of KF. The **general principles of treatment** include: strict control of sodium and water intake, maintenance of normovolaemia; nutritional support to minimize protein catabolism; prevention of metabolic complications, such as hyperkalaemia and acidosis, and prevention of infection. Care should be taken to avoid the use of potentially nephrotoxic drugs.

When kidney injury is short-lived, and in non-oliguric AKI, conservative measures alone may suffice. However, many patients will require **renal replacement therapy** (e.g. haemofiltration, haemodiafiltration or haemodialysis). The decision to start such treatment is usually primarily clinical, although laboratory data are also informative. In general, renal replacement should be started sooner rather than later. Factors that will prompt the decision include any of evidence of uraemic encephalopathy, pericarditis, pulmonary oedema, severe hyperkalaemia (e.g. plasma potassium >7.0 mmol/L) or severe acidosis (e.g. $[HCO_3^-]$ <12 mmol/L, $[H^+]$ >70 nmol/L).

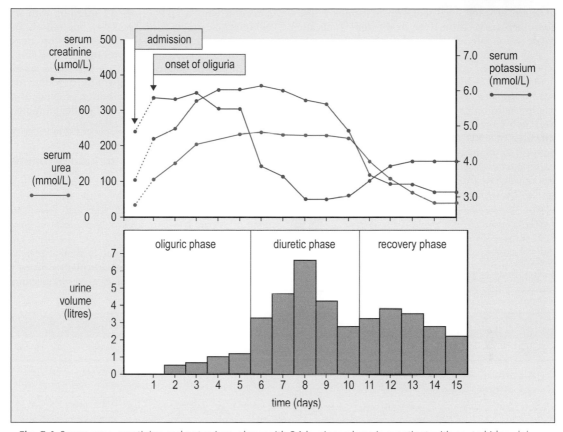

Fig. 5.4 Serum urea, creatinine and potassium, along with 24-h urine volume in a patient with acute kidney injury.

Dialysis or haemofiltration may have to be continued into the early part of the diuretic phase until the GFR has recovered sufficiently for the plasma concentration of creatinine to start falling. The main problem during the diuretic phase is to supply sufficient water and electrolytes to compensate for the excessive losses. Fluid replacement should not automatically be isovolaemic, because the diuresis is partly due to mobilization and excretion of excess ECF. From the onset of AKI until its resolution, it is essential to monitor the patient's plasma creatinine, sodium, potassium, bicarbonate, calcium and phosphate concentrations and urine volume.

The general principles of management are similar whatever the cause of AKI. In addition, specific measures may be indicated for certain diseases, for example the control of infection or hypertension and the use of immunosuppressive drugs in immunologically mediated kidney disease. **The importance of recognizing the circumstances that put patients at risk of AKI (e.g. sepsis, hypovolaemia, the use of x-ray contrast media in dehydrated patients or those with already impaired renal function, and the use of potentially nephrotoxic drugs) and of attempting to prevent renal damage by appropriate measures cannot be overemphasized.**

Chronic kidney disease
Causes, natural history and screening

Many disease processes can lead to progressive, irreversible impairment of kidney function. Glomerulonephritis, diabetes mellitus, hypertension, pyelonephritis, renovascular disease and polycystic kidneys account for the majority of cases where a cause can be determined. In effect, all these conditions lead to a decrease in the number of functioning nephrons. Patients may remain asymptomatic until the GFR falls to <15 mL/min. In some people, the natural history is of progression to **kidney failure**, the state when conservative measures are no longer sufficient and renal replacement therapy (dialysis or transplantation) becomes necessary to save the patient's life. The time between presentation and KF is very variable: it may be a matter of weeks or many years, depending on several factors, including how early CKD is detected, the aetiology, and the adequacy of measures to prevent further deterioration such as blood pressure control and avoidance of nephrotoxic drugs. In most patients, a graph of the reciprocal of serum creatinine concentration plotted against time approximates to a straight line. Such plots allow the prediction of when renal replacement therapy is likely to become necessary. An increase in the slope (indicating an increase in the rate of deterioration of kidney function) should alert the physician to a potentially treatable cause (e.g. hypovolaemia or infection).

Calculation of the eGFR provides a basis for screening for CKD. In the absence of other evidence of kidney disease (e.g. proteinuria or a structural abnormality), values ≥60 mL/min are regarded as normal. Values less than this are indicative of CKD and require further investigation and appropriate management. Table 5.4 shows the internationally agreed classification of CKD. The glomerular filtration rate (GFR) and albuminuria stages are combined to describe the CKD stage, for example, G3aA1 denotes

> If a patient is found to have an eGFR of <60 mL/min/1.73 m² and has not been tested before or has had normal kidney function previously, measurement of eGFR should be repeated within two weeks to check for rapidly deteriorating kidney function.

someone with a GFR of 45–59 mL/min with a urine albumin: creatinine ratio (ACR) <3 mg/mmol. There is an increased risk of adverse outcomes with increasing stages of both GFR and albuminuria. A new finding of CKD should be confirmed within two weeks to identify patients with accelerated progression of kidney disease. The frequency of subsequent monitoring depends on the stage of CKD, with lower eGFR and higher albumin excretion requiring more intensive follow-up.

Metabolic consequences of kidney failure

The major pathological and clinical features are similar in all patients with KF, whatever the cause. The metabolic features are summarized in Box 5.5. Although there is impairment of urinary concentration, polyuria is never gross (not >4 L/day), because the GFR is so low. The urine tends to be of constant osmolality, similar to that of plasma. The lack of urinary concentration is particularly noticed by the patient at night, and **nocturia** is a common complaint.

Table 5.4 **Classification of chronic kidney disease**			
GFR stage	**Description**	**GFR (mL/min/1.73 m²)**	**Comments**
G1	kidney damage with normal or raised GFR	>90	requires presence of proteinuria, haematuria or other kidney abnormality, e.g. on imaging
G2	kidney damage with mildly decreased GFR	60–89	requires presence of proteinuria, haematuria or other kidney abnormality, e.g. on imaging
G3a	mild to moderate reduction in GFR	45–59	increased risk of cardiovascular complications as GFR decreases
G3b	moderate to severe reduction in GFR	30–44	many patients still asymptomatic
G4	severe reduction in GFR	15–29	most patients symptomatic
G5	kidney failure	<15	renal replacement therapy usually required
Albuminuria stage	**Description**	**ACR (mg/mmol Creatinine)**	
A1	normal to mildly increased	<3	reference range: <3.0 mg/mmol
A2	moderately increased	3–30	commonly referred to as 'microalbuminuria'
A3	severely increased	>30	detectable using conventional dipsticks

Box 5.5 Metabolic and biochemical consequences of kidney failure

Metabolic features	Biochemical changes in plasma	
	Increased	Decreased
impairment of urinary concentration and dilution	potassium	sodium
impairment of electrolyte and hydrogen ion homoeostasis	urea	bicarbonate
retention of waste products of metabolism	creatinine	calcium
decreased calcitriol synthesis	hydrogen ion	
decreased erythropoietin synthesis	phosphate	
dyslipidaemia	magnesium	
reduced degradation of insulin and insulin resistance		
other endocrine abnormalities		

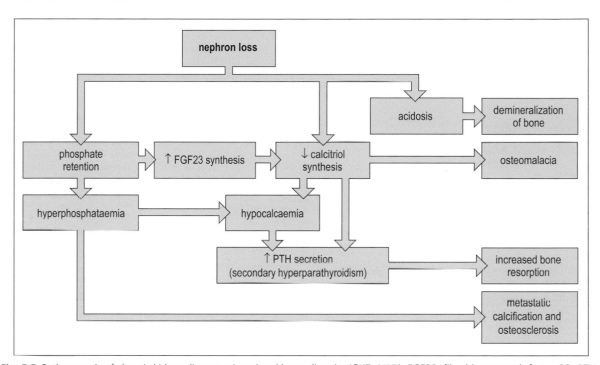

Fig. 5.5 Pathogenesis of chronic kidney disease–mineral and bone disorder (CKD–MBD). FGF23, fibroblast growth factor 23; PTH, parathyroid hormone.

The ability to dilute the urine may also be impaired late in the course of CKD, and patients become very sensitive to the effects of either fluid loss or overload. Eventually, the patient becomes oliguric as the GFR falls.

Sodium balance is usually maintained until the GFR falls to <20 mL/min. The majority of patients tend to retain sodium, but severe renal sodium wasting is occasionally seen. This syndrome of 'salt-losing nephritis' occurs most often in patients whose kidney disease particularly affects the tubules, for example, analgesic nephropathy, polycystic disease and chronic pyelonephritis.

Hyperkalaemia is a late feature of KF: it may be precipitated by a sudden deterioration in kidney function or by the injudicious use of potassium-sparing diuretics.

Patients with KF tend to be **acidotic**. The urinary buffering capacity is impaired as a result of decreased phosphate excretion and ammonia synthesis. The ability of individual nephrons to reabsorb filtered bicarbonate is often impaired. However, although plasma hydrogen ion concentration increases and bicarbonate decreases, these changes progress only slowly, because of buffering of excess hydrogen ions in bone.

Case history 5.3

History

A 56-year-old man presented to his family doctor with weight loss, generalized weakness and lethargy of 6 months' duration. During this time, he had been passing more urine than usual, particularly at night. He had become impotent.

Examination

He looked anaemic and had a blood pressure of 180/112 mmHg. His urine contained protein but no glucose.

Results

Serum:	sodium	130 mmol/L
	potassium	5.2 mmol/L
	bicarbonate	16 mmol/L
	urea	43.0 mmol/L
	creatinine	640 µmol/L
	eGFR	8 mL/min/1.73 m^2
	calcium (adjusted)	1.92 mmol/L
	phosphate	2.42 mmol/L
	alkaline phosphatase	205 U/L
Plasma:	glucose (random)	6.4 mmol/L
Blood:	haemoglobin	91 g/L

Summary

Very low eGFR, with low sodium, calcium, bicarbonate and haemoglobin. High phosphate. Normal glucose.

Interpretation

The results are consistent with kidney failure causing retention of phosphate and hydrogen ions. Mild hyponatraemia is a common finding but rarely requires specific treatment.

Discussion

The doctor's first thought was that this patient had diabetes mellitus, but the absence of glycosuria made this unlikely, and the results are typical of CKD. Failure of the kidneys to concentrate urine adequately results in polyuria and nocturia. Oliguria is a late feature of CKD. The history suggests slowly progressive, rather than acute, kidney disease. The presence of anaemia and the raised alkaline phosphatase (caused by CKD–MBD, see Fig. 5.5) are consistent with the diagnosis, although they are not specific findings.

The kidneys are small in most patients with CKD (unless because of amyloid or polycystic disease), and the demonstration of small kidneys by radiography or ultrasonography is another indicator of chronicity. So, too, is the presence of hypertension.

Many other clinical features may be present in patients with KF (Box 5.6). The causes of many of these features are unknown, but they are presumably related to the retention of toxins that cannot be excreted. These 'uraemic toxins' include phenolic acids, polypeptides, polyamines and many other substances.

Most patients with CKD become **hypocalcaemic** and, in time, many develop a **mineral and bone disorder (CKD–MBD)**, previously known as 'renal osteodystrophy'. This comprises secondary hyperparathyroidism or osteomalacia, or both ('mixed lesion'). A fourth type, **adynamic bone disease**, characterized by reduced trabecular bone formation and resorption, is increasingly being recognized, particularly in patients given calcitriol or other 1α-hydroxylated derivatives of vitamin D.

The pathogenesis of CKD–MBD is complex (Fig. 5.5). Retention of phosphate causes a tendency towards hyperphosphataemia, inhibiting calcitriol synthesis (mediated by increased production of fibroblast growth factor 23 [FGF23]) and leading to hypocalcaemia through a reduction in intestinal calcium absorption. PTH concentrations are elevated in CKD, secondary to hypocalcaemia, low calcitriol concentrations and down-regulation of the calcium-sensing and vitamin D receptors, activation of which normally reduces PTH secretion. Decreased concentrations of calcitriol may also contribute to the resistance to the action of PTH on bone that occurs in KF. High concentrations of PTH decrease the reabsorption of phosphate from each nephron, but eventually the falling GFR becomes the limiting factor in phosphate excretion and persistent hyperphosphataemia ensues. If the concentration of phosphate becomes so high that the solubility product of calcium and phosphate ($[Ca^{2+}] \times [Pi]$) is exceeded, metastatic calcification may occur. This is seen particularly in blood vessels and may in part contribute to the sclerotic deposits that can occur in bone. With advanced KF, the decrease in functioning kidney tissue also contributes to the decrease in calcitriol production. Another factor of importance is buffering of hydrogen ions by bone, which leads to demineralization. Aluminium can cause osteomalacia. In the past, the presence of aluminium in softened water used to prepare dialysis fluid has caused problems, as has the absorption of aluminium from orally administered salts given to bind phosphate in the gut and prevent hyperphosphataemia. Although overall exposure is now much lower, the few patients on dialysis still taking aluminium-containing medication require regular (three monthly) monitoring of serum aluminium concentrations.

In addition to the effect on calcitriol synthesis, **other endocrine consequences** of KF include decreased testosterone and

<table>
<tr><td>

Box 5.6 Clinical features of kidney failure

Neurological

lethargy
peripheral neuropathy

Musculoskeletal

growth failure
bone pain
myopathy

Gastrointestinal

anorexia
hiccough
nausea and vomiting
gastrointestinal bleeding

Cardiovascular

anaemia
hypertension
pericarditis

Dermal

pruritus
pallor
purpura

Genitourinary

nocturia
impotence

</td></tr>
</table>

oestrogen synthesis, abnormalities of thyroid function tests (not usually associated with clinical thyroid disease, although the incidence of both goitre and primary hypothyroidism is significantly increased in CKD), and abnormal glucose tolerance with hyperinsulinaemia caused by insulin resistance. However, insulin-treated diabetic patients who develop renal disease often have decreased insulin requirements, because insulin is metabolized in the kidney.

A normochromic normocytic **anaemia** is usual in KF, because of depression of bone marrow function by retained toxins and a decrease in the renal production of erythropoietin. A bleeding tendency may also be present, and bleeding may exacerbate the anaemia. Iron deficiency may also contribute to the anaemia and should be considered if the severity of the anaemia is disproportionate to the degree of renal insufficiency. Ferritin is often increased in patients with KF as a result of an inflammatory stimulus, which limits its use as a diagnostic marker for iron deficiency.

Other complications include **dyslipidaemia** (hypertriglyceridaemia and an increased plasma concentration of remnant particles), which contributes to the high risk of cardiovascular disease characteristic of CKD.

Management of chronic kidney disease

If the cause of CKD can be determined, appropriate treatment may reduce the rate of further loss of kidney function but may not prevent it completely. Some patients progress inexorably to KF, but considerable alleviation of symptoms and biochemical abnormalities can be obtained by conservative measures before renal replacement therapy becomes necessary.

As the kidneys become unable to control water and sodium balance, it is essential that intake is matched to obligatory losses. Diuretics can be used to promote sodium excretion if dietary salt restriction is inadequate, but excessive use can worsen kidney function. Volume depletion must be avoided: it decreases renal blood flow and thus the GFR.

Hypertension is a frequent complication of CKD and also exacerbates it. Angiotensin-converting enzyme inhibitors (ACEIs) and angiotensin II receptor blockers (ARBs) reduce the rate of progression of renal impairment in patients with CKD, especially in those with proteinuria, independently of their effect on blood pressure. However, in patients with renal artery stenosis or advanced CKD, ACEIs, ARBs and direct renin antagonists can cause deterioration in function and hyperkalaemia. Patients' plasma creatinine and potassium concentrations should be checked 1–2 weeks after starting treatment or increasing the dose.

Bicarbonate can be given orally to control acidosis. Treatment of hyperkalaemia is usually less urgent in CKD than in AKI because it develops more slowly. It can usually be controlled with loop diuretics or oral **ion-exchange compounds,** combined with dietary potassium restriction. Hyperphosphataemia can be controlled by giving oral phosphate binders (e.g. calcium carbonate, which also helps correct acidosis) and avoiding phosphate-rich foods.

Adequate **nutrition is critical** in patients with CKD but may be difficult to maintain because of poor appetite. Patients require specialist dietary advice to balance potassium and phosphate restriction with adequate protein intake to avoid negative nitrogen balance. In patients who are not candidates for maintenance dialysis or transplantation, a very low protein intake can give considerable symptomatic relief in the terminal stage of KF but an adequate intake of essential amino acids and carbohydrate is still required. Iron deficiency is common and often requires intravenous therapy. Vitamin D deficiency is also common, although guidelines take different approaches to the benefits of screening and treatment with cholecalciferol in patients with CKD.

Treatment of anaemia with recombinant erythropoietin or erythropoietin analogues has considerably improved the quality of life for patients with KF, before and while on replacement treatment. It is usually started when haemoglobin falls to <110 g/L. It is an effective treatment in the presence of adequate iron stores and has additional beneficial effects (e.g. on myocardial ischaemia). Adverse effects include hypertension and increased haematocrit with consequent hyperviscosity.

Bone disease should be monitored by regular measurements of plasma calcium, phosphate and PTH concentrations, alkaline phosphatase activity and bone densitometry. The basis of prevention and treatment is avoidance of hyperphosphataemia and hypocalcaemia. This usually requires a combination of an oral phosphate binder and oral calcitriol or another active form of vitamin D. PTH concentrations should ideally be maintained at two to nine times normal, reflecting the resistance to PTH that is characteristic of severe CKD or KF. Lower values indicate an increased risk of adynamic bone disease. Occasionally, the parathyroid glands become autonomous (tertiary hyperparathyroidism): the massively elevated concentrations of PTH can produce severe hypercalcaemia. Treatment is either with calcimimetic drugs (which suppress PTH secretion) or by parathyroidectomy.

The major cause of death in patients with CKD is cardiovascular disease. In addition to treating hypertension, other cardiovascular risk factors should be managed appropriately. Treatment of dyslipidaemia can both reduce the risk of cardiovascular disease and help to preserve renal function.

Renal replacement therapy

Renal replacement therapy may be required for patients with AKI (see p. 88) and for patients with KF. Techniques include dialysis, haemofiltration and combinations of the two and, in patients with KF, transplantation. Dialysis-related techniques do not replace the endocrine functions of the kidney: patients on long-term dialysis require treatment with erythropoietin and vitamin D derivatives. Patients who successfully undergo kidney transplantation are free of these restrictions but must take immunosuppressive drugs to prevent rejection.

The principle of **dialysis** is that blood is exposed to dialysis fluid from which it is separated by a semipermeable membrane. In **haemodialysis**, an extracorporeal circuit and artificial membrane are used and substances move from the plasma to the dialysate by diffusion. A controlled pressure gradient can be used to remove fluid. In **peritoneal dialysis**, dialysate is instilled into the peritoneal cavity, and the peritoneum acts as the semipermeable membrane. Haemodialysis is usually performed intermittently; peritoneal dialysis is often performed continuously but sometimes only overnight.

In **haemofiltration**, a membrane capable of a high rate of fluid transfer is used, but there is no dialysis fluid. A pressure gradient drives fluid and solutes across the membrane by a process called 'convection'. Fluid and electrolyte balance is maintained by infusion of a suitable fluid into the extracorporeal circuit. Haemofiltration is usually performed continuously. The technique of **haemodiafiltration** removes fluid and solutes by a combination of diffusion and convection, and provides greater urea and middle molecule (molecular mass >1000 Da) clearance than haemodialysis alone. Accumulation of middle molecules, such as β_2-microglobulin, can lead to widespread deposition in tissues, causing a form of amyloidosis.

The factors that govern the choice of renal replacement technique are complex. In AKI, the preferred technique is usually semicontinuous haemofiltration or haemodiafiltration. Patients with KF who require long-term renal replacement are offered intermittent haemodiafiltration or haemodialysis (typically three times weekly), or peritoneal dialysis. Peritoneal dialysis is usually performed continuously (continuous ambulatory peritoneal dialysis [CAPD]) and typically involves exchanges of 2 L fluid four times daily. It is a relatively simple technique and can be performed without specialized equipment. Automated peritoneal dialysis (APD) allows overnight fluid exchanges, leaving the daytime free. In peritoneal dialysis, the dialysate is made hypertonic with glucose to facilitate removal of fluid, but diffusion of this glucose into the bloodstream can lead to diabetes and hypertriglyceridaemia. Peritoneal dialysis can also lead to loss of protein. All renal replacement techniques can lead to loss of amino acids, trace minerals and vitamins.

Clearance rates by diffusion fall off rapidly with increasing molecular mass, but convection, which more nearly reflects normal glomerular function, allows fairly uniform clearance of all substances that can pass through the semipermeable membrane, typically decreasing significantly only with molecular masses exceeding 10 kDa. Haemodiafiltration, which combines both modalities, is therefore becoming the preferred option in appropriate patients. However, because the 'uraemic toxins' are primarily low-molecular-weight substances, dialysis is still an effective technique for renal replacement.

Patients who have undergone **transplantation** require careful clinical and biochemical monitoring to assess graft function and to provide warning of incipient graft rejection. Features of graft rejection include oliguria and pyrexia, but these may not be present and a rise in plasma creatinine concentration may be the first sign. However, an increase in creatinine can also occur with nephrotoxicity caused by ciclosporin, a frequently used immunosuppressive drug. Indicators of tubular damage—for example, the urinary activity of the tubular enzyme N-acetyl-β-D-glucosaminidase—have been studied as possible indicators of early rejection, but none is specific to the process and they are not widely used.

Proteinuria and the nephrotic syndrome

The glomeruli normally filter 7–10 g of protein per 24 hours, but almost all is reabsorbed by endocytosis and subsequently catabolized in the proximal tubules. Normal urinary protein excretion is <150 mg/24 h. Approximately half of this is uromodulin (Tamm–Horsfall protein), a glycoprotein secreted by tubular cells; <30 mg is albumin. The mechanisms of proteinuria are summarized in Box 5.7.

The presence or absence of proteinuria may be assessed using a reagent-impregnated strip (dipstick), which is dipped

Box 5.7 Mechanisms of proteinuria

Overflow

caused by presence in plasma of a high concentration of a low molecular weight protein, which is filtered in a quantity exceeding tubular reabsorptive capacity, e.g. Bence Jones protein, myoglobin

Glomerular

caused by increased glomerular permeability, e.g. albumin, immunoglobulins

Tubular

caused by impaired or saturated reabsorption of protein filtered by normal glomeruli, e.g. retinol-binding protein, α_1-microglobulin

Secretory

caused by secretion by kidneys or epithelium of urinary tract, e.g. uromodulin, immunoglobulins and other plasma proteins in presence of urinary tract infections or bladder tumours

---

into the urine. This reliably detects albumin at concentrations >200 mg/L but is less sensitive to other proteins. False-positive results are obtained with urine that is alkaline, contaminated by various antiseptics or contains x-ray contrast media. It should be appreciated that for a given protein excretion rate, protein concentration will be higher if the urine volume is low. UK guidelines therefore recommend formal laboratory testing, preferably using urinary albumin measurement, with results expressed as a ratio to creatinine concentration in a 'spot' urine sample to overcome these problems. Healthy adults excrete <3 mg albumin/mmol creatinine, which is equivalent to <15 mg protein/mmol creatinine. A value >30 mg albumin/mmol creatinine or >50 mg protein/mmol creatinine (approximately equivalent to 500 mg/24 h) reliably predicts significant proteinuria and requires referral for specialist assessment. However, any degree of proteinuria predicts an increased future risk of cardiovascular as well as kidney disease, and patients with microalbuminuria (3–30 mg/mmol creatinine) require good control of blood pressure and regular monitoring for progression of proteinuria.

Investigation of proteinuria

Patients known to be at risk of CKD (see Box 5.2) should be offered annual testing for proteinuria. Patients with documented CKD may require more frequent monitoring, depending on the stage of CKD. A high result requires confirmation on a second specimen, unless the albumin concentration is already >70 mg/mmol creatinine. Proteinuria discovered on dipstick testing also requires confirmation with laboratory quantitation on two separate specimens. If Bence Jones proteinuria is suspected (see Chapter 16), a specific test must be used, because this protein is not detectable by dipstick or by urine albumin measurement. Before investigating kidney function, incidental extrarenal causes of proteinuria, such as fever, strenuous exercise and burns, should be excluded: such proteinuria is usually not of long-term significance. Orthostatic proteinuria (see later) should also be excluded.

When the presence of proteinuria has been confirmed and infection excluded, simple tests of kidney function and renal ultrasound should be performed. If the results are all normal, there is no haematuria and albumin excretion is <30 mg/mmol creatinine (or protein excretion <50 mg/mmol), the patient need not be subjected to further investigation but should be followed up. With protein excretion in excess of this, or with other abnormal test results, further investigation, often including renal biopsy, is necessary to determine the cause. Albuminuria >70 mg/mmol (or proteinuria >100 mg/mmol) is virtually always pathological and usually signifies glomerular disease.

Orthostatic proteinuria is a benign condition in which proteinuria is present only when subjects are upright. It occurs in approximately 5% of young adults. The prevalence decreases with increasing age. Orthostatic proteinuria is thought to occur as a result of an increase in the hydrostatic pressure in the renal veins caused by anatomical variations. It is of no clinical significance and can confidently be diagnosed if two samples of urine collected immediately on rising in the morning on separate days are protein-free.

Electrophoresis of a concentrated specimen of urine may help to distinguish between the various types of proteinuria. In tubular proteinuria, for example, the predominant proteins are of low molecular mass, being filtered proteins that are incompletely reabsorbed. In glomerular proteinuria, higher-molecular-weight proteins are present. Electrophoresis of urine is also used for the detection of Bence Jones proteinuria.

In minimal change glomerulonephritis, the proteinuria is typically highly selective (i.e. proteins larger than albumin are mostly retained), whereas in most other causes of significant proteinuria, higher-molecular-weight proteins are also excreted (low selectivity).

The nephrotic syndrome

Hypoproteinaemia with oedema may develop if large amounts of protein are excreted in the urine. For this to occur, proteinuria must usually exceed 300 mg/mmol creatinine (~3 g/24 h). Although the ability of the liver to synthesize protein is greater than this, much of the filtered protein is catabolized after endocytosis by renal tubular cells and is thus lost from the circulation, even though it is not excreted in the urine. Conditions in which the nephrotic syndrome may occur are shown in Box 5.8.

The amount of proteinuria is not necessarily a useful guide to the severity of kidney disease. For example, in

Box 5.8 **The nephrotic syndrome: causes and clinical and biochemical features**

Causes	Clinical and biochemical features	
	Feature	**Mechanism**
minimal change glomerulonephritis	proteinuria	glomerular damage
membranous glomerulonephritis	oedema	low plasma albumin
idiopathic		secondary hyperaldosteronism
associated with carcinoma, drugs or	increased susceptibility to infection	low plasma immunoglobulins and
infection, e.g. malaria, hepatitis B		complement
systematic lupus erythematosus	thrombotic tendency	hyperfibrinogenaemia and low
diabetic nephropathy other forms of		antithrombin III
glomerulonephritis, e.g. focal sclerosing	hyperlipidaemia	increased apolipoprotein synthesis
glomerulosclerosis, AL amyloid		

minimal change glomerulonephritis, which has a good prognosis, the proteinuria may exceed that seen in patients with more aggressive glomerular lesions (see Case history 5.4).

The **clinical and biochemical features** of the nephrotic syndrome are summarized in Box 5.8. There are two aspects to **management**: treatment of the underlying disorder, where this can be identified and treatment is possible; and treatment of the consequences of protein loss. Minimal change glomerulonephritis, the most frequent cause of nephrotic syndrome in children, often responds to corticosteroids or immunosuppressive drugs. Other types of glomerulonephritis, more often seen in adults, are generally much less responsive to treatment.

General measures to counteract the consequences of protein loss include a high-protein, low-salt diet, although decreased appetite and impaired absorption of nutrients caused by oedema of the gut may be limiting factors. A high protein intake must be introduced with caution when there is concurrent KF. Removal of excess fluid should be undertaken with caution, because too rapid a diuresis can lead to hypovolaemia and thus impair kidney function; potassium depletion must also be avoided. Spironolactone is the diuretic of first choice, but thiazides or loop diuretics may be necessary in addition. Prevention of infection is vital, and hypertension requires careful control. The risk of thrombosis, especially renal vein thrombosis, which may cause a rapid increase in proteinuria, may warrant the prophylactic use of anticoagulants.

Renal tubular disorders

Renal tubular disorders can be congenital or acquired; they can involve single or multiple aspects of tubular function.

Box 5.9 **Causes of renal Fanconi syndrome**

Inherited metabolic disease

cystinosis (Lignac–Fanconi disease)
galactosaemia
fructose intolerance
tyrosinaemia
Wilson disease, Dent disease, Lowe syndrome

Nephrotoxins

heavy metals (e.g. cadmium)
drugs

Paraproteinaemia

Amyloid

The congenital conditions are inherited and all are rare: their clinical sequelae relate to the consequences of loss of substances that are normally completely or partially reabsorbed by the tubules. Some are discussed here; others (e.g. Liddle syndrome, a cause of hypertension) are included in accounts of their consequences in other chapters.

Renal Fanconi syndrome

The renal Fanconi syndrome is a generalized disorder of tubular function characterized by **glycosuria, amino aciduria, phosphaturia** and **acidosis**. It may be idiopathic or may occur secondarily to a variety of conditions (Box 5.9). One of these is cystinosis, a rare autosomal recessive disease in which there is a defect in the transport of cystine out of lysosomes due to an inactivating mutation in the

Case history 5.4

History

An 8-year-old girl presented to her family doctor with puffy eyes and swelling of her legs. She had noticed that her urine had become frothy.

Examination

She had generalized oedema. Dipstick testing showed significant proteinuria.

Results

Serum:		
	sodium	130 mmol/L
	potassium	3.6 mmol/L
	bicarbonate	32 mmol/L
	urea	2.0 mmol/L
	creatinine	18 µmol/L
	calcium (total)	1.70 mmol/L
	total protein	35 g/L
	albumin	15 g/L
	triglyceride	16 mmol/L
	cholesterol	12 mmol/L
	the serum was lipaemic	
Urine:	total protein : creatinine ratio	1200 mg/mmol

Summary

Nephrotic range proteinuria, grossly raised lipids, very low albumin, low creatinine and urea, normal bicarbonate. Mild hyponatraemia. Potassium is at the low end of the normal range.

Interpretation

The presence of proteinuria, hypoalbuminaemia and oedema constitutes the nephrotic syndrome. There is a secondary mixed hyperlipidaemia.

Discussion

The oedema is, in part, a result of redistribution of ECF between the vascular and interstitial compartments in response to a very low plasma albumin concentration; secondary aldosteronism, with evidence of potassium depletion, is often present as a consequence.

Loss of protein is not confined to albumin. Plasma concentrations of hormone-binding proteins, transferrin and antithrombin III are also reduced. On the other hand, there is usually an increase in the concentrations of high-molecular-weight proteins such as α_2-macroglobulin, coagulation factors (fibrinogen, factor VIII, etc.) and the apolipoproteins, which are too large to be lost even through the damaged glomeruli. The increase in apolipoprotein synthesis causes secondary hypercholesterolaemia and hypertriglyceridaemia (and thus lipaemia), and these may in turn cause pseudohyponatraemia (see p. 42). In adults with persistent nephrotic syndrome, accelerated atherosclerosis may develop. Changes in the concentrations of coagulation factors can predispose to venous thrombosis, particularly in the renal veins. Total calcium concentration is low due to reduced albumin concentration, although ionized calcium is usually within the reference range, despite renal loss of vitamin D metabolites bound to vitamin D-binding globulin. Note that adjusted calcium concentration (see Box 14.1) is not reported when albumin is so low, as the calculation is invalid. Loss of immunoglobulins and complement components renders patients with nephrotic syndrome very susceptible to infection.

The GFR may be low, normal or increased in patients with the nephrotic syndrome. In minimal change glomerulonephritis, it is often increased, and the low urea and creatinine concentrations in this patient reflect this. The quantity of protein excreted must be judged in relation to the GFR. A decrease in excretion usually heralds improvement as the glomeruli become less permeable, but it may occur because of a decrease in GFR. This may be because of the underlying disease or a decline in plasma volume.

---

gene for cystinosin, a lysosomal membrane protein. This leads to cystine accumulation and the deposition of cystine crystals in many body tissues, including the kidneys. Affected infants fail to thrive, develop rickets and polyuria with dehydration, and eventually progress to KF. Treatment with cysteamine, which depletes lysosomal cystine, may slow progression of the disease. Cystinosis should not be confused with cystinuria, a disorder of tubular transport.

Renal tubular acidosis

The defect in proximal (type 2) RTA is impairment of bicarbonate reabsorption. Proximal RTA may be a component of Fanconi syndrome but can also occur as an isolated phenomenon. A transient form can occur in infants. Bicarbonate can be completely reabsorbed if the plasma bicarbonate concentration is low, and thus patients may excrete normal amounts of acid but at the expense of systemic acidosis. Treatment consists of administering large amounts of bicarbonate, for example 10 mmol/kg body weight per 24 hours.

Distal (type 1 or classical) RTA occurs more frequently. It can be either inherited or acquired, for example secondarily to hypercalcaemia or autoimmune diseases. There is a defect in hydrogen ion excretion, and the urine cannot be acidified. Consequences include hypercalciuria, nephrocalcinosis, renal calculi and often hypokalaemia. In general, it is more usual for acidotic states to be associated with hyperkalaemia, but in these types of RTA, the impaired ability of the kidneys to excrete hydrogen ions necessitates increased potassium excretion when sodium is reabsorbed in the distal tubules, and this may cause potassium depletion and hypokalaemia. Treatment of distal RTA involves the administration of potassium supplements and bicarbonate in sufficient quantities to buffer normal hydrogen ion production (1–3 mmol/kg body weight per 24 h).

The most frequently encountered type of RTA is type 4, which is usually acquired. It is associated with hypoaldosteronism, either secondary to adrenal disease or to kidney disease in which there is decreased renin secretion (hyporeninaemic hypoaldosteronism, e.g. in diabetic nephropathy) or resistance to aldosterone (e.g. in obstructive nephropathy). In contrast with the other types of RTA, there is hyperkalaemia. The urine can be maximally acidified, but only at the expense of a systemic acidosis. The clinical features are primarily those of the underlying cause. Management is directed at the underlying cause and correction of the hyperkalaemia.

The diagnosis of RTA requires a high index of suspicion. Typically, there is hyperchloraemia and a normal anion gap. Other causes of this combination (e.g. loss of alkaline fluid from the gut or treatment with carbonic anhydrase inhibitors) must be excluded. Measurement of urine pH and plasma potassium concentration will usually indicate the correct diagnosis. Confirmation of the diagnosis of distal RTA may require a formal urinary acidification test using a combination of fludrocortisone and furosemide. Failure to acidify urine to pH 5.3 or less indicates an acidification defect. Ammonium chloride loading is an alternative test but is very unpleasant for the patient and the drug is difficult to source. Diagnosis of proximal RTA may occasionally require determination of the renal threshold for bicarbonate.

Defects of urinary concentration

Impairment of urinary concentration is a feature of nephrogenic diabetes insipidus, a group of primary tubular disorders. It is also a feature of cranial diabetes insipidus and CKD, and can occur with hypercalcaemia, hypokalaemia and certain drugs, notably lithium. In inherited nephrogenic diabetes insipidus, vasopressin secretion is normal, but there is a mutation affecting either its receptor (the V2 receptor) or aquaporin 2. Hypercalcaemia and hypokalaemia interfere with the intracellular cyclic adenosine monophosphate-mediated signalling pathway that leads to the insertion of aquaporins into the cell membranes of the collecting ducts.

Glycosuria and amino aciduria

Benign renal glycosuria is discussed on p. 245. Renal glycosuria can also occur in association with other tubular abnormalities, for example, as part of the renal Fanconi syndrome.

Amino aciduria can occur in combination with normal plasma concentrations of amino acids as a result of defective tubular reabsorption, e.g. in Hartnup disease and cystinuria. Overflow amino aciduria occurs secondarily to elevated plasma concentrations when the tubular transport mechanism is saturated, e.g. in phenylketonuria.

Cystinuria has an incidence of about 1 in 7000 live births. Defective tubular reabsorption of cystine, ornithine, arginine and lysine leads to their excretion in the urine. The loss of these amino acids would alone be of little consequence, but cystine is relatively insoluble, and cystinuria predisposes the patient to urinary calculus formation. The management of cystinuria is discussed on p. 348.

Hypophosphataemic rickets

Hypophosphataemic rickets, also known as vitamin D–resistant rickets, has a dominant X-linked pattern of inheritance and is associated with a defect in the PHEX protein, which regulates FGF23 (see Table 15.2). Failure of tubular phosphate reabsorption in response to high concentrations of FGF23 leads to severe rickets and growth retardation. This does not respond to treatment with vitamin D alone, even if administered in massive doses, but can be treated effectively with a combination of oral phosphate supplements and vitamin D, usually given as a 1α-hydroxylated derivative. An autosomal dominant variety has also been described, in which circulating FGF23 is resistant to normal proteolysis.

Hypophosphataemic rickets should not be confused with inherited vitamin D-dependent rickets type I, an autosomal recessive condition. The defect is in the 1α-hydroxylation of 25-hydroxycholecalciferol. This condition can be treated with 1α-hydroxylated derivatives of vitamin D alone and is discussed, together with vitamin D-dependent rickets type II, in Chapter 15 (p. 274).

Urinary calculi
Pathogenesis

Stones (or calculi) can form in urine when it is supersaturated with the crystalloid components of the calculus. Predisposing factors, and the commoner types of calculus that occur clinically, are shown in Box 5.10. Most stones form within the collecting system of the kidneys, although some form in the bladder. Stones can remain clinically silent for many years, but if they start moving,

Box 5.10 **Urinary tract stones**

Predisposing factors to formation

dehydration
urinary tract infection
persistently alkaline urine
persistently acidic urine (e.g. with diabetes mellitus)
hypercalciuria
hyperuricosuria
hyperoxaluria
urinary stagnation (caused by obstruction)
lack of urinary inhibitors of crystallization (e.g. hypocitraturia)

Composition

calcium oxalate (±phosphate)
calcium phosphate
uric acid
magnesium ammonium phosphate ('struvite')
cystine

Biochemical investigations

analysis of stone
plasma:
    calcium
    bicarbonate
    phosphate
    urate
urine:
    pH
    amino acids
    24-h volume
    24-h excretion of sodium, calcium, oxalate, urate and citrate
    consider urine acidification test for RTA

RTA, renal tubular acidosis.

they typically cause severe colicky pain (ureteric colic) and sometimes visible haematuria. The presence of stones increases the risk of urinary infection and, conversely, urinary infections increase the risk of developing stones.

Hypercalciuria is present in up to 30% of patients with calcium oxalate/phosphate stones. It may be associated with hypercalcaemia, for example, caused by primary hyperparathyroidism. Frequently, however, hypercalciuria is idiopathic: patients are normocalcaemic, and the primary abnormality is usually either an increase in intestinal absorption or a renal leak of calcium, although reabsorption from bone may also be a factor. A high dietary salt intake may exacerbate hypercalciuria because there is a link between sodium and calcium excretion by the kidneys.

Hyperoxaluria predisposes to renal calculus formation. Primary hyperoxaluria is a rare inherited metabolic disorder. Three types have been described: increased hepatic oxalate synthesis is common to all. In type 1, there is deficiency of the enzyme alanine–glyoxylate aminotransferase, leading to increased urinary excretion of oxalic, glyoxylic and glycolic acids; KF develops in the majority of cases, and calcium oxalate crystals develop in many body issues. In type 2 there is increased urinary excretion of oxalic and glyceric acids; although it has been considered to be a milder condition, there have been reports of patients progressing to KF. In type 3, hyperoxaluria is the only metabolic abnormality detected.

Secondary hyperoxaluria is much more common and is usually caused by increased intestinal absorption of dietary oxalate, with or without increased oxalate ingestion. This may be seen in patients with a variety of gastrointestinal disorders, in particular with inflammatory bowel diseases and conditions associated with malabsorption. In these circumstances, non-absorbed free fatty acids bind to calcium. This limits the amount of calcium available to combine with oxalate to form calcium oxalate, which is insoluble and is normally excreted in the faeces. As a result, an increased amount of oxalate remains in solution and can be absorbed into the bloodstream.

Citrate forms soluble complexes with calcium and is an endogenous inhibitor of calcium precipitation. Urine citrate excretion depends to a considerable extent on the composition of the diet but is decreased in acidosis and potassium depletion, both of which increase its renal reabsorption. Hypocitraturia increases the risk of calcium phosphate and oxalate stone formation.

Uric acid stones may be associated with **hyperuricosuria** and hyperuricaemia, but they are most commonly caused by production of persistently acid urine, particularly in patients with diabetes mellitus. The incidence of uric acid stones has increased in line with the increased prevalence of diabetes and glucose intolerance.

Investigation

The history and examination may suggest an underlying cause for urinary calculi, such as inadequate fluid intake. Biochemical tests that should be performed on plasma and urine are shown in Box 5.10. If a stone is available, it should be analyzed, because the composition may indicate a specific treatment. The urine must be examined for evidence of infection in all patients presenting with urinary calculi. The radiographic appearance of a retained stone may be characteristic; for example, 'staghorn' calculi often contain mixed phosphates and may be related to chronic infection; pure uric acid stones (not containing calcium) are radiolucent. Many calculi can be detected by ultrasound, although

Case history 5.5

History

A 38-year-old man developed severe acute pain radiating from his left kidney to his groin. He had no fever but noticed that his urine was red. He had developed similar symptoms 4 and 10 years previously: after each of these episodes he had passed a urinary stone without any intervention. His father had also been treated for kidney stones in the past.

Examination

He was distressed and sweating but apyrexial. He had gross haematuria.

Investigations

An abdominal x-ray showed a 3-mm stone in the lower third of his left ureter.

Progress

He was given pain relief and tamsulosin tablets and advised to drink plenty of water. The stone passed spontaneously three days later. He was referred to a metabolic clinic six weeks later.

Results

Serum:	calcium (adjusted)	2.45 mmol/L
	phosphate	0.98 mmol/L
	creatinine	93 µmol/L
	eGFR	89 mL/min/1.73 m²
	bicarbonate	26 mmol/L
24-h urine:	calcium	9.8 mmol (<7.5)
	oxalate	280 µmol (<450)
	sodium	230 mmol
	citrate	3.2 mmol (2–6)
	volume	1.2 L
Stone analysis:	calcium oxalate	100%

Summary

Normal kidney function, hypercalciuria with normocalcaemia and high sodium excretion.

Interpretation

Hypercalciuria is a risk factor for the formation of calcium oxalate stones and can be exacerbated by a high salt intake, reflected in the high urine sodium output. The 24-h urine volume is well below that recommended for someone with a history of kidney stone formation.

Discussion

The pain on presentation is typical of renal colic, when a stone moves from the renal pelvis into the ureter and towards the bladder. If the stone is small enough, it may pass out of the body spontaneously. Tamsulosin, an alpha-blocker, relaxes the smooth muscle of the urinary tract and increases the chance that the stone will pass. Haematuria is often present in patients with urinary stones, and 'red urine' may be the presenting complaint.

People with recurrent urinary stones are at high risk of developing further stones, especially if there is also a positive family history, so identification of an underlying metabolic cause is helpful to direct preventive treatment. Calcium oxalate is the commonest type of stone, but an underlying cause for such stones is not always apparent.

This patient had hypercalciuria, high urine sodium excretion and a low urine volume, all of which promote the development of calcium-containing stones. His urine citrate and serum bicarbonate were normal, which exclude an underlying renal tubular disorder. An abnormality of oxalate metabolism or absorption is unlikely with normal urine oxalate excretion.

He was advised to drink at least another litre of water a day and to reduce his salt intake. He was started on indapamide, which reduces urine calcium excretion. Three months later, his urine calcium excretion had fallen to 5.4 mmol/24 h and the volume had increased to 2.5 L. His kidney function was checked annually thereafter, given his increased risk of developing CKD.

---

low-dose CT scanning is the preferred first-line investigation, especially if surgical intervention or lithotripsy is being considered.

Management

Small stones are often passed spontaneously or with the help of oral alpha-blockers, which relax the smooth muscle of the ureters. Larger calculi may require surgical removal (often endoscopically) or disintegration by ultrasound (lithotripsy). Any urinary tract infection should be treated. Identifying the cause of urinary calculus formation enables the design of a regimen to reduce further stone formation (see Case History 5.5). This is particularly important in patients in whom stones form recurrently; they are at increased risk of developing CKD and require long-term monitoring of kidney function.

The management of cystinuria is considered on p. 348. Hyperuricaemia should be treated with allopurinol if stones are composed of uric acid (see p. 282).

Alkalinisation of the urine with potassium citrate increases the solubility of both cystine and uric acid but may be difficult to achieve. A high fluid intake is appropriate in all patients with a tendency to form urinary calculi.

If patients who form calcium stones are hypercalcaemic, the underlying cause should be treated. In the normocalcaemic majority, dietary manipulation to correct excessive intake of sodium, calcium or oxalate is appropriate. However, calcium restriction below the recommended daily intake is contraindicated because oxalate absorption is likely to increase and there may be adverse effects on the skeleton. In patients who do not respond to such measures, thiazide diuretics (which decrease urinary calcium excretion) and potassium citrate supplementation can be effective at preventing recurrence.

SUMMARY

- **The kidneys have three major functions:** the control of extracellular fluid volume and composition (including hydrogen ion homoeostasis), excretion of waste products of metabolism and hormone production.
- The most widely used test of overall kidney function is the **plasma creatinine concentration**. It may be used in calculations, with additional data such as age, race and sex, to generate an **estimated glomerular filtration rate (eGFR)**. The presence of **proteinuria** is a sensitive, although not specific, indicator of damage to the kidneys.
- **Acute kidney injury (AKI)** is a life-threatening condition in which there is a potentially reversible deterioration in kidney function. Causes include renal hypoperfusion, specific kidney diseases, obstruction to urine flow and nephrotoxic drugs. When hypoperfusion is responsible, it may be possible to prevent the development of intrinsic kidney damage by restoration of normal perfusion. Biochemical features of AKI include increases in plasma urea and creatinine concentrations, hyperkalaemia, hyperphosphataemia, acidosis and fluid retention. Patients are often oliguric and require renal replacement therapy until kidney function recovers.
- In **chronic kidney disease (CKD)**, kidney function is irreversibly lost; patients may eventually require transplantation or long-term dialysis. Causes include diabetes, vascular diseases, glomerulonephritis and pyelonephritis. CKD usually develops slowly and, because the kidneys have considerable functional reserves, patients may present late in the course of the illness. Retention of urea, creatinine and other waste products, and disturbance of sodium and water homoeostasis, are characteristic; severe acidosis and hyperkalaemia are late features of the condition. Bone disease, with hypocalcaemia and hyperphosphataemia, and anaemia result from impairment of renal endocrine function. Screening populations at risk of CKD allows early intervention to decrease the rate of progression.
- The **nephrotic syndrome** comprises proteinuria, hypoproteinaemia and oedema, and can be a result of a variety of diseases that affect the glomeruli. The clinical and biochemical features stem from the loss of protein from the body. The loss of albumin and other proteins leads to oedema and increased susceptibility to infection. The increased synthesis of other, larger, proteins leads to hypercoagulability and hyperlipidaemia. Uraemia may or may not be present, depending on the nature of the underlying glomerular damage.
- **Disorders of renal tubular function** can lead to decreased excretion of substances that are excreted by the tubules (e.g. hydrogen ions) or to increased excretion of substances that are normally reabsorbed (e.g. glucose). They can be inherited or acquired.
- The formation of **urinary calculi** is essentially the result of supersaturation of the urine. Factors that predispose to calculus formation include the excretion of high solute loads (e.g. of calcium, oxalate or urate), inadequate water intake, production of persistently acidic urine and infection.

Chapter | 6 |

The liver

Introduction

The liver is of vital importance in intermediary metabolism and in the detoxification and elimination of toxic substances (Box 6.1). Damage to the organ may not obviously affect its activity, because the liver has considerable functional reserve, and as a consequence, simple **tests of liver function** (e.g. plasma bilirubin and albumin concentrations) are insensitive indicators of liver disease. Tests that reflect liver cell damage (particularly the measurement of the activities of hepatic enzymes in plasma) are often superior in this respect, although it is not strictly correct to call them 'liver function' tests.

The results of the **standard biochemical liver function tests rarely provide a precise diagnosis** on their own because they reflect the basic pathological processes common to many conditions. However, these tests are relatively inexpensive, widely available and non-invasive. They are of value in detecting the presence of liver disease, following its progress and indicating the need for other, more complex tests, particularly imaging and liver biopsy. Serological tests (e.g. for autoantibodies and evidence of viral infection) are also important in the investigation of liver disease.

The liver has a dual blood supply: approximately two-thirds from the portal vein, which drains much of the gut and through which most of the nutrients absorbed from the gut reach the liver; and the remainder from the hepatic artery, which supplies most of the liver's oxygen. This anatomy allows for first-pass metabolism where drugs or other toxic agents absorbed from the gut must pass through the liver (where they are metabolized) before reaching the systemic circulation. Blood leaves the liver through hepatic veins, which drain into the inferior vena cava.

The metabolic activity of the liver takes place within the parenchymal cells, which constitute 80% of the organ mass; the liver also contains Kupffer (reticuloendothelial) cells and stellate cells (vitamin A storing cells, which are responsible for fibrosis). Parenchymal cells are contiguous with the venous sinusoids, which carry blood from the portal vein and hepatic artery, and with the biliary canaliculi, the smallest ramifications of the biliary system (Fig. 6.1). Substances destined for excretion in the bile are secreted from hepatocytes into the canaliculi, pass through the intrahepatic ducts and reach the duodenum via the common bile duct.

The most common disease processes that affect the liver are:

- **hepatitis**, which may be acute or chronic, or a combination of both, in which there is damage to and destruction of liver cells
- **cirrhosis**, in which fibrosis leads to shrinkage of the liver, decreased numbers of hepatocytes and hence decreased hepatocellular function, hypertension in the portal venous system and cholestasis (obstruction of bile flow)
- **tumours**, both primary but, more frequently, secondary; for example, metastases from cancers of the large bowel, stomach and bronchus.

Patients with liver disease often present with characteristic symptoms and signs, particularly **jaundice**, the yellow-orange discolouration of the skin caused by a high plasma concentration of bilirubin, but the clinical features may be non-specific, and in many patients, liver disease is discovered incidentally. Because of the intimate relationship between the liver and biliary system, extrahepatic biliary disease may present with clinical features suggestive of liver disease or may have secondary effects on the liver. For instance, obstruction to the common bile duct may cause jaundice and, if prolonged, a form of cirrhosis.

Bilirubin Metabolism

Bilirubin is derived mainly from the haem moiety of haemoglobin molecules. Haem is liberated when senescent red cells are removed from the circulation by the

Box 6.1 Major functions of the liver

Carbohydrate metabolism

gluconeogenesis
glycogen synthesis and breakdown

Fat metabolism

fatty acid synthesis
cholesterol synthesis and excretion
lipoprotein synthesis
ketogenesis
bile acid synthesis
25-hydroxylation of vitamin D

Protein metabolism

synthesis of plasma proteins (including some coagulation
     factors but not immunoglobulins)
urea synthesis from ammonia

Metabolism and excretion

bilirubin
steroid hormones
drugs and foreign compounds

Storage

glycogen
vitamin A
vitamin B_{12}
iron

reticuloendothelial system (Fig. 6.2); the iron in haem is reutilized, but the tetrapyrrole ring is degraded to bilirubin. Other sources of bilirubin include myoglobin and the cytochromes.

Unconjugated bilirubin is not water soluble: it is transported in the bloodstream bound to albumin and taken up by a specific carrier protein on hepatocytes. It is then transported to the smooth endoplasmic reticulum, where it undergoes conjugation, principally with glucuronic acid, to form monoglucuronides and diglucuronides; this process is catalysed by the enzyme uridine diphosphate (UDP)-glucuronosyltransferase. The resulting **conjugated bilirubin is water soluble,** and most is secreted into the biliary canaliculi, this being the rate-limiting step in bilirubin metabolism. The small proportion that diffuses back into the bloodstream is rapidly taken up again by the liver.

The secreted bilirubin eventually reaches the small intestine via the ducts of the biliary system. In the gut, bilirubin is converted by bacterial action into urobilinogen, a colourless compound. Some urobilinogen is absorbed from the gut into the portal blood. Hepatic uptake of this is incomplete: a small quantity reaches the systemic circulation and is excreted in the urine. Most of the urobilinogen in the gut is oxidized in the colon to a brown pigment, stercobilin, which is excreted in the stool.

Less than 500 mg bilirubin is produced daily, but the healthy liver can metabolize and excrete more than three

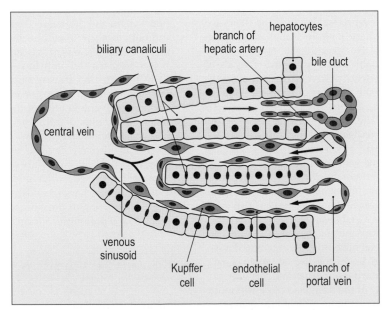

Fig. 6.1 Microstructure of the liver. The liver consists of acini in which sheets of hepatocytes, one cell thick, are permeated by sinusoids carrying blood (black arrow) from the portal venules and hepatic arterioles to the central vein. Bile (red arrow) is secreted from the hepatocytes into canaliculi, which drain into the bile ducts.

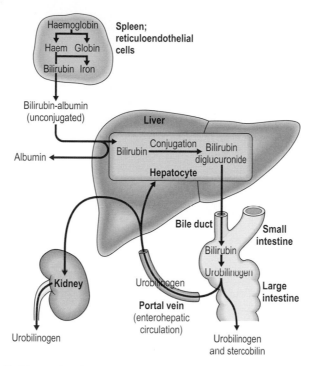

Fig. 6.2 Bilirubin metabolism. Bilirubin, produced primarily from haemoglobin breakdown, is taken up into hepatocytes, where it is conjugated in the smooth endoplasmic reticulum and excreted via the bile ducts into the gut, where it is converted to urobilinogen. Most of the urobilinogen is oxidized to stercobilin in the colon, but some is absorbed from the small intestine and enters the enterohepatic circulation to be re-excreted in the bile; some reaches the systemic circulation and is excreted in the urine.

> ⚠ Bilirubinuria, bilirubin detected in urine with a dipstick, reflects an increase in the plasma concentration of conjugated bilirubin and is always pathological.

times this amount. The measurement of plasma bilirubin concentration is thus an insensitive test of liver function: it is frequently normal in early or mild liver disease.

The bilirubin normally present in the plasma is mainly (~95%) unconjugated; because it is protein bound, it is not filtered by the kidney glomeruli, and in health, bilirubin is not detectable in the urine.

Although jaundice is a frequent feature of liver disease, it may not be obvious clinically unless the plasma bilirubin concentration is more than twice the upper reference limit (URL), that is, >50 µmol/L. It becomes obvious to lay observers when the concentration exceeds 100 µmol/L. Hyperbilirubinaemia can be caused by increased production of bilirubin, impaired metabolism, decreased excretion or a combination of these. The causes of jaundice are listed in Box 6.2.

Biochemical Assessment of Liver Function

Plasma bilirubin concentration

Hyperbilirubinaemia can be caused by an excess of either conjugated or unconjugated bilirubin, or both. The separate measurement of these entities is useful in the diagnosis of neonatal jaundice, where there may be some doubt as to the relative contribution of defective conjugation and other causes; it is less often required in adults. If the plasma bilirubin concentration is <100 µmol/L and other tests of liver function are normal, it is likely that the raised values are due to the unconjugated form of the pigment. The urine can be tested to confirm this because with unconjugated hyperbilirubinaemia there is no bilirubin in the urine. In adults, severe jaundice is almost always a result of conjugated hyperbilirubinaemia.

Hyperbilirubinaemia is not always present in patients with liver disease, nor is it exclusively associated with liver disease. For example, it is not usually present in patients

Box 6.2 Classification and major causes of jaundice (see Figs. 22.3 and 22.4 for newborns)

Pre-hepatic	Posthepatic
haemolysis	gallstones
ineffective erythropoiesis	biliary stricture
	carcinoma of pancreas or
	biliary tree
	cholangitis

Hepatic

premicrosomal	postmicrosomal
drugs, e.g. rifampicin, which interfere with bilirubin uptake	impaired excretion
	hepatitis
	drugs, e.g. methyl-testosterone, rifampicin
	Dubin–Johnson syndrome
microsomal	Rotor syndrome
prematurity	intrahepatic obstruction
hepatitis, e.g. viral or drug induced	hepatitis
	cirrhosis
Gilbert syndrome	infiltrations, e.g.lymphoma, amyloid biliary atresia
Crigler–Najjar syndrome	tumours
	extrahepatic sepsis

Box 6.3 Laboratory findings that may be present in haemolytic jaundice

plasma bilirubin	unconjugated rarely >100 µmol/L except in neonates
plasma enzymes	aspartate aminotransferase (but not alanine aminotransferase) and lactate dehydrogenase slightly increased
plasma haptoglobin	decreased
urine urobilinogen	increased
peripheral blood	increased reticulocyte count decreased haemoglobin abnormal red cell morphology on blood film positive Coombs (direct antiglobulin) test

and in the Crigler–Najjar syndrome, there may be a massive rise in the plasma concentration of unconjugated bilirubin. If bilirubin concentration exceeds 300 µmol/L in infants, its uptake into the brain may cause severe, irreversible brain damage (kernicterus).

Conjugated hyperbilirubinaemia

Conjugated hyperbilirubinaemia is due to leakage of conjugated bilirubin from either hepatocytes or the biliary system into the bloodstream when its normal route of excretion is blocked. The water-soluble conjugated bilirubin entering the systemic circulation is excreted by the kidneys, as a result of which **the urine develops a deep orange-brown colour**. In complete biliary obstruction, no bilirubin reaches the gut, no stercobilin is formed and the **stools are pale in colour**. The differential diagnosis of jaundice caused by conjugated bilirubin is considered on p. 114.

A **third fraction of bilirubin**, delta bilirubin, consisting of conjugated bilirubin bound covalently to albumin, is found in the plasma of patients with long-standing conjugated hyperbilirubinaemia. This substance has a half-life similar to that of albumin. Its persistence in the plasma during the resolution of liver disease or after the relief of obstruction explains the persistence of jaundice in the absence of bilirubinuria that can occur in these circumstances.

Plasma enzymes

Enzyme activity measurements used in the assessment of the liver include **aspartate** and **alanine aminotransferases** (formerly called 'transaminases' and still abbreviated AST and ALT, respectively), **alkaline phosphatase** (ALP) and

with well-compensated cirrhosis, but it is found in patients with advanced pancreatic carcinoma blocking the common bile duct.

Unconjugated hyperbilirubinaemia

When an excess of bilirubin is unconjugated, the concentration in adults rarely exceeds 100 µmol/L. In the absence of liver disease, unconjugated hyperbilirubinaemia is most often due either to haemolysis or to Gilbert syndrome, an inherited abnormality of bilirubin metabolism (see p. 115).

In a patient with haemolysis, hyperbilirubinaemia results from increased production of bilirubin, at a rate that exceeds the capacity of the liver to remove and conjugate the pigment. Nevertheless, more bilirubin is excreted into the biliary canaliculi and then into the gut, the amount of urobilinogen entering the enterohepatic circulation is increased and urinary urobilinogen is increased. Laboratory findings in haemolytic (prehepatic) jaundice are summarized in Box 6.3.

Activity of the hepatic conjugating enzymes is usually low at birth but increases rapidly thereafter; the transient 'physiological' jaundice of the newborn reflects this. With excessive haemolysis, as in Rhesus incompatibility, or a lack of conjugating enzyme activity, as occurs in prematurity

γ-**glutamyltransferase** (γGT). In general, these enzymes are not specific indicators of liver dysfunction. The hepatic iso-enzyme of ALP is an exception, and ALT is more specific to the liver than AST.

Increased aminotransferase activities reflect cell damage; they may be >20 times the URL in patients with hepatitis. **In cholestasis** (obstruction to the flow of bile), **plasma ALP activity is increased**. This is due mainly to increased enzyme synthesis (enzyme induction), stimulated by cholestasis. In severe cholestatic jaundice, plasma ALP activity may be up to 10 times the URL.

In practice, however, increases in the plasma activities of both the aminotransferases and ALP are often present in patients with liver disease, although one may predominate. In predominantly cholestatic disease, there may be secondary hepatocellular damage. The reverse is also true: cholestasis frequently occurs in primarily hepatocellular disease. Increased γGT activity is found in both cholestasis and hepatocellular damage: this enzyme is a very sensitive indicator of hepatobiliary disease but is non-specific. Thus, although certain patterns of plasma enzyme activities are frequently observed in various types of liver disease, they are not reliably diagnostic.

The enzymes AST and ALT provide essentially the same information, and most laboratories measure only one in a standard profile of liver function tests. The ratio of AST to ALT is used in some prognostic scoring systems (for example Fibrosis-4 [FIB-4] scoring in non-alcoholic fatty liver disease [NAFLD], see p. 113) and is often high in ethanol-related liver disease.

Plasma enzyme activities are very useful in following the progress of liver disease once the diagnosis has been made. Falling aminotransferase activity suggests a decrease in hepatocellular damage, and falling ALP activity suggests a resolution of cholestasis. However, in severe acute liver failure, a decrease in aminotransferase activity may misleadingly suggest an improvement when it is actually due to almost complete destruction of parenchymal cells.

It is important to appreciate that there are many extrahepatobiliary causes of increased plasma activities of the aminotransferases, γGT and ALP. These are discussed in Chapter 16.

Plasma proteins

Albumin is synthesized in the liver, and its concentration in the plasma is in part a reflection of the liver's functional capacity. Plasma albumin concentration tends to decrease in chronic liver disease but is usually normal in the early stages of acute hepatitis because of its long half-life (~20 days). There are many other causes of hypoalbuminaemia, as discussed in Box 16.1 in, but a normal plasma albumin concentration in a patient with chronic liver disease implies adequate synthetic function; a fall may signify a significant deterioration.

The **prothrombin time**, usually expressed as a ratio to a control value (the international normalized ratio [INR]), is a test of plasma clotting activity and reflects the activity of vitamin K-dependent clotting factors synthesized by the liver. An increase in the prothrombin time is often an early feature of acute liver disease, but a prolonged prothrombin time may also reflect vitamin K deficiency (in which case, a single parenteral dose of vitamin K should normalize the prothrombin time within 18 h).

A polyclonal increase in **immunoglobulins** is a frequent finding in patients with chronic liver disease (particularly of autoimmune origin) and may cause an increase in plasma total protein concentration even when albumin concentration is decreased. Some laboratories measure both albumin and total protein as part of a liver function test profile and derive a parameter called 'globulin' (total protein minus albumin), which mostly comprises immunoglobulin. Plasma immunoglobulin A (IgA) is often increased in alcoholic liver disease, IgG in autoimmune hepatitis and IgM in primary biliary cirrhosis, but these findings are non-specific. More useful diagnostic information may be obtained from measuring individual **autoantibodies**: antimitochondrial antibody is increased in 95% of patients with primary biliary cirrhosis, and anti–smooth muscle, anti-liver–kidney microsomal or antinuclear antibodies in many patients with autoimmune hepatitis (Table 6.1). Viral infection, an important cause of both acute and chronic liver disease, can be detected by measurement of viral antigens and antibodies to them.

Diagnostically useful changes in the concentrations of other plasma proteins are shown in Table 6.2.

Other tests of liver function

Given the imperfections of the simple tests of liver function that were discussed earlier, it is not surprising that many tests have been devised with a view to providing greater diagnostic sensitivity and specificity. Various dynamic function tests (which measure clearance of substances such as aminopyrine, antipyrine, indocyanine green and caffeine) are available but infrequently used. These tests are more sensitive than conventional tests but are time-consuming; their use is likely to remain limited to special situations (e.g. the monitoring of novel treatments). Thus, the standard panel of biochemical tests in hepatobiliary disease continues to be albumin and total bilirubin concentrations and the activities of an aminotransferase, ALP and γGT, together with the INR.

Plasma bile acid concentrations are increased in liver disease, but, although this is a highly specific finding, bile acid measurements are in general no more sensitive than conventional tests. They do, however, have a special role in liver disease developing during pregnancy (see p. 121).

Table 6.1 Typical frequencies (%) of occurrence of autoantibodies in autoimmune liver diseases

	Antinuclear or smooth muscle	Antimitochondrial	Anti-liver–kidney microsomal	Perinuclear antineutrophil cytoplasmic (pANCA)
autoimmune hepatitis	80	0	<5	up to 90
primary biliary cirrhosis	~30	>95	0	rare
sclerosing cholangitis	~25	0	0	~75

Table 6.2 Plasma proteins of diagnostic value in liver disease

Protein	Condition	Change in concentration
albumin	chronic liver disease	↓
γ-globulins	cirrhosis, especially autoimmune	↑
α_1-antitrypsin	cirrhosis caused by α_1-antitrypsin deficiency	↓
caeruloplasmin	Wilson disease	↓
α-fetoprotein	primary hepatocellular carcinoma	greatly ↑
transferrin	haemochromatosis	normal but >50% saturated with iron
ferritin	haemochromatosis	greatly ↑

The use of biochemical tests to detect hepatic fibrosis is discussed on p. 111.

Non-biochemical investigation of hepatobiliary disease

Many other types of investigation can provide valuable information in patients suspected of having hepatobiliary disease. **Imaging techniques provide primarily anatomical information.** Transcutaneous ultrasound examination, inexpensive and safe, is widely used as a first-line imaging investigation. It can reveal gallstones, dilatation of the biliary system, tumours and the characteristic hyperechoic nature of hepatic fatty infiltration. Endoscopic ultrasound is particularly good for visualizing the pancreas and portal vein. Doppler ultrasonography is used to assess blood flow and patency of blood vessels supplying the liver. Elastography, an ultrasound-based technique, can be used to determine the degree of liver fibrosis: liver elasticity decreases with increasing fibrosis. Cholangiography is used to examine the biliary system using an x-ray contrast medium given either endoscopically (endoscopic retrograde cholangiopancreatography), intraoperatively or percutaneously into the liver (percutaneous transhepatic cholangiography). Magnetic resonance cholangiopancreatography (MRCP) is tending to replace contrast cholangiography. Arteriography can reveal the typical pathological circulation in hepatic tumours. Various techniques of computed tomography (CT) and magnetic resonance imaging can demonstrate structural abnormalities and space-occupying lesions in the hepatobiliary system. Isotopic scanning (nuclear medicine) techniques are of limited use but may help with the evaluation of tumours and to assess the patency of the cystic duct. The gold standard of diagnosis, particularly in chronic liver disease and cancer, is histology, usually of tissue obtained by percutaneous biopsy.

Liver Disease

Acute hepatitis

Acute hepatitis is usually caused by viral infection (particularly with hepatitis viruses A, B, C, D and E, but also Epstein–Barr virus and cytomegalovirus) or toxins (e.g. ethanol, carbon tetrachloride, various fungal toxins and a host of drugs, of which the most frequently implicated is probably paracetamol [acetaminophen]). There is considerable variation in the severity and time course of the disease, but the pattern of changes in

Table 6.3 **Typical biochemical changes during acute hepatitis**		
	Pre-icteric	**Icteric**
plasma bilirubin	N/↑	↑↑
plasma aminotransferases	↑↑↑	↑
plasma alkaline phosphatase	N	N/↑
urine bilirubin	↑	↑
urine urobilinogen	↑	absent
N, normal.		

the standard liver function tests reflects the common underlying pathological process and is similar whatever the cause. Typically, the transaminase activities increase early, with rises in bilirubin concentrations owing to cholestasis occurring at a later stage as the hepatitis is resolving.

Patients may present with jaundice, but there is often a pre-icteric stage with relatively non-specific symptoms such as anorexia and malaise. Infection with hepatitis A most commonly occurs in children and is often asymptomatic (it is less likely to be so in adults). When symptoms do develop, they coincide with maximal aminotransferase activities and tend to improve before jaundice appears. Hepatitis E is endemic in many areas of the world but is infrequently acquired in the UK.

Early in the course of acute hepatitis, bilirubin and urobilinogen are usually readily detectable in the urine by a simple dipstick technique. For as long as the plasma bilirubin is raised, bilirubin continues to be excreted in the urine. Urobilinogen may disappear from the urine at the height of the jaundice, when, because of cholestasis, no bilirubin reaches the gut, but it reappears as the hepatitis resolves and biliary excretion returns to normal. These changes (Table 6.3) are of no practical value in the management of hepatitis, but the detection of bilirubin in the urine is a simple and valuable diagnostic pointer to hepatitis in the pre-icteric stage of the illness.

Many cases of viral hepatitis resolve completely. In severe cases, liver failure may develop (fulminant hepatitis), but most patients who survive the acute illness eventually recover completely, with aminotransferase activities falling to normal in 10–12 weeks. In some patients with hepatitis B or C infections, aminotransferase activities remain elevated; antigenaemia persists and chronic liver disease ensues. Infection with hepatitis A or E does not

Case history 6.1

History

A 20-year-old student developed a flu-like illness with loss of appetite, nausea and pain in the right hypochondrium.

Examination

The liver was just palpable and tender. Two days later, he developed jaundice, his urine became darker in colour and his stools became pale.

Results (see Appendix for reference ranges)

		On presentation	1 week later
Serum:	bilirubin	38 µmol/L	230 µmol/L
	albumin	40 g/L	38 g/L
	ALT	450 U/L	365 U/L
	ALP	70 U/L	150 U/L
	γGT	60 U/L	135 U/L
Urine:	bilirubin	positive	positive
	urobilinogen	positive	negative

Summary

Significantly raised ALT on presentation, followed by a rise in bilirubin, ALP and γGT.

Interpretation

The history and results are consistent with an acute viral hepatitis. The first set of results shows early hepatitis; impairment of the hepatic secretion of conjugated bilirubin and of urobilinogen uptake from the portal blood causes both of these substances to be excreted in the urine.

The second set of results shows high serum bilirubin but with a fall in ALT as the phase of maximum cellular damage has passed. An increase in ALP, usually of not more than three times the URL, is common at this stage, the ALP and γGT indicating the subsequent development of cholestasis.

Discussion

In hepatitis, the bilirubin in plasma is both conjugated and unconjugated, with the former predominating. Conjugated bilirubin is excreted in the urine and the pale stool reflects the decreased biliary excretion (as does the subsequent absence of the urobilinogen in the urine). The albumin concentration has remained normal in this acute illness.

progress to chronic disease, although some patients experience prolonged cholestasis with hepatitis E. Infection with hepatitis E carries a particular risk (to the mother and the fetus) during pregnancy.

Chronic hepatitis

Chronic hepatitis is defined as **hepatic inflammation persisting for more than 6 months**. There are many causes. Autoimmune hepatitis, chronic infection with hepatitis B or C, and ethanol are particularly important.

Autoimmune hepatitis can occur at any age; it occurs three times more frequently in women than in men. It can also present (in ~40%) as acute hepatitis. The aetiology is unknown, although there is a strong association with other autoimmune diseases. There is no single pathognomonic test but a viral aetiology must always be excluded. Autoantibodies (antinuclear and anti–smooth muscle) are frequently present in the plasma in high titre, and plasma IgG concentrations are often markedly elevated. Anti-liver–kidney microsomal antibodies are characteristic of a type of autoimmune hepatitis that more frequently presents in childhood and is more often acute in onset with a more aggressive course. However, none of these antibodies may be detectable at first presentation in up to 10% of patients, and autoantibodies (particularly anti–smooth muscle) are present in 10–15% of patients with viral hepatitis.

Plasma aminotransferase activities are usually elevated in chronic hepatitis, but other liver function tests are often normal unless cirrhosis develops. Although the natural history of autoimmune hepatitis is of progression to cirrhosis, this is often preventable if immunosuppressive treatment (usually with azathioprine and/or corticosteroids) is started early in the course of the condition.

Acute liver failure

The term 'acute liver failure' encompasses a range of clinical syndromes of severe liver dysfunction and encephalopathy (neuropsychiatric dysfunction) developing within 6 months of the first clinical evidence of disease. It is also referred to as 'fulminant liver failure'.

Acute liver failure can be hyperacute (encephalopathy developing within 7 days of the onset of jaundice), acute (7–28 days) or subacute (jaundice preceding encephalopathy by 5–12 weeks). It is a rare condition; **toxins and drugs** (e.g. paracetamol) **and viral hepatitis are the most frequent causes**. The underlying hepatic lesion is usually potentially reversible, because the liver has a considerable capacity for regeneration, but the metabolic disturbance is profound and the prognosis poor.

Metabolic features of acute liver failure include severe hyponatraemia, hypocalcaemia and hypoglycaemia. Hydrogen ion homoeostasis is frequently disturbed. Lactic acidosis may develop as a result of the failure of hepatic gluconeogenesis from lactate, but may be masked by a respiratory alkalosis caused by toxic stimulation of the respiratory centre. Generalized depression of the brainstem may lead to respiratory arrest. In some cases (although not usually with paracetamol poisoning), a metabolic alkalosis predominates: this is in part related to excessive urinary potassium loss, because of intracellular potassium depletion and secondary aldosteronism, and in part to the accumulation of basic substances, such as ammonia, in the blood.

The prothrombin time is greatly prolonged as a result of impaired hepatic synthesis of clotting factors, and bleeding is an almost universal clinical problem.

Acute liver failure is often accompanied by acute kidney injury (AKI). However, plasma urea concentrations are often relatively low, reflecting decreased hepatic synthesis. Plasma creatinine concentration is theoretically a more reliable guide both to kidney function and to whether the patient requires haemodialysis, although high bilirubin can interfere in some older methods for measuring creatinine.

Hepatic encephalopathy is the term used to describe the reversible neuropsychiatric syndrome that can occur in both acute and chronic liver failure: it is discussed on p. 111. Patients with acute liver failure are at particular risk of developing raised intracranial pressure, which should be managed in a specialist liver unit and for which the first-line treatment is osmotic therapy with intravenous mannitol or hypertonic saline.

Management involves support of vital functions, correction of the metabolic imbalances and aggressive management of sepsis and bleeding. Respiratory failure may necessitate artificial ventilation, and renal replacement treatment may be required if kidney injury occurs. There are currently no techniques available for artificial hepatic support and as yet tissue engineering solutions have not progressed beyond clinical trials. In severe disease, the liver may be damaged to an extent that prevents regeneration, and only liver transplantation offers a prospect of long-term survival.

The use of liver transplantation as treatment for acute liver failure has highlighted a need for good prognostic information. Factors that are considered include the cause of the liver failure, rapidity of onset, severity of encephalopathy, organ availability and any relative or absolute contraindications. Prognosis can be evaluated using a variety of scores such as the Acute Physiology and Chronic Health Evaluation (APACHE II) and King's College Criteria. The most useful laboratory features are raised INR (with a value >10 indicating a very poor prognosis), acidosis and presence of AKI.

Cirrhosis

Cirrhosis is a process in which death of liver cells with regeneration leads **to fibrosis, scarring and destruction of the normal liver architecture**. Causes of cirrhosis include chronic excessive ethanol intake, autoimmune disease (e.g. autoimmune hepatitis and primary biliary cirrhosis), chronic infection with hepatitis B or C virus and various inherited metabolic diseases, including Wilson disease, haemochromatosis and α_1-antitrypsin deficiency. Consequences (see later) include cholestasis and impaired hepatic function progressing to liver failure. The latter is often precipitated by a specific event, such as bleeding into the gut (particularly from oesophageal varices, see later) and infection.

Primary biliary cirrhosis is a progressive autoimmune disease characterized by destruction of intrahepatic bile ducts that typically affects middle-aged women. Although the presence of antimitochondrial antibodies in the plasma is characteristic of the disease, exceptions do occur; other autoantibodies may also be present, and there are overlap syndromes with other autoimmune liver diseases.

Biochemical investigation

Because of the great functional capacity of the liver, **metabolic and clinical abnormalities may not become apparent until late in the course of the disease**; until this time, the cirrhosis is said to be 'compensated'. There are no reliable, simple biochemical tests to diagnose subclinical disease. There has been considerable interest in the development of non-invasive methods of **detecting hepatic fibrosis** in patients at risk of cirrhosis (e.g. patients with hepatitis C, or alcoholic fatty liver disease or NAFLD), with a view to instituting treatment to slow or prevent disease progression. Biopsy has been considered to be the definitive technique for this purpose but is invasive, has a low but significant morbidity and mortality, and may cause false-negative results because of sampling error. Efforts have therefore been made to develop biochemical tests to indicate the presence of fibrosis.

Procollagen type 3 peptide (P3NP) is a peptide produced during collagen synthesis: its concentration in plasma reflects the rate of development of fibrosis, although it can also be increased by inflammation and necrosis. Its measurement has a role in the monitoring of patients being treated with methotrexate (a cytotoxic drug that can induce fibrosis, see p. 370). It is recommended that P3NP concentration is measured annually in dermatology patients (false positives occur in rheumatology patients) being treated with methotrexate, and that liver biopsy be considered in patients with persistently high values.

Several indicators of hepatic fibrosis have been described involving combinations of various test results to produce a fibrosis index. Examples include the FibroTest (FibroSure in the USA) and the Enhanced Liver Fibrosis (ELF) test based on plasma measurements of standard and more esoteric tests. The NAFLD fibrosis score and FIB-4 index use easily available demographic and routine laboratory data to predict prognosis. In combination with elastography (see p. 108), these may prove superior to biopsy for the detection of early fibrosis.

Case history 6.2

History

A 56-year-old woman, who worked in a pub, was admitted to hospital because of drowsiness and jaundice. One year earlier she had been treated for oesophageal varices after an episode of haematemesis. She had no further bleeding. The patient had been advised to abstain from ethanol.

Examination

She was obviously jaundiced with clinical signs of chronic liver disease. Her urine was very dark.

Results

		Current results	1 year ago
Serum:	albumin	25 g/L	36
	bilirubin	260 µmol/L	12
	ALP	315 U/L	95
	ALT	134 U/L	25
	γGT	360 U/L	245
Plasma:	INR	3.3	1.1

Summary

Predominantly raised ALP and γGT, with significantly raised INR and low albumin.

Interpretation

The low serum albumin, raised serum bilirubin, and prolonged prothrombin time (INR, see p. 107) are due to reduced synthetic or excretory function, whereas the enzyme changes are markers of cholestatic liver cell damage. The raised γGT 1 year previously could have been due to either cholestasis or ethanol induction.

Discussion

The patient had continued to drink and the resulting liver damage eventually affected hepatic function. Hepatic decompensation may be precipitated in chronic liver disease by sepsis, bleeding into the gut, for example, from varices, erosions and ulcers, and by various drugs, including diuretics.

Complications

Both the decreased hepatic function and disturbances of liver architecture can create numerous complications. **Hepatic encephalopathy**, a potentially reversible neuropsychiatric syndrome characterized by a decrease in consciousness and impairment of higher functions, is often present in decompensated cirrhosis and can also be a feature of acute liver failure. Its pathogenesis is uncertain, but accumulation of neurotoxins, including ammonia, and false

Case history 6.3

History

A 40-year-old woman presented with jaundice. There was no history of exposure to viral hepatitis, recent foreign travel, injections or transfusions. She did not drink ethanol. She had been well in the past but had suffered from increasingly intense pruritus during the previous 18 months.

Results

Serum:		
	total protein	85 g/L
	albumin	28 g/L
	bilirubin	340 µmol/L
	ALP	522 U/L
	ALT	98 U/L
	γGT	242 U/L

Summary

Markedly raised bilirubin and ALP, low albumin and raised total protein, small rise in ALT.

Interpretation

The very high ALP and bilirubin indicate cholestatic jaundice. The low albumin is consistent with chronic liver disease but with the high total protein also indicates an increase in immunoglobulin concentrations, often seen in autoimmune liver disease.

Discussion

Further investigations revealed a high titre of antimitochondrial antibodies, characteristic of primary biliary cirrhosis, and this was confirmed by percutaneous liver biopsy. Tiredness, pruritus and jaundice are common features of primary biliary cirrhosis, with pruritus often preceding the development of jaundice. Pruritus in chronic liver disease is thought to be due to the accumulation of bile salts.

! Decompensation of chronic liver disease is indicated by jaundice, coagulopathy (e.g. INR >1.5), ascites, variceal bleeding and/or hepatic encephalopathy. Therefore, the development of jaundice (or any of these other features) in those with cirrhosis even with normal or low transaminases may indicate decompensation and should be investigated urgently.

---

factors such as gastrointestinal bleeding and the provision of enemas or laxatives (e.g. lactulose) to empty the bowels of nitrogen-containing material. Lactulose also inhibits replication of ammoniagenic bacteria. Non-absorbable antibiotics can be used to sterilize the gut to reduce the production of toxins by bacteria. Dietary protein restriction is no longer recommended because it risks exacerbating or causing malnutrition, but replacing animal with vegetable proteins may help by reducing the intake of aromatic amino acids, which accumulate in liver failure. An adequate energy intake is essential, and fluid and electrolyte balance must be maintained.

Ascites is the accumulation of free fluid in the peritoneal cavity: cirrhosis causes portal hypertension, inducing splanchnic vasodilatation, which leads to a decrease in effective arterial blood volume, triggering the activation of the renin–angiotensin–aldosterone system, the sympathetic nervous system and the release of vasopressin, resulting in hyponatraemia. Hypoalbuminaemia may also contribute. Sodium restriction is required, and there are roles both for diuretics, such as spironolactone with furosemide, and low-salt albumin infusions in the management of ascites.

Acute kidney injury is a recognized complication of chronic liver disease, particularly end-stage alcoholic cirrhosis. It may take the form of acute tubular necrosis, due, for example, to haemorrhage or infection, but more frequently is functional in nature; that is, the kidneys are histologically normal and tubular function is intact, the urine being concentrated and having a low sodium concentration. There is, however, no sustained benefit from extracellular fluid volume expansion. This 'hepatorenal syndrome' may arise spontaneously or be precipitated by fluid loss (diarrhoea, inappropriate use of diuretics). Response to treatment is generally poor, and there is progressive decline in kidney function, fluid retention and severe hypotension, although death is usually from liver rather than kidney failure. The pathogenesis is incompletely understood: intense renal vasoconstriction, probably secondary to systemic arterial underfilling, is an important factor.

Disturbances of endocrine function are common in patients with chronic liver disease. The most obvious is the feminization of males, with gynaecomastia, impotence, decreased body hair and testicular atrophy. Altered metabolism of both androgens and oestrogens and an increase in the plasma concentration of sex hormone binding globulin (see p. 212) are thought to be responsible.

neurotransmitters, are thought to contribute. However, there is a poor correlation between their blood concentrations and the severity of encephalopathy. Ammonia is normally metabolized by the liver, and the increase is a result of both decreased metabolism and shunting of ammonia-rich blood from the portal system directly into the systemic circulation. In the brain, the increased supply of ammonia promotes the production of glutamine from glutamate, increasing intracellular osmolality and causing astrocyte swelling. **Bleeding** from oesophageal varices (distended connections between the portal and systemic venous systems) can precipitate encephalopathy as a result of the absorption of amino acids from digested blood.

The treatment of hepatic encephalopathy is thus directed at measures to reduce the absorption of ammonia from the gut. These include appropriate management of any precipitating

Management

Once established, **hepatic cirrhosis is irreversible**. If possible, any underlying cause should be treated appropriately. Specific complications, including ascites, bleeding (e.g. from oesophageal varices) and malabsorption, may also be amenable to treatment. Causes of death include hepatic encephalopathy, uncontrollable bleeding and septicaemia.

The use of liver transplantation as treatment for cirrhosis has brought about a need for accurate prognostic tests. Several prognostic indices (e.g. the Child–Pugh and MELD [model for end-stage liver disease] or its UK variant UKELD scores) have been developed based on a combination of clinical features and the results of laboratory tests such as the INR and plasma albumin and bilirubin concentrations. Surgery should not be undertaken while the short-term prognosis for the patient is still good, nor should it be delayed until the patient is moribund.

Ethanol and the liver

Ethanol is a common cause of liver disease. There are three main categories. First, fat accumulation in the liver (**hepatic steatosis**) occurs frequently in people who abuse ethanol; it may cause asymptomatic hepatomegaly, with modest increases in plasma aminotransferases, a more marked increase in γGT activity, but a normal bilirubin concentration. This is a reversible condition if patients abstain completely from ethanol. Second, frank **alcoholic hepatitis** often develops after a bout of heavy drinking in patients with a history of excessive ethanol ingestion; this can be a life-threatening condition. Third, chronic ethanol ingestion is a common cause of **cirrhosis**. This risk is greater for women than for men, but cirrhosis is not inevitable even in heavy drinkers: only about 10% of heavy drinkers develop cirrhosis. Risk factors include obesity and diabetes; there is also a genetic component. The most important aspect of management, apart from general supportive measures and treatment of any complications, is to persuade the patient to abstain totally from ethanol. If this can be achieved, the prognosis in alcoholic cirrhosis is better than in cirrhosis due to other causes. The pathogenesis of alcoholic liver disease is multifactorial. Fat accumulation is secondary to inhibition of fatty acid oxidation, increased hepatic uptake and synthesis of fatty acids and accumulation of triglycerides; the development of hepatitis involves oxidative stress and activation of cytokines, leading to damage to intracellular membranes, and an immunological response to antigens created from adducts of acetaldehyde and products of lipid peroxidation to proteins.

There are no specific **biochemical diagnostic markers** of alcoholic liver disease, although in patients known to have liver disease, the presence of an elevated γGT (disproportionate to any increases in other liver enzymes), a ratio of the plasma activities of AST to ALT of >2, hypertriglyceridaemia, increased plasma IgA concentration and red cell macrocytosis are highly suggestive. An increase in the concentration of a variant form of transferrin (carbohydrate-deficient transferrin) is often present in the plasma of heavy drinkers, although both false-negative and false positive results occur. Measurements of specific ethanol metabolites (ethyl glucuronide and ethyl sulphate) in urine show promise for the detection of ethanol use but are not widely available. Other aspects of ethanol toxicity are considered in Chapter 21.

Non-alcoholic fatty liver disease

The term 'non-alcoholic fatty liver disease' (NAFLD) encompasses a range of conditions from simple hepatic steatosis (fat deposition alone) to non-alcoholic steato-hepatitis (in which inflammation is present), which can lead to cirrhosis. It is frequently seen in patients with the **metabolic syndrome** (insulin resistance, truncal obesity and hyperlipidaemia, see p. 152) and the population prevalence is rising. Other causes include parenteral feeding (particularly with an excess of energy substrates, see p. 149), starvation, some inherited metabolic disorders (e.g. glycogen storage disease type 1) and drugs, particularly amiodarone, an antiarrhythmic agent.

Patients may complain of discomfort in the right upper quadrant of the abdomen but are usually asymptomatic. Plasma bilirubin and albumin concentrations are normal, but aminotransferase activities can be up to two to four times the URLs, with the AST:ALT ratio typically being ≤1 (a higher ratio indicates increased risk of progression to cirrhosis); γGT activity is usually elevated, to an extent that reflects the amount of fat deposition. Plasma ferritin concentration is found to be elevated in >50% of patients: this usually reflects liver damage rather than iron overload.

Liver biopsy shows fatty infiltration, but, as with the patient in Case history 6.4, the diagnosis is usually made on the basis of the clinical features and the elimination of other causes. In the majority of patients, the prognosis is good, and the condition resolves if the underlying cause can be treated effectively. In some, however, there is progression through steatohepatitis to fibrosis, impaired liver function and, eventually, cirrhosis. The NAFLD fibrosis score (see p. 111) can be used to predict which patients are at risk of progression.

Management includes diet and exercise to achieve weight loss, abstention from ethanol to avoid additional hepatic stress and appropriate treatment of cardiovascular risk factors. NAFLD can recur in a transplanted liver if weight loss is not achieved.

Case history 6.4

History

A 54-year-old woman with newly diagnosed diabetes was referred to a diabetes clinic for initial investigation and treatment. She drank very little ethanol.

Examination

Unremarkable except for a body mass index of 36 kg/m^2 (ideal 19–25 kg/m^2).

Results

Serum:	creatinine	83 µmol/L
	eGFR	69 mL/min/1.73 m^2
	bilirubin	16 µmol/L
	ALT	72 U/L
	ALP	110 U/L
	γGT	98 U/L
	albumin	43 g/L
	cholesterol	5.2 mmol/L
	triglyceride (fasting)	7.4 mmol/L
Blood:	HbA$_{1c}$	78 mmol/mol (9.2%) (treatment target <59 mmol/mol)

Summary

Raised HbA$_{1c}$ with hypertriglyceridaemia and mildly elevated ALT and γGT.

Interpretation

The raised triglyceride concentration is typical of poorly controlled diabetes, indicated by the high HbA$_{1c}$, and is associated with fat deposition in (and disruption of) the liver.

Discussion

The abnormal liver function tests prompted serological tests for hepatitis viruses and autoantibodies (negative) and iron studies for haemochromatosis (normal). Ultrasound examination of the liver showed hyperechogenicity typical of fatty infiltration. A presumptive diagnosis of NAFLD was made; she was given dietary advice and prescribed metformin. Six months later, her body mass index had fallen to 31 kg/m^2 and her glycaemic control had improved (HbA$_{1c}$ 53 mmol/mol [7%]). Repeat liver function tests were normal, but the fasting triglyceride concentration was 3.2 mmol/L suggesting further weight loss was required.

Tumours and infiltrations

The liver is a common site for tumour metastasis. Primary liver tumours are uncommon in the western world but occur frequently in other geographic areas. Primary tumours are associated with cirrhosis, persistence of hepatitis B and C, and various carcinogens, including aflatoxins. Plasma α-fetoprotein is elevated at diagnosis in ~70% of patients with primary hepatocellular carcinomas and is a valuable marker for this tumour, although it can also be increased, usually to a lesser extent, in acute and chronic hepatitis and in cirrhosis. Infiltrative conditions that can affect the liver include lymphomas and amyloidosis. Patients with such conditions, and with intrahepatic tumours, are often not jaundiced. The only biochemical abnormality may be an increase in plasma ALP activity.

Jaundice in adults

The common causes of jaundice are shown in Box 6.2. In adults, jaundice caused by unconjugated hyperbilirubinaemia is usually mild. Gilbert syndrome, haemolysis and interference with hepatic bilirubin uptake by drugs are the major causes. Other liver function tests are normal and bilirubin is absent from the urine. Diagnosis is usually straightforward. Gilbert syndrome (see p. 115) is usually diagnosed by exclusion of other causes; features of haemolytic jaundice are summarized in Box 6.3.

Cholestasis is obstruction to the normal flow of bile. It can be a feature of intrahepatic disease (particularly cirrhosis) and extrahepatic disease (e.g. carcinoma of the head of the pancreas, causing obstruction of the common bile duct). In addition to clinical features related to its cause, consequences include fatigue, malabsorption (particularly of fat-soluble vitamins) and osteoporosis (more particularly in males). Although invariably present in severe cholestasis, jaundice may not be present in the early stages. In cholestatic jaundice, the majority of the excess bilirubin is conjugated, even in liver disease when there may also be decreased uptake and conjugation of bilirubin.

The differential diagnosis of cholestatic jaundice includes primarily hepatocellular disease and biliary obstruction, both intrahepatic and extrahepatic (see Box 6.2). Valuable diagnostic information may be provided by the history and examination. **Biochemical tests** can also give useful information; for example, a high plasma aminotransferase activity suggests the presence of hepatocellular damage, whereas a very high ALP activity suggests cholestasis. Serology for detection of autoantibodies is essential, as well as for viral infection if transaminase activity is elevated.

It is rarely possible to distinguish reliably between intrahepatic and extrahepatic cholestasis from the results of biochemical tests alone. The next step is usually ultrasound examination, followed by further imaging or liver biopsy depending on the level of the obstruction (see p. 108).

The causes and investigation of jaundice that develops after surgery are discussed in Case history 6.7. Cholestasis, sometimes leading to jaundice, is a recognized complication of parenteral nutrition (see p. 150).

Case history 6.5

History

An elderly woman consulted her general practitioner because of weight loss, 8 kg over 2 months, loss of appetite and new constipation.

Examination

She was anaemic and had obviously lost weight. The liver was enlarged and had an irregular edge; a mass was palpable in the right iliac fossa.

Results

Serum:

	albumin	30 g/L
	ALP	314 U/L
	γGT	119 U/L
	bilirubin	16 μmol/L
	ALT	39 U/L
Blood:	haemoglobin	87 g/L

Summary

Raised ALP and γGT associated with low albumin and anaemia.

Interpretation

The clinical findings and results are highly suspicious of bowel cancer with metastases. The raised ALP and γGT activities suggest liver involvement, cholestatic pattern, although increased ALP activity can also be associated with bone metastases. Hypoalbuminaemia is common in malignant disease and is usually multifactorial, being caused by poor nutrition, increased catabolism (cancer cachexia) and replacement of normal hepatic tissue by tumour. Anaemia is also common and may be caused by direct suppression of haematopoiesis, malnutrition or chronic bleeding from the primary tumour.

Discussion

Colonoscopy demonstrated a carcinoma of the caecum; ultrasound examination of the liver showed several lesions, characteristic of tumour deposits. With hepatic metastases, there is often no increase in plasma bilirubin concentration unless lymph nodes at the porta hepatis are involved and obstruct the major bile ducts. Although tumour deposits within the liver can cause obstruction of small bile ducts, which is reflected by the increase in ALP and γGT, bilirubin leaking into the bloodstream can be taken up and excreted by parts of the liver not affected by tumour.

Carcinoma of the caecum is often clinically silent and may not present until extensive secondary spread has occurred.

Inherited abnormalities of bilirubin metabolism

There are four conditions in which jaundice is caused by an inherited abnormality of bilirubin metabolism: Gilbert, Crigler–Najjar, Dubin–Johnson and Rotor syndromes. Their characteristics are summarized in Table 6.4. Gilbert syndrome affects ~7% of the population, but the others are rare. It is most commonly caused by a mutation in the promoter for the UDP-glucuronosyltransferase gene (*UGT1A1*), which leads to decreased enzyme activity and hence decreased conjugation of bilirubin. In some cases, there is also decreased hepatic uptake of bilirubin.

The jaundice of **Gilbert syndrome** is typically mild (<100 μmol/L) and present only intermittently. It is often noticed during an infection or a period of decreased food intake, possibly because fasting increases plasma concentrations of free fatty acids, which compete with bilirubin for transport by albumin and uptake into liver cells. There may be mild malaise and abdominal discomfort, the only physical sign being the intermittent jaundice (scleral icterus). The liver is histologically normal and there are no significant sequelae.

Gilbert syndrome is usually diagnosed on the basis of the clinical features and the exclusion of other causes of hyperbilirubinaemia, including haemolysis. Genetic testing for the commonest mutant allele (*UGT1A1*28*) is available, although rarely necessary.

Isolated abnormalities of 'liver enzymes'

With the widespread use of biochemical investigations, often for no clear clinical purpose, abnormalities of liver enzymes are frequently discovered incidentally, that is, in the absence of clinical evidence of hepatobiliary disease. The following should be considered:

- **an isolated increase in ALP** is usually due to bone disease (particularly Paget disease): hepatic causes usually result in an increase in γGT and the combination should prompt further investigation
- **an isolated increase in γGT** is usually due to enzyme induction (e.g. by ethanol or drugs) and not to liver damage
- **isolated increases in aminotransferases** are common. They may indicate clinically silent hepatitis (e.g. viral or autoimmune), which must be excluded, although NAFLD (see p. 113) is a more frequent cause. The possibility that drugs (whether prescribed, over the counter, recreational or contained in herbal remedies) are responsible should always be considered
- abnormalities of liver function tests are seen frequently in acutely ill patients: causes include intrahepatic cholestasis secondary to sepsis and hepatic congestion secondary to heart failure.

Case history 6.6

History

A retired publican presented to his general practitioner with a 3-month history of epigastric pain radiating into the back and not related to meals. He was given a proton pump inhibitor, but returned one month later with more severe pain, weight loss and jaundice. Over the past week, his urine had become dark in colour and his stools pale.

Examination

Apart from the jaundice and signs of recent weight loss, no abnormality was found.

Results

Serum:		
	total protein	72 g/L
	albumin	40 g/L
	bilirubin	380 µmol/L
	ALP	510 U/L
	ALT	80 U/L
	γGT	115 U/L

Summary

Markedly raised bilirubin and ALP activity with smaller increases in ALT and γGT activities.

Interpretation

The results of the biochemical tests (predominantly elevated ALP with very high bilirubin) suggest that the jaundice is due to biliary obstruction and militate against, although do not exclude, the presence of liver disease.

Discussion

Ultrasound examination demonstrated the presence of dilated bile ducts and a CT scan of the abdomen demonstrated a tumour within the head of the pancreas. The clinical features are very suggestive of a carcinoma of the head of the pancreas obstructing the common bile duct as it enters the duodenum. However, the biochemical results could also be caused by a calculus obstructing the common bile duct, a metastatic tumour involving lymph nodes at the hilum of the liver or intrahepatic cholestasis.

Pancreatic carcinoma often presents late as painless cholestatic jaundice, by which point it may be too advanced for treatment to be curative. Although the plasma concentration of the tumour marker CA19-9 is often elevated, it is not specific for pancreatic cancer and is therefore not an effective diagnostic or screening test (see p. 360), especially since a proportion of the population do not produce it at all.

Table 6.4 **Inherited disorders of bilirubin metabolism**

Syndrome	Defect	Clinical features
Gilbert	decreased conjugation of bilirubin (autosomal recessive or dominant)	mild, fluctuant unconjugated hyperbilirubinaemia that increases on fasting, normal liver biopsy and normal life span
Crigler–Najjar	type 1 (autosomal recessive) total absence of conjugating enzyme function	severe unconjugated hyperbilirubinaemia, early death caused by kernicterus, partial response to phototherapy, none to phenobarbital
	type 2 (mostly autosomal recessive) partial defect (<20%) of conjugating enzyme function	severe unconjugated hyperbilirubinaemia but good response to phenobarbital and phototherapy, often survive to adulthood
Dubin–Johnson	decreased hepatic excretion of bilirubin (autosomal recessive)	mild, fluctuant conjugated hyperbilirubinaemia, hepatic pigment deposition (melanin-like), increased coproporphyrin I/III ratio in urine, bilirubinuria, normal life span
Rotor	decreased reuptake of conjugated bilirubin from the bloodstream (autosomal recessive, both copies of *SLCO1B1* and *SLCO1B3* need to be altered)	mild, fluctuant conjugated hyperbilirubinaemia but no hepatic pigmentation, increased total urine porphyrin, very rare, normal life span

Case history 6.7

History

An elderly man had been admitted to hospital with acute abdominal pain with generalized peritonitis. Imaging had suggested a perforated viscus found, at laparotomy, to be due to a ruptured diverticulum of the sigmoid colon. A defunctioning colostomy had been constructed. Some 72 hours later he was still very ill.

Examination

He was hypotensive despite adequate fluid replacement and treatment with inotropic drugs; faeculent material was leaking from his wound, and he was slightly jaundiced.

Results

Serum: bilirubin   103 µmol/L
              ALT   124 U/L
              ALP   152 U/I

Summary

Jaundice with mildly elevated ALT and ALP

Interpretation

The elevated ALP with raised bilirubin is consistent with cholestasis, but the elevated aminotransferase could be caused by damage to other tissues besides the liver (see p.297).

Discussion

Postoperative jaundice is a common clinical problem. Causes include:
- increased bilirubin formation (e.g. caused by haemolysis of transfused stored blood or resorption of haematomas)
- hepatocellular damage (e.g. caused by drugs, shock, transfusion-transmitted or coincidental hepatitis)
- intrahepatic cholestasis (e.g. caused by sepsis, hypotension, drugs or parenteral nutrition)
- extrahepatic obstruction (e.g. caused by calculi or perioperative damage to the bile ducts).

Postoperative jaundice is often multifactorial, as in this patient who was both hypotensive and septic. The cause of cholestasis in septic patients is uncertain: impaired hepatic secretory capacity, obstruction caused by swelling of Kupffer cells and changes in the composition of bile may all play a part.

Case history 6.8

History

A medical student recovering from an attack of influenza was noticed to be slightly jaundiced. He was worried that he might have hepatitis.

Results

Serum: bilirubin   60 µmol/l
              ALP   74 U/L
              ALT   35 U/L
Blood: haemoglobin   160 g/L
              reticulocytes   1% (<2%)
Urine: bilirubin   negative

Summary

Isolated mild hyperbilirubinaemia with no bilirubinuria.

Interpretation

The negative urine bilirubin indicates that the excess bilirubin in the serum is unconjugated. There is no evidence of hepatocellular damage, and the normal haemoglobin and reticulocyte count indicate that haemolysis is unlikely to be the cause of the raised bilirubin. By elimination, the diagnosis is Gilbert syndrome.

Discussion

The pattern of inheritance depends on the mutation type, and can be autosomal recessive or dominant. Family members may have recognized episodes of asymptomatic jaundice in themselves or other relatives.

If there is no apparent cause for an isolated increase in one of these 'liver enzymes', and the increase is modest (up to twice the URL), it is usually recommended that the test is repeated after a short period (e.g. two months). If it remains elevated or increases, further investigation is indicated, but if it has fallen, the patient can be reassured.

Uncommon liver diseases

Wilson disease is an inherited abnormality (autosomal recessive) of copper metabolism, characterized by decreased biliary excretion of copper and decreased incorporation of copper into caeruloplasmin, a plasma protein. It is caused by mutations in the *ATP7B* gene that codes for an ATPase responsible for the transport of copper across intracellular membranes, particularly in hepatocytes. More than 200 mutations have been identified, and most patients are compound heterozygotes. The average prevalence worldwide is 1 in 30,000 (carrier rate is approximately 1 in 90). Copper is deposited in the liver, the basal ganglia of the brain and in the corneas of the eyes. Patients with Wilson disease may present at almost any age but most frequently either in childhood with acute liver disease, accompanied in many cases by haemolysis and a kidney tubular defect (because of the toxicity of the free copper released from hepatocytes), or in young adulthood with cirrhosis or manifestations of disease of the basal ganglia (e.g. dysarthria, tremor and choreiform movements, see p. 329). There may also be psychiatric manifestations.

The biochemical features of Wilson disease are a reduced plasma caeruloplasmin concentration and low–normal or low plasma copper (with increased binding to albumin). The decrease in caeruloplasmin is not unique to Wilson disease but is also seen in chronic hepatitis and malnutrition. Basal urinary copper excretion is increased (>0.75 µmol/24 h) and there is a striking increase (typically to >25 µmol/24 h) after the administration of D-penicillamine, which chelates free copper. The definitive diagnostic test is the demonstration of a high copper content in liver tissue obtained by biopsy; increased hepatic copper deposition is also seen to a lesser extent in primary biliary cirrhosis and in neonatal biliary atresia, but these conditions have other distinguishing features. Advances in DNA sequencing technology, which allows the detection of numerous mutations, have increased the potential for genetic diagnosis, especially in asymptomatic siblings.

Wilson disease is treated initially with a chelating agent, penicillamine or trientine, which increases the urinary excretion of copper and often halts the progress of the disease. Zinc can then be used for maintenance, since it induces metallothionein in enterocytes, which binds dietary copper and reduces its absorption. Lifelong monitoring with liver function tests and urine copper measurements is required. When patients present with acute liver disease, the only effective treatment is liver transplantation. Because the genetic defect is expressed in the liver, transplantation effectively cures the disease.

α_1-**Antitrypsin deficiency** (see p. 288), an inherited condition characterized either by the absence of this protein from the plasma or by the presence of an abnormal form of the protein, is another rare cause of cirrhosis.

Haemochromatosis

Haemochromatosis is characterized by excessive intestinal iron absorption resulting in iron overload as a result of mutations in genes involved in iron metabolism. The most frequent mutations affecting adults are in the hereditary haemochromatosis (*HFE*) gene (haemochromatosis type 1, classic haemochromatosis). The gene product (HFE protein) binds to transferrin receptor 1 (a regulator of intestinal iron absorption, see p. 145), and the most frequent mutation (C282Y) prevents the formation of a disulphide bond required for the transport of HFE protein to the cell surface. The resulting reduction in hepatic hepcidin production causes inappropriately high intestinal iron absorption and contributes to the excess iron uptake by the liver.

The mode of inheritance is **autosomal recessive**. The *HFE* gene is located on chromosome 6, closely linked to the class 1 HLA locus. In the UK, 90% of patients with haemochromatosis are **homozygous for C282Y mutation** and most of the remainder for the **H63D mutation**. The prevalence of the homozygous state for haemochromatosis is about ~1 in 200 in northern European populations, making it possibly the most common of the inherited metabolic diseases. A different form of haemochromatosis, in which the mutation directly affects the transferrin receptor, occurs in southern Europe. There are also rare forms that present in children or neonates. Heterozygotes have increased plasma ferritin concentrations but are not at risk of developing tissue damage (with the possible exception of a very low risk in women).

The phenotypic expression in homozygotes depends on the availability of dietary iron and overall iron turnover. Thus, the condition occurs clinically in men more frequently than in women (because of menstrual iron loss), and when it does occur in women, it does so on average at a later age. Even in men it is uncommon before the age of 40 years; although the defect is present from birth, it is only when the body becomes massively overloaded with iron that clinical features develop. Furthermore, the prevalence in homozygotes in countries with a high dietary content of available iron is greater than where the dietary content is low.

Excess iron deposits in liver, joints and endocrine glands and its presenting clinical features are non-specific. Haemochromatosis is therefore underdiagnosed but it should be considered in all patients with **chronic liver disease** (unless some other obvious cause is apparent) and in **non-obese people developing diabetes in middle life**. Other typical features include bronzing of the skin, arthropathy, especially in the hands, and

> A patient with north European ancestry and evidence of iron overload, ferritin concentration >300 µg/L (>200 µg/L in females) and a transferrin saturation >50% (>40% in females), with no obvious cause and a normal full blood count should have molecular testing for haemochromatosis.

erectile impotence or loss of libido. It may be detected incidentally by elevated markers of iron status including raised iron and ferritin concentrations and transferrin saturation.

Liver biopsy is no longer recommended for diagnosis; however, if the plasma ferritin concentration is >1000 µg/L or there is biochemical evidence of liver damage (increased plasma ALT activity), referral to gastroenterology for the exclusion of fibrosis is indicated.

Management and prognosis. The mainstay of treatment is repeated venesection; with each 500 mL blood, 200–250 mg iron is removed from the body. It is often possible to do this as frequently as once a week without rendering the patient anaemic. Once plasma ferritin concentration is reduced to 20–30 µg/L and transferrin saturation to <50%, further accumulation can be prevented by less frequent (2- to 3-monthly) venesection. Diabetes and heart failure are treated by conventional means, and hormonal deficiencies by appropriate replacement. Untreated, the prognosis is poor, but it is considerably improved by removal of the excess iron. There is often an improvement in cardiac and hepatic function, but the diabetes, hypogonadism and joint disease are not affected.

Desferrioxamine, an iron-chelating agent, is valuable in patients receiving multiple blood transfusions for refractory anaemia, who are at risk of developing iron overload. It has to be infused intravenously or subcutaneously: unless this is performed daily, the rate of removal of iron is much slower than with venesection.

Other causes of iron overload. Iron overload can also occur with increased intestinal absorption of iron, either acutely, as in iron poisoning (see Chapter 21), or chronically, as occurs, for example, in African iron overload (Bantu siderosis) in which people with an inherited predisposition to increased intestinal iron absorption consume beer brewed using iron vessels. Increased parenteral iron administration occurs unavoidably in patients given repeated blood transfusions for the treatment of refractory anaemias, which can also lead to overloading of the body's iron stores (haemosiderosis or acquired hae-

mochromatosis). The excess iron is deposited mainly as haemosiderin in reticuloendothelial cells in the liver and spleen, where it is relatively innocuous, but with time, parenchymal deposition may lead to hepatic fibrosis and myocardial damage.

Liver transplantation

Liver transplantation is now increasingly used for the treatment of irreversible, severe liver disease, both acute and chronic. Donor organs are scarce and careful patient selection is vital. The left and right lobes can be transplanted into separate recipients. Although in the past only cadaveric livers were used, there is now an active living donor programme, which utilizes the huge regenerative capacity of healthy liver. Auxiliary partial transplantation is also being used to support patients with acute liver failure pending a hoped-for recovery of function of the native liver.

After surgery, the major complications include bleeding, AKI, immediate non-function of the graft, infection and rejection. Long term, the original liver disease may recur in the transplanted organ. The results of measurements of plasma aminotransferases and other liver function tests may suggest the development of complications, but diagnosis usually rests on imaging techniques or biopsy. Most immunosuppressive drugs can have adverse effects; monitoring of immunosuppressive treatment is discussed in Chapter 21 (see p. 365).

Gallstones and biliary tract disease

Gallstones are composed primarily of cholesterol with varying amounts of bilirubin and calcium salts. Cholesterol is maintained in solution in bile by virtue of the surface-active properties of bile salts and lecithin, but although a change in the proportion of these components may predispose to stone formation, other factors are also involved. Stones consisting primarily of bilirubin diglucuronide may develop in patients with chronic haemolytic anaemia.

Gallstones may be clinically silent. They can, however, cause biliary colic and obstruction and predispose to cholecystitis, cholangitis and pancreatitis. Biochemical tests may be of value in the management of these conditions, but the analysis of biliary calculi is of no importance in the routine diagnosis or surgical management of patients with gallstones.

Primary sclerosing cholangitis (PSC) is a cholestatic liver disease characterized by inflammation and progressive fibrosis of the biliary system, leading to cirrhosis and liver failure. The condition is of unknown aetiology.

Case history 6.9

History

A 45-year-old man presented with weight loss, lassitude, weakness, loss of libido and impotence. There was no history of travel.

Examination

His skin was noticeably bronzed, although it was winter, and he had hepatosplenomegaly, rather sparse body hair and small testes.

Results

Blood:	HbA$_{1c}$	62 mmol/mol (7.8%) (≥48 mmol/mol consistent with diabetes)
Serum:	ALT	135 U/L
	ALP	100 U/L
	iron	67 µmol/L
	iron-binding capacity	70 µmol/L
	transferrin saturation	95.7%
	ferritin	5000 µg/L
	testosterone (9 a.m.)	9 nmol/L
	luteinizing hormone (LH)	2 IU/L

Summary

Markedly raised ferritin and transferrin saturation with raised ALT activity, HbA$_{1c}$ and low–normal testosterone.

Interpretation

Significant iron overload with biochemical evidence of liver damage, glucose intolerance and possibly hypogonadotrophic hypogonadism. The very high transferrin saturation and ferritin concentrations are typical of severe haemochromatosis.

The HbA$_{1c}$ is consistent with a diagnosis of diabetes mellitus, although this would need to be confirmed by a repeat test given the lack of symptoms of diabetes.

Abnormalities of liver enzymes are very common in haemochromatosis, which should be considered in any patient with a chronic increase in plasma ALT activity. Parenchymal iron deposition in the liver leads to cirrhosis, which may be complicated by the development of hepatocellular carcinoma; the liver disease can be exacerbated by excessive ethanol ingestion.

Iron can deposit in any gland causing either secondary or primary gland failure. In this case, the low–normal testosterone with a low LH concentration suggests that the hypogonadism is at least in part due to pituitary damage. Deposition of iron in the pancreas causes islet cell destruction and diabetes.

Discussion

The joints are often involved as well and deposition of iron in the myocardium can cause arrhythmias and cardiac failure. Skin pigmentation is virtually always present in idiopathic haemochromatosis, although it develops insidiously and may go unnoticed by the patient. It is a result of increased melanin deposition (and haemosiderin in advanced cases).

The families of patients with haemochromatosis should be screened to detect homozygotes, who are at risk of developing the condition. Prophylactic treatment before the onset of overt disease has been shown to prevent the development of cirrhosis and reduce the (otherwise considerable) risk of hepatocellular carcinoma.

Although it can occur at any age, most patients are young men, and some two–thirds have inflammatory bowel disease (usually ulcerative colitis). The majority (60–80%) of patients are positive for perinuclear antineutrophil cytoplasmic antibodies, but these are by no means specific to this condition, occurring, for example, in up to 90% of patients with autoimmune hepatitis. The presence of increased IgG4 indicates a more rapidly progressive subtype but one that responds to corticosteroid treatment. Patients with PSC have a 10–15% lifetime risk of developing **cholangiocarcinoma**, an aggressive tumour of bile ducts. Although plasma CA19-9 concentrations may increase markedly in cholangiocarcinoma, they are also elevated in PSC and reflect disease activity. However, up to 10% of the population lack the antigen completely. There is no curative medical treatment, although symptomatic management (e.g. cholestyramine for pruritus) can be beneficial. Liver transplantation is performed, but there is a risk of the disease recurring.

Liver disease in children

Jaundice is common in neonates and is frequently physiological (see p. 384). Such jaundice is due to unconjugated bilirubin and does not persist beyond 2 weeks after birth. Separate measurement of conjugated bilirubin ('split bilirubin') can be helpful. If >25% of plasma bilirubin is conjugated, hepatobiliary disease should be considered (see Boxes 22.3 and 22.4). **Clinical features that suggest liver disease** include pale stools and dark urine, bruising or bleeding, hepatomegaly, failure to thrive and (rarely) dysmorphic features. The causes of conjugated hyperbilirubinaemia in neonates include neonatal hepatitis (caused by intrauterine infection, e.g. with cytomegalovirus, rubella or toxoplasmosis, or perinatal infection, e.g. with herpes simplex), biliary abnormalities (biliary atresia, choledochal cysts) and metabolic disorders (α_1-antitrypsin deficiency, tyrosinaemia type 1, galactosaemia, cystic fibrosis, etc.). There are several forms of progressive familial intrahepatic cholestasis (PFIC). PFIC-1 (Byler disease or FIC1) and PFIC-2 (bile salt export pump deficiency) are characterized by low plasma activities of γGT, but the activity of this enzyme is increased in a third type, PFIC-3 (a deficiency of the class III multidrug resistance permeability glycoprotein). Some cases of these rare conditions appear to be sporadic. Alagille syndrome is another rare (inherited) cause of chronic cholestasis, in which there is characteristic facial dysmorphism and often cardiac abnormalities.

Beyond the neonatal period, the causes of liver disease include viral hepatitis, autoimmune disease and metabolic disorders. In contrast with infants presenting in the neonatal period, older children with liver disease may not be jaundiced.

Liver disease in pregnancy

Pregnancy can reveal previously undiagnosed liver disease or exacerbate known pre-existing disease, particularly primary biliary cirrhosis. Some liver diseases, however, occur only during pregnancy.

Two conditions typically cause cholestasis: hyperemesis gravidarum and intrahepatic cholestasis of pregnancy. In **hyperemesis gravidarum**, severe vomiting, usually in the first trimester, can cause dehydration and undernutrition. There may be mild jaundice, and plasma liver enzyme activities may be increased up to four times normal. Fat accumulation in the liver has been demonstrated on biopsy and is probably related to undernutrition, because the abnormalities can be reversed by improving nutrient intake. **Intrahepatic cholestasis of pregnancy** typically occurs in the last trimester. The major clinical feature is pruritus, which may later be accompanied by mild jaundice, although plasma bilirubin concentration rarely exceeds 100 μmol/L; plasma ALP activity can be increased up to 10-fold, but interpretation is complicated by the contribution from placental ALP. Bile acid concentrations may be increased up to 100-fold and this may be the only biochemical abnormality. The condition resolves rapidly after delivery but is associated with an increased risk of premature labour and stillbirth. The cause is unknown, but there is evidence that it has a genetic basis.

There are also hepatic syndromes specific to pregnancy. **Acute fatty liver of pregnancy** is a severe, uncommon condition, which typically presents late in pregnancy, with malaise, anorexia, vomiting and abdominal pain, followed by jaundice and a substantial risk of progression to acute liver failure and biochemical findings typical of that condition. Hyperuricaemia is an early biochemical abnormality. Untreated, the mortality rate is up to 20%, but rapid resolution usually follows delivery. A greater than expected number of cases are associated with a genetic defect of long-chain fatty acid oxidation in the infant.

Pregnancy-induced hypertension (pre-eclampsia, see p. 222) is characterized by the development of hypertension, proteinuria and oedema, typically in the third trimester or late in the second. A small number of patients progress to eclampsia, with severe hypertension, seizures and coma. Treatment of hypertension may be required, but delivery is usually curative. In the **HELLP syndrome** (haemolysis, elevated liver enzymes [aminotransferases up to 10 × normal] and low platelet count [<100 × 10^{12}/L]), pre-eclampsia is associated with nausea, vomiting, abdominal pain and disseminated intravascular coagulopathy. There is moderate, and mainly unconjugated, hyperbilirubinaemia, but (in contrast with acute fatty liver of pregnancy) encephalopathy does not occur. The pathogenesis of pregnancy-induced hypertension is uncertain, but there is increasing evidence that implicates disordered immune responses to fetal tissue and endothelial dysfunction.

Drugs and the liver

The liver plays a central role in the metabolism of many drugs, converting them to polar, water-soluble metabolites, which can be excreted in bile and urine. The enzymes involved are located in the smooth endoplasmic reticulum of the hepatocytes. Metabolism usually involves two types of reaction: phase 1 metabolism, for example, oxidation or demethylation by cytochrome P450–linked enzymes; and phase 2 metabolism, in which phase 1 metabolites are conjugated with polar molecules, for example glucuronic acid or glutathione. Drugs can cause primarily steatosis, necrosis or cholestasis, acutely or chronically. Mixed damage can also occur.

Drug-induced liver damage may be predictable, arising when a toxic metabolite is produced by a phase

1 reaction at a rate that exceeds the detoxicating capacity of the phase 2 reaction, as occurs, for example, in a paracetamol overdose. However, many drugs may have toxic effects when used in therapeutic doses; this response **(idiosyncratic hepatotoxicity) is unpredictable** and is independent of the dose of the drug administered. Some idiosyncratic reactions to drugs, such as halothane-induced liver damage, have an immunological basis: the binding of a metabolite to a liver cell protein alters its antigenicity and provokes an immune response.

Paracetamol overdosage is an important cause of severe acute liver disease (see p. 372). Aspirin can cause acute liver failure with steatosis in susceptible infants (Reye syndrome). Other frequently used drugs that can cause liver damage include sodium valproate, phenytoin and methotrexate, but there are many others, and the list in Box 6.4 is not intended to be exhaustive. Minor degrees of hepatic dysfunction occur relatively frequently as a result of idiosyncratic responses, but overt hepatotoxicity is fortunately rare. The simple tests of liver function and damage are important for the detection of hepatotoxicity during trials of new drugs.

Other adverse effects of drugs on the liver include hepatic fibrosis or cirrhosis (particularly with methotrexate), granuloma formation, vascular disease and the development of tumours. Drugs, including herbal and alternative remedies, should always be considered in the diagnosis of patients presenting with jaundice or abnormal liver function tests.

Box 6.4 **Some drugs that cause liver disease**

Dose-dependent hepatotoxicity

paracetamol (in overdose)
tetracyclines (high doses only)
azathioprine
methotrexate

Idiosyncratic hepatotoxicity

isoniazid[a]
halothane
methyldopa[a]
rifampicin[b]
dantrolene[a]

Steatosis

aspirin
tetracyclines
sodium valproate
amiodarone[a]

Dose-dependent cholestasis

methyltestosterone
oestrogens

Idiosyncratic cholestatic hepatitis

chlorpromazine
erythromycin estolate
chlorpropamide
carbimazole
nitrofurantoin[a]

---

[a]Signifies that chronic hepatitis can occur.
[b]Rifampicin also impairs bilirubin uptake and excretion, and induces hepatic enzymes involved in drug metabolism.

Table 6.5 Typical patterns of abnormalities of simple liver function tests in various liver diseases

	Acute hepatitis	Chronic hepatitis	Cirrhosis	Cholestasis	Malignancy and infiltrations
bilirubin	N to ↑↑	N to ↑	N to ↑	↑ to ↑↑↑	N
aminotransferases	↑↑↑	↑	N to ↑	N to ↑	N to ↑
alkaline phosphatase	N to ↑	N[a]	N to ↑↑	↑↑↑	↑↑
albumin	N	N to ↓	N to ↓	N	N to ↓
γ-globulins	N	↑	↑	N	N
prothrombin time	N to ↑[b]	N to ↑	N to ↑[b]	N to ↑[c]	N

[a]May be increased if cirrhosis is present.
[b]Not corrected by parenteral vitamin K.
[c]Corrected by parenteral vitamin K.
N, normal.

SUMMARY

- **The liver has a central role in intermediary metabolism and is also responsible for the detoxification of many foreign compounds, deamination of amino acids and synthesis of urea, synthesis and excretion of bile, metabolism of some hormones, synthesis of plasma proteins and storage of certain vitamins.**
- Because of its considerable functional reserve, **biochemical tests tend to be insensitive indicators of hepatic function, although they can be highly sensitive indicators of damage to the liver.** The results of biochemical tests often indicate the nature of a liver disease (Table 6.5), but less often indicate a specific diagnosis. They are, however, invaluable in monitoring the course of liver disease and the response of patients to treatment. **Imaging techniques and biopsy are more often diagnostic.**
- The most frequently performed biochemical tests are the measurement of plasma **bilirubin** and **albumin** concentrations and **aminotransferase** (ALT or AST), alkaline phosphatase [in bold], (ALP) and [gamma]-glutamyltransferase [in bold] ([gamma]GT) activities.
- A raised plasma bilirubin concentration is a frequent but not invariable finding in patients with liver disease. However, **conjugated hyperbilirubinaemia can result from extrahepatic biliary obstruction, and a mild, unconjugated hyperbilirubinaemia is often a result of haemolysis.**
- Greatly increased plasma aminotransferase activities are characteristic of hepatocellular damage; greatly increased ALP activity is characteristic of biliary obstruction. However, the aminotransferases may be increased irrespective of either the nature or cause of hepatocellular damage, and ALP may be increased with both intrahepatic and extrahepatic obstruction. In many patients with liver disease, moderate increases in both enzymes are observed.

Furthermore, changes in neither of these enzymes are specific to liver disease.
- Plasma γGT activity is frequently increased in liver disease, but an isolated increase may indicate excessive ethanol consumption; the finding of an increase in γGT in a patient with an increased plasma ALP activity implies a hepatic origin for the latter.
- **Albumin** is synthesized by the liver but, because of its long plasma half-life, plasma albumin concentration tends to be decreased only in chronic liver disease. Many other factors can also affect albumin concentration. Blood clotting factors are synthesized in the liver, and the prothrombin time (often expressed as INR) provides a sensitive and rapidly responsive index of hepatic synthetic capacity.
- **Serological** tests for specific **autoantibodies** are valuable in the differential diagnosis of chronic liver disease. Serology for evidence of **viral infection** is valuable in both acute and chronic liver disease. Other tests which may be useful in specific liver diseases include the measurement of α-fetoprotein (liver cancer), α_1-antitrypsin (α_1-antitrypsin deficiency), ferritin and transferrin saturation (haemochromatosis) and copper and caeruloplasmin (Wilson disease).
- **Haemochromatosis**, a genetically determined disorder characterized by excessive absorption of dietary iron and subsequent iron overload, is an important cause of liver disease and cirrhosis due to iron deposition in the parenchymal cells of the liver. Iron can deposit in many other tissues including skin, heart and endocrine glands resulting in clinical features such as skin pigmentation, cardiomyopathy and impaired endocrine function. The condition is best treated by repeated venesection to remove iron from the body.

Chapter | 7 |

The gastrointestinal tract

Introduction

The digestion and absorption of food represent a complex process, which depends on the integrated activity of the organs of the alimentary tract. Food is mixed with the various digestive fluids, which contain enzymes and cofactors, and is broken down into small molecules that are absorbed by the intestinal epithelium. Polymeric carbohydrates, such as starch, undergo incomplete conversion to monosaccharides and disaccharides, the latter undergoing further hydrolysis by intestinal brush border disaccharidases (e.g. lactase) to allow absorption of the constituent monosaccharides. Proteins are broken down by proteases (secreted as inactive precursors) and peptidases to oligopeptides and amino acids. The absorption of fat is necessarily more complex because most fats are immiscible with water. Mechanical mixing and the action of bile salts create an emulsion of triglycerides (strictly, triacylglycerols; see Chapter 17), which are a substrate for pancreatic lipase. This enzyme converts triglycerides to free fatty acids and monoglycerides. These are then incorporated with bile salts into mixed micelles and are absorbed from these into intestinal epithelial cells, where they are re-esterified.

All these processes require the intimate mixing of enzymes, cofactors and substrates, and the maintenance of the optimum [H+] (pH) for enzyme activity. Disorders of the stomach, pancreas, liver and small intestine can each result in the malabsorption of nutrients. The assessment of nutritional status is covered in Chapter 8.

In addition to its importance in the absorption of water and nutrients, the mucosal lining of the gastrointestinal tract has an important barrier function, providing protection against the action of hydrogen ions and enzymes, and preventing invasion of its wall by its normal bacterial flora. However, the gut microbiota is being increasingly recognized as physiologically important in health as well as in disease. The small intestine also contributes to this protective function through its immune function. In gastrointestinal disease, this barrier function may be compromised, and bacteria may gain access to the circulation and cause septicaemia.

The gut also secretes numerous hormones: many of these hormones act on the gut itself or its related organs; others are involved in signalling hunger and satiety to the brain, and thus in appetite control.

The Stomach

In the stomach, food mixes with **acidic gastric juice**, which contains the proenzyme of **pepsin** (pepsinogen), and **intrinsic factor**, essential for the absorption of vitamin B_{12} in the terminal ileum. Secretion of gastric juice is under the combined control of the vagus nerve and the hormone gastrin.

Gastrin is secreted by G cells in the antrum of the stomach (Table 7.1), stimulating gastric motility, acid secretion and mucosal growth and pepsinogen secretion from the chief cells. Negative feedback is provided by the acid itself as well as gastrointestinal hormones, e.g. somatostatin, secretin, gastric inhibitory peptide (GIP), vasoactive intestinal peptide (VIP), calcitonin and glucagon. Gastrin is a polypeptide hormone, present in the bloodstream in various forms; the physiological significance of this heterogeneity is not known. All the variants have an identical C-terminal amino acid sequence, and, importantly, analytical methods should be based on recognition of this epitope, otherwise results may be misleading.

Gastric disorders and investigation of gastric function

Biochemical investigations are of limited use in the diagnosis of gastric disorders: the stomach can be directly

Table 7.1 Some physiological, pharmacological and pathological causes of hypergastrinaemia

Physiological	Increased gastric acid	Achlorhydria
increased vagal discharge	Zollinger–Ellison syndrome	atrophic gastritis
food, particularly amino acids and peptides in stomach	hypersecretion of gastrin by antral G cells	drugs: proton pump inhibitors and H_2 antagonists
gastric distension	idiopathic peptic ulcer disease	pernicious anaemia
increase in extracellular calcium	gastro-oesophageal reflux disease	
	Helicobacter pylori	
	gastric cancer	
	short bowel syndrome	
	chronic kidney disease	

inspected by endoscopy, and contrast radiography can also provide valuable information. Biochemical tests can be used to investigate conditions in which it is suspected that gastric acid secretion may be abnormal, particularly in atypical or recurrent peptic ulceration. The investigation of pernicious anaemia is discussed in Chapter 8.

Most **peptic ulceration** is associated either with non-steroidal anti-inflammatory drug use or with colonization of the stomach with *Helicobacter pylori*. This organism is able to survive in an acid environment and, although it provokes an immunological response in the host, it also has mechanisms for evading host immunity. Once infection has occurred, it tends to persist with consequences ranging from asymptomatic infection to gastric and duodenal ulceration or gastric adenocarcinoma, depending on host, bacterial and environmental factors. The infection can be eradicated with appropriate combinations of antibiotics and an inhibitor of H^+, K^+-ATPase (i.e. a proton pump inhibitor).

Diagnosis of *H. pylori* infection is by serology, ^{13}C urea breath test or stool antigen test. Patients should stop taking proton pump inhibitors for at least 2 weeks before testing. Plasma antibody measurements have poor sensitivity due to a variety of factors including host immune response and antigenic variation; they also remain positive for a considerable time after eradication therapy. The stool antigen test has similar performance to breath testing. However, multiple factors can result in false negatives, such as low bacterial levels, antigen degradation in the intestinal tract, watery stool and storage temperature, and in the UK, the test is not recommended for monitoring eradication. *H. pylori* can split urea to form ammonia and carbon dioxide, therefore if isotopically labelled (^{13}C or ^{14}C) urea is given orally, the isotope can be measured in expired breath to indicate infection. The sensitivity of this test is 96% and specificity virtually 100%, but the specialist equipment required limits its availability.

If a patient requires gastroscopy, a rapid urease test can be performed. A biopsy specimen of the stomach mucosa is placed in a medium containing urea and an indicator; this will change colour in the presence of *H. pylori*. The sensitivity is approximately 90% but reduces after eradication therapy. Other tests include culture (successful in only 50–70% of infected biopsies) and histology which are limited by the fastidious nature of the bacteria, patchy colonization, similar morphology to other species and the long time frame. Improvements in histological stains and genetic techniques may provide more efficient alternatives in the future.

Atypical peptic ulceration

In a small number of patients, peptic ulceration is atypical: for example, duodenal ulcers are resistant to medical treatment or recur, or there are multiple or jejunal ulcers. Atypical peptic ulceration is a feature of **Zollinger–Ellison syndrome**, a rare condition in which hypergastrinaemia is caused by a gastrinoma of the pancreas, duodenum or, less frequently, the G cells of the stomach. Approximately 60% of gastrinomas are malignant, and in ~25% of cases they occur as part of a syndrome of multiple endocrine neoplasia (see Chapter 20). Plasma gastrin concentrations typically exceed 400 ng/L (normal <100 ng/L) and do not discriminate between sporadic and genetic tumours. In addition to having recurrent or atypical peptic ulceration, patients sometimes have steatorrhoea, caused by inhibition of pancreatic lipase by the excessive gastric acid.

The first-line biochemical test in such patients is the measurement of **fasting plasma gastrin concentration**. H_2 inhibitors should be stopped 3 days, and proton pump inhibitors 2 weeks, before taking blood for gastrin measurement, because these drugs result in achlorhydria, which increased gastrin secretion. Because the hormone is very labile, blood samples must be centrifuged, separated and frozen as quickly as possible. Although most patients with gastrinomas have hypergastrinaemia, some do not, probably because they produce variants of gastrin that are not detected by standard gastrin immunoassays. Other conditions associated with hypergastrinaemia are shown in Table 7.1. Chronic kidney disease results in hypergastrinaemia for a range of reasons including hypochlorhydria, G cell hyperplasia, hyperparathyroidism and lack of renal gastrin metabolism. If the cause of hypergastrinaemia is in doubt, it may be helpful to measure plasma gastrin concentration after the administration of secretin. This hormone increases gastrin secretion from most gastrinomas (dependent on secretin receptor status) but reduces it or has no effect in hypergastrinaemia from other causes.

Patients with Zollinger–Ellison syndrome may be kept under surveillance if their tumour is small. Other patients may benefit from surgical removal of the tumour, radiotherapy, chemotherapy or hormonal therapy in disseminated malignant disease. Long-term treatment with inhibitors of gastric acid secretion may also be necessary even if the tumour has been resected.

The Pancreas

The pancreas is an essential endocrine organ that produces insulin, glucagon, pancreatic polypeptide and other hormones; its **endocrine functions** are discussed in Chapter 13. The **exocrine secretion** of the pancreas is an alkaline, bicarbonate-rich fluid containing various enzymes essential for normal digestion: the proenzyme forms of the proteases, trypsin, chymotrypsin, carboxypeptidase and elastases; the lipolytic enzyme lipase; colipase; the starch hydrolase, amylase; the sterol hydrolase, cholesterol esterase and others including phospholipase and nucleases.

The secretion of pancreatic fluid is primarily under the control of two hormones secreted by the small intestine: **secretin**, a 27 amino acid polypeptide, which stimulates the secretion of an alkaline fluid, and **cholecystokinin** (CCK), which stimulates the secretion of pancreatic enzymes and contraction of the gallbladder, and induces satiety. The structure of CCK is very similar to gastrin, CCK circulates at lower concentrations and demonstrates molecular heterogeneity making measurement difficult. Both secretin and CCK are secreted in response to the presence of acid, amino acids and partly digested proteins in the duodenum.

Pancreatic disorders and their investigation

The major disorders of the exocrine pancreas are acute pancreatitis, chronic pancreatitis, pancreatic cancer and cystic fibrosis. Biochemical investigations are essential in the diagnosis and management of the first of these, of limited use in the second and of little use in the third. Cystic fibrosis, an inherited metabolic disease that causes progressive loss of pancreatic function, is discussed in Chapter 19. Clinical evidence of impaired exocrine function is usually only seen in advanced pancreatic disease; 90% of acinar tissue must be lost before symptoms appear. Endocrine function is usually well preserved, although glucose intolerance or frank diabetes can develop in severe or advanced disease. Endocrine disease of the pancreas is discussed in Chapter 13.

Acute pancreatitis

Acute pancreatitis presents as an **acute abdomen**, with severe pain and variable degrees of shock. The most frequent known causes are excessive ethanol ingestion, gallstones and as a complication of endoscopic retrograde pancreatography (ERCP); many cases are idiopathic. Less common causes include infection (usually viral), hypertriglyceridaemia and hypercalcaemia. The pancreas becomes acutely inflamed and, in severe cases, haemorrhagic.

The initial lesion involves intracellular activation of enzyme precursors, leading to the generation of oxygen free radicals and an acute inflammatory response. This may extend beyond the pancreas as a systemic inflammatory response syndrome and lead to adult respiratory distress syndrome, circulatory failure and acute kidney injury. Sepsis, probably as a result of bacterial translocation from the gut, is a life-threatening complication. Some degree of organ failure occurs in ~25% of patients, and the mortality rate is 5–10%.

The **clinical diagnosis** is confirmed by finding **a high plasma amylase or lipase** activity (>3 times the upper reference limit [URL]) as well as a typical appearance on computed tomography (CT) scanning (Case history 7.1). Amylase (see p. 299) is secreted by salivary glands and the exocrine pancreas. Its activity in plasma is usually (although not invariably) raised in acute pancreatitis, often to >10 times the URL. However, the increase may not be so great, and elevated activities may be seen in other conditions presenting with acute abdominal pain, particularly perforated duodenal ulcer (Box 7.1). Amylase is a relatively small molecule and is rapidly excreted by the kidneys (hence the increase in plasma activity in kidney failure); in mild pancreatitis, rapid clearance may be reflected by a normal plasma value but increased urinary amylase (amylase/creatinine clearance ratio >5%). Extraabdominal causes of raised plasma amylase activity rarely result in increases of more than five times the URL.

Measurement of the pancreas-specific isoenzyme of amylase can improve the diagnostic specificity of plasma

Macroamylasaemia

Proteins can become complexed with another protein (e.g. immunoglobulin) to form an entity of much greater apparent molecular mass; renal clearance is reduced as a result. This has no direct clinical sequelae but can misleadingly suggest the presence of organ damage and lead to unnecessary investigations and treatment. Macroamylasaemia is an example of a high plasma enzyme activity caused by reduced clearance (amylase/creatinine clearance ratio <1%). Other examples include macro-AST, macro-ALT, macroprolactin (see Chapter 9, p. 158 and Case history 9.4), macrotroponin, macro-LDH and macro-CK. Gel filtration or precipitation with polyethylene glycol can detect macro-complexes if required.

amylase determinations. Measurement of plasma lipase activity has been advocated as a more specific test for acute pancreatitis but is not as widely available. It is particularly useful when a raised amylase activity is thought to be of non-pancreatic origin or due to macroamylasaemia: the lipase activity should be normal. A combination of lipase and amylase measurement is reported to have specificity

and sensitivity of ~90%. Serial measurements of these enzymes are not usually helpful because they may not reflect disease activity.

The plasma of patients with pancreatitis may be lipaemic (because of hypertriglyceridaemia), and there may be a small increase in bilirubin concentration and alkaline phosphatase activity. Hypertriglyceridaemia can result in spuriously low amylase activity; lipase measurement is preferable if available in a timely fashion.

Several **prognostic scoring systems** that include biochemical data have been developed for acute pancreatitis to identify patients at greatest risk who should be managed in an intensive care facility. Three or more positive findings within 48 hours of onset using the modified Glasgow criteria (Box 7.2) constitute severe pancreatitis: mortality rate is <2% if only one or two signs are present, but >40% with five or more. The APACHE-II scoring system (applicable to many acute conditions) is more complicated but more powerful: it is based on the measurement of 12 physiological variables, the patient's age and evidence of chronic illness on admission. A plasma C-reactive protein concentration >150 mg/L is also a good marker of disease severity.

Case history 7.1

History

A 53-year-old man developed severe abdominal pain radiating through to the back 18 hours before admission to hospital. He had no previous history of gastrointestinal disease but admitted to a heavy ethanol intake over many years.

Examination

He was mildly shocked, and his abdomen was tender in the epigastric region, with slight guarding.

Investigations

No evidence of either intestinal obstruction or perforation of a viscus on radiographic examination.

Results (see Appendix for reference ranges)

Serum:		
	urea	10 mmol/L
	creatinine	90 µmol/L
	eGFR	84 mL/min/1.73 m^2
	total calcium	1.95 mmol/L
	adjusted calcium	2.15 mmol/L
	albumin	30 g/L
	amylase	5000 U/L
Plasma:	glucose	12 mmol/L

Summary

Very high amylase with low calcium, high glucose and urea.

Interpretation

The finding of a very high serum amylase activity is suggestive of acute pancreatitis but is not diagnostic because many other conditions can cause elevated activity.

Discussion

The diagnosis of pancreatitis is based on the clinical history, evidence of inflammation (usually by CT scanning) and the finding of a high plasma amylase or lipase activity. In this case, the history is suggestive of pancreatitis, and the clinical findings, although non-specific, are consistent. The radiological findings militate against, but do not exclude, intestinal obstruction and perforation, two important differential diagnoses.

The slightly raised urea, with normal creatinine, can be explained by kidney hypoperfusion caused by shock. Loss of protein-rich exudate into the peritoneal cavity frequently causes a fall in plasma albumin concentration and contributes to the hypocalcaemia that is often present, especially in severe cases of acute pancreatitis. The formation of insoluble calcium salts of fatty acids, released within and around the inflamed pancreas by pancreatic lipase, also contributes to the hypocalcaemia. Hyperglycaemia may occur but is usually transient.

Box 7.1 Causes of increased plasma amylase activity (with estimate of usual degree of increase)

>10 × URL

acute pancreatitis

>5 × URL

perforated duodenal ulcer
intestinal obstruction
other acute abdominal disorders
acute kidney injury
diabetic ketoacidosis
ruptured fallopian tube

Usually <5 × URL

salivary gland disorders, e.g. calculi and inflammation
(including mumps)
chronic kidney disease (late stages)
macroamylasaemia
morphine administration (spasm of sphincter of Oddi)

URL, upper reference limit.

Box 7.2 Modified Glasgow score for assessing the severity of pancreatitis

Within 48 h of onset of symptoms

age >55 years
white blood cell count >15 × 10^9/L
blood glucose >10 mmol/L
serum lactate dehydrogenase >600 U/L
serum urea >16 mmol/L
serum adjusted calcium <2.00 mmol/L
serum albumin <32 g/L
Po_2 <7.9 kPa

The **management** of severe acute pancreatitis is essentially conservative. Patients should be given nothing by mouth. Fluid and electrolyte balance should be maintained by intravenous infusion and adequate analgesia provided. Enteral (nasojejunal) feeding may be introduced once pain and nausea have subsided and is to be preferred to parenteral nutrition. Antibiotics are recommended only if there is evidence of infection. ERCP and sphincterotomy may be of benefit if gallstones are present. Some complications, for example pseudocyst, may require surgery.

Chronic pancreatitis

Chronic pancreatitis is an uncommon condition, which usually presents with abdominal pain or malabsorption, and occasionally with impaired glucose tolerance. The malabsorption is due to impaired digestion of food, but there is considerable functional reserve, and pancreatic lipase output must be reduced to only 10% of normal before steatorrhoea occurs. Such a reduction only occurs in extensive disease or if the main pancreatic duct is obstructed. **Ethanol is an important causative factor** and there may be a history of recurrent acute pancreatitis.

Tests of exocrine function (see later) are unhelpful in the investigation of pain thought to be of pancreatic origin, but they are sometimes used to establish that pancreatic insufficiency is present in patients who present with malabsorption. Measurements of plasma amylase and lipase activities are of no value: they are normal or low in patients with chronic pancreatitis and even sometimes with acute exacerbations (particularly if alcoholic pancreatitis). Measurements of faecal enzymes are discussed later in this chapter. Pancreatic calcification is frequently visible on plain abdominal radiograph of patients with advanced chronic pancreatitis. Ultrasound imaging will exclude gallstones or a dilated biliary system, and show the morphology of the pancreas. If abnormal, it should be followed by CT scanning. Magnetic resonance cholangiopancreatography (MRCP) is capable of revealing the characteristic anatomical changes of chronic pancreatitis long before the results of functional tests become abnormal. Where available, this technique has replaced ERCP, which has a high (~10%) rate of complications. Percutaneous pancreatic biopsy (CT or ultrasound guided) is feasible but requires considerable skill.

The damage to the organ in chronic pancreatitis is irreversible. **Management** involves treatment of the underlying cause, if known, pain relief and avoidance of alcohol. Oral pancreatic enzyme supplements are indicated when features of malabsorption are present. Diabetes is treated with insulin. Surgery may be required when there is intractable pain.

Tests of pancreatic function

Pancreatic **elastase** and **chymotrypsin activities in faeces** are reduced in chronic pancreatic insufficiency (see Case history 7.2). Measurements of both enzymes have been used as tests for this condition: both show high sensitivity and specificity, with elastase being slightly superior in both respects. Measurement of faecal elastase is now widely used to distinguish between diarrhoea of pancreatic and nonpancreatic origin. The measurement of faecal fat excretion is regarded as obsolete in the UK.

Other tests of pancreatic function that have been used in the past are now rarely performed. They include

129

Case history 7.2

History

A middle-aged publican presented with flatulence and abdominal distension. Further questioning revealed that he had lost weight and was passing frequent, bulky, foul-smelling bowel motions that were difficult to flush away.

Investigations

A plain abdominal radiograph revealed pancreatic calcification, which was confirmed by CT scanning.

Results

Serum:	calcium (adjusted)	2.10 mmol/L
	phosphate	0.70 mmol/L
	alkaline phosphatase	264 U/L
	albumin	40 g/L
	vitamin D	22 nmol/L
Plasma:	glucose (fasting)	12 mmol/L
	parathyroid hormone	17 pmol/L
Faeces:	elastase	52 µg/g
	(normal >500 µg/g; severe pancreatic insufficiency <100)	

Summary

Hypocalcaemia and hypophosphataemia with a raised alkaline phosphatase. Hyperparathyroidism, low vitamin D and a very low faecal elastase activity.

Interpretation

The clinical, and biochemical, features are characteristic of malabsorption (Table 7.2). With gross steatorrhoea, further investigations to establish malabsorption are not necessary, but the cause must be determined. The low faecal elastase activity suggests pancreatic insufficiency.

The presence of pancreatic calcification is very suggestive of ethanol-induced chronic pancreatitis. The raised fasting concentration of glucose (if confirmed) is consistent with diabetes mellitus and reflects deficiency of insulin caused by destruction of the endocrine pancreas. Hyperparathyroidism is likely secondary to vitamin D deficiency caused by the malabsorption.

Discussion

The patient was advised to abstain from alcohol. He was treated for diabetes and given pancreatic enzyme supplements to add to his food and the symptoms regressed. This therapeutic response provides further confirmation of the diagnosis of pancreatic insufficiency.

---

direct and indirect tests. The former includes the measurement of bicarbonate concentration and amylase or trypsin activity directly in duodenal fluid after either a test meal (Lundh test) or the administration of secretin and CCK. Bicarbonate concentration and enzyme activities are decreased in chronic pancreatic insufficiency. Indirect tests measure the excretion of an orally administered substance that requires pancreatic enzyme activity for its absorption, e.g. the fluorescein dilaurate and *p*-aminobenzoic acid (PABA) tests. They are no longer available in the UK.

Carcinoma of the pancreas

Pancreatic carcinoma can be difficult to diagnose (see Case history 6.6). Presentation often occurs as a result of metastases rather than as a direct effect of the primary tumour. Other presentations include obstructive jaundice, when a tumour in the head of the pancreas obstructs the common bile duct, and malabsorption. Biochemical tests of pancreatic function are rarely of any use in diagnosis, and other techniques, particularly imaging, are far more powerful diagnostic tools. The plasma concentration of the tumour markers carcinoembryonic antigen (CEA) and CA 19-9 (see Chapter 20 p. 359-360) are elevated in up to 80% of patients with pancreatic malignancy, but they can be elevated with other (particularly colorectal) cancers and sometimes in non-malignant disease. Unfortunately, pancreatic cancer often presents late; by the time it is diagnosed, metastases are often present and only palliative surgical procedures are feasible.

The Small Intestine

The small intestine is the site of absorption of all nutrients; most of this absorption takes place in the duodenum and jejunum, but vitamin B_{12} and bile salts are absorbed in the terminal ileum (see Chapter 8). Approximately 8 L of fluid enters the gut every 24 hours. This is derived from ingested food and water and from the digestive juices, including those secreted by the small intestine itself. Most of this fluid, including the salts it contains, is reabsorbed in the jejunum, ileum and large intestine.

The small intestine can be affected by many disease processes, but their major effects on function relate to the consequences of impaired absorption of nutrients and fluid, and to disruption of its barrier function.

Table 7.2 Malabsorption: clinical features, common causes and tests

Clinical features	Investigations
Retention in the bowel of non-absorbed nutrients	
diarrhoea[a], steatorrhoea abdominal discomfort and distension[a] flatulence[a]	
Decreased absorption of nutrients	
anaemia[a] (iron, folate and vitamin B_{12} deficiency)	full blood count, red cell indices (mean corpuscular volume (MCV)), mean corpuscular haemoglobin (MCH), plasma iron, ferritin, vitamin B_{12}, folate
glossitis, angular stomatitis[a] (iron deficiency)	plasma iron, ferritin
osteomalacia and rickets (vitamin D deficiency)	plasma calcium, phosphate, alkaline phosphatase, 25-hydroxycholecalciferol
oedema, (hypoalbuminaemia)	plasma albumin
bleeding tendency (vitamin K deficiency)	INR (prothrombin time)
weight loss[a], growth failure in children[a]	weight, height and growth charts
Causes	
pancreatic enzyme deficiency, e.g. chronic pancreatitis and cystic fibrosis	faecal elastase
bile salt deficiency, e.g. biliary obstruction and hepatic disease	
intestinal, e.g. coeliac disease, tropical sprue, Crohn disease and partial resection	coeliac serology and duodenal biopsy[b], faecal calprotectin, imaging[b]
bacterial overgrowth, e.g. gastric surgery, internal fistulae, strictures and jejunal diverticulosis	breath tests[b]

[a]Indicates the most common features.
[b]Second-line tests.
INR, international normalized ratio.

Investigation of intestinal function
Tests for gut permeability

Some conditions of the small intestine, including inflammatory bowel diseases (IBDs), cause **increased gut permeability**. This can be assessed by measuring the faecal concentration of the neutrophil protein, **calprotectin**. This is increased in almost all patients with IBD, often to >10 times the URL, correlates well with disease activity and is predictive of relapse in patients in remission. Of great practical importance is the fact that faecal calprotectin is usually normal in patients with irritable bowel syndrome (IBS), so that the demonstration of a normal value obviates the need for more extensive investigation of patients in whom a diagnosis of IBD or IBS is being considered. Lactoferrin is another white cell protein that is released into the faeces during active inflammatory conditions of the bowel. Its measurement is thought to give similar information to that of calprotectin, but it has not been as extensively investigated. Faecal excretion of both proteins is increased during bacterial or parasitic bowel infections and also with bowel cancers.

Tests of carbohydrate absorption

A variety of tests involving the ingestion of carbohydrates and the measurement of their plasma concentrations or urinary excretion were developed for the investigation of small intestinal function, before the widespread use of endoscopic biopsy. The best known is the **xylose absorption test** which has been rendered obsolete because of non-specificity and improvement in other diagnostic modalities.

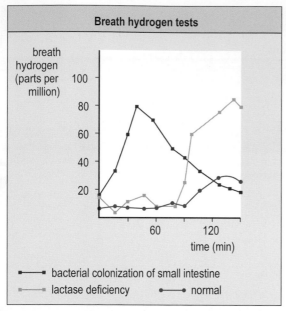

Breath hydrogen tests

breath hydrogen (parts per million)

- bacterial colonization of small intestine
- lactase deficiency
- normal

Fig. 7.1 Breath hydrogen tests. Hydrogen is not produced by mammalian cells; its presence in expired air is due to bacterial fermentation of unabsorbed carbohydrate. Typical results are shown from the test performed in a patient with bacterial colonization of the small intestine when challenged with oral lactulose (10 g), where the lactulose acts as a substrate for bacterial metabolism, and in a patient with intestinal lactase deficiency when challenged with oral lactose (50 g), compared with a healthy individual given lactose. Hydrogen is generated by the fermentation of unabsorbed lactose in the colon, with the result that the increase in breath hydrogen occurs later than with small intestinal bacterial overgrowth.

Suspected intestinal **disaccharidase deficiency** can be investigated by administering the appropriate disaccharide (50 g) orally and measuring the blood glucose response. The test is unphysiological because of the large oral load of, for example, lactose, although patients who do not develop symptoms during the test are not lactose intolerant. A more reliable but difficult-to-perform test is to measure urine excretion ratios of hydrolysable and non-hydrolysable disaccharides after oral administration, e.g. lactose and lactulose. Normally, very little lactose reaches the urine because it is hydrolysed in the small intestine. With lactase deficiency, more lactose is available for absorption and eventual excretion in the urine. The absorption and excretion of lactulose are unaffected by enzyme deficiencies.

A much more common approach is to measure breath hydrogen after giving the disaccharide (Fig. 7.1): because it is not absorbed, the disaccharide reaches the colon, where one of the products of bacterial fermentation is hydrogen. However, results can be affected by intestinal transit time and bacterial overgrowth in the small intestine. Another approach to the investigation of disaccharidase deficiencies is measurement of the appropriate enzyme in a biopsy sample.

The most common disaccharidase deficiency affects lactase. It may be acquired; it often occurs transiently when there is damage to gut mucosa, such as after gastroenteritis. However, it is most often constitutional, as it is normal for lactase activity to decrease after an infant has been weaned. It may be more correct to say that the persistence of activity commonly seen in Caucasians is the 'abnormal' state. Less common are sucrase–isomaltase and maltase deficiencies.

Tests of amino acid absorption

Tests of amino acid absorption from the gut are used only as research procedures. Generalized malabsorption of amino acids occurs only with extensive small bowel disease. Malabsorption of specific amino acids occurs in certain inherited metabolic disorders: for example, deficiency of tryptophan can occur in Hartnup disease, an inherited disorder of the transport of neutral amino acids. In cystinuria, there is impaired intestinal transport of the dibasic amino acids lysine, cystine, ornithine and arginine (see p. 98), but this condition is not associated with a deficiency syndrome.

Loss of protein from the gut in a protein-losing enteropathy can be assessed by measuring faecal radioactivity after parenteral administration of isotopically labelled proteins (e.g. ^{51}Cr-albumin), or by measuring faecal α_1-antitrypsin (which resists enzymatic proteolysis on its passage through the bowel). Such investigations are not frequently performed, however, because the cause of any hypoproteinaemia is usually obvious in such conditions.

Tests of fat absorption

Because the absorption of fat is a complex process, the effects of fat malabsorption are often a prominent feature of generalized malabsorption. For this reason, and because fat malabsorption can occur with gastric, pancreatic, hepatic and intestinal disease, tests of fat absorption can be used to diagnose generalized malabsorption. However, the presence of generalized malabsorption can often be reliably inferred from clinical findings (particularly steatorrhoea) and the results of simple tests (see p.131). Further investigations will then be required to determine the cause of malabsorption, but formal tests to confirm its presence are now required only infrequently.

Measurement of faecal fat excretion is now rarely performed in the UK because it is unpleasant for all concerned and is difficult to perform correctly. The **triolein breath test,** developed as an alternative, has also largely fallen into disuse. The principle of the test is that, when isotopically

---

Case history 7.3

History

A 3-year-old boy was referred for the investigation of failure to thrive: he was below the third centile for height and the tenth for weight, although both parents were tall. He had frequent diarrhoea and did not appear to enjoy his food.

Examination

He was anaemic and had abdominal distension; there was obvious wasting of the muscles of the limbs, buttocks and shoulder girdle.

Results

Serum:	albumin	30 g/L
	anti-tissue transglutaminase antibodies	strongly positive
Blood:	haemoglobin	97 g/L
	blood film	hypochromic, microcytic red cells

Summary

Low albumin and haemoglobin, positive for anti-tissue transglutaminase (TTG) antibodies.

Interpretation

Hypoproteinaemia and a hypochromic, microcytic anaemia, characteristic of iron deficiency, are common in patients with malabsorption. The positive serology suggests coeliac disease.

Discussion

Coeliac disease was confirmed by high titres of endomysial antibodies and HLA-DQ8 positivity on genetic testing, which obviates the need for an intestinal biopsy in children. A gluten-free diet was started and the boy's symptoms regressed. Twelve months later he was growing normally and had low titres of anti-TTG, as expected if patients adhere to a gluten-free diet.

---

labelled ^{13}C- or ^{14}C-triolein (a triglyceride) is given orally, digested and absorbed, some of the label appears in the breath as isotopically labelled carbon dioxide, which can be measured.

Tests for bacterial overgrowth

Bacterial overgrowth in the small intestine can occur in a number of conditions, particularly when there is decreased gastric acid production or stasis of gut contents, for example as a result of a stricture or in jejunal diverticulosis. Bacterial deconjugation of bile acids leads to failure of mixed micelle formation and malabsorption of fat.

The most reliable diagnostic test for bacterial overgrowth is aspiration and culture of small bowel contents. However, this method has disadvantages: it is an invasive procedure, and the cultures are sometimes negative even when other evidence of bacterial overgrowth is overwhelming.

Breath tests can be used to diagnose bacterial overgrowth. Bacteria metabolize carbohydrates in the gut, releasing hydrogen, which is absorbed into the bloodstream and excreted through the lungs. Breath hydrogen content can be measured either after a test dose of glucose or after administration of a non-absorbable carbohydrate (see Fig. 7.1).

Non-biochemical tests of intestinal function

A biopsy of the mucosa of the small intestine can be performed endoscopically under direct vision. **Wireless capsule endoscopy** can also be used to visualize the inside of the small intestine. **Small intestinal biopsy** is the definitive procedure for the diagnosis of coeliac disease (gluten-induced enteropathy, Case history 7.3).

Characteristic radiographic appearances are seen in patients with certain intestinal diseases, for example, Crohn disease (Case history 7.4).

Disorders of intestinal function

Malabsorption

The term **malabsorption** strictly refers to impaired absorption of the products of digestion, whereas **maldigestion** is failure of digestion, which may be responsible for non-absorption of nutrients, for example, in pancreatic insufficiency. In practice, because the resultant clinical syndromes are basically the same, the term **malabsorption is commonly used to encompass both disorders**.

The **clinical features** of malabsorption are varied and stem from either deficiency of nutrients or retention of nutrients within the bowel lumen. The clinical features and common causes of malabsorption are shown in Table 7.2.

More than one mechanism can be responsible for malabsorption in individual cases. After gastric surgery, for example, impaired mixing of food with digestive juices, decreased stimuli to their secretion, rapid transit and bacterial colonization of a blind afferent loop may all contribute to malabsorption.

Investigations are required for two purposes: to diagnose malabsorption and **to determine its cause**. If the diagnosis is obvious clinically (e.g. if steatorrhoea is present), only tests to determine the cause are required. If the

History

A 35-year-old woman presented with diarrhoea, weight loss and abdominal pain. She had had two previous episodes of the same symptoms, lasting for several weeks on each occasion in the preceding 2 years but had not sought medical advice.

Examination

She was clinically anaemic.

Results

Serum:	albumin	28 g/L
	anti-parietal cell antibodies	negative
	folate	5 µg/L (3—20)
	vitamin B$_{12}$	95 ng/L (200–910)
Blood:	haemoglobin	85 g/L
	red cell volume	110 fL (84–98)
Faeces:	calprotectin	910 µg/g (<60)

Summary

Low albumin, macrocytic anaemia with vitamin B$_{12}$ deficiency and significantly raised faecal calprotectin.

Interpretation

Weight loss is a common feature of gastrointestinal disease. The low albumin and anaemia are consistent with malabsorption. The macrocytosis is consistent with vitamin B$_{12}$ deficiency. Pernicious anaemia is unlikely with normal serology and the symptoms of pain and diarrhoea. Faecal calprotectin is typically high in active inflammatory bowel disorders such as Crohn disease or ulcerative colitis. The terminal ileitis of Crohn disease prevents vitamin B$_{12}$ absorption.

Discussion

A colonoscopy revealed no pathology, which excluded ulcerative colitis, but a barium meal and follow-through showed narrowing and ulceration of the terminal ileum, with an ileo–ileal fistula. These radiographic appearances are typical of Crohn disease, an inflammatory disease of the gut in which ulceration and fibrosis occur and may lead to the formation of strictures and fistulae. Although the condition can affect any part of the gut, the ileum is most often involved. The course is often one of remission and exacerbation.

In the acute illness, mesalazine, steroids or tumour necrosis factor-α inhibitors such as infliximab may be used and nutritional support may be necessary. Surgery may be required for intestinal obstruction or fistulae, or if medical treatment fails. Azathioprine can be used to maintain remission. Malabsorption in Crohn disease may be because of either damage to the ileum or bacterial overgrowth in a stagnant loop, a possible consequence of internal fistula formation.

---

diagnosis is uncertain, simple tests (see Table 7.2) should be performed first; if the results of these are normal, malabsorption is unlikely and further expensive or invasive tests often can be avoided.

Coeliac disease

Coeliac disease, also known as gluten-sensitive enteropathy, is the commonest cause of malabsorption in the UK. The malabsorption is a consequence of villous atrophy, affecting particularly the mucosa of the proximal small intestine. Coeliac disease is a result of sensitivity to gliadin, a component of gluten, a protein present in wheat and other cereal flours. It varies considerably in severity. It may present in infancy (typically on weaning with severe failure to thrive, apathy, muscle wasting and steatorrhoea), in later childhood (with growth failure, anaemia or bone disease; see Case history 7.3) or in adults (typically with diarrhoea and often a long history of being unwell). It is strongly associated with the human leucocyte antigen (HLA) alleles DQ2 and DQ8 and has an increased incidence in patients with type 1 diabetes mellitus, dermatitis herpetiformis and autoimmune thyroid disease. Complete withdrawal of gluten from the diet leads to regrowth of villi and eventual resolution of symptoms.

Although serology is usually the first investigation, definitive diagnosis is by **intestinal biopsy**, especially in adults. The characteristic villous atrophy resolves on exclusion of gluten from the diet and recurs after a gluten challenge. Biopsy can be avoided in children with typical symptoms and positive serology, who are found to be positive for the associated HLA alleles. Various **antibodies** (e.g. against gliadin, reticulin, endomysium and tissue transglutaminase [TTG]) are present in the plasma in active disease. The detection of TTG antibody provides the most sensitive (~89%) and specific (~98%) serological screening test for coeliac disease and is the recommended first-line test in the UK. If the result is equivocal, endomysial antibody detection should be the next investigation. Serum total immunoglobulin A (IgA) concentration is also measured as part of the analytical protocol: most laboratories measure the IgA antibody to TTG and endomysium, and false-negative tests occur in IgA deficiency (seen in 10% of patients). In these circumstances, measurements of IgG antibody to TTG or endomysium can be used. In adults, measurement of endomysial antibodies is usually restricted to those with IgA deficiency and if an IgG TTG assay is not available; HLA typing is only used in adults who are unlikely to have a positive duodenal biopsy because they have already excluded gluten from their diet and refuse to reintroduce it.

Intestinal failure

Intestinal failure is a condition in which the ability of the intestine to absorb fluids and nutrients threatens a person's nutritional status and hence health. Unless very short-lived, it is an indication for **nutritional support**. Acute, reversible intestinal failure can be a complication of surgery (e.g. as a result of sepsis or fistula formation), chemotherapy or irradiation. Chronic intestinal failure is most frequently a consequence of the short bowel syndrome, when a large segment of small intestine has been resected because of, for example, ischaemia after vascular occlusion. Other causes of chronic intestinal failure include Crohn disease, radiation enteritis, systemic sclerosis and amyloid.

The gut has considerable reserve capacity, and the **severity of dysfunction** in short gut syndrome is related to the site of resection, the length of the segment resected and the extent to which adaptation (an increase in the absorptive capacity of the remaining gut) occurs. Adaptation can occur to a greater extent in the ileum than in the jejunum. The volume of fluid lost through an ileostomy decreases with time: little or no reduction occurs with a jejunostomy. Less dysfunction follows resection of midjejunum than of proximal small intestine (essential for the absorption of most nutrients) or of ileum (essential for bile acid and vitamin B_{12} absorption). Preservation of the ileocaecal valve reduces colonization of the small intestine by colonic bacteria and increases the transit time of gut contents, allowing more time for absorption. In practice, patients with <75 cm of residual small intestine after bowel resection almost invariably require long-term parenteral nutrition. Patients with up to 200 cm usually require oral or enteral supplementation. Most patients will require parenteral nutrition initially, but the early introduction of at least some enteral nutrition promotes adaptation and helps protect the barrier function of the gut. Provided that it does not cause a significant increase in fluid loss, enteral provision can be gradually increased and parenteral support decreased, with care being taken to ensure that the patient's nutritional requirements are fully met. The provision of nutritional support is discussed in Chapter 8.

The major problem in the first few days after gut resection is **fluid and electrolyte loss**; accurate measurement and replacement of the losses are essential. These losses may decrease as adaptation occurs, or be controllable with drugs. Some patients, however, require long-term supplements of fluids and electrolytes (e.g. magnesium), even if they can absorb sufficient nutrients.

> ### Box 7.3 **Some common causes of chronic diarrhoea (lasting for >4 weeks)**
>
> intestinal infections, especially after travel abroad
> inflammatory bowel disease
> irritable bowel syndrome
> laxative use
> colorectal cancer
> pancreatic insufficiency
> small bowel disease, e.g. coeliac disease
> surgical resection of small bowel
> thyrotoxicosis
> dietary, e.g. lactose in patients with lactase deficiency, xylose or sorbitol in 'low-sugar' foods

Long-term complications of the short-bowel syndrome include persistent diarrhoea, nutrient deficiencies, gallstones (caused by bile salt wasting) and urinary tract stones (caused by hyperoxaluria, see p. 99). Deficiencies of some nutrients are commoner than of others. Vitamin B_{12} deficiency can complicate ileal resection; zinc and magnesium deficiency are common with persistent diarrhoea; and malabsorption of vitamin D and calcium can cause metabolic bone disease. Persisting lactase deficiency may limit milk intake, further compromising calcium status.

The metabolism of dietary carbohydrate as a result of abnormal microbial colonization of the gut can cause metabolic acidosis because of the production of lactic acid. The cause of the acidosis may go unrecognized because the lactate produced is the $D(-)$-isomer rather than the $L(+)$-isomer, which is formed during glycolysis. The $D(-)$-isomer is not measured in most assays for lactate.

Other intestinal disorders

Given the amount of fluid that enters the gut each day, there is considerable potential for **fluid and electrolyte depletion** in situations of impaired reabsorption. Dehydration can complicate prolonged vomiting and diarrhoea and enterocutaneous fistulae. Magnesium and potassium depletion are also frequently associated with excessive loss of fluid from the gastrointestinal tract.

In some patients, there is **increased secretion of fluid** into the gut; for example, in cholera, massive fluid loss can occur very rapidly. Secretory diarrhoea also occurs with villous adenomata of the rectum (tumours that secrete large volumes of potassium-rich mucus), and with tumours that secrete VIP, which cause profuse, watery diarrhoea, the **Verner–Morrison syndrome**.

Chronic diarrhoea (lasting >4 weeks) is a common presenting complaint in primary care. The commoner causes are listed in Box 7.3.

Table 7.3 Some gastrointestinal hormones, their locations and principal functions (see also Box 8.2 and Table 20.2)

Hormone	Location	Function
gastrin	gastric antrum	stimulates gastric acid secretion and growth of gastric and intestinal mucosa
cholecystokinin (CCK)	duodenum, jejunum	stimulates pancreatic enzyme secretion and gallbladder contraction
secretin	duodenum, jejunum	stimulates pancreatic bicarbonate secretion
pancreatic polypeptide (PP)	pancreas	inhibits exocrine pancreatic secretion
gastric inhibitory polypeptide (GIP)	duodenum, jejunum	releases insulin in response to glucose (hence also known as glucose-dependent insulinotropic polypeptide)
vasoactive intestinal polypeptide (VIP)	entire gastrointestinal (GI) tract	neurotransmitter; regulates GI motility and secretion
motilin	stomach, small intestine and colon	stimulates GI motility

Colorectal cancer is one of the commonest cancers in the developed world, and a number of countries now screen defined age groups with a high risk of development of the disease (often >60 years, see p. 361). The screening test detects occult blood in the faeces: most cancers will bleed small amounts before they cause symptoms. The guaiac faecal occult blood (FOB) test that has been in use for many years is now being supplanted by the more sensitive and specific faecal immunochemical test (FIT) for haemoglobin. The prognosis depends on the stage at which the disease is detected, hence the emphasis on early diagnosis. Localized tumours that can be fully resected surgically have an excellent prognosis. Individuals with a strong family history of colorectal cancer are screened at a much earlier age, usually by endoscopy. These include patients with genetic mutations known to predispose to the development of colorectal cancer, e.g. familial adenomatous polyposis. Patients with symptoms that could be attributable to colorectal cancer should be investigated directly, usually by endoscopic examination; faecal occult blood testing is of little value in such settings. Many colorectal cancers produce CEA (see p.359), and plasma concentrations are useful in monitoring treatment but not in diagnosis.

Gastrointestinal Hormones

The principal gastrointestinal functions of gastrin, secretin, CCK, insulin and glucagon have been understood for some time. In recent years, a large number of other gastrointestinal polypeptide hormones have been discovered (Table 7.3). Some of these are known to influence the function of the exocrine (and endocrine) pancreas and the gastrointestinal tract; others are involved in signalling hunger and satiety to the central nervous system, and these are of importance in the control of appetite (see Chapter 8). Currently, assays for these hormones are available only in specialized laboratories, and the indication for measuring them for diagnostic purposes is largely confined to patients with suspected hormone-secreting tumours, for example, with Verner–Morrison syndrome. Table 20.2 shows the clinical symptoms and signs encountered with some of these neuroendocrine tumours.

SUMMARY

- **The gastrointestinal tract is responsible for the digestion and absorption of food.** This process also depends on normal hepatic and pancreatic function and is controlled by both neural and humoral mechanisms.
- Formal assessment of gastric acid secretion is now seldom required, but measurement of the hormone gastrin, which stimulates **gastric acid** secretion, is valuable in patients with atypical peptic ulceration, because this may be caused by a gastrin-secreting tumour.
- Many other **gut hormones** have been described. The measurement of some of them may similarly be useful in the investigation of patients suspected of having a hormone-secreting tumour.
- The **malabsorption syndrome** can be a result of intestinal, pancreatic or hepatic dysfunction. Significant malabsorption can readily be excluded by simple tests on blood or serum. If malabsorption is obvious clinically—for instance, because of weight loss and gross steatorrhoea— tests for malabsorption add nothing to the diagnosis, although measurement of specific nutrients may be helpful for monitoring treatment. Once a diagnosis of malabsorption has been made, investigations are required to determine the cause if this is not obvious clinically. Biochemical, histological and radiological data may all be useful in this context.
- **Acute pancreatitis** typically presents as an acute abdomen. Increased plasma amylase or lipase activity is characteristic of, although not specific to, this condition. Shock, acute kidney injury, hypocalcaemia and hyperglycaemia may be complicating factors. The major predisposing factors are gallstones, alcohol and following ERCP. When severe, acute pancreatitis has a poor prognosis.
- **Chronic pancreatitis** usually presents with pain or malabsorption, or both. Ethanol is the commonest cause. The pancreatic damage is irreversible; treatment is aimed at relieving symptoms.
- Approximately 8 L of fluid is secreted into the gut each day, the great majority of which is reabsorbed. **The loss of fluid and salts from the gut** because of vomiting, diarrhoea or a fistula can lead to severe salt and water depletion.
- **Intestinal failure** most frequently complicates resection of the small intestine or Crohn disease. Excessive fluid loss is a common problem, and nutritional support is required, sometimes in the long term.

Chapter | 8 |

Clinical nutrition

Introduction

An adequate intake of nutrients is essential for normal growth and development and for the maintenance of health. These nutrients include proteins, to supply amino acids, energy substrates (carbohydrates and fat), inorganic salts, micronutrients (vitamins and trace elements) and other essential nutrients such as essential fatty acids. The daily requirements for these nutrients are determined by many factors, including age, sex, physical activity and the presence of disease; if an individual's requirements are not met, a clinical deficiency syndrome may develop.

This chapter discusses the pathology of some **specific deficiency syndromes**, with particular reference to the role of the laboratory in their diagnosis and management. This role is also discussed in relation to patients suffering from, or at risk of, **generalized malnutrition**. **Nutritional support** for these patients can be provided enterally (i.e. into the alimentary tract, either by mouth or through a feeding tube) or parenterally (intravenously, bypassing the gut). Such treatment requires close cooperation between the clinician and the laboratory, particularly when the patients are also acutely ill, and when such support is required in the long term.

Excessive intake of nutrients can also be harmful. **Obesity** is a common condition in the developed world (two-thirds of the adult population of the UK are overweight or obese), and its prevalence is increasing. Its ultimate cause is an intake of energy substrates in excess of requirements; the factors that contribute to this are complex, but at a population level the main determinants are usually reduced levels of physical exercise and increased availability of energy-rich foods. Much evidence links several common diseases, including coronary heart disease, hypertension and some cancers (e.g. breast, colon), with a relative excess or insufficiency of one or more components of the diet.

Vitamin Deficiencies

Vitamin deficiency states can arise as a result of:
- inadequate intake (with normal requirements)
- impaired absorption
- impaired metabolism (if metabolism is necessary for function)
- increased requirements
- increased losses.

The biochemical functions of most vitamins are well understood, but although the deficiency syndrome may obviously relate to a specific known function (e.g. osteomalacia in vitamin D deficiency), this is not always the case (e.g. beriberi and Wernicke encephalopathy in thiamin deficiency). Although the clinical presentation of individual vitamin deficiency states is usually characteristic, in generalized malnutrition multiple deficiencies can occur and cause a complex clinical presentation.

The classic deficiency syndromes are the end result of a process in which deficiency of a vitamin leads first to mobilization of body stores, then to tissue depletion, biochemical impairment (subclinical deficiency) and, eventually, frank deficiency.

The actions of vitamins are almost entirely intracellular, and their plasma concentrations do not necessarily reflect intracellular concentrations and thus functional availability. It follows that plasma concentrations of vitamins may be unreliable as indicators of the body's vitamin status. In deficiency states, plasma concentrations tend to fall before tissue concentrations. In contrast, if a vitamin is administered to a patient with deficiency, a rise in plasma concentration to normal is not necessarily indicative of adequate replacement.

The best means of assessing a patient's vitamin status depends on the vitamin in question. The range of techniques that can be used is illustrated by the examples given in the following sections.

Water-Soluble Vitamins

Vitamin B$_1$ (thiamin)

Thiamin pyrophosphate is a cofactor in the metabolism of pyruvate to acetyl coenzyme A (CoA), 2-oxoglutarate to succinyl CoA, and in a reaction of the pentose shunt pathway catalysed by the enzyme transketolase. The body contains only about 30 times the daily requirement of this vitamin. Diets high in carbohydrate require more thiamin for their assimilation than diets high in fat, and thus, for example, subclinical thiamin deficiency may be unmasked in malnourished patients when their carbohydrate intake is increased rapidly (refeeding syndrome, see p. 149).

Deficiency of vitamin B$_1$ causes a primarily sensory polyneuropathy (**dry beriberi**), cardiac failure (**wet beriberi**), **Wernicke encephalopathy**, characterized by ophthalmoplegia and ataxia and which may progress rapidly to stupor and death, and **Korsakoff psychosis**, of which memory loss is usually the most obvious feature. These can occur alone or in combination. In the UK, the most frequent manifestation is encephalopathy, seen chiefly in patients with chronic alcoholism whose diet is poor.

Wernicke encephalopathy responds rapidly to thiamin and, because the vitamin is cheap and non-toxic, this therapeutic response can be used to make the diagnosis. Laboratory tests for deficiency are seldom necessary. It may, however, be necessary formally to document deficiency in nutritional research. Thiamin concentration can be measured directly in whole blood. Before direct measurements became available, a functional assay was used in which **red cell transketolase** activity was measured both with and without the addition of its cofactor thiamin pyrophosphate to the reaction mixture. Basal enzyme activity is low in clinically obvious deficiency; it may be normal in subclinical deficiency but is increased by the addition of the cofactor.

Direct whole blood assays of **riboflavin** (vitamin B$_2$) and **pyridoxine** (vitamin B$_6$) are now also available. Deficiency of each of these vitamins (manifest in both cases principally by angular stomatitis, cheilosis and dermatitis) is uncommon in developed countries but may sometimes be seen in alcoholics and grossly malnourished individuals.

Nicotinic acid (niacin, vitamin B$_3$)

Nicotinic acid is the precursor of nicotinamide. This is a constituent of the coenzymes **nicotinamide adenine dinucleotide (NAD)** and its **phosphate (NADP)**, which are essential to glycolysis and oxidative phosphorylation.

Part of the body's nicotinic acid requirement is met by endogenous synthesis from tryptophan. The deficiency syndrome, **pellagra** (comprising an erythematous skin rash that leads to desquamation, gastrointestinal disturbance, particularly diarrhoea, and dementia), can result from either an inadequate dietary intake of nicotinic acid or decreased synthesis. The latter may be a feature of the **carcinoid syndrome** (see p. 355), in which there is increased metabolism of tryptophan to hydroxyindoles, with consequently less being available for nicotinic acid synthesis, and of **Hartnup disease**, a rare inherited disorder of the epithelial transport of neutral amino acids, in which there is decreased intestinal absorption of tryptophan from the gut.

Nicotinic acid status can be assessed by measurement of its urinary metabolites, although this is rarely necessary.

Folic acid

A derivative of folic acid is vital to **purine** and **pyrimidine** (and hence nucleic acid) synthesis. Folic acid deficiency is relatively common: its most usual manifestation is as a **macrocytic anaemia** with **megaloblastic marrow changes**. The concentration in red cells reflects the body's folate reserves, whereas plasma concentrations reflect recent dietary intake: however, most laboratories only measure folate in serum or plasma. Body stores in the liver become depleted after about 3 months of a low-folate diet. Folates occur naturally in many foods, particularly dark green, leafy vegetables. In some countries, cereals and flours are fortified with folate.

It is essential to diagnose the cause of megaloblastic anaemia before it is treated. Giving folate alone to patients with vitamin B$_{12}$ deficiency risks precipitating or exacerbating the neurological manifestations of vitamin B$_{12}$ deficiency.

The use of folate supplements in pregnancy to reduce the risk of **neural tube defects** is discussed in a later section.

Vitamin B$_{12}$

Vitamin B$_{12}$ comprises a number of closely related substances called **cobalamins**, which are essential to nucleic acid synthesis. Deficiency can cause **megaloblastic anaemia** and **neurological manifestations**, either alone or together. The neurological features, which may be caused by demyelination, include peripheral neuropathy, subacute combined degeneration of the spinal cord, dementia and optic atrophy.

Dietary deficiency of this vitamin is rare except in vegans: considerable amounts are stored in the liver, with the result that deficiency is not common even with severe malabsorption (unless of very long standing). Vitamin B$_{12}$ deficiency is most frequently seen in disorders of the gastrointestinal system, particularly **pernicious anaemia**. This is an autoimmune disease, resulting in failure of production in the stomach of **intrinsic factor**, which is essential for the absorption of the vitamin from the terminal ileum. Autoantibodies to intrinsic factor are present in 50% of patients with pernicious anaemia and are specific for the condition, whereas parietal cell antibodies, although present in 90% of patients, also occur in many older people with gastric atrophy. Patients require treatment with parenteral vitamin B_{12}, because oral supplements cannot be absorbed.

Three carrier proteins are involved in the transport of vitamin B_{12}, but the only form used by the tissues is that bound to transcobalamin. Measurements of the transcobalamin complex (active vitamin B_{12}, holotranscobalamin) are said to be more specific and sensitive for detecting deficiency than assays for total vitamin B_{12}. Subclinical deficiencies of both folate and vitamin B_{12} increase plasma concentrations of homocysteine, which is a risk factor for cardiovascular disease. Decreased availability of vitamin B_{12} also increases the plasma concentration of methylmalonic acid, whose measurement may be helpful in diagnosing borderline deficiency of the vitamin.

Vitamin C (ascorbic acid)

Ascorbic acid is essential for the hydroxylation of proline residues in **collagen**, and thus for the normal structure and function of this protein. It is a powerful antioxidant and acts by maintaining iron in the hydroxylating enzyme in the reduced (Fe^{2+}) state. Vitamin C also **facilitates the intestinal absorption of dietary non-haem iron** by keeping it in the Fe^{2+} state. Subclinical deficiency of ascorbic acid is quite often present in elderly housebound people. The concentration of ascorbate in plasma reflects recent dietary intake and is a poor index of tissue stores of the vitamin. These are better assessed by determination of ascorbate concentration in leukocytes. In practice, this is seldom necessary, because ascorbic acid is cheap and non-toxic, so a therapeutic trial of vitamin supplementation is the simplest procedure to confirm suspected vitamin C deficiency. (See Case history 8.1.)

Fat-Soluble Vitamins

Vitamin A

Vitamin A is a constituent of the retinal pigment **rhodopsin**. It is also essential for the normal synthesis of **mucopolysaccharides** and growth of **epithelial tissue**. Mild deficiency causes **night blindness**, but in more severe cases degenerative changes in the eye may lead to complete **loss of vision**. The normal liver contains considerable stores of the vitamin, and deficiency is rarely seen in affluent societies. It is, however, an important cause of blindness in many areas of the world.

Vitamin A is present in the diet and can also be synthesized from dietary **carotenes**. It can be measured in plasma, in which it is transported bound to prealbumin and a

---

Case history 8.1

History

An 80-year-old widow was admitted to hospital with bronchopneumonia and obvious self-neglect. She lived alone but had several cats, and a neighbour who had called the doctor said that most of the woman's pension was spent on her pets.

Examination

She had widespread perifollicular haemorrhages.

Management

A clinical diagnosis of scurvy was made. She was given ascorbic acid (500 mg/day) as well as antibiotics. After her pneumonia resolved, she was transferred to a care home where she was given a balanced diet. Her condition improved rapidly, with disappearance of the perifollicular haemorrhages and weight gain.

Discussion

Clinically obvious deficiency of vitamin C is rare, and its development requires a very restricted diet for prolonged periods, without any fresh fruit or vegetables. It is usually associated with more generalized malnutrition, especially in those who live alone or are reclusive. One portion of fresh fruit or vegetables a day is more than enough to prevent scurvy (cooking destroys much of the vitamin C). Some breakfast cereals and drinks are fortified with vitamin C.

---

specific retinol-binding globulin. A low binding protein concentration can cause the plasma concentration of vitamin A to be low and impair its delivery to tissues even when hepatic stores of the vitamin are adequate. Measurements of vitamin A status are rarely required in practice, because deficiency is rare in the western world, but they may be useful (together with vitamin E) for monitoring adequacy of pancreatic enzyme replacement in children with cystic fibrosis (see Chapter 19). In areas of the world where deficiency is endemic, the facilities required to provide laboratory confirmation of the diagnosis are often not available, although the diagnosis is usually obvious clinically.

Vitamin D

Vitamin D is obtained both from endogenous synthesis, by the action of ultraviolet light on 7-dehydrocholesterol in the skin to form cholecalciferol (vitamin D_3) and from the diet. In most individuals, endogenous synthesis is the major source of vitamin D, although in regions such as northern Europe, sunlight exposure is only sufficient to enable synthesis to occur during summer months, with reliance on vitamin D stores and dietary vitamin D in winter. Dietary sources include oily fish, eggs and milk. Some plants, and in particular mushrooms, contain ergocalciferol (vitamin D_2); processed foods including margarine and some breakfast cereals are fortified with this form of the vitamin. Vitamin D supplements may contain either vitamin D_2 or vitamin D_3. The two forms of vitamin D undergo the same metabolic changes in the body and have identical physiological actions, and the term 'vitamin D' is frequently used to refer to both forms of the vitamin.

Vitamin D itself has little physiological activity. It is hydroxylated first in the liver to 25-hydroxyvitamin D (calcidiol) and then in the kidneys to 1,25-dihydroxyvitamin D (calcitriol) (see Fig. 14.4). These metabolites are transported in the circulation by a specific binding protein. 25-Hydroxyvitamin D is the main storage form of the vitamin, principally in adipose tissue. Most of the physiological actions of vitamin D are mediated by calcitriol; its effects on calcium homeostasis and bone metabolism are discussed in Chapter 14.

Vitamin D status can be assessed in the laboratory by measurement of the plasma concentration of 25-hydroxyvitamin D. This undergoes seasonal variation, being higher in the summer than in the winter. The definition of vitamin D sufficiency has been much debated. Concentrations at which there is no biochemical evidence of disturbed calcium homeostasis such as a secondary rise in plasma parathyroid hormone concentrations, and no clinical evidence of adverse effects of insufficiency, are often taken to be optimal. Most authorities worldwide now recommend that a value of >50 nmol/L is **sufficient** for the population as a whole. Plasma 25-hydroxyvitamin D concentrations of <25 nmol/L are associated with an increased risk of rickets or symptomatic osteomalacia and are termed **deficient**. 25-hydroxyvitamin D concentrations in the range 25–50 nmol/L are suboptimal for healthy calcium, muscle and bone metabolism and are termed **insufficient**.

Vitamin D deficiency is seen most frequently in people who have a low dietary intake of the vitamin and decreased endogenous synthesis, such as the elderly who are housebound or institutionalised. It is also seen in the UK in people of south Asian origin, particularly women, in whom the effects of low intake may be exacerbated by decreased production in the skin because of both limited skin exposure to sunlight and darker pigmentation. Binding of calcium in the gut by dietary phytates may also contribute to the osteomalacia to which they are prone. Breast milk contains relatively little vitamin D, and infants are at risk of vitamin D deficiency particularly if premature (the vitamin is transported across the placenta mainly in the last trimester of pregnancy) or if the mother is vitamin D deficient (Case history 8.2).

Vitamin D deficiency due to a combination of decreased synthesis and dietary deficiency is the commonest cause of **rickets** in children and **osteomalacia** in adults, and is frequently associated with muscle pain and weakness as well as bone disease. Other causes include disordered metabolism of vitamin D and malabsorption. The clinical biochemistry of rickets and osteomalacia is considered in more detail in Chapter 15.

Vitamin D insufficiency is increasingly being recognized as a public health concern in Europe and North America, particularly amongst the elderly, pregnant women and some social and ethnic groups, in whom its prevalence has been reported to be as high as 80%. Vitamin D insufficiency (and indeed frank deficiency) is so common in the general population that many authorities now recommend that people who are at risk (e.g. pregnant women, breast-fed babies, people with a dark skin, and the elderly and institutionalised) should take a daily vitamin D supplement; routine measurement of plasma vitamin D concentration is not necessary in most of these people.

Vitamin D insufficiency is strongly associated with decreased bone density and an increased risk of fractures, especially in women. The role of vitamin D is not confined to calcium and bone metabolism: it is also involved in cellular differentiation, particularly of immunocompetent cells. Vitamin D insufficiency has been linked with an increased risk of developing cardiovascular disease, diabetes mellitus, breast and gastrointestinal cancers, infections such as tuberculosis and influenza, autoimmune disorders such as rheumatoid arthritis and possibly multiple sclerosis. Whether vitamin D insufficiency is a direct cause of these disorders is debatable (supplements do not ameliorate the risks), but there is a definite inverse association between vitamin D concentrations and all-cause mortality in the general population.

Vitamin E

Vitamin E (tocopherol) is an important **antioxidant**, particularly in cell membranes, protecting unsaturated fatty acid residues against free radical attack. Clinical deficiency may occur in **severe malabsorption**, particularly in infants. Manifestations include **haemolytic anaemia** and **neurological dysfunction**.

Vitamin K

Vitamin K is required for the γ-carboxylation of glutamate residues in **coagulation factors II (prothrombin), VII, IX and X**. This process confers physiological activity by permitting the binding of calcium to the proteins. Vitamin K deficiency results in an increase in the **prothrombin time**, a functional assay of relevant coagulation

Case history 8.2

A 15-month-old boy, whose parents are of Asian origin, was admitted for investigation of failure to thrive. He was below the tenth centile for length and below the fifth centile for weight. He was not yet walking. He had been exclusively breast-fed because he had refused solid food. There was no history of diarrhoea or vomiting. He had a 26-month-old sister who was fit and well.

Examination

He was very thin but had no organomegaly or other abnormal findings.

Results (see Appendix for reference ranges)

Blood:

haemoglobin	82 g/L
mean corpuscular volume (MCV)	68 fL (78–94)

Plasma:

calcium	1.81 mmol/L
albumin	37 g/L
adjusted calcium	1.87 mmol/L
phosphate	0.86 mmol/L
ferritin	<7 µg/L
25-hydroxyvitamin D	17 nmol/L

Summary

Microcytic anaemia with a low ferritin. Hypocalcaemia, phosphate low for age. Very low 25-hydroxyvitamin D.

Interpretation

The microcytic anaemia is typical of iron deficiency, which is confirmed by the finding of a very low ferritin concentration. The low calcium concentration is a direct result of vitamin D deficiency. The phosphate concentration is low for a child of this age and is a consequence of the secondary hyperparathyroidism that develops with severe vitamin D deficiency.

Discussion

He was given multivitamin and mineral supplements, with extra iron and vitamin D, and was weaned onto appropriate food for his age, after which he began to gain weight.

His mother was investigated subsequently and was also found to be severely iron and vitamin D deficient. She had very little exposure to sunlight. Her first pregnancy probably depleted her of iron and vitamin D and with a second pregnancy a few months after the first, she did not have time to replenish her stores. She had not taken any supplements during pregnancy.

Breast milk may not contain enough vitamin D and iron to provide adequate quantities beyond the first few months of life, especially if the mother is already deficient in these nutrients. In the UK, women are advised to take vitamin D supplements throughout pregnancy, which should provide adequate stores for breastfeeding the baby for the first 6 months after birth. It is common practice to give supplements of vitamins A, C and D to children from the age of 6 months to 5 years.

---

factor activity, although the most frequent use of measurements of prothrombin time (often expressed as the **international normalized ratio (INR)**) is in the monitoring of patients on anticoagulant treatment with antagonists of vitamin K (e.g. warfarin). These clotting factors are synthesized in the liver, and the prothrombin time is also used as a test of liver function.

Vitamin K is produced by gut flora, so deficiency is rarely seen in adults unless there is severe malabsorption. Neonates are at higher risk before gut colonization, and in many places it is routine practice to give vitamin K to newborns.

Vitamins as Drugs

In addition to their long-appreciated role as essential micronutrients, there is evidence that taking some vitamins in supraphysiological amounts may be beneficial. The term 'nutraceuticals' has been used to describe nutrients used pharmacologically. For example, folic acid supplements taken very early in pregnancy have been proven to reduce (although not abolish) the risk of the fetus having a neural tube defect.

Vitamins C and E and β-carotene are antioxidants. Oxidative damage by free radicals may play a role in a range of diseases including cardiovascular disease and cancer. However, clinical trials of vitamin supplements have not consistently shown evidence of benefit. Furthermore, a high intake of vitamins may not be without risk: vitamins A and D are toxic in excess, and even water-soluble vitamins (an excess of which can be excreted in the urine) may be harmful in high amounts. For example, pyridoxine, which has been used in the prophylaxis of premenstrual tension, can be neurotoxic when taken in large doses. High concentrations of biotin (vitamin B_7) in plasma are a cause of spurious results in some immunoassays, such as those used to measure hormones (see p. 2).

The role of high doses of vitamins in the management of some inherited metabolic diseases, is discussed in Chapter 19.

Table 8.1 Trace elements in the human body

Element	Function
chromium	component of chromodulin, (potentiates insulin)
cobalt	component of vitamin B_{12}
copper	cofactor for cytochrome oxidase[b]
fluorine[a]	present in bone and teeth, function unknown
iodine	component of thyroid hormones
iron	component of haem pigments
manganese	cofactor for several enzymes
molybdenum	cofactor for xanthine oxidase
selenium	cofactor for glutathione peroxidase[b]
silicon[a]	present in cartilage, function unknown
zinc	cofactor for many enzymes

[a]Indicates elements that are present but are not known to be essential.
[b]And other enzymes.

Trace Elements

The maintenance of normal health requires provision in the diet not only of adequate protein, energy substrates and vitamins but also of various inorganic salts and trace elements. Trace elements in the body are, by definition, present in concentrations of <100 parts per million (ppm); the elements are listed in Table 8.1. None is required in more than milligram quantities each day, and the daily requirement for some is measurable in micrograms. Consequently, the 'essential' status of some of these trace elements is difficult to confirm.

Trace element deficiency

Deficiencies of trace elements can occur for the same general reasons as vitamin deficiencies. These include severe malnutrition, artificial feeding (especially if prolonged), prematurity and the presence of excessive losses (such as with enterocutaneous fistulae or severe diarrhoea). Multiple deficiencies may occur in these conditions, confusing the clinical picture and making diagnosis difficult.

Trace element toxicity

Toxicity from trace elements is rare but may be found in factory workers exposed to individual elements such as chromium. Excessive oral zinc ingestion causes copper deficiency because it inhibits copper absorption. Long-term parenteral administration of trace elements requires careful monitoring as it bypasses the normal control mechanisms involved in absorption from the gut (see later). Manganese toxicity sometimes occurs during long-term parenteral nutrition (PN), especially in patients with reduced capacity for manganese excretion because of cholestasis. The measurement of plasma chromium and cobalt concentrations in patients with metal-on-metal joint replacements is discussed on p. 376.

Laboratory assessment

The laboratory assessment of the body's trace element status presents a range of difficulties. The concentration of trace elements in plasma is low (μmol/L or lower), and care must be taken to avoid environmental contamination, for example by use of special 'trace element' blood tubes. For some elements, for example manganese, whole blood is preferred because concentrations are higher than in plasma.

The metabolic response to illness, including the acute-phase response (see p. 289), results in a change in the concentration of plasma proteins to which some trace elements are bound, or redistribution of elements into cells, so interpretation must take this into account (see next sections for zinc, copper and selenium). Furthermore, plasma or whole blood concentrations may not accurately reflect the concentration of a trace element at its (usually intracellular) site of action. Trace element deficiency should be anticipated in patients at risk and steps taken to prevent the occurrence of a deficiency syndrome.

Zinc

Zinc is essential for the activity of many enzymes, including several involved in nucleic acid and protein synthesis. The clinical manifestations of **zinc deficiency** include **dermatitis** and **delayed wound healing**; there is, however, no evidence that zinc supplementation accelerates wound healing in patients who are not deficient. Zinc deficiency is a well-recognized potential complication of artificial (particularly parenteral) nutrition if insufficient supplementation is provided. Patients who are catabolic—for example, after trauma or major surgery—**lose large amounts of zinc in the urine** and are at risk of becoming depleted. Severe deficiency is seen in the condition **acrodermatitis enteropathica**, in which there is an inherited defect in intestinal zinc absorption.

Plasma zinc concentrations must be interpreted with caution. Low plasma concentrations are not exclusive to zinc deficiency: they are also seen in conditions such as malignant disease and chronic liver disease without associated clinical evidence of tissue deficiency. Plasma zinc concentrations fall by up to 20% after a meal and also during an acute-phase response, as a result of uptake by the liver. Measurement of C-reactive protein (see p. 289) as an indicator of the acute-phase response may help with the interpretation of plasma zinc concentrations. Because zinc is extensively bound to albumin, plasma zinc concentration should also be considered in relation to that of albumin.

Copper

Copper is essential for the activity of certain enzymes, notably cytochrome oxidase and superoxide dismutase. In the blood, 80% to 90% of copper is present in **caeruloplasmin**. The latter is an acute-phase protein, so plasma concentrations will rise with an inflammatory response. Copper deficiency is uncommon: manifestations include **anaemia** and **leukopenia**. **Wilson disease**, a disorder characterized by excessive tissue deposition of copper, is discussed in Chapter 6.

Selenium

Selenium is required as a prosthetic group for several enzymes, including **glutathione peroxidase**. This, together with the tocopherols (vitamin E), is part of the antioxidant system that protects membranes and other vulnerable structures from oxidative attack by free radicals. These highly reactive species can be generated, for example, as a result of the activation of phagocytic cells or exposure to ionizing radiation. Selenium deficiency is usually only seen as a result of a low intake: it is endemic in some parts of China that have a low soil selenium content, where it has been linked to Keshan disease (cardiomyopathy) and Kashin-Beck disease (osteoarthropathy). It has also been reported in patients on long-term PN. Selenium can be measured in plasma, but results must be interpreted in relation to C-reactive protein, since concentrations fall during the acute-phase response owing to uptake into cells. Measurement of **red cell glutathione peroxidase activity** may provide a better measure of tissue selenium status.

Iodine

Iodine deficiency causes goitre and, if severe, hypothyroidism; it is now uncommon in the developed world, where iodine is sometimes added to salt and dairy products are plentiful, but it is still a problem in some areas. Subclinical iodine deficiency has been identified more recently as a problem in schoolgirls and pregnant women in the UK.

Nutritional Aspects of Anaemia

Anaemia is a reduction in the haemoglobin concentration in the blood, which may be due to reduced or defective red blood cell production, increased red blood cell destruction or loss of cells due to bleeding. One important group of causes of defective red cell production is deficiency of the nutrients iron, vitamin B_{12} and folate, which are collectively termed haematinics. The effects of haematinic deficiencies are, however, not confined to red blood cells; each also has other specific metabolic consequences.

Iron

The total iron content of the adult body is approximately 4 g (70 mmol), of which some two-thirds is in **haemoglobin**. Iron stores (mainly spleen, liver and bone marrow) contain about one-quarter of the body's iron. Most of the remainder is in **myoglobin** and other haemoproteins; only 0.1% of the total body iron is in the plasma, where it is almost all bound to a transport protein, **transferrin**.

Iron absorption and transport

The mean daily intake of iron is about 20 mg (0.36 mmol), but <10% of this is absorbed. The regulation of iron absorption is complex. There are three major influences:

* the state of the body's iron stores (absorption being increased when they are depleted and decreased when they are replete)
* erythropoiesis (absorption is increased when erythropoiesis is increased, irrespective of the state of the iron stores)
* recent iron intake (a dietary iron bolus decreases iron absorption for several days).

The main site of iron absorption is the proximal small bowel (Fig. 8.1). Iron is more readily absorbed in the Fe^{2+} form, but dietary iron is mainly in the Fe^{3+} form. Gastric secretions are important in iron absorption in that they liberate iron from food (although haem can be absorbed intact) and promote the conversion of Fe^{3+} to Fe^{2+}. Ascorbic acid and other reducing substances facilitate iron absorption, whereas phytic acid (in cereals), phosphates and oxalates form insoluble complexes with iron and decrease its absorption.

Iron is transported into enterocytes by the protein divalent metal transporter 1. Once absorbed, it is either transported directly into the bloodstream on the protein **ferroportin 1**, or bound to **apoferritin**, a complex iron-binding protein, to form **ferritin**, which remains within the enterocyte. This iron is lost into the lumen of the gut when mucosal cells are shed. Iron absorption is regulated by **hepcidin**, a peptide hormone that binds to ferroportin and inhibits its

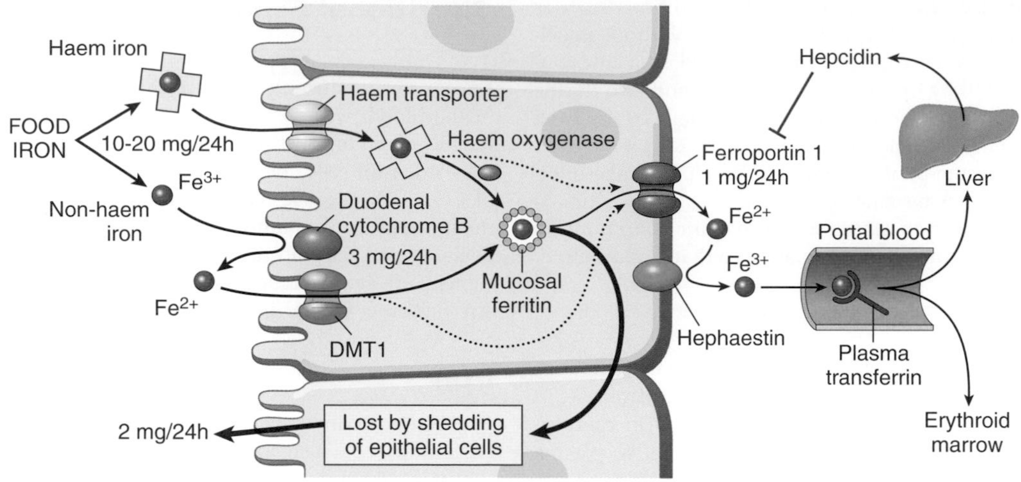

Fig. 8.1 Proximal intestinal iron absorption. Within the lumen, duodenal cytochrome B catalyses the reduction of dietary ferric iron (Fe^{3+}) to ferrous iron (Fe^{2+}); this is facilitated by the presence of gastric acid. Fe^{2+} is absorbed via the divalent metal transporter 1 (DMT1). Haem is absorbed directly across the brush border before release of its iron by haemoxygenase. Intracellular iron is either transported into the blood via ferroportin 1 or converted to mucosal ferritin. After oxidation by hephaestin back to Fe^{3+}, iron is transported to bone marrow or the liver bound to transferrin. Iron absorption is regulated by hepcidin, which is produced by the liver and inhibits ferroportin. Mucosal iron that is not absorbed via ferroportin 1 is ultimately lost back into the intestine in shedding epithelial cells. Modified from Kumar, V., Abbas, A., Aster, J: *Robbins Basic Pathology*. Philadelphia, PA, 2012, Elsevier.

ability to transport iron, thereby increasing the proportion of iron that is shed as ferritin. In iron deficiency, the apoferritin content of mucosal cells decreases and a greater proportion of absorbed iron reaches the bloodstream.

In the blood, iron is transported mainly bound to transferrin, each molecule of which binds two Fe^{2+} ions. Transferrin is normally about one-third saturated with iron. In tissues, iron is bound in ferritin and in haemosiderin, which is an aggregate of partially degraded ferritin particles. Free iron is very toxic, and protein binding allows iron to be transported and stored in a non-toxic form.

Iron is lost from the body in faeces (non-absorbed and shed mucosal iron), by desquamation of skin and, in women, by menstrual blood loss. Endogenous iron loss in men is about 2 mg (36 µmol)/24 h. Very little iron is excreted in the urine.

Investigation of iron deficiency

Iron deficiency may be caused by inadequate intake, impaired absorption, excessive loss or a combination of these. The anaemia that develops is **hypochromic** and **microcytic**. The percentage of red cells that are hypochromic is a particularly useful test for iron deficiency and can be measured by many modern automated haematology analyzers. **Plasma ferritin concentration** is the best non-invasive test for iron deficiency; its use and limitations are described below. Transferrin receptor concentration is another useful test, although it is not widely available. Measurement of plasma iron concentration has only limited clinical value, even when combined with total iron binding capacity in order to calculate transferrin saturation. Ultimately, a diagnosis of iron deficiency is confirmed by demonstrating a response of these parameters to iron therapy.

Plasma iron

Normal plasma iron concentration in men is 9–29 µmol/L; it is marginally lower in women. However, measurement of plasma iron concentration is of little value in the investigation of iron metabolism, except in relation to haemochromatosis and in the diagnosis and management of iron poisoning. A decline in plasma iron concentration is a late feature of iron deficiency, although a raised plasma iron is usually present in iron overload. The concentration of iron in the plasma fluctuates considerably; differences of >20% can occur within a few minutes, and of >100% from one day to the next. Considerable catamenial variation occurs in women. Many conditions, including infection, trauma, chronic inflammatory disorders (especially rheumatoid arthritis) and neoplasia, are associated with low plasma iron concentrations (but normal iron stores), whereas others, for example hepatitis, cause an increase in concentration.

Total iron-binding capacity

Plasma total iron-binding capacity (TIBC) is a functional measure of the total capacity of transferrin to transport iron. The transferrin saturation can then be calculated by dividing the plasma iron concentration by the TIBC: normal values lie between approximately 25% and 45% in adults. Although plasma TIBC is increased in iron deficiency, many other factors can affect it, and transferrin saturation, dependent as it is on the (highly variable) plasma iron concentration, is also highly variable. Although a low saturation is characteristic of iron deficiency, it also occurs in other conditions, such as pregnancy and chronic disease, in the absence of iron deficiency. Transferrin saturation is consistently increased in iron overload, which is the main indication for its measurement.

Plasma ferritin

Measurement of plasma ferritin concentration is superior to plasma iron and iron-binding capacity for the assessment of body iron stores. In healthy individuals, plasma ferritin concentrations are usually within the range 20–300 µg/L. The only known cause of a low concentration is a decrease in body iron stores. Concentrations <20 µg/L indicate depletion, and concentrations <12 µg/L suggest a complete absence of stored iron. However, plasma ferritin concentration is increased during an acute-phase inflammatory response, and patients with iron deficiency may have plasma ferritin concentrations within the reference range (e.g. up to 50–60 µg/L) when they are acutely ill. The same applies to patients with chronic inflammatory conditions (e.g. rheumatoid disease) and chronic kidney disease (CKD). Patients with CKD frequently develop anaemia as a result of impaired utilization of stored iron, but this can coexist with iron deficiency. In CKD, iron deficiency should be considered in any patient with a plasma ferritin concentration of <100 µg/L but results should be interpreted in combination with transferrin saturation; alternative tests, such as the percentage of hypochromic red cells, are superior markers of iron deficiency in this group of patients.

The plasma ferritin concentration is increased in iron overload, for example in haemochromatosis (see p. 118), but may also be increased in some patients with liver disease and certain types of cancer, because of release of the protein from tissues, as well as during an acute-phase inflammatory response. Elevated concentrations should thus be interpreted with caution, although iron overload is excluded if plasma ferritin concentration is normal.

Transferrin receptor

The uptake of transferrin-bound iron into cells is facilitated by a transferrin receptor that is present on the surface of all iron-requiring cells in the body, with the highest number on the surface of erythrocyte precursors in the bone marrow. Receptor binding leads to internalization and uptake into vesicles where the iron is released. Transferrin receptor synthesis is controlled by iron: it is increased in iron deficiency. The plasma concentration increases to two to three times normal when anaemia is present, but the rise occurs only after iron stores become functionally depleted, whereas ferritin concentrations fall earlier, as iron stores fall. The concentration is also increased in conditions in which there is chronically increased erythroid proliferation, for example sickle cell disease and hereditary spherocytosis. Transferrin receptor concentration does not increase significantly in patients with the anaemia of chronic disease; it may have a particularly valuable role in the diagnosis of iron deficiency in chronic inflammatory disease and CKD. However, the test has not been shown to be better than the standard tests of iron status in general clinical practice.

Vitamin B$_{12}$ deficiency

Deficiency of vitamin B$_{12}$ causes **megaloblastic anaemia**, which is characterized by increased red cell mean corpuscular volume (MCV) and mean corpuscular haemoglobin (MCH). Other characteristic haematological findings include hypersegmented nuclei in granulocytes. Other clinical manifestations of vitamin B$_{12}$ deficiency, and its diagnosis, are discussed in more detail on pp. 140–141.

Folate deficiency

Folate deficiency presents with a similar haematological picture to vitamin B$_{12}$ deficiency, although it has a different range of non-haematological manifestations (see p. 140).

Provision of Nutritional Support

Patients who have, or are at risk of developing, nutritional deficiencies require nutritional support. In the case of specific deficiencies, for example of vitamin D, dietary supplementation may be all that is required. Generalized undernutrition, usually encompassing an inadequate intake of protein, energy substrates and micronutrients, requires generalized nutritional support. This should be provided **enterally** (using the gut) wherever possible, but in patients with intestinal failure (see Chapter 7), **parenteral (intravenous) nutrition** is required.

Undernutrition increases the morbidity and mortality of patients in hospitals, yet it is a relatively frequent finding. **Nutritional assessment** should be a routine part of any medical examination, and nutritional support considered for any patient who cannot eat normally. In the

UK, guidelines recommend that outpatients in high-risk groups and all inpatients should be screened for malnutrition using a validated rapid assessment tool, for example, the Malnutrition Universal Screening Tool (available at www.bapen.org.uk).

All forms of nutritional support require careful biochemical monitoring. Laboratory data may contribute to the decision to initiate nutritional support and are essential to the assessment of requirements and for monitoring to ensure adequate provision and avoidance of metabolic complications. Nutritional support is best provided by a multidisciplinary team, including, for example, a clinician, pharmacist, dietitian, specialist nurse and often a clinical biochemist. Such teams are sometimes involved in the care of patients receiving nutritional support in the community as well as in hospital.

Nutritional assessment

Various techniques are available for nutritional assessment, including recording of recent food intake, anthropometric measurements (body height and weight, skinfold thicknesses, midarm muscle circumference), functional measurements (e.g. grip strength) and laboratory measurements, particularly of plasma protein concentrations. Screening tools for malnutrition have been developed that include:

- body mass index (BMI) (weight [kg]/height [m]^2)
- percentage unintentional weight loss
- the time over which nutrient intake has been unintentionally reduced
- the likelihood of impaired nutrient intake in the future.

The diagnosis of severe malnutrition does not require laboratory tests because it is clinically obvious. Neither are they required to confirm a need for nutritional support in patients at risk, for example, after resection of most or all of the small intestine. A plasma albumin concentration <30 g/L is often mistakenly taken as evidence of malnutrition, but plasma albumin concentrations are affected by many pathological processes, and this is a non-specific finding and an insensitive test. In simple starvation, plasma albumin concentrations may remain within reference limits for several weeks (decreased synthesis is accompanied by

a decrease in the rate of catabolism), whereas in septic or catabolic patients the plasma albumin concentration can fall rapidly as a result of increased breakdown and redistribution out of the vascular compartment. Other plasma proteins (e.g. transferrin, retinol-binding protein) show no advantage over albumin as indices of nutritional status in an individual, although they may be useful in population studies. Even combinations of biochemical and anthropometric measurements in 'prognostic nutritional indices' are no better than careful, informed, clinical assessment in determining which patients are likely to benefit from nutritional support.

Techniques for generalized nutritional support

Enteral nutrition is safer, cheaper and usually more convenient for the patient than parenteral feeding. If patients are unable to eat (e.g. cannot swallow as a result of stroke or neurological disease), nutritionally complete liquid feeds can be administered either through a nasogastric tube or, when enteral feeding is likely to be required in the long term, through a **gastrostomy** or **jejunostomy**.

If a patient's complete nutritional requirements cannot be met enterally, parenteral supplementation will be required. Patients with **intestinal failure** will require **parenteral nutrition (PN)**, in which most or all nutritional requirements are met using an intravenously administered admixture of amino acids, glucose, fat, vitamins and minerals. PN is less physiological than enteral nutrition because it bypasses the stomach and delivers nutrition directly into the systemic rather than the hepatic portal circulation. It is good practice, therefore, to provide a small amount of enteral feed if it is tolerated, even if a patient is receiving PN, because it helps maintain **gut barrier function**, preventing the translocation of gut bacteria into the circulation and providing some energy directly to the mucosal cells. Some patients with intestinal failure can absorb sufficient nutrients but not enough water and minerals, particularly if they have fluid losses through an ileostomy. Such patients may require periodic infusion of intravenous fluids such as 0.9% saline with added potassium or magnesium, or both, if necessary. The causes of intestinal failure are summarized in Chapter 7.

In a patient who has previously been well nourished, short-term loss of intestinal function (e.g. caused by ileus after abdominal surgery) is not an indication for PN, but, in general, nutritional support should be instituted if a patient is unlikely to meet his or her calorific requirements for a period longer than 5 days. Preoperative nutritional support in malnourished patients (e.g. before surgery for carcinoma of the oesophagus) should be for at least 7–10 days if it is to improve outcome. However, each patient

All patients admitted to hospital acutely should be screened for malnutrition within 24 hours. The commonly used MUST screening tool is a simple 5-step method that produces a score using body mass index (BMI), unintentional weight loss and presence of acute illness with cessation of normal nutritional intake. Patients with a score of 2 or more should be referred for specialist nutritional support.

must be assessed individually. Patients with irreversible intestinal failure require lifelong PN support and, although this will be initiated in hospital, it can be continued in the patient's home.

Parenteral nutrition

In PN, most or all of a patient's nutritional requirements are compounded together under sterile conditions in a single bag and infused at a steady rate using a pump. The high osmolality of feeds containing high concentrations of glucose as the major source of energy causes irritation to the vascular endothelium. They are therefore usually infused via a central venous catheter with its tip sited in the **superior vena cava**, to allow rapid dilution of the feed with a large volume of blood. This technique is preferred for long-term feeding, but short-term PN can be provided through a **peripheral vein**, particularly if the feed can be compounded using an isotonic fat emulsion as the major energy source. Feeds are usually infused initially over 24 hours, but this limits patients' mobility; patients on PN at home typically infuse their feeds overnight.

Patients' **nutritional requirements** must be assessed individually. Energy requirements can be based on an assessment of basal requirements (e.g. as given by the Harris–Benedict equation) modified to take into account such factors as whether the patient is mobile, pyrexial, catabolic, etc. (all these increase energy expenditure). Energy is usually provided as a mixture of glucose solution and fat emulsion; the latter also provides essential fatty acids. Nitrogen requirements are provided as a balanced mixture of essential and non-essential L-amino acids: maintenance requirements are typically 0.15 g/kg body weight, but more is often appropriate in malnourished or severely ill patients. It is essential to supply sufficient energy as glucose or fat to enable the infused amino acids to be synthesized into protein. The provision of amino acids in excess of metabolic requirement or with insufficient energy may be harmful, increasing the amount of nitrogen that has to be excreted by the kidneys and causing an increase in plasma urea concentration. Typical requirements for the major minerals are indicated in Table 8.2, but many of these can be affected by numerous factors. For example, patients with significant nasogastric aspirates, diarrhoea or fistulae will have increased sodium requirements, whereas these may be decreased in patients with liver disease or kidney failure. Micronutrients are usually provided using commercially prepared mixtures that contain the typical daily requirement, but these may require supplementation, for example, with thiamin, zinc, etc. according to the needs of the individual patient.

Special formulations are available for patients with specific problems, such as high concentrations of branched chain amino acids for patients with liver disease

Table 8.2 Daily composition of a typical parenteral feed for a 60 kg adult

energy	1800 kcal (1000 mL 20% dextrose, 500 mL 20% fat emulsion)
nitrogen	9 g (as L-amino acids)
sodium	60–100 mmol
potassium	40–100 mmol
calcium	5–10 mmol
magnesium	5–10 mmol
phosphate	15–30 mmol
total volume	2.5 L

Note: precise requirements must be determined individually from clinical assessment and laboratory tests. Vitamins and trace elements are usually added in accordance with reference nutritional intake values.

and glutamine-rich feeds for patients in intensive care. Lipid formulations made with mixtures of medium- and long-chain fatty acids may be cleared more rapidly from the circulation and decrease potentially harmful lipid peroxidation. Formulations using a mixture of soya bean and fish oils are less likely to cause cholestasis and long-term liver complications than those with soya bean lipids alone.

Complications of parenteral feeding can be divided into **catheter-related** and **metabolic** complications. Catheter-related complications include damage to nearby structures during placement, infection, venous thrombosis and catheter blockage. Scrupulous adherence to sterile technique is essential during catheter placement and when the feed is changed. Metabolic complications are summarized in Box 8.1. **Refeeding syndrome** can occur in previously malnourished individuals as metabolism changes from a catabolic to an anabolic state, resulting in potentially fatal transcellular shifts of fluids and electrolytes. Cardiac dysrhythmias, respiratory muscle weakness and seizures can ensue. The risk of refeeding syndrome should be assessed before nutritional support is started: those at high risk require a gradual introduction of feeds over several days, ensuring adequate provision of vitamins and electrolytes. An example is given in Case history 8.3.

Severely ill patients sometimes have insulin resistance and become hyperglycaemic if glucose is infused in excess of the capacity for its metabolism. Rebound hypoglycaemia can occur if a feed is stopped suddenly. Hypokalaemia or hyperkalaemia can occur if input is inappropriate: this must be guided by regular monitoring. Mild hyponatraemia (sodium concentration 125–135 mmol/L) is frequent in patients receiving PN. It is often multifactorial and is not on its own an indication for increasing the amount of

Box 8.1 Metabolic complications of parenteral nutrition

hyperglycaemia
hypokalaemia/hyperkalaemia
hyponatraemia/hypernatraemia
hypophosphataemia
hypomagnesaemia
abnormal liver function tests
acidosis
hypoglycaemia on stopping (rarely significant)

Long-term parenteral nutrition

metabolic bone disease
deficiency states
cholestatic liver disease
hepatic steatosis

sodium in the feed. True sodium depletion is rare: it results in intravascular volume depletion and is indicated by the finding of a low urine sodium concentration (provided that renal function is normal). Inadequate clearance of infused triglycerides results in lipaemia, with plasma appearing milky; plasma triglyceride concentrations should be monitored. Liver function tests may become abnormal either because of the underlying disease process or as a direct consequence of PN: a cholestatic pattern is usually due to the lipid component of the infusion, but raised plasma aminotransferase activities may indicate hepatic steatosis, driven by an inappropriately high rate of glucose infusion. These are usually reversible findings, but occasionally patients on long-term PN develop irreversible liver damage.

Laboratory monitoring

Careful clinical monitoring, especially of **weight, fluid status** and **temperature**, is essential during PN. The catheter entry site must be inspected daily for signs of infection. For these reasons, PN should only be provided in areas where nursing staff are trained in its safe administration. The frequency of laboratory monitoring will depend on individual circumstances, including the patient's illness and the requirement to monitor the provision of PN. Monitoring will need to be more frequent during the first few days of PN, if major deficiencies are identified and if a patient's clinical condition is unstable. In stable patients, monitoring can be less frequent; patients on home PN require monitoring only every 6–8 weeks. A guide to the frequency of monitoring, based on UK NICE (National Institute for Health and Care Excellence) guidelines (https://www.nice.org.uk/guidance/cg32), is given in Table 8.3.

If patients are being fed adequately, they will be in neutral (if previously adequately nourished) or positive (if undernourished) nitrogen balance. Albumin has a long half-life and its concentration increases only slowly in response to improved nutrient intake. It is important to be aware that plasma albumin concentrations will remain low in spite of adequate nutrition in patients who have an inflammatory response to their underlying illness or sepsis.

Eating Disorders

Anorexia nervosa is a body dysmorphic disorder characterized by weight loss to <85% of ideal weight, achieved by deliberate food avoidance and sometimes excessive exercise. Females are more commonly affected than males. Patients can become severely emaciated, and treatment requires both psychological and nutritional support. They are at increased risk of developing refeeding syndrome, and thus require close monitoring, especially at the start of treatment. Typical endocrine and biochemical abnormalities associated with anorexia nervosa are shown in Table 8.4. Bulimia nervosa is also characterized by an abnormal body image, but patients tend to alternate between binge eating and periods of starvation to counteract the weight gain. The biochemical abnormalities are similar but tend to be milder than those found in patients with anorexia nervosa.

Obesity

Contrary to a widely held belief among lay people, obesity (defined as a **BMI** [weight/height^2] **exceeding 30 kg/m^2**, the ideal BMI being 18.5–25 kg/m^2) is rarely a consequence of a specific endocrine disorder. Rare hypothalamic disorders can cause hyperphagia as a result of interference with the satiety and appetite centres, but although patients with Cushing syndrome, hypothyroidism and sometimes hypogonadism tend to be **overweight** (BMI 25–30 kg/m^2), they are not usually obese. **Obesity is a common disorder** in developed countries (current prevalence 26% of adults in the UK, with an additional 40% of the population being overweight). Its prevalence is increasing in both developed and developing countries, particularly among children.

Overweight and obesity are a consequence of an intake of energy substrates in excess of requirements, and numerous factors, including genetic, socioeconomic and behavioural, may contribute to this. Elucidation of the mechanisms responsible for controlling food intake may help in our understanding of this common clinical

Case history 8.3

History

A 30-year-old woman with Crohn disease was admitted to hospital with severe diarrhoea and weight loss of 7 kg over the preceding month. Her weight on admission was 36 kg. She was prescribed loperamide and prednisolone, and a tunnelled subclavian catheter was inserted for parenteral feeding. She was started on a PN regimen designed to meet her full estimated nutritional requirements, including 60 mmol potassium and 30 mmol phosphate per 24 h.

Results

Serum:		On admission	After 24 h PN
Serum:	sodium	136 mmol/L	132 mmol/L
	potassium	4.2 mmol/L	2.9 mmol/L
	phosphate	0.9 mmol/L	0.32 mmol/L
	creatinine	48 µmol/L	46 µmol/L
Plasma:	glucose	4.6 mmol/L	9.2 mmol/L

Summary

Acute fall in plasma potassium and phosphate concentrations.

Interpretation

She had normal electrolyte concentrations on admission, but developed acute hypokalaemia and hypophosphataemia consistent with the onset of refeeding syndrome after the rapid increase in carbohydrate input. The rise in glucose was consistent with a degree of glucose intolerance. The low–normal serum creatinine concentration reflects her low muscle bulk.

Discussion

Falls in potassium and phosphate concentrations despite apparently adequate provision in the feed are often seen when PN is started, particularly if the patient's nutritional status is poor. Hypokalaemia and hypophosphataemia are a result of rapid intracellular uptake of these ions, the former in part stimulated by insulin secreted in response to the glucose load and the latter by repletion of cellular high-energy phosphate compounds. Other features of the refeeding syndrome include hypomagnesaemia, hyperglycaemia and circulatory overload; deficiency of thiamin can lead to the Wernicke–Korsakoff syndrome.

Daily biochemical monitoring is essential when patients are first started on PN, both to ensure the adequacy of provision of fluid volume and electrolytes and to detect complications. Glucose intolerance is frequent in catabolic patients and those treated with corticosteroids, and insulin may need to be given to prevent hyperglycaemia.

problem. The **hypothalamus** plays a central role in the regulation of appetite, and a variety of polypeptides and proteins are known that increase or decrease food intake. A selection is shown in Box 8.2; some are hormones, some are neurotransmitters and some appear to fulfil either role depending on where they are synthesized. How these (and other) factors work together to regulate appetite and food intake in the short and long term is an active area of research, not least in the hope of developing acceptable pharmacological approaches to management where dietary and lifestyle intervention fails.

Only one drug is currently licensed for the treatment of obesity in the UK. **Orlistat** is an inhibitor of pancreatic lipase, which decreases the digestion and hence the absorption of dietary fat, allowing modest weight loss. A number of centrally acting drugs that enhance satiety have been used in the past but have been withdrawn from the market because of unacceptable side effects. Replacement treatment with leptin, a peptide produced by fat cells that is involved in appetite control, has proved to be effective in a few obese children with leptin deficiency, but the majority of obese people have high leptin concentrations (reflecting their high fat mass), to which they appear to be resistant, and do not respond to such treatment. One of the more promising recent approaches is the use of glucagon-like peptide-1 (GLP-1) agonists (see p. 225 and 236) which suppress appetite and promote satiety.

Counselling regarding modification of the diet and of eating habits and encouragement of an appropriate level of aerobic exercise are central to the management of obesity. Such modification must be long term: weight lost rapidly is almost inevitably regained. A high degree of personal motivation on the patient's part is essential. Successful lifestyle management requires a multidisciplinary approach, for example, involving physicians, dietitians, psychologists and nurses. Many patients need a continuing high level of support, and the financial implications are considerable.

Surgical intervention can be effective in patients with severe obesity: procedures are of two types: purely restrictive procedures to reduce the size of the stomach and those that also cause a degree of malabsorption (e.g. partial small-intestinal bypass). Part of the effect of the latter may be a reduction in appetite mediated by changes in the secretion of gut hormones. Massive intestinal bypass procedures to produce malabsorption have been abandoned because of unacceptable side effects.

Patients with obesity frequently have hepatic steatosis with abnormal liver function tests (especially an increase

> Patients are at increased risk of refeeding syndrome if their BMI is <16 kg/m^2; they have undergone unintentional weight loss of >15% in the preceding 3–6 months; they have had very little or no nutrient intake for >10 days; they have a history of alcohol abuse; they are oncology patients receiving chemotherapy, or if they have low plasma concentrations of potassium, phosphate or magnesium before initiation of feeding. In such patients, nutritional input must be started at a low rate and built up to full requirements over 4–7 days, with appropriate supplementation of thiamin, other vitamins and trace elements, together with potassium, phosphate and magnesium as required. It is sometimes appropriate to delay feeding until supplementation is underway and electrolyte disturbances have been corrected.

Table 8.3 Frequency of laboratory monitoring in patients receiving parenteral nutrition

Analyte (in plasma/blood)	Frequency
sodium, potassium, glucose[a], magnesium, phosphate, urea, creatinine	daily
liver function tests (including prothrombin time), CRP	twice weekly
calcium, albumin, full blood count, red cell indices	weekly
zinc, copper, folate, vitamin B$_{12}$	2- to 4-weekly
selenium, manganese, vitamin D, iron, ferritin	3- to 6-monthly

All analytes (with the exception of vitamins and minerals, unless there is longstanding undernutrition) should be measured before parenteral nutrition is started, as a guide to the formulation of the feed. The frequency of monitoring can be reduced in patients on long-term parenteral nutrition.
[a]In patients with hyperglycaemia, more frequent measurement of glucose is required.
CRP, C-reactive protein.

Table 8.4 Biochemical and endocrine abnormalities found in patients with anorexia nervosa

Abnormality	Mechanisms
hypokalaemia	vomiting, use of diuretics and laxatives
hypomagnesaemia	as above
hypochloraemic metabolic alkalosis	as above
hyponatraemia	water loading to increase weight before clinic visits
elevated aminotransferase activities	possibly from glutathione depletion
hypothalamo-pituitary axis disturbance amenorrhoea, with low FSH and oestradiol concentrations	suppression of gonadotrophin-releasing hormone
low free T4, T3 concentrations	metabolism diverted to reverse free T3 production
high cortisol concentration	stress response

FSH, follicle-stimulating hormone.

Box 8.2 Some proteins and polypeptides know to modulate appetite

Increase food intake (orexigenic)	Decrease food intake (anorexigenic)
agouti-related peptide	cholecystokinin
ghrelin	cocaine- and amfetamine-related transcript (CART)
neuropeptide Y	glucagon-like peptide 1
	leptin
	melanocortins (α-MSH)
	pancreatic polypeptide
	peptide YY
	oxyntomodulin

in aminotransferases, see p. 113). Other associated abnormalities include hyperuricaemia, hyperlipidaemia and glucose intolerance. Obesity (particularly visceral or abdominal) is a major risk factor for the development of type 2 diabetes mellitus. Obesity causes insulin resistance, probably through multiple and incompletely understood mechanisms, including secretion of adipokines by visceral adipose tissue and a direct toxic effect of lipid accumulation in liver and muscle. There is a clear association between insulin resistance, fasting hypertriglyceridaemia (mainly in very low-density lipoproteins), low plasma high-density lipoprotein–cholesterol concentration and hypertension. This clustering is known as **the metabolic syndrome** and is a major risk factor for coronary heart disease.

SUMMARY

- **Nutritional deficiency syndromes** include those caused by the lack of a single nutrient and those in which there is generalized deficiency.
- Specific laboratory methods are available for the diagnosis of **deficiencies of individual water-soluble vitamins** but, with the exception of those for folic acid and vitamin B_{12}, they are rarely required in clinical practice. Among the **fat-soluble vitamins**, vitamin A deficiency is rare in the developed world, but vitamin D deficiency, leading to rickets and osteomalacia, occurs relatively frequently, particularly in the elderly, premature infants, patients with malabsorption and in certain racial groups. Vitamin D insufficiency is very common. Vitamin K deficiency leads to impairment of blood clotting, with prolongation of the prothrombin time.
- **Deficiencies of trace elements,** such as zinc, copper and selenium, are sometimes difficult to diagnose because plasma concentrations may not accurately reflect tissue status with regard to these elements and are affected by changes in plasma protein concentrations or the inflammatory response to disease.
- **Iron deficiency** is a cause of microcytic anaemia. It is most readily diagnosed by demonstrating a low plasma ferritin concentration, although ferritin concentrations are raised during both acute-phase and chronic inflammatory responses. Deficiencies of **vitamin B_{12}** and **folate** are also nutritional causes of anaemia.
- Patients with **generalized malnutrition** show characteristic, although not specific, biochemical abnormalities, for example, low plasma concentrations of albumin, transferrin and certain other proteins. There may also be evidence of specific deficiencies of vitamins or minerals. These patients require **nutritional support.** This should be enteral wherever possible, that is, using the gut, either by supplementation of the diet or by tube feeding.
- In patients with **intestinal failure**, feeding must be parenteral, i.e. the infusion of nutrients intravenously. There is a risk of metabolic complications—for example, hyperglycaemia, hyperkalaemia or hypophosphataemia and hypokalaemia (**refeeding syndrome**)—but these should be preventable by judicious choice of nutritional regimen and frequent biochemical monitoring. Both biochemical and clinical monitoring are necessary to follow the patient's response to treatment.
- Some essential nutrients can be harmful if taken in excess; if an individual's total energy intake is greater than requirements, obesity will develop. **Obesity** can cause hepatic steatosis and hyperlipidaemia, and is a major risk factor for the development of type 2 diabetes and cardiovascular disease.

Chapter | 9 |

The hypothalamus and the pituitary gland

Introduction

The pituitary gland consists of two parts: the **anterior pituitary**, or adenohypophysis; and the **posterior pituitary**, or neurohypophysis. Although closely related anatomically, they are embryologically and functionally quite distinct. The anterior pituitary comprises primarily glandular tissue, whereas the posterior pituitary is of neural origin. The pituitary gland is situated at the base of the brain, in close relation to the hypothalamus (Fig. 9.1), which has an essential role in the regulation of pituitary function.

Anterior Pituitary Hormones

The anterior pituitary secretes several hormones, some of which are trophic; that is, they stimulate the activity of other endocrine glands (Table 9.1). The secretion of hormones by the anterior pituitary is controlled by hormones secreted by the hypothalamus, which reach the pituitary through a system of portal blood vessels. The secretion of hypothalamic hormones is influenced by higher centres in the brain, and the secretion of both hypothalamic and pituitary hormones is regulated by feedback from the hormones whose production they stimulate in target organs. Most of the blood supply of the anterior pituitary gland is derived from the hypothalamus, ensuring that it is exposed to high concentrations of the hypothalamic hormones. However, the concentrations of these hormones in the systemic circulation are low.

Growth hormone

Growth hormone (GH, somatotrophin) is a 191–amino acid polypeptide hormone. It is **essential for normal growth**, although mainly it acts indirectly by stimulating the liver to produce **insulin-like growth factor-1** (IGF-1), also known as somatomedin-C. IGF-1 has considerable amino acid sequence homology with insulin and shares some of its actions. GH also has a number of **metabolic effects**, which are summarized in Box 9.1. The release of GH is controlled by two hypothalamic hormones: growth hormone-releasing hormone (GHRH) and somatostatin (also known as somatotrophin release-inhibiting factor). IGF-1 exerts negative feedback at the level of the pituitary, where it modulates the actions of GHRH, and at the level of the hypothalamus, where, together with GH itself, it stimulates the release of somatostatin.

The concentration of GH in the blood varies widely through the day and may at times be undetectable (<0.3 µg/L) with currently available assays. Physiological **secretion occurs in sporadic bursts**, lasting for 1–2 hours, mainly during deep sleep. Peak concentrations may be as high as 13 µg/L. The rate of secretion increases from birth to early childhood and then remains stable until puberty, when a massive increase occurs, stimulated by testosterone in males and oestrogens in females; thereafter, the rate of secretion declines to a steady level, before falling to low levels in old age. **Secretion can be stimulated** by stress, exercise, hypoglycaemia, fasting and ingestion of certain amino acids. Such stimuli can be used in provocative tests for diagnosing GH deficiency. GH secretion is inhibited by an increase in blood glucose, and this effect provides the rationale for the use of the oral glucose tolerance test in the diagnosis of excessive GH secretion. **Excessive secretion** (usually caused by a pituitary tumour) causes gigantism in children and acromegaly in adults; **deficiency** causes growth retardation in children, and can cause fatigue, loss of muscle strength, impaired psychological well-being and an adverse cardiovascular risk profile (elevated plasma total and low-density lipoprotein cholesterol concentrations and hyperfibrinogenaemia) in adults.

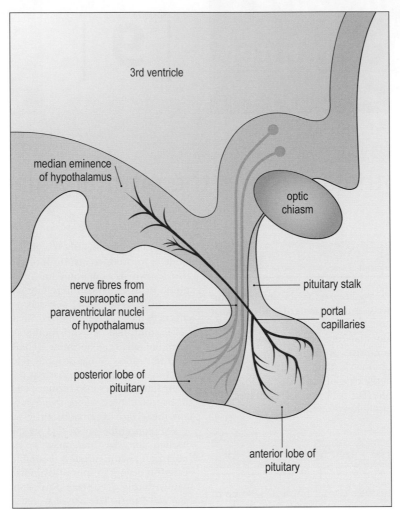

Fig. 9.1 Diagrammatic sagittal section through part of the brain to show the anatomical relationship of the pituitary gland and hypothalamus. The portal blood vessels, through which hypothalamic hormones reach the anterior pituitary, and nerve fibres, which transport hypothalamic hormones to the posterior pituitary, are shown.

Somatostatin, the 14–amino acid hypothalamic peptide that inhibits GH secretion, has many other actions, both within the hypothalamo-pituitary axis and elsewhere. For example, it inhibits the release of thyroid-stimulating hormone (TSH) in response to thyrotrophin-releasing hormone (TRH), and it is present in the gut and pancreatic islets, where it inhibits the secretion of many gastrointestinal hormones, including gastrin, insulin and glucagon. The physiological significance of these actions is poorly understood. Rare somatostatin-secreting tumours of the pancreas have been described, and somatostatin secretion can also occur from medullary carcinomas of the thyroid and small cell carcinomas of the lung. Somatostatin analogues are used therapeutically to stop bleeding from oesophageal varices (an unlicensed indication in the UK), to inhibit hormone secretion by tumours and to treat acromegaly. A third hormone, ghrelin, also affects GH secretion. The main site of its production is the stomach, and it is involved in the regulation of appetite (see Box 8.2), but it is also produced in the hypothalamus and stimulates GH secretion.

Prolactin

Prolactin is a 199–amino acid polypeptide hormone, which circulates in monomeric and various polymeric forms. Its principal physiological action is to initiate and sustain lactation. It also has a role in breast development in females; at high concentrations, it inhibits

Table 9.1 Anterior pituitary hormones and their actions

Hormone	Target organ	Action
growth hormone (GH)	liver others	IGF-1 (somatomedin-C) synthesis, hence growth stimulation metabolic regulation
prolactin	breast	lactation
thyroid-stimulating hormone (TSH)	thyroid	thyroid hormone synthesis and release
follicle-stimulating hormone (FSH)	ovary, testis	oestrogen synthesis oogenesis spermatogenesis
luteinizing hormone (LH)	ovary, testis	ovulation corpus luteum, hence progesterone production testosterone synthesis
adrenocorticotrophic hormone (ACTH)	adrenal cortex skin	glucocorticoid synthesis and release pigmentation
β-lipotropin		precursor of endorphins

IGF-1, insulin-like growth factor-1.

Box 9.1 Metabolic actions of growth hormone

increases lipolysis (hence ketogenic)
increases hepatic glucose production and decreases tissue glucose uptake (hence diabetogenic)
increases protein synthesis (hence anabolic)

---

the synthesis and release of gonadotrophin-releasing hormone (GnRH) from the hypothalamus, and thus gonadotrophins from the pituitary, inhibiting ovulation in females and spermatogenesis in males. Prolactin secretion is controlled by the hypothalamus through the release of dopamine, which normally exerts an inhibitory effect. There is no known specific hypothalamic prolactin-releasing hormone in humans. Although both TRH and vasoactive intestinal polypeptide (VIP) stimulate prolactin secretion, it is not thought that this is physiologically important. The principal **physiological stimuli** to prolactin secretion are pregnancy and suckling. **Increased prolactin secretion** occurs with prolactin-secreting tumours and is also frequently seen with other pituitary tumours if they obstruct blood flow from the hypothalamus, and thus the dopamine-dependent inhibition of prolactin secretion. In the absence of dopamine, prolactin secretion is autonomous.

The secretion of prolactin is pulsatile, increases during sleep, after meals, after exercise and with stress (both physical and psychological), and, in females, is dependent on oestrogen status, making it difficult to define an upper reference limit for plasma prolactin concentration. A plasma prolactin concentration of ~700 mIU/L is often regarded as a threshold above which further investigation may be necessary, but this may vary between laboratories depending on the analytical method in use. There is no useful lower reference value for plasma prolactin concentration. Its secretion increases during pregnancy, but concentrations fall to normal within approximately 7 days after birth if a woman does not breast-feed. With breast-feeding, concentrations start to decline after about 3 months, even if breast-feeding is continued. The consequences of hyperprolactinaemia are discussed on p. 168. Prolactin deficiency is uncommon but does occur, for example, with pituitary infarction: its principal manifestation is failure of lactation.

Thyroid-stimulating hormone

TSH (thyrotrophin) is a glycoprotein (molecular mass, 28 kDa) composed of an α- and a β-subunit; the amino acid composition of the α-subunit is common to TSH, the pituitary gonadotrophins and human chorionic gonadotrophin (hCG), but the β-subunit is unique to TSH.

The reference range for plasma TSH concentrations is ~0.3–4.0 mIU/L. TSH binds to specific receptors on thyroid cells and in doing so stimulates the synthesis and secretion of thyroid hormones. Secretion of TSH is stimulated by the hypothalamic tripeptide TSH-releasing (or thyrotrophin-releasing) hormone (TRH); this effect, and probably the release of TRH itself, is inhibited by high circulating concentrations of thyroid hormones (see Fig. 11.2).

Macroprolactin

Macroprolactin is a macromolecular complex of prolactin and IgG antibody. The prolactin in the macroprolactin complex is not biologically active, but it is detected by most prolactin immunoassays and, therefore, contributes to the total measured plasma concentration of prolactin. Macroprolactin remains in the plasma for longer than uncomplexed (monomeric) prolactin and, therefore, results in an increase in plasma prolactin concentration even though the patient has no clinical consequences of hyperprolactinaemia.

Approximately 15% of cases of hyperprolactinaemia are a result solely of the presence of macroprolactin, although its presence does not rule out a true increase in monomeric prolactin. Laboratories can detect the presence of macroprolactin by methods that remove macromolecular complexes from plasma by precipitation. By such means it is possible to estimate the amount of biologically active monomeric prolactin present. Many laboratories automatically screen for macroprolactin when a patient is found to have an increased plasma prolactin concentration for the first time, but if not, the clinician should request this if the reported prolactin result is not consistent with the clinical findings.

Thus, **thyroid hormone secretion is regulated by a negative feedback** system: if plasma concentrations of thyroid hormones decrease, TSH secretion increases, stimulating thyroid hormone synthesis; if they increase, TSH secretion is suppressed. TSH can take up to 12 weeks to respond fully to changes in plasma thyroid concentration. In primary hypothyroidism, TSH secretion is increased; in hyperthyroidism, it is decreased. TSH deficiency can cause hypothyroidism, but hyperthyroidism caused by TSH-secreting tumours is rare (see Chapter 11).

Gonadotrophins

Follicle-stimulating hormone (FSH) and luteinizing hormone (LH) are both glycoproteins with a molecular mass of ~30 kDa, consisting of two subunits, α and β. The β-subunits are unique to each hormone, but the α-subunits are the same and are also present in TSH and hCG. The **synthesis and release** of both hormones are stimulated by the hypothalamic decapeptide GnRH, with these effects being modulated by circulating gonadal steroids. GnRH is secreted episodically, resulting in pulsatile secretion of gonadotrophins with peaks in plasma concentration occurring at approximately 90-min intervals.

In **males**, LH stimulates testosterone secretion by Leydig cells in the testes. Some of the testosterone is converted to oestradiol in the Leydig cells and in adipocytes. Both testosterone and oestradiol feed back to block the action of GnRH on LH secretion. FSH, in concert with high intra-testicular testosterone concentrations, stimulates spermatogenesis; its secretion is inhibited by inhibin (Fig. 9.2), a hormone produced during spermatogenesis.

In **females**, the relationships are more complex. Oestrogen (mainly oestradiol) secretion by the ovaries is stimulated primarily by FSH during the first part of the menstrual cycle; both hormones are necessary for the development of Graafian follicles. As oestrogen concentrations in the blood rise, FSH secretion declines until oestrogens trigger a positive feedback mechanism, causing an explosive release of LH and, to a lesser extent, FSH. The increase in LH stimulates ovulation and development of the corpus luteum, but rising concentrations of oestrogens and progesterone then inhibit FSH and LH secretion; inhibin from the ovaries also appears to inhibit FSH secretion. If conception does not occur, declining concentrations of oestrogens and progesterone from the regressing corpus luteum trigger menstruation and the release of LH and FSH, initiating the maturation of further follicles in a new cycle (Fig. 9.3). Before puberty, plasma concentrations of LH and FSH are very low and unresponsive to exogenous GnRH. With the approach of puberty, FSH secretion increases before that of LH.

Increased concentrations of gonadotrophins are seen in ovarian failure in females, whether pathological or after the natural menopause. FSH is the preferred test for menopause, if one is required, as the FSH rise is both higher than and precedes that of LH. High concentrations of FSH are seen in azoospermic males, and LH is increased if testosterone secretion is decreased.

Gonadotrophin-secreting tumours (secreting either LH or FSH) of the pituitary are rare. **Decreased gonadotrophin secretion**, leading to secondary gonadal failure, is more common. It can be either an isolated phenomenon, caused by hypothalamic dysfunction, or occur with generalized pituitary failure (see Chapter 12).

Adrenocorticotrophic hormone

Adrenocorticotrophic hormone (ACTH) is a polypeptide (molecular mass, 4500 Da), comprising a single chain of 39 amino acids. Its **biological function**, which is to stimulate adrenal glucocorticoid (but not mineralocorticoid) secretion, is dependent on the N-terminal 24 amino acids. ACTH is a fragment of a much larger precursor, **proopiomelanocortin** (POMC; molecular mass, 31 kDa) (Fig. 9.4), which is the precursor not only of ACTH but also of β-lipotropin, itself the precursor of endogenous opioid peptides (endorphins), and melanocyte-stimulating hormones. Melanocyte-stimulating hormones stimulate melanin production by melanocytes; genetic variability in the melanin pathway is associated with the diversity of human pigmentation and susceptibility to melanoma. ACTH release is controlled by a hypothalamic peptide, corticotrophin-releasing hormone

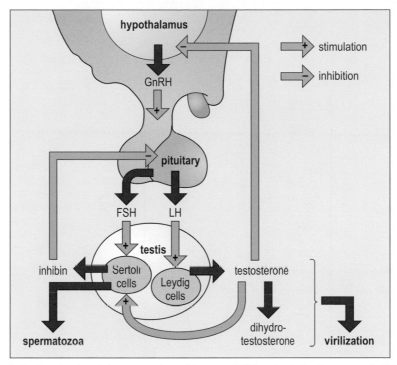

Fig. 9.2 Control of testicular function by pituitary gonadotrophins. FSH, follicle-stimulating hormone; GnRH, gonadotrophin-releasing hormone; LH, luteinizing hormone.

(CRH). ACTH secretion is pulsatile and also shows **diurnal variation**, the plasma concentration being highest at approximately 8:00 a.m. and lowest at midnight. Secretion is greatly increased by stress and is inhibited by cortisol. Thus, cortisol secretion by the adrenal cortex is controlled by negative feedback, but this and the circadian variation can be overcome by the effects of stress. The normal value for plasma ACTH concentration at 9:00 a.m. is <50 ng/L.

Increased secretion of ACTH by the pituitary is seen with pituitary tumours (Cushing disease) and in primary adrenal failure (Addison disease). The hormone may also be secreted ectopically by non-pituitary tumours. Excessive ACTH synthesis is associated with increased pigmentation, because of the melanocyte-stimulating action of ACTH and other POMC-derived peptides. **Decreased secretion** of ACTH may be an isolated phenomenon but is more commonly associated with generalized pituitary failure.

Measurement of Anterior Pituitary Hormones

Measurements of pituitary hormone concentrations are required in both suspected hypofunction and hyperfunction

(the latter is usually the result of a pituitary tumour and is often accompanied by partial hypofunction of other pituitary cell types). **The investigation of suspected pituitary hypofunction should begin with measurement of pituitary and target organ hormones in a blood sample taken at 09:00 a.m.** TSH deficiency will be apparent from a low free thyroxine concentration without the elevation of TSH characteristic of primary hypothyroidism. Plasma TSH concentration may be normal or low in hypopituitarism: it is rarely undetectable.

In males with hypopituitarism, plasma testosterone concentration is low, and LH and FSH concentrations are normal or low. Like cortisol, testosterone demonstrates diurnal variation so should only be measured soon after waking. In premenopausal females, amenorrhoea with a low plasma oestradiol concentration and normal or low gonadotrophins suggests hypothalamic or pituitary dysfunction. A normal ovulatory plasma progesterone concentration (see p. 220) indicates the integrity of the hypothalamo–pituitary–ovarian axis without the need for further testing; a history of regular, normal menstrual cycles also effectively excludes gonadotrophin deficiency. In healthy postmenopausal women, plasma gonadotrophin concentrations increase markedly in response to decreasing ovarian function; in hypopituitarism, they are normal or low.

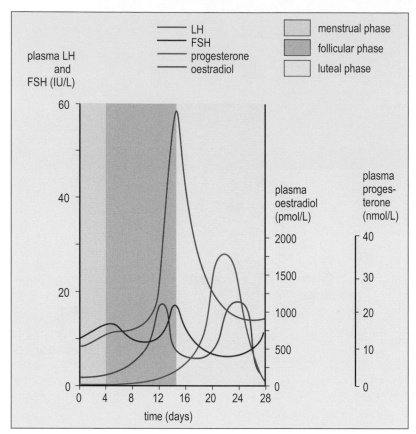

Fig. 9.3 Changes in the plasma gonadotrophin concentrations during the menstrual cycle, together with the resultant changes in oestradiol and progesterone concentrations. FSH, follicle-stimulating hormone; LH, luteinizing hormone.

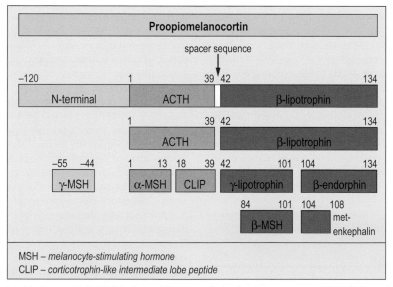

Fig. 9.4 Adrenocorticotrophic hormone (ACTH) is derived by proteolysis of a precursor, proopiomelanocortin, as are β-lipotropin, itself the precursor of endorphins and enkephalins, and melanocyte stimulating hormone.

Releasing hormone tests

Tests involving the administration of TRH and GnRH followed by measurement of TSH and gonadotrophins have traditionally been used in the investigation of pituitary disease, often combined with the insulin hypoglycaemia test (IHT). However, the use of these tests has been criticized on the grounds that the responses to these releasing hormones reflect only the readily releasable pituitary pools of the hormones concerned and do not assess the physiological integrity of the pituitary. Normal responses can occur in spite of other evidence of pituitary hypofunction. The response to the releasing hormones is often delayed in patients with hypothalamic, as opposed to pituitary, dysfunction, but such delayed responses can also occur in pituitary disease. In practice, the releasing hormone tests often add little to what can be deduced from clinical observation and the results of basal hormone measurements; furthermore the pharmacological preparations can be difficult to source.

Insulin hypoglycaemia test

In the IHT, the stress of insulin-induced hypoglycaemia is used to assess the secretion of GH and ACTH by the pituitary (in practice, cortisol is usually measured for the reasons explained earlier and because the assay of ACTH is technically more demanding). The test is **potentially hazardous** because of the possible sequelae of hypoglycaemia; hence it requires medical supervision and is contraindicated in patients with a history of fits or ischaemic heart disease. It should not be performed in patients whose 9:00 a.m. plasma cortisol concentration is low. In children, it should only be performed in specialized units. Concentrated dextrose solution must be available for immediate administration should severe hypoglycaemia develop, but this does not invalidate the results of the test. The stress needs to be only very brief to be effective. It is important that hypoglycaemia is achieved, because if it does not occur, a lack of response might be because of the inadequacy of the stimulus rather than pituitary failure. If hypoglycaemia does not develop, a further dose of insulin must be given. The test can be combined with releasing hormone tests, although, as discussed, the results of these tests often provide little additional useful information. When the induction of hypoglycaemia is contraindicated, glucagon can be used to stimulate cortisol and GH secretion instead of insulin. The protocol for a combined anterior pituitary hormone test using both releasing hormones and hypoglycaemia is given in Fig. 9.5 and the interpretation discussed below.

Tests for growth hormone deficiency

Because GH is secreted sporadically, it may be undetectable in the plasma of healthy individuals. Thus, even though a concentration >5 μg/L in a single sample excludes significant deficiency, a low concentration is not necessarily indicative of deficiency. GH secretion can be assessed using the IHT: a peak plasma concentration <5 μg/L after adequate hypoglycaemia (blood glucose concentration <2.2 mmol/L) is reliable evidence of GH deficiency.

Because the IHT is potentially hazardous, various other tests of GH secretion have been devised, involving the administration of, for example, GHRH with arginine, glucagon or L-DOPA, although the relevance of these pharmacological stimuli to the physiological secretion of GH is questionable. GH concentrations >5 μg/L are usually regarded as excluding GH deficiency, but lesser responses are not conclusive evidence of deficiency. Vigorous exercise also stimulates GH secretion, but even with standardized protocols an apparently subnormal response may not indicate GH deficiency. More reliable information may be provided by serial measurement of GH secretion over a 24-h period, through an indwelling cannula, but there are obvious practical drawbacks to this procedure.

Measurements of IGF-1 have a role in conjunction with GH stimulation tests in the investigation of suspected GH deficiency but are not reliable on their own. A low plasma concentration of IGF-1, together with an impaired or absent GH response to stimulation, confirms GH deficiency. Some patients who appear clinically to have GH deficiency have normal or elevated plasma GH concentrations but, because of a receptor or intracellular signalling defect, are resistant to its action. This condition is known as Laron syndrome (or Laron-type dwarfism): patients have low plasma IGF-1 concentrations. Notably, although plasma IGF-1 concentrations are much less variable than those of GH, they do vary with age and nutritional status: measured values should always be assessed with reference to age- and sex-matched reference values. The IGFs are carried in the plasma bound to IGF-binding proteins (IGFBPs), and measurement of IGFBP-3, whose synthesis is stimulated by GH, may be a better marker of GH deficiency in children.

Tests for adrenocorticotrophic hormone deficiency

The integrity of the hypothalamo–pituitary–adrenal axis can also be tested using the IHT (see Fig. 9.5). A rise in plasma cortisol concentration to at least 550 nmol/L after adequate hypoglycaemia is generally considered to indicate a normal axis (thresholds are laboratory specific due to differences between the analytical method used). It has been shown that if the basal (9:00 a.m.) plasma cortisol concentration is <100 nmol/L, the cortisol response to hypoglycaemia is never normal, whereas it invariably is normal if the basal concentration is >500 nmol/L. A formal IHT

161

Combined test of anterior pituitary function

Procedure

1. Fast patient overnight and weigh

2. Insert and heparinize i.v. cannula

3. Draw and discard 1 mL of blood before collecting each sample and heparinize cannula after each sample is drawn

4. After 30 min take basal blood sample and analyze for glucose, cortisol (or ACTH), FSH, LH, TSH, free thyroxine, GH and testosterone/oestradiol

5. Give 200 µg TRH, 100 µg GnRH and 0.15 U/kg body weight soluble insulin

6. Take blood samples for analysis as follows:

time (min)	assay				
	glucose	cortisol	FSH, LH	TSH	GH
0	*	*	*	*	*
15	*				
20			*	*	
30	*	*			*
45	*				
60	*	*	*	*	*
90	*	*			*
120	*	*			*

7. Repeat insulin dose at 45 min if patient has not become clinically hypoglycaemic (plasma glucose <2.2 mmol/L) and extend sampling accordingly

Normal response

cortisol	increment peak	>200 nmol/L >550 nmol/L (the same criteria apply if glucagon is used)
GH	peak	>5 µg/L
FSH	peak	>1.5 times basal concentration
LH	peak	>5 times basal concentration
TSH	increment	≥2 mIU/L (elderly) ≥5 mIU/L (young adults)

Fig. 9.5 Combined test (triple-bolus test) of anterior pituitary function. Note that hormone concentrations constituting a normal response may vary depending on assay used. In patients thought very likely to be hypopituitary, the insulin dose should be 0.1 U/kg body weight; in patients with Cushing disease or acromegaly, a dose of 0.3 U/kg may be needed. When glucagon (1 mg i.m.) is used instead of insulin, blood samples for cortisol and growth hormone (GH) should be taken at 30-min intervals from 90 to 240 min after the injection (GH and cortisol responses occur later than when insulin is used). ACTH, adrenocorticotrophic hormone; FSH, follicle-stimulating hormone; GnRH, gonadotrophin-releasing hormone; i.v., intravenously; LH, luteinizing hormone; TRH, thyrotrophin-releasing hormone; TSH, thyroid-stimulating hormone.

Table 9.2 **Main clinical features of hypopituitarism**		
Hormone	**Features of deficiency**	
GH	children:	growth retardation
	adults:	decreased muscle bulk and strength, impaired psychological well-being, osteopenia, atherogenic lipid profile, increased abdominal fat, any tendency towards hypoglycaemia may be accentuated
prolactin	failure of lactation	
gonadotrophins	children:	delayed puberty
	women:	oligomenorrhoea, infertility, atrophy of breasts and genitalia
	men:	impotence, azoospermia, testicular atrophy
	both sexes:	decreased libido, loss of body hair, fine wrinkling of skin, skin flushing
ACTH	weight loss, weakness, hypotension, hypoglycaemia and other features of glucocorticoid deficiency, usually of insidious onset unless stressed; decreased skin pigmentation; loss of pubic and axillary hair in women	
TSH	weight gain, cold intolerance, fatigue, constipation and other features of hypothyroidism	
vasopressin	thirst, polyuria	
ACTH, adrenocorticotrophic hormone; GH, growth hormone; TSH, thyroid-stimulating hormone.		

therefore may not be necessary in patients whose basal plasma cortisol concentrations are outside the range of 100–500 nmol/L. The short ACTH stimulation test (tetracosactide or Synacthen test, see p. 179), used primarily in the investigation of adrenal failure, has also been advocated as a test for ACTH deficiency. This may seem illogical, but the rationale is that ACTH deficiency causes adrenal atrophy and thus decreases adrenal responsiveness to ACTH. The results of the IHT and short ACTH stimulation tests correlate well: a plasma cortisol concentration >550 nmol/L 60 min after the administration of synthetic ACTH (250 μg intravenously [i.v.]) excludes ACTH deficiency.

Prolactin secretion is increased by stress, but in practice, the measurement of prolactin in an IHT adds nothing to the information provided by a single basal measurement.

Imaging the pituitary

Once a pituitary disorder has been diagnosed on the basis of the clinical findings and laboratory investigations, imaging techniques are used to provide essential anatomical information. Computed tomography (CT) allows visualization of the bony structures in the vicinity of the pituitary, but magnetic resonance imaging (MRI) is superior for imaging the soft tissues. Formal assessment and documentation of the visual fields are also essential, because pituitary tumours can extend to damage the optic pathways.

Disorders of Anterior Pituitary Function

Hypopituitarism

Hypopituitarism can result from **hypothalamic or pituitary disease** (Table 9.2 and Case history 9.1). Tumours of the pituitary are the more common cause. Partial hypopituitarism is seen more frequently than complete loss of pituitary function. When the tumour cells are functional, clinical features of hormone excess may also be present. The presenting features depend on several factors, including the extent and severity of the hormone deficiencies. Decreased GH secretion is an early feature of pituitary failure, but although its effects can be dramatic in children, they are less obvious in adults. In general, **GH and gonadotrophin secretion (LH before FSH) are affected before that of ACTH.** It is uncommon for hypothyroidism to be the presenting feature of pituitary failure. Isolated deficiency of some of the anterior pituitary hormones can occur, but this is usually congenital and in most instances is due to failure of secretion of the relevant hypothalamic hormone. Haemorrhage into a pituitary tumour can cause 'pituitary apoplexy'. The onset is sudden, usually with headache, signs of meningism, loss of vision and reduced consciousness. Immediate treatment with intravenous fluids and hydrocortisone is required, often followed by surgery. Some of the many causes and clinical features of hypopituitarism are indicated in Box 9.2 and Table 9.2.

163

Box 9.2 Main causes of hypopituitarism

Infection
meningitis (especially tuberculous)
syphilis

Tumours
pituitary (adenoma, craniopharyngioma)
cerebral (primary, secondary)

Vascular disease
postpartum necrosis (Sheehan syndrome)
infarction (especially of tumours)
severe hypotension
cranial arteritis

Infiltration/deposition/inflammation
granulomatous disease (sarcoidosis, histiocytosis X)
haemochromatosis
lymphocytic hypophysitis

Trauma

Iatrogenic
surgery
therapeutic skull irradiation (in malignancy)
prolonged treatment with glucocorticoids or thyroid
    hormones (isolated ACTH and TSH suppression
    respectively)

Hypothalamic disorders
functional disturbances e.g. anorexia nervosa
    and starvation (reversible hypogonadotrophic
    hypogonadism)
all of the above (e.g. tumours, deposition, trauma,
    radiotherapy)
genetic (isolated releasing hormone deficiencies e.g. GHRH)

Suspected anterior pituitary hypofunction is investigated using the tests described previously. It may be accompanied by hypofunction of the posterior pituitary (causing diabetes insipidus); the investigation of this condition is discussed on p. 170. Diabetes insipidus is uncommon, except with large pituitary tumours that invade the hypothalamus, but can develop, often transiently, after surgery. Even in patients with impaired vasopressin (antidiuretic hormone [ADH]) secretion, diabetes insipidus may not be apparent if ACTH secretion is also impaired, because cortisol, the secretion of which is dependent on ACTH, is necessary for normal water excretion. The role of the laboratory in the monitoring of GH replacement is discussed later; replacement treatment in gonadotrophin, ACTH and TSH deficiency is discussed in the chapters dealing with their respective target organs.

Anorexia nervosa, a disorder characterized by self-imposed starvation as a result of a preoccupation with (and impaired perception of) body size, may clinically resemble hypopituitarism (see p.150). Amenorrhoea, caused by decreased gonadotrophin secretion, is common to both conditions. However, pubic and axillary hair, which may be lost in hypopituitarism, is normal in anorexia nervosa, and there may even be additional (lanugo) hair on the body. The weight loss of anorexia nervosa is usually severe in comparison with that which typically occurs in hypopituitarism. Plasma cortisol and GH concentrations tend to be elevated in anorexia nervosa (see Table 8.4).

Growth hormone deficiency

GH deficiency is an uncommon but important cause of growth retardation; other causes are summarized in Chapter 22. GH may be undetectable in the plasma in normal children, which means that, although a random concentration >5 µg/L excludes significant deficiency, a low concentration in a random blood sample is of no diagnostic value: dynamic testing (see earlier) is essential for this.

GH deficiency is treated with regular injections of biologically synthesized human GH. In adults with GH deficiency, treatment with GH improves body composition (increased muscle mass and decreased adipose tissue) and general quality of life. It results in improvements in bone mineral density, cardiovascular risk profile and psychological well-being. In the UK, treatment of adults with GH is recommended only in severe deficiency, and should be discontinued if it is of no demonstrable benefit. GH status should be monitored by regular measurement of plasma IGF-1 concentrations, which should be maintained within their age-adjusted reference range. Clinical assessment should comprise both physiological measurements, including blood pressure, weight and waist/hip ratio, and assessment of quality of life. A plasma lipid profile and fasting glucose or HbA_{1c} should be measured annually. Bone mineral density should be monitored regularly, especially if low at diagnosis. GH is not recommended to promote anabolism in patients with critical illness; increased mortality has been reported in some studies of such treatment. Its use to increase muscle mass in the absence of evidence of deficiency (e.g. in weightlifters) is inadvisable, because harmful side effects can result.

Pituitary tumours

Pituitary tumours may be purely destructive but are often functional, producing **excessive quantities of a hormone.**

Case history 9.1

History

A 50-year-old man was brought in by ambulance having tripped and fallen down a flight of stairs, losing consciousness for a few seconds. He frequently felt dizzy when getting out of bed in the morning. Over the preceding 12 months he had suffered loss of libido and found it necessary to shave less frequently than before; he had also noticed some loss of axillary and pubic hair.

Examination

There was no sign of physical injury.

Imaging investigations

A CT head scan showed enlargement of the pituitary fossa.

Results (see Appendix for reference ranges)

Serum:	cortisol (9:00 a.m.)	200 nmol/L
	GH	<0.3 µg/L
	free thyroxine	9.8 pmol/L
	TSH	2 mIU/L
	Testosterone	4 nmol/L
	LH	<1.5 IU/L
	FSH	<1.0 IU/L
	Prolactin	<50 mIU/L

Combined glucagon, TRH and GnRH stimulation test:

Serum:	cortisol (maximum)	350 nmol/L at 120 min
	LH, FSH	no increment over basal values
	GH	no increment over basal value
	TSH	suboptimal increment

Summary

GH, gonadotrophin, testosterone and prolactin concentrations are all low; the cortisol and thyroxine concentration are in the lower part of the normal range. These hormones show little or no response to appropriate stimuli.

Interpretation

Typical clinical and biochemical features of hypopituitarism (see Table 9.2). (Note that the addition of TRH and GnRH to glucagon stimulation has added little extra information.) The low testosterone is secondary to the lack of gonadotrophins.

Discussion

Cortisol replacement therapy was started immediately, followed by testosterone and thyroxine. Within a few hours, the patient became polyuric and signs of water depletion developed. His serum sodium concentration, which was low on admission (128 mmol/L), rose to 149 mmol/L. Diabetes insipidus, caused by impaired release of vasopressin, can be masked by simultaneous cortisol deficiency and revealed when replacement therapy is started. Synthetic vasopressin was given, which controlled his polyuria.

He subsequently underwent surgery, and a chromophobe adenoma was successfully removed. On follow-up, there was no evidence of recovery of pituitary function and he remained on replacement therapy.

Even tumours that appear to be non-functional may secrete small (clinically insignificant) quantities of the glycoprotein pituitary hormones or just the α-subunit. Non-functional tumours usually present in patients older than 60 years. The order of frequency with which increased hormone secretion occurs in patients with pituitary tumours is **prolactin** (about 25% of all tumours), **GH** and **ACTH**; **gonadotrophin** or **TSH**-secreting tumours are rare. Any pituitary tumour may cause clinical features because of the destruction of normal pituitary tissue (i.e. hypopituitarism) and the effects of intracranial space-occupying lesions, resulting in headache, vomiting and papilloedema. Visual field defects (often bitemporal hemianopia) may develop when an upward-growing tumour impinges on the optic chiasm; occasionally a patient's sight may be threatened.

Growth hormone excess: acromegaly and gigantism

Acromegaly and gigantism are usually (95% of cases) the result of **excessive GH secretion** by a pituitary tumour. Acromegaly is an occasional feature of multiple endocrine neoplasia type 1 (see Box 20.2). Approximately 5% of cases are the result of ectopic secretion of GHRH (e.g. by a bronchial carcinoid tumour). Excessive GH secretion causes increased growth of soft tissues and bone. If this occurs before the epiphyses have fused, continued growth of long bones occurs, leading to gigantism. More commonly, GH-secreting tumours occur in adults, producing acromegaly, with increased growth of soft tissues, hands, feet, jaw and internal organs. The GH concentration in a random

165

History

A 10-year-old boy was referred to hospital for investigation of short stature. He had always been small, but his parents became worried when his 7-year-old brother overtook him in height. He had only grown 3 cm since his height had been measured 3 years previously but was otherwise well.

Examination

Normal apart from his short stature.

Results

Serum: GH: 1.5 µg/L (after vigorous
                                     exercise)

                                     1.3 µg/L (after glucagon
                                     stimulation)

             IGF-1   40 µg/L (70–458)

             IGFBP-3   1.5 mg/L (2.1–7.7)

             Other appropriate tests were normal (see p. 386).

Summary

Subnormal growth velocity and subnormal plasma GH concentrations.

Interpretation

The diagnosis of GH deficiency depends on the demonstration of both the previously mentioned features.

Discussion

A normal plasma GH concentration (>5 µg/L), either at random or after exercise, obviates the need to perform the more invasive glucagon stimulation test. Exercise should be according to a standard protocol to ensure that it provides a sufficient stimulus to GH secretion. In this case the response was subnormal, and the glucagon stimulation test was performed to confirm GH deficiency. The low IGF-1 and IGFB3 concentrations provide additional support for this diagnosis, although they may also be low in other conditions, including malnutrition, hypothyroidism, liver disease and GH resistance (Laron syndrome, see p. 164).

Sex steroids are important in determining the magnitude of the response. Equivocal responses in children with pubertal delay require that the test is repeated after priming with sex steroids.

There was no other evidence of pituitary hypofunction in this boy and no evidence of a destructive pituitary lesion. A diagnosis of idiopathic GH deficiency was made. He began treatment with GH and grew at a normal rate thereafter, although he was always shorter than his peers. Typically, the lost height is not completely restored when GH deficiency is treated.

plasma sample is usually raised, but because GH secretion is normally episodic, the clinical diagnosis should be confirmed biochemically by demonstrating a failure of GH suppression in response to an oral glucose tolerance test. In healthy subjects, plasma GH concentration falls to <0.3 µg/L during this procedure. In acromegaly and gigantism, GH fails to suppress normally, and there may even be an increase in concentration. The glucose response may indicate impaired glucose tolerance (~25% of patients) or, less frequently (10%), diabetes mellitus, because GH stimulates glycogenolysis.

Plasma IGF-1 concentrations are elevated in patients with acromegaly and are used both in diagnosis and to follow the response of patients to treatment; there is less fluctuation in its concentration than in that of GH, although it is affected by nutritional status, insulin resistance, age and other factors.

The **clinical features** of excessive GH secretion are related to both the somatic (body structure) and the metabolic effects of the hormone (Table 9.3 and Case history 9.3). In addition, features directly caused by the presence of the pituitary tumour are often present. Hyperprolactinaemia, caused either by interference with the normal inhibition of prolactin secretion or (less frequently) by cosecretion with GH by

the tumour itself, occurs in 30% of patients with acromegaly, but there may be impaired secretion of other pituitary hormones.

Treatment of acromegaly and gigantism is aimed at reducing excessive GH secretion, preventing or treating deficiencies of other pituitary hormones and preventing damage to surrounding structures, particularly the optic nerves, by the tumour. In practice, it is often difficult to achieve all these goals. The main modes of treatment are surgery, external irradiation and medical therapy. Transsphenoidal resection of the pituitary tumour is the treatment of choice in the majority of cases. Occasionally, with large tumours with suprasellar extension, transfrontal craniotomy is necessary. If there is continuing evidence of excessive GH secretion, external irradiation or, more frequently, medical therapy can be used. The most effective drugs are octreotide and lanreotide, which are long-acting analogues of somatostatin. Dopamine agonists (e.g. bromocriptine, cabergoline), which stimulate GH secretion in healthy subjects but inhibit it in many patients with acromegaly, are also used. A GH receptor antagonist (pegvisomant) is now available, and appears, on the basis of its ability to normalize plasma IGF-1 concentrations, to be highly effective, albeit expensive.

Table 9.3 Clinical features of excessive growth hormone (GH) secretion

Somatic	Metabolic	Local effects of tumour

increased growth of:
  skin, subcutaneous tissues skull, jaw
  hands, feet
  long bones, if before fusion of
    epiphyses
  nerve compression (particularly
    carpal tunnel syndrome)
excessive sweating, greasy skin, acne
goitre
cardiomegaly, hypertension
increased risk of colon cancer
	elevated, non-suppressible plasma GH
	  concentration
	glucose intolerance
	clinical diabetes mellitus
	hypercalcaemia
	hyperphosphataemia
		headache
		visual field defects
		hypopituitarism
		diabetes insipidus

Case history 9.3

History

A 40-year-old man was referred to an endocrine clinic with new-onset impotence and excessive sweating in the absence of exertion. His wife thought that his facial features had become coarser, and he had recently had to buy a larger pair of shoes than normal because his old ones had become uncomfortable.

Examination

Mild hypertension and subtle bitemporal hemianopia.

Results

Oral glucose tolerance test:

	baseline	120 min glucose/ minimum GH
plasma glucose	8.5 mmol/L	11.5 mmol/L
serum GH	7.3 µg/L	6.7 µg/L
9:00 a.m. serum:	prolactin	800 mIU/L
	testosterone	11 nmol/L
	LH	2.0 IU/L
	FSH	1.5 IU/L
	free T4	16 pmol/L
	TSH	0.8 mU/L

Short ACTH stimulation test:

	baseline	60 min
serum cortisol	400 nmol/L	700 nmol/L

Investigations

Visual field testing demonstrated partial bitemporal hemianopia, and an MRI scan showed a pituitary tumour with suprasellar extension.

Summary

High basal GH concentration, which fails to suppress in response to glucose. Fasting and 2-h glucose results are high. The basal prolactin concentration is elevated.

Interpretation

The results are consistent with acromegaly, caused by a pituitary tumour (confirmed on MRI), with associated hyperprolactinaemia, diabetes mellitus, and possible hypogonadism; testosterone concentration is low–normal secondary to low gonadotrophin secretion. The pituitary–thyroid and pituitary–adrenal axes appear normal.

Discussion

The optic chiasm lies immediately above the pituitary and compression of it can either cause visual field defects, characteristically a bitemporal hemianopia or quadrantanopia, or threaten complete visual failure.

All patients with acromegaly and gigantism must be followed up and reassessed regularly for evidence of either recurrence (indicated by an increase in plasma IGF-1 concentrations) or further loss of normal pituitary function. HbA$_{1c}$ should be monitored for evidence of glucose intolerance or development of diabetes, and blood pressure should be measured regularly.

Box 9.3 Causes and clinical features of hyperprolactinaemia

Causes

Physiological

stress, sleep, pregnancy, suckling

Drugs

dopamine antagonists, e.g. phenothiazines, butyrophenones, risperidone, metoclopramide
dopamine-depleting agents, e.g. methyldopa, reserpine
others, e.g. oestrogens, verapamil

Pituitary disorders

prolactin-secreting tumour (prolactinoma)
tumours blocking dopaminergic inhibition of prolactin secretion
pituitary stalk section and surgery

Others

hypothyroidism, ectopic secretion, chronic kidney disease

Macroprolactinaemia

(biologically active prolactin concentration normal)

Clinical features

Females

oligomenorrhoea, amenorrhoea
infertility
galactorrhoea

Males

impotence
infertility
gynaecomastia

Hyperprolactinaemia

Hyperprolactinaemia is a common endocrine abnormality. It is an important cause of infertility in both males and females, impotence in males and menstrual irregularity in females. These effects are thought to be mediated through inhibition of the pulsatility of GnRH secretion by prolactin. The causes and clinical features of hyperprolactinaemia are summarized in Box 9.3. There may also be features related to the cause of the hyperprolactinaemia. The causes include various drugs, which either block pituitary dopaminergic receptors or deplete the brain of dopamine, in addition to pituitary tumours (prolactinomas) and destructive pituitary lesions that interfere with the normal inhibition of prolactin secretion. Prolactinomas are usually small (microadenomas, <10 mm diameter): 10% are larger tumours (macroadenomas)

that erode the pituitary fossa and extend outside its confines. Overall, prolactinomas occur more frequently in women, but affected men are more likely to have a macroadenoma.

Prolactin secretion is stimulated by stress, and plasma concentrations also depend on oestrogen status. It is therefore difficult to define an upper reference limit for plasma prolactin concentration. Slightly elevated prolactin concentrations are less likely to be of significance in well-oestrogenized women. If no physiological or drug-related cause can be found (see later), further investigation is usually indicated if a patient is found to have a confirmed plasma prolactin concentration >700 mIU/L. Plasma prolactin concentrations in patients with microadenomas are usually <5000 mIU/L. Prolactin-secreting tumours >10 mm in diameter are usually associated with plasma prolactin concentrations >5000 mIU/L. Lower concentrations in patients with large pituitary tumours are usually a result of disruption of the delivery of dopamine to the pituitary. Prolactin-secreting tumours often respond rapidly to medical treatment, which is important if a large tumour is associated with visual failure.

Drugs, hypothyroidism and, in women with amenorrhoea, pregnancy must be excluded as causes of hyperprolactinaemia. Apparently high concentrations of the hormone (up to 5000 mIU/L) can sometimes be caused by **macroprolactin** (see p. 158), which is a complex of prolactin with an immunoglobulin that is detected by immunoassays but is not biologically active. The possibility that a high prolactin concentration is due to macroprolactin should be excluded before further investigation is undertaken (Case history 9.4).

Numerous dynamic tests have been proposed to aid in the diagnosis of suspected prolactin-secreting tumours. One is the demonstration of the diminished response of prolactin to TRH. However, this is not a consistent or specific finding, and neither the TRH nor any other dynamic test is of established value in the diagnosis of prolactinomas. If a tumour is diagnosed, the secretion of other anterior pituitary hormones must be tested to detect possible subclinical deficiency. With small tumours, other pituitary functions are usually normal. Formal assessment of visual fields is mandatory in patients with macroprolactinomas.

Microprolactinomas only rarely grow, and if the patient is asymptomatic, no treatment may be necessary. **Treatment with a dopamine agonist** (e.g. cabergoline or bromocriptine) is indicated in patients with a macroprolactinoma or a symptomatic microprolactinoma (including women who wish to regain fertility). Plasma prolactin concentration usually falls to normal and tumour shrinkage occurs. Treatment usually has to be continued long term but can sometimes be successfully tapered and discontinued after the plasma prolactin concentration has been normal for at least 2 years and if there is no visible tumour remnant on MRI. Patients who do not respond to, or are intolerant of, medical treatment are treated by transsphenoidal surgery, but this is less

Case history 9.4

History

A couple underwent investigation for infertility, having been unable to conceive after 18 months without using contraception. Semen analysis showed normal numbers of motile sperm. Blood was taken from the female partner for hormone analysis 7 days before her next menstrual period was due.

Results

Serum:		
	FSH	8.2 IU/L
	LH	11.2 IU/L
	progesterone	35 nmol/L
	prolactin	1040 mIU/L

Summary

The gonadotrophin concentrations are normal and the prolactin concentration is elevated.

Interpretation

The progesterone concentration suggests that ovulation (see p. 220) has occurred. The prolactin is raised but there is no obvious suppression of the gonadal axis.

Discussion

A similar result was obtained on a repeat blood sample. Further analysis in the laboratory demonstrated that 59% of the plasma prolactin was present as macroprolactin and the estimated concentration of biologically active monomeric prolactin was 440 mIU/l (within the reference range). The woman missed her next menstrual period and a pregnancy test performed shortly after it had been due was positive. The initial results are not suggestive of pregnancy, as the gonadotrophins would be suppressed.

---

successful for macroprolactinomas than for microprolactinomas. External radiotherapy may be necessary in patients who do not respond adequately to dopamine agonists or surgery, but there is risk of damage to adjacent structures. There is only a low risk that a microadenoma will enlarge during pregnancy, so dopamine antagonists can usually be stopped for the duration. Monitoring of plasma prolactin concentration during pregnancy is of little value because of the normal pregnancy-associated increase.

Cushing disease

Cushing disease, in which increased secretion of cortisol by the adrenal cortex is secondary to increased secretion of ACTH by the anterior pituitary, is discussed in Chapter 10. Treatment is usually with transsphenoidal surgery. Before this technique was in use, some patients were treated by adrenalectomy: these patients may later develop hyperpigmentation and the clinical features of a large pituitary tumour (Nelson syndrome). The pigmentation is due to the melanocyte-stimulating activity of ACTH and its precursors.

Other conditions related to pituitary tumours

Tumours that secrete TSH or gonadotrophins are rare. The finding of a high plasma α-subunit concentration may provide a clue to their presence. Approximately 30% of pituitary tumours, usually chromophobe adenomas, are non-functioning. They can present with features of hypopituitarism because of the physical presence of the tumour or because of destruction of normal pituitary tissue by the tumour.

Even apparently non-functioning tumours may secrete small, clinically insignificant quantities of hormones. Some secrete only the α-subunit of the glycoprotein hormones, and measurement of plasma α-subunit concentration may be useful in assessing the success of treatment in such cases.

Asymptomatic pituitary tumours may be discovered incidentally on a skull radiograph or head CT scan taken for some other purpose ('incidentalomas'). If pituitary function is demonstrably normal and there are no mass effects, no intervention is required.

Posterior Pituitary Hormones

The posterior pituitary secretes two hormones: vasopressin (ADH) and oxytocin. They are synthesized in the hypothalamus and pass down nerve axons into the posterior pituitary, from where they are released into the circulation. Oxytocin is involved in the control of uterine contractility and of milk release from the lactating breast. Disorders of its secretion are uncommon and not clinically important. In contrast, vasopressin is essential to life, and disorders of its secretion are well recognized.

Vasopressin

Vasopressin has a vital role in the **control of the tonicity of the extracellular fluid**, and hence indirectly of the intracellular fluid, and of water balance. Excessive secretion results in dilutional hyponatraemia, with a risk of water intoxication; decreased secretion results in diabetes insipidus, a condition in which there is uncontrolled excretion of water with a tendency towards severe dehydration. The consequences of excessive secretion of vasopressin (syndrome of inappropriate antidiuresis) are discussed on p. 39–40; in some patients, vasopressin secretion is from tumour cells rather than the

Box 9.4 **Causes of diabetes insipidus**

Cranial

tumours:
  craniopharyngioma
  secondary tumours
  pituitary tumours with suprasellar extension
granulomatous disease
meningitis and encephalitis
vascular disorders
trauma (may be transient)
surgery (often transient)
idiopathic
familial (~5% of cases)

Nephrogenic

familial
metabolic:
  hypokalaemia
  hypercalcaemia
drugs:
  lithium
  demeclocycline
postobstructive uropathy
renal tubular disease:
  pyelonephritis
  polycystic disease
  amyloid
  sickle cell disease

hypothalamus. **Diabetes insipidus**, in contrast, is a rare condition; it is usually a result of pituitary or hypothalamic disease (cranial diabetes insipidus (CDI)) (Box 9.4 and Case history 9.5), although it can also be due to a failure of the kidneys to respond to the hormone (nephrogenic diabetes insipidus [NDI]). The most common causes of NDI are hypokalaemia, hypercalcaemia and lithium toxicity. In about 5% of patients, it is inherited: in X-linked familial NDI, there is a defect in the vasopressin receptor; in autosomal recessive familial NDI, the defect is in the water channel protein, aquaporin-2. Partial NDI can also occur in patients who have an inappropriately high water intake, which dilutes medullary hypertonicity and therefore prevents the formation of normally concentrated urine.

Diabetes insipidus is characterized by polyuria (typically >3 L urine/24 h in adults) and thirst. Unless the hypothalamic thirst centre is also damaged, thirst leads to increased fluid intake (polydipsia). The differential diagnosis includes other conditions that cause polyuria and polydipsia, particularly diabetes mellitus, hypercalcaemia and chronic kidney disease. Children with diabetes insipidus

may present with enuresis. CDI can become worse during pregnancy, because of degradation of residual vasopressin by placental vasopressinase.

A compulsive desire to drink (psychogenic or primary polydipsia) also causes polyuria. However, in this case polyuria is secondary to increased fluid intake, whereas in diabetes insipidus the opposite applies, with polydipsia being a response to polyuria. In both conditions, the urine is dilute. An early-morning urine osmolality >750 mmol/kg excludes diabetes insipidus. Plasma sodium concentration and osmolality are usually normal in both conditions, although they may be high–normal in diabetes insipidus (and frankly elevated if patients are denied water) and low–normal in primary polydipsia.

If there is doubt about the diagnosis, a **water deprivation test** should be performed (Box 9.5). This is effectively a biological assay for vasopressin. Patients with diabetes insipidus may become dangerously dehydrated if denied access to fluid; both they and patients with psychogenic polydipsia may also exercise considerable ingenuity to obtain fluid. Close supervision is therefore essential.

In a healthy subject, the urine becomes concentrated in response to water deprivation and plasma osmolality does not exceed 295 mmol/kg. In diabetes insipidus, the urine does not become concentrated and plasma osmolality rises. In patients who are water overloaded before the test is started, the urine may not become concentrated: plasma osmolality is usually low and may remain so thus inhibiting vasopressin secretion which is stimulated only if the osmolality rises to >285 mmol/kg. If water overload is suspected, it may be necessary to carefully control water intake for a few days before the water deprivation test is performed.

At the end of the 8-h period, the patient is allowed to drink water and is given 1-desamino-D-arginine-vasopressin (desmopressin), a synthetic analogue of vasopressin. In CDI, the urine will become concentrated; in patients with NDI, it remains dilute. If the water deprivation test is to be carried out on a patient with known or suspected anterior pituitary disease, adequate cortisol replacement must be provided.

If the results of a water deprivation test are equivocal (as in practice they often are), the plasma vasopressin response to hypertonic saline infusion can be assessed. The response is normal (i.e. an increase in vasopressin) in patients with NDI or primary polydipsia, but blunted or absent in patients with CDI (Fig. 9.6). The former two conditions can be distinguished by comparing plasma vasopressin concentration with urine osmolality after a period of fluid deprivation (Fig. 9.7). In NDI, plasma vasopressin is much higher than normal. Copeptin, a peptide derived from the C-terminal of the precursor molecule prepro-vasopressin,

Case history 9.5

History

A middle-aged woman, who had undergone mastectomy and local radiotherapy for carcinoma of the breast 2 years previously, attended her regular outpatient appointment. There was no sign of recurrence, but she complained of increasing thirst over the previous months and that she was passing copious amounts of urine. The thirst became intolerable if she went without water for more than a few hours, and her sleep was disturbed by the frequent need to pass urine and have a drink. She was admitted for investigation.

Examination

Normal.

Results

Plasma: osmolality   296 mmol/kg
              sodium   144 mmol/L
Urine: osmolality   90 mmol/kg

Water deprivation test: after 6 h of water deprivation, her weight had fallen from 60 to 57 kg; the test was therefore stopped. At end of test:

Plasma: osmolality   307 mmol/kg
Urine: osmolality   220 mmol/kg

There was no glycosuria. Plasma creatinine, potassium and calcium concentrations were all normal.

She was then allowed to drink and was given a dose of desmopressin. After this her urine osmolality rose to 810 mmol/kg.

Summary

History of intolerable thirst with a slightly raised plasma osmolality yet dilute urine that concentrated on administration of desmopressin.

Interpretation

Diabetes insipidus is confirmed by the failure to conserve water and concentrate the urine during water deprivation. The response to desmopressin indicates vasopressin deficiency, CDI, rather than kidney insensitivity, NDI.

Discussion

She was treated successfully with regular administration of desmopressin, and her symptoms resolved. A CT scan revealed a small lesion in the region of the hypothalamus presumed to be a metastatic deposit from her breast carcinoma.

Box 9.5 **Water deprivation test procedure**

allow fluids overnight before test and light breakfast with no fluid; no smoking permitted
weigh patient
allow no fluid for 8 h; patient must be under constant supervision during this time
every hour:
    weigh patient (stop test if weight falls by >5% initial body weight[a])
    patient empties bladder: measure urine volume and osmolality
every 2 h:
    measure plasma osmolality (stop test if osmolality >300 mmol/kg[a])
after 8 h:
    if plasma osmolality ≤295 mmol/kg and urine osmolality >750 mmol/kg, normal response: end of test, allow patient to drink (test can be terminated earlier if this urine osmolality is exceeded)
    if plasma osmolality >295 mmol/kg, give 2 μg desmopressin intramuscularly and measure urine osmolality every hour for a further 3 h (and restrict water intake to <500 mL over next 8 h)
For interpretation of results, see Fig. 9.8.

[a]End-point diagnostic of diabetes insipidus; allow access to fluid and assess response to desmopressin.

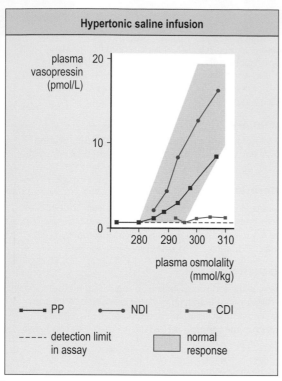

Fig. 9.6 Hypertonic saline infusion. Typical responses to the intravenous infusion of 5% saline are shown for patients with nephrogenic diabetes insipidus (NDI), cranial diabetes insipidus (CDI) and primary polydipsia (PP).

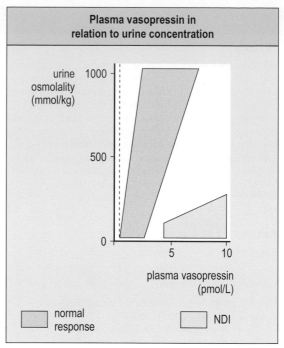

Fig. 9.7 Plasma vasopressin in relation to urine concentration during water deprivation. In nephrogenic diabetes insipidus (NDI), vasopressin concentrations are inappropriately high in relation to urine osmolality.

is cosecreted on an equimolar basis with vasopressin; it is considerably more stable and easier to measure and therefore may form a suitable alternative to vasopressin measurement. An algorithm for the investigation of polyuria is given in Fig. 9.8. As vasopressin is both unstable in vitro and difficult to measure, a closely supervised therapeutic trial of desmopressin treatment can be used instead. This causes an improvement in CDI, has no effect in NDI and causes increasing hyponatraemia in primary polydipsia.

Management of diabetes insipidus

Patients must always have access to adequate fluid and, whenever possible, the underlying disease should be treated.

CDI is usually treated with desmopressin, given orally or as a nasal spray. If polyuria is only mild (i.e. urine volume <4 L/24 h), specific treatment may not be necessary. Patients must learn to monitor their fluid output and input to avoid water intoxication. This may be a particular problem if the sensation of thirst is blunted.

Patients with NDI, because they do not respond to vasopressin, must maintain an adequate water intake to avoid dehydration. Hydronephrosis and hydroureter secondary to bladder distension may occur and lead to kidney impairment. Thiazide diuretics, which induce a state of sodium depletion, stimulating renal sodium and water retention, may reduce the polyuria. Potassium supplements or the concomitant use of a potassium-sparing diuretic may be necessary to prevent hypokalaemia.

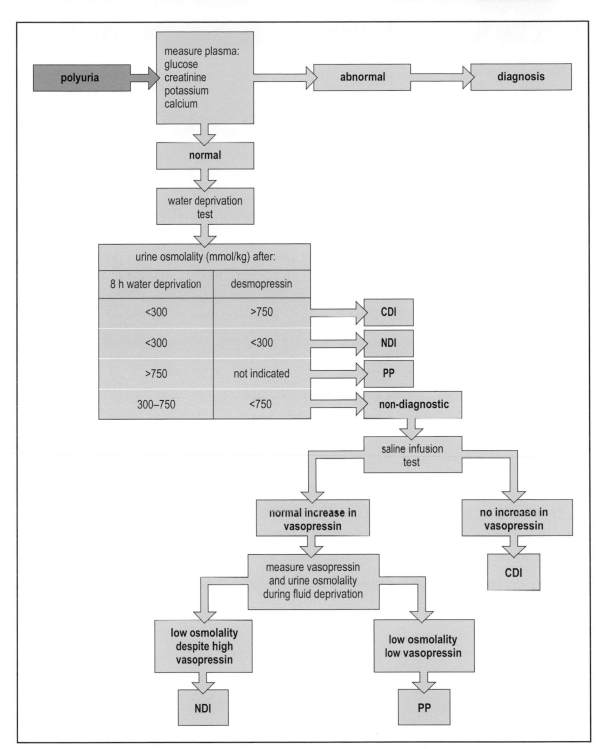

Fig. 9.8 Algorithm for the investigation of polyuria. CDI, cranial diabetes insipidus; NDI, nephrogenic diabetes insipidus; PP, primary polydipsia.

SUMMARY

- The **anterior pituitary gland** secretes **growth hormone** (GH) and **prolactin**, and trophic hormones that control the activity of the gonads (**luteinizing hormone** (LH) and **follicle-stimulating hormone** (FSH)), thyroid (**thyroid-stimulating hormone** (TSH)) and the adrenal cortex (**adrenocorticotrophic hormone** (ACTH)). The secretion of all these hormones is regulated by **hypothalamic hormones**, which reach the pituitary through a portal system of blood vessels. The trophic hormones are, in addition, controlled by feedback mechanisms involving the hormones produced by the respective target organs.

- **Anterior pituitary hypofunction** (hypopituitarism) can result in the inadequate production of one or more hormones; the clinical manifestations depend on the particular pattern of deficiency. Hypopituitarism may either be the result of disease affecting the pituitary itself or be secondary to hypothalamic disease, with failure of production of hypothalamic hormones. Hypopituitarism is investigated by measuring basal and stimulated concentrations of pituitary hormones.

- **Pituitary tumours** can cause hypopituitarism by destroying normal pituitary tissue, but may be functional and produce syndromes related to excessive hormone secretion. Pituitary tumours producing prolactin, GH and ACTH are well recognized, but secretion of gonadotrophins or TSH is rare. In addition to their endocrine effects, both functional and non-functional tumours can cause clinical features related to their space-occupying effects.

- The **posterior pituitary gland** secretes **oxytocin** and **vasopressin.** Both are synthesized in the hypothalamus and reach the posterior pituitary through nerve axons. Because of this, damage to the posterior pituitary may cause only temporary failure of hormone secretion. Oxytocin stimulates uterine contraction during labour but does not otherwise appear to be an essential hormone.

- **Vasopressin** is essential to life because it controls water excretion by altering the permeability of the kidney collecting tubules to water in response to changes in extracellular fluid osmolality.

- **Excessive vasopressin secretion** produces **water retention** with a dilutional hyponatraemia. Defective vasopressin secretion results in diabetes insipidus, with uncontrolled renal water loss. Diabetes insipidus also can be caused by renal insensitivity to vasopressin; the two types can be distinguished from each other, and from psychogenic polydipsia, by assessing the response to a water deprivation test or the infusion of hypertonic saline.

Chapter | **10** |

The adrenal glands

Introduction

The adrenal glands have two functionally distinct parts: the cortex and the medulla. The **adrenal cortex** is essential to life; it produces three classes of steroid hormone: glucocorticoids, mineralocorticoids and androgens. The **medulla**, which is functionally part of the sympathetic nervous system, is not essential to life, and its pathological importance is related mainly to the occurrence of rare catecholamine-secreting tumours.

Glucocorticoids, of which the most important is **cortisol**, are secreted in response to adrenocorticotrophic hormone (ACTH), which is itself secreted by the pituitary in response to the hypothalamic corticotrophin-releasing hormone (CRH). Cortisol exerts negative feedback control on ACTH release through inhibiting the action of CRH; it also inhibits CRH secretion. Glucocorticoids have many actions (Box 10.1) and are particularly important in mediating the body's response to stress. Corticosterone, a precursor of aldosterone, is a weak glucocorticoid (30% of the activity of cortisol).

The most important **mineralocorticoid** is **aldosterone**. This is secreted in response to angiotensin II (a potent and short-lived vasoconstrictor), produced as a result of the activation of the renin–angiotensin system by a decrease in renal blood flow and other indicators of decreased extracellular fluid (ECF) volume (Fig. 10.1). Secretion of aldosterone is also directly stimulated by hyperkalaemia. The main action of aldosterone is to stimulate the reabsorption of sodium and the excretion of potassium and hydrogen ions in the distal convoluted tubules of the kidneys; its effect on sodium results in having a central role in the determination of the ECF volume and its effect on potassium and hydrogen accounts for the hypokalaemia and metabolic alkalosis seen in hyperaldosteronism. ACTH does not have a major physiological role in aldosterone secretion, although it has a role in its synthesis through stimulating cholesterol desmolase, the first step in the biosynthetic pathway of the adrenal steroids. Curiously, the secretion of aldosterone by adrenal tumours is affected by ACTH (see p. 189). Both cortisol and aldosterone have a high affinity for mineralocorticoid receptors, and the considerably higher plasma concentration of cortisol has the potential to overwhelm these receptors. However, the renal tubular cells contain 11β-hydroxysteroid dehydrogenase, which converts cortisol to cortisone. The latter has low affinity for mineralocorticoid receptors, thus allowing them to respond primarily to aldosterone.

The adrenal cortex is also a source of **androgens**, including dehydroepiandrosterone (DHEA), DHEA sulphate (DHEAS) and androstenedione. These stimulate libido and the development of pubic and axillary hair in females, but are weak androgens in comparison with testosterone and have only a minor physiological function in males. The clinical effects of excessive adrenal androgens can be a prominent feature of adrenal disorders in females.

Adrenal Steroid Hormone Biosynthesis

The hormones secreted by the adrenal cortex are synthesized from cholesterol by a sequence of enzyme-catalysed reactions (Fig. 10.2). An awareness of these pathways is important for the understanding of congenital adrenal hyperplasia (CAH), a group of conditions each caused by a lack of one of these enzymes.

Measurement of Adrenal Steroid Hormones

Adrenal steroid hormones can all be measured by immunoassays, although cross-reactivity occurs between steroids in some assays (e.g. between 11-deoxycortisol and cortisol); mass spectrometry is a much more specific alternative method. The plasma concentrations of steroid hormones can fluctuate for various reasons, and thus single results must be interpreted with caution.

The measurement of urinary cortisol excretion is valuable in the investigation of Cushing syndrome. **Urinary 'steroid profiling'**, in which steroids are separated and quantified by gas–liquid chromatography, often combined with mass spectrometry, is particularly valuable in the investigation of suspected CAH; it may also be helpful in the investigation of suspected adrenal carcinoma.

Box 10.1 Principal physiological functions of glucocorticoids

increase protein catabolism
increase hepatic glycogen synthesis
increase hepatic gluconeogenesis
inhibit ACTH secretion (negative feedback mechanism)
sensitize arterioles to action of noradrenaline, hence involved in maintenance of blood pressure
have permissive effect on water excretion; required for initiation of diuresis in response to water loading
inhibit the inflammatory and immune responses
inhibit bone formation (through inhibition of type 1 collagen synthesis)

ACTH, adrenocorticotrophic hormone.

Cortisol

Some 95% of cortisol in the blood is bound to protein, principally to the cortisol-binding globulin, **transcortin**. Free cortisol concentration, and thus the amount of cortisol that can be excreted unchanged in the urine, is very low. Transcortin is almost fully saturated at normal cortisol concentrations. Because of this, if cortisol production increases, the concentration present in the plasma in the free form, and thus the amount that is excreted, increases to a disproportionately greater extent than the total. For this reason, measurement of the 24-h urinary excretion of cortisol, provided that an accurate urine collection can be made, is a sensitive way of detecting increased, but not decreased, secretion of the hormone. Transcortin concentration is affected by numerous other factors, not least by oestrogens, which increase the concentration. The possibility of falsely 'normal' plasma resulting in cortisol deficiency states should be considered in women on contraceptive pills or hormone-replacement therapy.

Plasma cortisol concentrations show diurnal variation, being highest in the morning and lowest at night (Fig. 10.3). Blood for cortisol measurement should usually be drawn between 8:00 and 9:00 a.m.; however, samples can be taken at 11:00 p.m. to detect loss of the diurnal variation, an early feature of adrenal hyperfunction (Cushing syndrome). Random measurements are rarely of any value in the diagnosis of adrenal disease,

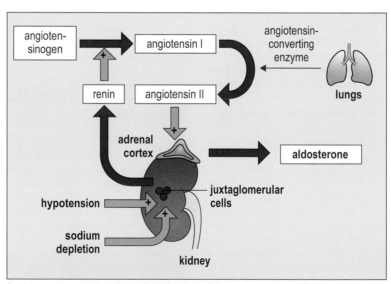

Fig. 10.1 Stimulation of aldosterone secretion through activation of the renin–angiotensin system. Renin, released into the plasma from the juxtaglomerular cells of the kidney in response to various stimuli, catalyses the formation of angiotensin I from the protein angiotensinogen. Angiotensin I is metabolized to an octapeptide, angiotensin II, by ACE during its passage through the lungs. Angiotensin II stimulates the release of aldosterone from the adrenal cortex; it is a powerful pressor agent and also stimulates thirst and the secretion of vasopressin.

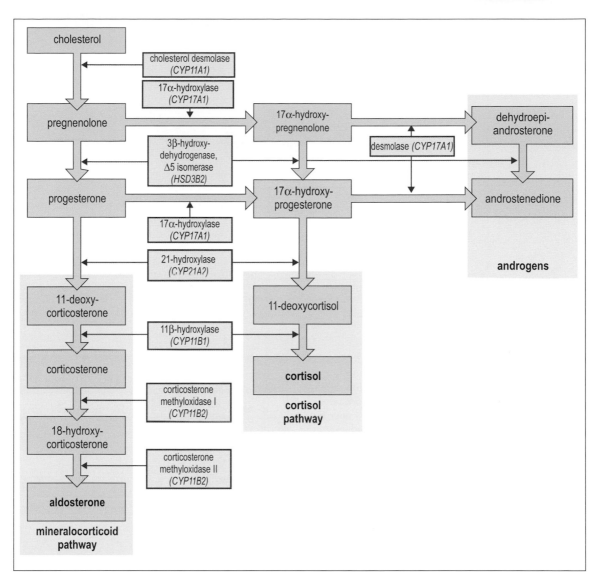

Fig. 10.2 Biosynthesis of adrenal steroid hormones. Cortisol and the androgens are synthesized in the zona reticularis and zona fasciculata of the adrenal glands. Corticosterone methyloxidase II, required for the synthesis of aldosterone, is present only in the zona glomerulosa. Androstenedione can be converted to testosterone in peripheral tissues, but in adult males, adrenal androgens and the testosterone derived from them make only a minor contribution to total androgenic activity.

except that a high concentration may reasonably be taken to exclude adrenal failure.

Cortisol is secreted in response to stress, mediated through ACTH, further limiting the value of single cortisol measurements. Investigations of adrenal hypofunction or hyperfunction often involve measurement of cortisol after attempting to stimulate or suppress its secretion.

When interpreting plasma cortisol results, it should be remembered that the synthetic glucocorticoid prednisolone may cross-react with cortisol in immunoassays for the hormone. Cross-reaction does not occur with dexamethasone or with spironolactone, an aldosterone antagonist used as a diuretic.

Aldosterone

Aldosterone secretion is stimulated through the action of renin; therefore, it is often helpful to measure plasma renin at

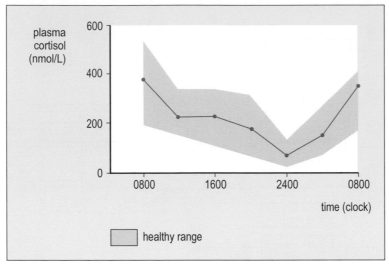

Fig. 10.3 Diurnal variation in plasma cortisol concentration. Plasma cortisol concentrations are at their highest shortly after waking and then decline throughout the day to reach a nadir in the late evening. Because of this variation, it is important that blood samples are taken at times that coincide with either the peak or the trough, with random samples being of little value. The graph shows mean values and the range in a sample of healthy people.

the same time as the concentration of aldosterone, to establish whether aldosterone secretion is autonomous or under normal control. Calculation of the plasma **aldosterone:renin ratio** in a random blood sample is a useful screening test for autonomous aldosterone secretion: this is excluded by a low value (see p.188). Plasma aldosterone concentration varies with posture: the use of samples taken from patients while they are recumbent or ambulant is discussed further in connection with the investigation of primary aldosteronism (see p. 187).

Androgens

Measurements of adrenal androgens are of value in the diagnosis and management of CAH (see p. 188) and in the investigation of virilization in women (see Chapter 12).

Disorders of the Adrenal Cortex

Patients with adrenal disorders can present with clinical features related to either hypofunction or hyperfunction. In CAH, a combination of features may be present.

Adrenal hypofunction (Addison disease)

Addison disease is an uncommon but life-threatening condition; the common causes and clinical features are listed in Table 10.1. The cases originally described by Addison

Table 10.1 Causes and clinical features of primary adrenal hypofunction

Causes	Clinical features
Common	
glucocorticoid treatment	tiredness, generalized weakness, lethargy
autoimmune adrenalitis	anorexia, nausea, vomiting,
tuberculosis	weight loss
	dizziness, postural hypotension
	pigmentation
	loss of body hair (women)
Less common	
adrenalectomy	hypoglycaemia
secondary tumour deposits	depression
amyloidosis	
haemochromatosis	
histoplasmosis	
adrenal haemorrhage	

were caused by tuberculosis, but **autoimmune disease** is now the major cause in the UK. In such patients, adrenal autoantibodies are usually present, and there may be associated autoimmune disease affecting other tissues (e.g. pernicious anaemia).

The commonest cause of adrenal hypofunction is suppression of the pituitary–adrenal axis by glucocorticoids used therapeutically. Although patients may develop features of Cushing syndrome during treatment, a sudden withdrawal of steroids or failure to increase the dose during stress (e.g. surgery) may precipitate acute adrenal failure. Normal pituitary–adrenal function is regained only slowly when steroids are withdrawn, and it is essential that the dosage is reduced gradually when steroid treatment is to be discontinued.

The majority of the **clinical features** of adrenal failure are due to the lack of glucocorticoids and mineralocorticoids. Increased pigmentation is a result of the high concentrations of ACTH, which occur because of the loss of negative feedback by cortisol: ACTH has some melanocyte-stimulating activity (see p. 158).

Adrenal failure usually has an insidious onset, with non-specific symptoms, but can develop acutely case 10.2. **Adrenal crisis** is a medical emergency. The clinical features include severe hypovolaemia, shock, hyperkalaemia and hypoglycaemia. It can be precipitated by stress (e.g. due to infection, trauma or surgery) in patients with incipient adrenal failure. Patients being treated with glucocorticoids, whether in physiological doses (replacement therapy) or pharmacological doses (e.g. in severe inflammatory conditions) are also susceptible to adrenal failure in these circumstances if the dosage is not increased. Acute adrenal failure may occur after haemorrhage into the adrenal glands as a complication of anticoagulant treatment and in meningococcal septicaemia. Although the adrenals are a relatively frequent site of tumour metastasis, this only occasionally results in adrenal insufficiency.

Adrenal failure can occur secondarily to **pituitary failure** as a result of decreased stimulation by ACTH. Other features of hypopituitarism may be present (see p.163). The abnormal pigmentation that is stimulated by ACTH in patients with primary adrenal failure does not occur. Hyponatraemia may be present, because the lack of cortisol reduces the ability of the kidneys to excrete a water load, but plasma potassium concentrations are normal and there is no renal salt wasting because aldosterone secretion is not dependent on ACTH. Hypotension may still be present, however, because the sensitivity of arteriolar smooth muscle to catecholamines is reduced by a lack of cortisol.

Unless a patient is being treated with synthetic corticosteroids, adrenal failure is highly likely if the plasma cortisol concentration is <100 nmol/L in a blood sample drawn at 9:00 a.m. and unlikely if it is >500 nmol/L. However, in the majority of patients with adrenal failure, whether primary or secondary, the plasma cortisol concentration lies between these extremes, and an **ACTH stimulation test** (also called the 'short Synacthen test') must be performed to confirm the diagnosis (Box 10.2). In both primary and secondary

> An early morning cortisol <100 nmol/L indicates a high likelihood of adrenal failure, if the individual is not already taking glucocorticoids, requiring urgent investigation and action.

Box 10.2 Adrenocorticotrophic hormone (ACTH) stimulation test (also known as tetracosactide or Synacthen tests) for the diagnosis of adrenal failure and subsequent tests to consider

Procedure	Results[b]
take blood sample at 9:00 a.m. for measurement of cortisol and ACTH inject 250 μg ACTH i.m. or i.v. after 60 min[a] take blood for cortisol measurement	normal adrenal function: if plasma cortisol after ACTH shows an increment of 200 to >550 nmol/L

Adrenal insufficiency confirmed

ACTH analysis (9:00 a.m. or basal sample from ACTH stimulation test)	primary adrenal insufficiency: greater than 2 × upper reference limit secondary adrenal insufficiency: low or low–normal

Further tests to consider if primary adrenal insufficiency confirmed:

infants, children and selected adults
   17-hydroxyprogesterone (17-OHP)
   urine steroid profiling if 17-OHP normal
>6 months old
   antiadrenal antibodies
   very long chain fatty acids in males
   imaging of adrenals for infiltrative disease, malignancy, haemorrhage and infections
any age
   aldosterone:renin ratio

[a]There is controversy regarding post stimulation sample timing and either 30 min or 60 min have been recommended by guidelines. There is a risk of falsely diagnosing adrenal insufficiency if a 60-min sample is not measured.
[b]Values are essay dependent.

---

adrenal failure, the response in the ACTH stimulation test is absent or blunted (Case history 10.1). It has been suggested that some patients with early adrenal failure may exhibit a normal response to 250 μg tetracosactide, because this is a supraphysiological dose or, in the case of secondary adrenal failure, the adrenal gland has yet to atrophy. The distinction between primary and secondary adrenal failure can usually be made from measurement of the plasma ACTH concentration at 9:00 a.m.: high values (a result of decreased negative feedback by cortisol) are typical of primary adrenal failure; low or low–normal values are typical of secondary adrenal failure. This is only required if the cause of adrenal failure is not known and is therefore not useful for those being investigated after prolonged glucocorticoid use.

Although, ideally, these tests should be done before starting treatment, when a **severely ill patient** is judged clinically to have adrenal failure, **treatment should not be delayed**. A blood sample taken before treatment can be helpful to confirm or refute the diagnosis because the patient is likely to be stressed and have a maximal endogenous ACTH response. Treatment with intravenous hydrocortisone and fluid replacement with 0.9% sodium chloride should be started while awaiting the cortisol result. Plasma potassium and glucose concentrations should be monitored and intravenous glucose provided if necessary.

An ACTH stimulation test, if not possible at presentation, should be performed within 2 weeks of starting glucocorticoid replacement to avoid misdiagnosis because of adrenal suppression by this steroid treatment. The administered steroid must be switched to dexamethasone 48 h before the test, because other synthetic steroids cross-react with laboratory immunoassays for cortisol (and hydrocortisone is identical to cortisol).

Once primary adrenal failure has been diagnosed, the cause should be sought, for example, by measuring antiadrenal antibodies (present in 90% of patients with autoimmune disease) and looking for evidence of tuberculosis (see Box 10.2). The most likely causes should be sought first, and, for example, 17-hydroxyprogesterone (17-OHP) for CAH should be limited to those presenting in infancy or with other suspicious features. Aldosterone:renin ratio can establish the functionality of the mineralocorticoid axis and the requirement for fludrocortisone replacement.

Case history 10.1

History

A 17-year-old woman presented with a 2-month history of tiredness and lethargy. She had noticed that she became dizzy when she stood up.

Examination

She had pigmentation of the buccal mucosa, palmar creases and an old appendicectomy scar. Her blood pressure was 120/80 mmHg lying down and 90/50 mmHg on standing.

Results (see Appendix for reference ranges)

Serum:	sodium	128 mmol/L
	potassium	5.4 mmol/L
	urea	8.5 mmol/L
Plasma:	glucose (fasting)	2.5 mmol/L

ACTH stimulation test:

Serum:	cortisol 9:00 a.m. (baseline)	150 nmol/L
	cortisol 60 min after ACTH	160 nmol/L
Plasma:	ACTH (9:00 a.m.)	500 ng/L

Antiadrenal antibodies detectable at high concentration

Summary

Postural hypotension, hyperpigmentation with hypotension, hyperkalaemia with failure of cortisol stimulation in short Synacthen test and high baseline ACTH; high urea.

Interpretation

Primary adrenal failure, with probable pre-renal acute kidney injury. The 9:00 a.m. cortisol is at the lower limit of the reference range, and there is virtually no response to ACTH. Except in severe cases, cortisol is measurable in the plasma, even though the concentration is low–normal or frankly low. However, this represents the maximal output of the adrenal glands, because they are already stimulated by the high concentration of endogenous ACTH.

Discussion

Postural hypotension is a common finding in adrenal failure: it is due to a decrease in ECF volume caused by a lack of aldosterone, leading to sodium loss, together with a decrease in arteriolar tone caused by loss of the permissive effect of cortisol on the action of catecholamines. This decrease in ECF volume may also cause a degree of pre-renal acute kidney injury, as demonstrated in this case. Hyponatraemia is not always present in adrenal failure, particularly in the early stages. Sodium is lost isotonically from the kidneys, but the lack of cortisol may cause water retention and, with severe hypovolaemia, vasopressin (antidiuretic hormone [ADH]) secretion is stimulated. Deficiency of aldosterone is also responsible for potassium retention, and thus hyperkalaemia.

The fasting plasma glucose concentration is at the low end of the reference range in this patient: the unopposed action of insulin may cause symptomatic hypoglycaemia.

The patient's symptoms resolved rapidly after starting glucocorticoid and mineralocorticoid replacement. Some 10 years later, the patient's periods ceased. Her premature menopause was due to autoimmune ovarian failure. There is a recognized association between autoimmune adrenal failure and other organ-specific autoimmune diseases such as ovarian and thyroid failure.

All patients with primary adrenal failure require **life-long replacement therapy**, usually with both hydrocortisone and fludrocortisone, a synthetic mineralocorticoid. Hydrocortisone replacement is usually given in three unequal doses (e.g. 10 mg in the morning and 5 mg at midday and in the early evening), although a once-daily modified-release formulation has been developed. The adequacy of replacement can be assessed clinically and by measuring plasma cortisol concentration at intervals throughout the day (cortisol 'day curve'): this allows detection of a concentration that is too high shortly after a dose or too low shortly before the next dose is due. Mineralocorticoid treatment can be assessed by measuring plasma renin activity: elevated activity implies inadequate replacement, and complete suppression implies excessive replacement (which can cause hypertension). Hydrocortisone has some intrinsic mineralocorticoid activity, and occasionally patients may be free of symptoms on hydrocortisone alone, particularly if they maintain a high salt intake. A trial of androgen replacement with DHEA is currently recommended in women with primary adrenal insufficiency and low libido, energy or depressive symptoms despite adequate mineralocorticoid and glucocorticoid replacement. If no benefit is obtained within 6 months the DHEA should be discontinued.

Long-term follow-up is essential to ensure the continuing adequacy of replacement treatment and to check for the development of other autoimmune endocrine disease. The dose of hydrocortisone should be increased during intercurrent illness, trauma, surgery and other stressful situations.

Adrenal hyperfunction

In Cushing syndrome, there is overproduction primarily of glucocorticoids, although mineralocorticoid and androgen production may also be excessive. In Conn syndrome, mineralocorticoids alone are produced in excess.

Cushing syndrome

The causes and clinical features of Cushing syndrome are listed in Box 10.3. **Cushing disease,** that is, adrenal hyperfunction secondary to a pituitary corticotroph adenoma, accounts for 60–70% of cases of spontaneously arising Cushing syndrome (i.e. not caused by treatment with steroids). The **clinical features** are caused primarily by the glucocorticoid effects of excessive cortisol, but cortisol precursors, and indeed cortisol itself, have some mineralocorticoid activity. Thus, sodium retention, leading to hypertension, and potassium wasting, causing a hypokalaemic alkalosis, are common findings, except in iatrogenic disease (synthetic glucocorticoids have little or no mineralocorticoid activity). Increased production of adrenal androgens may also contribute to the clinical presentation.

Pseudo-Cushing syndrome, in which patients appear cushingoid and may have some of the biochemical abnormalities of true Cushing disease, can occur in severe depression and in alcoholics. Alcohol-related pseudo-Cushing syndrome usually resolves rapidly on withdrawal of alcohol. Patients with severe obesity may also look cushingoid, but Cushing syndrome is a rare cause of obesity.

There are **two diagnostic steps** in the investigation of a patient with suspected Cushing syndrome: **the demonstration of increased cortisol secretion and subsequently the elucidation of the cause**. It is common to see patients who look cushingoid, but it is much less common that Cushing syndrome is the cause. It is, therefore, essential to exclude those patients who do not have adrenal disease and identify the small number who need further investigation. Tests used for this purpose (Table 10.2) are the measurement of **24-h urinary cortisol excretion**, the **overnight**

Box 10.3 **Causes and clinical features of Cushing syndrome**

Causes

corticosteroid or ACTH treatment
pituitary hypersecretion of ACTH (Cushing disease)
adrenal adenoma
adrenal carcinoma
ectopic ACTH secretion by tumours, e.g. carcinoma of bronchus and carcinoid tumours

Clinical features

truncal obesity ('moon facies', 'buffalo hump', protuberant abdomen)
facial plethora
thinning of skin
striae (typically red/purple and >1 cm wide)
excessive bruising
acne
skin pigmentation (only if ACTH elevated)
hirsutism (especially in adrenal carcinoma)
menstrual irregularities
hypertension
glucose intolerance
kidney stones
muscle weakness and wasting, especially of proximal muscles
back pain (osteoporosis and vertebral collapse)
psychiatric disturbances: euphoria, mania, depression, insomnia, short term memory loss, irritability
hypokalaemia
in children: loss of height velocity, weight gain, delayed puberty, pseudoprecocious puberty, short stature, virilisation

ACTH, adrenocorticotrophic hormone.

Case history 10.2

History

A 40-year-old woman, who had recently started treatment for hypothyroidism based on symptoms of tiredness, constipation and general malaise and a serum thyroid-stimulating hormone concentration of 60 mIU/L, presented shortly afterwards with abdominal pain, vomiting and diarrhoea after a meal including cold chicken. These symptoms persisted and were unusually severe, and her general practitioner referred her to the local hospital.

Examination

She was severely dehydrated and hypotensive.

Results

Serum:	sodium	120 mmol/L
	potassium	5.6 mmol/L
	urea	12.0 mmol/L
Plasma:	glucose	2.5 mmol/L

Summary

Hyponatraemia, hypokalaemia and hypoglycaemia with high urea.

Interpretation

The pattern of biochemical abnormalities is characteristic of adrenal insufficiency with probable pre-renal acute kidney injury.

Discussion

On more careful examination she had pigmentation over her knees and knuckles. Intravenous hydrocortisone, together with intravenous 0.9% saline and glucose were immediately started. The woman's condition improved rapidly; the laboratory later reported that the cortisol concentration was 65 nmol/L on the admission blood sample.

Adrenal failure often develops insidiously, but adrenal crisis can be precipitated at any time by stress. Another factor of relevance in this case is the hypothyroidism: treatment of hypothyroidism in a patient with coexistent incipient adrenal failure can cause this to become clinically overt. Multiple endocrinopathies may also raise the possibility of autoimmune polyendocrine syndrome (or pituitary insufficiency, but unlikely here as TSH was high).

This patient's increased skin pigmentation was a result of increased pituitary ACTH production, and this, together with the finding of an appropriately high TSH in response to thyroid failure, suggests that she had primary rather than secondary adrenal failure.

Table 10.2 Screening tests for Cushing syndrome[a]

Test	Normal result[b]
24-h urinary cortisol excretion	<300 nmol/24 h (at least twice)
1 mg overnight/0.5 mg every 6 h for 48 h low-dose dexamethasone suppression test	plasma cortisol <50 nmol/L at 9:00 a.m.
midnight salivary cortisol	<2 nmol/L (at least twice)

[a]Cushing syndrome is excluded by one normal result in the suppression tests or two normal results in the non-suppression tests.
[b]The values for cortisol concentration used for diagnosis may vary between laboratories.

or low–dose dexamethasone suppression test and late-night salivary cortisol. Isolated measurements of plasma cortisol concentration are of no value; they are often normal during the day in patients with Cushing syndrome.

Increased 24-h urinary cortisol excretion is characteristic of Cushing syndrome, but specificity is poor: increased excretion can also occur in pseudo-Cushing syndrome and severe obesity. Sensitivity is also poor but can be improved by making several urine collections. If the urine collection is incomplete, the true excretion will be underestimated. This problem can be obviated by expressing the results as a ratio to the urinary creatinine excretion.

Dexamethasone is a synthetic glucocorticoid that binds to cortisol receptors in the pituitary and suppresses ACTH release (and thus the secretion of cortisol by the adrenals) in healthy individuals. In the **overnight dexamethasone suppression test**, 1 mg is given at night and blood is drawn for measurement of cortisol at 9:00 the next morning. In healthy individuals, this should be <50 nmol/L. Failure of suppression is characteristic of Cushing syndrome but is not specific because it may also be seen in pseudo-Cushing syndrome, as a result of stress and accelerated dexamethasone metabolism in the presence of drugs such as phenytoin or carbamazepine that induce the CYP3A4 enzyme system. Fewer false-positive results occur with the **low-dose** dexamethasone suppression test, in which dexamethasone is given at a dose of 0.5 mg 6-hourly for 48 h, and cortisol is measured on the morning after the last dose. False-positive results (i.e. failure to suppress) rarely occur with the latter test but are still a possibility in patients taking CYP3A4 inducing drugs. It is important that, if urinary cortisol excretion is to be measured, the period of collection does not include the time when dexamethasone is being given.

Loss of diurnal variation of cortisol secretion is an early feature of Cushing syndrome, and the diagnosis is

24-h urine collections

Measurement of the amount of a hormone (or other analyte) excreted in the urine throughout a 24-h period is potentially a useful method of assessing its overall rate of secretion during that period. In endocrine disorders characterized by overproduction, for example Cushing syndrome and phaeochromocytoma, the hormone in question may have a diurnal variation or episodic secretion pattern that makes single measurements in plasma difficult to interpret. For electrolytes the excretion will depend on dietary intake and the body's requirements.

Accurate determination of 24-h urinary excretion depends first on obtaining a complete 24-h collection from the patient and second ensuring that, if the analyte is susceptible to degradation, or precipitation, an appropriate preservative is present in the container.

To **obtain a complete collection**, the patient must be provided with clear instructions. He or she should be instructed to empty their bladder completely and discard that urine immediately before starting the collection. All urine passed throughout the subsequent 24-h period must be collected into the bottle, using a funnel or other collection device if necessary, and the patient must completely empty the bladder into the bottle at exactly 24 h after the collection begins. Start and end time must be recorded. The volume, and creatinine excretion, can be measured by the laboratory and, if low, may suggest that not all the urine produced in 24 h was collected. Even with apparently meticulous attention to detail a 24-h urine collection provides a relatively imprecise estimate of true 24-h urine, and analyte, output.

Catecholamines are unstable in urine at physiological pH, so some laboratories add an **acid preservative** (e.g. hydrochloric acid) to the container before it is issued to the patient. Patients must be warned about the risk of burns if the acid comes into contact with their skin and also that they must not pour the acid away before making the collection. Conversely, cortisol is stable in non-acidified urine, and the presence of acid renders the sample unsuitable for analysis. Different preservatives are required for other urine tests: the laboratory should issue appropriate containers for the tests requested and can provide advice.

virtually excluded if the plasma cortisol concentration at 11:00 p.m. or midnight is normal (<100 nmol/L). Because the patient must be resting and not stressed, plasma cortisol measurement at night is not a practical outpatient procedure. It necessitates hospital admission, itself a stressful event, with the result that false-positive results are common. It has largely been replaced by measurement of salivary cortisol on a midnight sample, which can be collected by the patient at home. Salivary cortisol concentration is approximately equal to plasma free cortisol concentration,

which is much lower than total cortisol concentration because 95% of plasma cortisol is bound to cortisol-binding globulin (see earlier, p. 176).

Cyclical Cushing syndrome, in which the hypersecretion of cortisol varies with time (sometimes over several years), is uncommon but well recognized, and it can pose a considerable diagnostic problem.

Once increased cortisol secretion has been documented, **measurements of plasma ACTH** are used to determine how to investigate the patient further. However, the hormone is very labile and, if valid results are to be obtained, plasma must be separated rapidly, using a refrigerated centrifuge, and kept deep-frozen until the assay is performed. Low ACTH concentrations suggest an adrenal cause (requiring adrenal imaging), and very high concentrations, ectopic secretion of ACTH (Table 10.3 and Case history 10.3). More moderately elevated concentrations are usual in patients with pituitary-dependent Cushing disease and are sometimes found with ectopic secretion of ACTH, especially by small or occult tumours such as carcinoids. Further biochemical investigations used to elucidate the cause of Cushing syndrome include the **high-dose dexamethasone suppression test** and the **CRH test** (see pp. 183 and 184). The former involves giving 2 mg dexamethasone 6-hourly for 48 h; plasma cortisol concentration is measured at 9:00 on the morning after the last dose. In Cushing disease, the cortisol concentration characteristically decreases to <50% of the pretreatment value. Failure of suppression suggests ectopic ACTH secretion or an adrenal tumour. Exceptions to these typical results occur frequently. Many patients with ectopic ACTH secretion have a characteristic clinical presentation, with weight loss, severe muscle weakness, pigmentation, hypertension, hypokalaemic alkalosis and diabetes, but without the classic somatic manifestations of Cushing disease. In other cases, however (particularly when caused by carcinoid tumours), ectopic ACTH secretion may produce a clinical syndrome that is clinically and biochemically identical to Cushing disease. **Imaging techniques**, for example chest x-ray and pituitary and abdominal computed tomography (CT) scanning, may reveal a tumour, while **selective venous blood sampling** for ACTH measurement, to locate the source of ACTH secretion, can also be helpful.

In Cushing disease, the pituitary usually remains susceptible to feedback by glucocorticoids but is less sensitive than normal (Fig. 10.4A) (i.e. a higher concentration of cortisol is necessary to suppress ACTH; Fig. 10.4B). In Cushing syndrome caused by adrenal tumours, whether adenomas or carcinomas, and also in ectopic ACTH secretion, there is usually no response to dexamethasone, even at the higher dose, because pituitary ACTH secretion is already suppressed by the high plasma cortisol concentrations (Fig. 10.4C). With adrenal tumours, feedback of cortisol to the pituitary suppresses ACTH, whereas with ectopic ACTH

183

Table 10.3 Typical results of adrenal function tests in Cushing syndrome

Condition	BASAL CORTISOL (nmol/L)	DEXAMETHASONE SUPPRESSION TEST		CRH TEST	PLASMA ACTH (ng/L)
		Low dose	High dose		
Cushing disease	↑ (<1000)	no suppression	suppression	response	↑ (<200)
adrenal tumour	↑(variable)	no suppression	no suppression	no response	↓
ectopic ACTH[a] secretion	greatly ↑ (>1000)	no suppression	no suppression	no response	greatly ↑ (>200)

[a]With ectopic adrenocorticotrophic hormone (ACTH) secretion by carcinoid tumours, the results of these tests may be identical to those seen in Cushing disease, as the tumour may have glucocorticoid receptors that will respond to dexamethasone.
CRH, corticotrophin-releasing hormone.

secretion, ACTH concentrations are often (but not always) very high (Fig. 10.4D). The results of biochemical tests in the various forms of Cushing syndrome are summarized in Table 10.3.

The CRH test can be useful to differentiate between Cushing disease and ectopic ACTH secretion. In Cushing disease, CRH (100 μg i.v.) typically increases plasma ACTH concentration by 50% over baseline after 60 min, and cortisol concentration by 20%, whereas with ectopic ACTH secretion or an adrenal tumour there is typically no response.

The management of Cushing syndrome depends on the cause. Adrenal adenomas and, if possible, carcinomas should be resected. The treatment of choice for Cushing disease is transsphenoidal hypophysectomy (pituitary resection), but when pituitary surgery is not possible, or is unsuccessful, bilateral adrenalectomy is necessary. Bilateral adrenalectomy must always be followed by treatment to the pituitary (usually external irradiation) to prevent continued growth of the pituitary tumour. If this is not done, the tumour may increase in size and give rise to clinical symptoms and signs, including pigmentation resulting from the secretion of excessive quantities of ACTH (Nelson syndrome). Patients who have undergone hypophysectomy or bilateral adrenalectomy will require appropriate steroid replacement therapy for life. When surgery is not possible, and in all patients pending surgery, symptomatic relief may ensue from the use of drugs that block cortisol synthesis, such as metyrapone, which inhibits steroid 11-hydroxylase.

Conn syndrome

This condition is characterized by **excessive production of aldosterone**. The principal causes and the clinical features are shown in Box 10.4. In about two-thirds of patients, the cause is an adrenal adenoma; these occur three times more frequently in women than in men.

Most other cases are a result of diffuse hypertrophy of the zona glomerulosa of the adrenal cortex (uncommon in age <40 years). A rare cause is glucocorticoid-remediable aldosteronism, an inherited (autosomal dominant) condition in which aldosterone synthesis is under the control of ACTH. These conditions are collectively classified as **primary aldosteronism**. The **clinical features** of Conn syndrome are **hypokalaemic alkalosis**, a consequence of aldosterone-induced increased renal potassium and hydrogen ion excretion, and **hypertension**, a consequence of sodium retention. Many patients are diagnosed when hypokalaemia is found during the investigation of hypertension: diagnosing Conn syndrome is important because it is usually curable by surgery. Its prevalence is 5–10% of patients with hypertension, increasing to approximately 20% in those with resistant hypertension, many of whom are normokalaemic.

Primary aldosteronism may be mimicked by treatment with carbenoxolone and by the ingestion of liquorice. Both of these substances have metabolites that inhibit 11β-hydroxysteroid dehydrogenase. This enzyme converts cortisol to an inactive metabolite, cortisone, but does not affect aldosterone. Its inhibition in mineralocorticoid-sensitive tissues in effect potentiates the action of cortisol as a mineralocorticoid. For the same reason, an inherited defect in this enzyme (which mimics the effect of inhibition) is the cause of the syndrome of apparent mineralocorticoid excess, a rare cause of hypertension and hypokalaemic alkalosis. It, and related conditions, are discussed on p. 321.

High aldosterone concentrations are also seen in patients whose plasma renin activity is increased. This is **secondary aldosteronism**, because the adrenal glands are responding to their normal trophic stimulus, in contrast with the autonomous secretion of aldosterone in Conn syndrome.

Secondary aldosteronism is far more common than the primary form and is associated with a variety of conditions

Case history 10.3

History

A 35-year-old male scaffolder presented with muscle weakness. This mainly affected his thighs, with the result that he sometimes had to use his hands to help himself up from a sitting position. He was also finding it difficult to walk up a flight of stairs. He had no other complaints.

Examination

He had a cushingoid appearance, with truncal obesity, proximal muscle wasting, violaceous abdominal striae and a plethoric 'moon face'. His blood pressure was 182/108 mmHg. He admitted that he had noticed the changes in his appearance developing over the past 9 months. He was admitted to hospital for further investigation.

Results

Serum:	sodium	136 mmol/L
	potassium	3.2 mmol/L
	bicarbonate	33 mmol/L
	cortisol (9:00 a.m.)	930 nmol/L
Plasma:	glucose (fasting)	6.5 mmol/L
	ACTH (9:00 a.m.)	130 ng/L
Urine cortisol excretion		840 nmol/24 h
Salivary cortisol (midnight)		9 nmol/L (<2)

Dexamethasone suppression test:

| 9:00 a.m. serum cortisol after 0.5 mg dexamethasone four times daily for 2 days (low dose) | 880 nmol/L |
| 9:00 a.m. serum cortisol after 2.0 mg dexamethasone four times daily for 2 days (high dose) | 320 nmol/L |

Summary

High urinary cortisol excretion and high midnight salivary cortisol concentration with a raised plasma ACTH.

Interpretation

The lack of diurnal variation and high cortisol excretion suggest adrenal hyperfunction. The diagnosis is Cushing disease. The clinical features and results of the two-stage test are typical of Cushing disease, with no change after the low dose but decreased cortisol secretion after the high-dose dexamethasone test, and a raised ACTH (see Table 10.3).

Discussion

This patient has a hypokalaemic alkalosis, a result of renal potassium and hydrogen ion wasting, and hypertension, a result of sodium retention. The fasting blood glucose is elevated: impaired fasting glycaemia or impaired glucose tolerance are common in Cushing syndrome, but frank diabetes is uncommon, except in ectopic ACTH secretion. If the patient is coincidentally diabetic, there may be a marked deterioration in glycaemic control.

A brain magnetic resonance imaging (MRI) scan in this patient showed a normal pituitary fossa: in Cushing disease, the pituitary tumour secreting ACTH is usually very small but may be revealed by MRI. CT scanning may be used if MRI is contraindicated or not available.

(Box 10.5) in which renin secretion is increased. Patients may or may not be hypertensive, depending on the underlying condition.

When investigating a patient with hypokalaemia and hypertension, many possible causes of secondary aldosteronism can be eliminated, either on clinical grounds or on the basis of simple tests. Plasma sodium concentration is usually high–normal or slightly elevated in primary aldosteronism; in secondary aldosteronism, the concentration is usually <138 mmol/L. If necessary, measurement of plasma renin activity or mass under appropriate conditions (see later) will distinguish between primary and secondary aldosteronism. It is low in the former condition but elevated in the latter.

Primary aldosteronism should be suspected in any hypertensive patient who has a low plasma potassium concentration, but the commonest cause of this association is treatment with loop or thiazide diuretics. In these circumstances, plasma potassium concentration should be checked after withdrawal of the diuretic for 2 weeks before proceeding to further investigations. Other causes of hypokalaemia should be excluded. However, in early disease or in patients on a low sodium intake (as is often recommended in hypertension), plasma potassium concentration may be normal or only slightly low; it may even be slightly increased if hypertension has been treated with an angiotensin-converting enzyme (ACE) inhibitor. The hypokalaemia of Conn syndrome is a result of excessive renal potassium excretion. Hypokalaemia from other causes (apart from diuretic therapy) should lead to maximal renal potassium retention. Thus, in a patient with hypokalaemia who is not taking a diuretic, renal potassium excretion of >30 mmol/24 h is very suggestive of aldosteronism.

There should be **three stages to the diagnosis of primary aldosteronism**: screening, diagnosis and establishment of the cause. **Screening** involves measuring aldosterone and renin in the same plasma sample, with calculation of the ambulant aldosterone:renin ratio. The

Cushing syndrome

(A) Normal

Production of cortisol by adrenal cortex stimulated by ACTH

Cortisol exerts a negative feedback effect on release of ACTH by pituitary

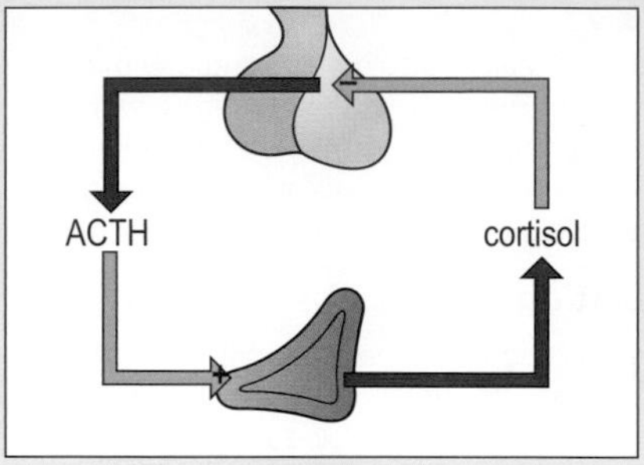

(B) Cushing disease

ACTH secretion increased

Pituitary insensitive to feedback by normal levels of cortisol

Higher levels of cortisol required to produce negative feedback effect on ACTH secretion

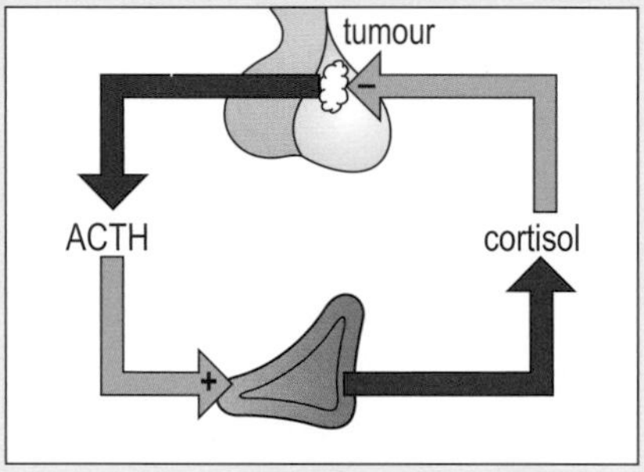

(C) Adrenal tumours

Autonomous cortisol production

High circulating cortisol inhibits ACTH secretion

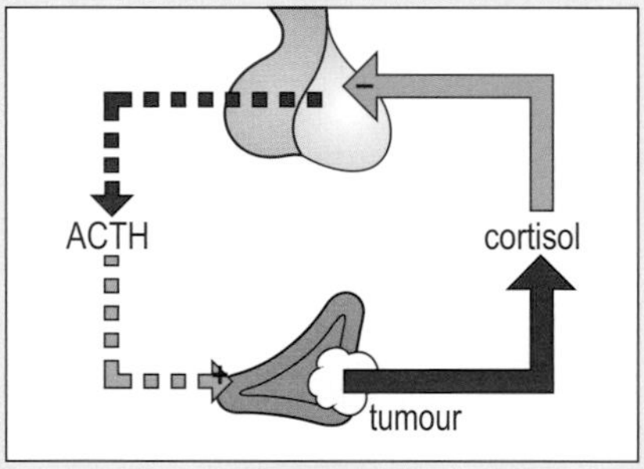

(D) Ectopic ACTH secretion

High level of ACTH secreted by tumour stimulates excessive cortisol production

Inhibition of secretion of ACTH by pituitary

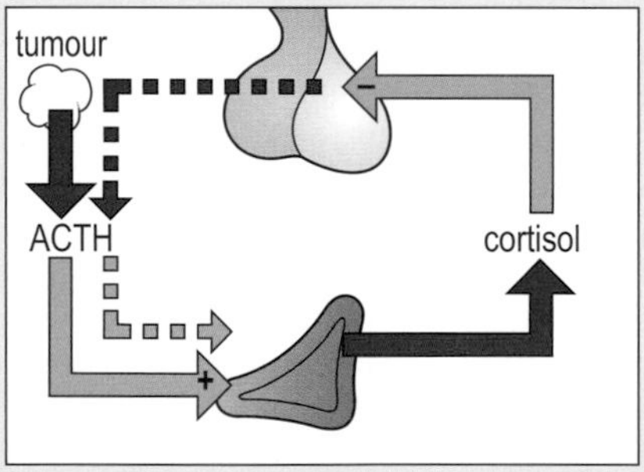

Fig. 10.4 Pituitary–adrenal relationships in Cushing syndrome. ACTH, adrenocorticotrophic hormone.

Box 10.4 **Causes and clinical features of Conn syndrome**

Causes

adrenal adenoma[a]
bilateral hypertrophy of zona glomerulosa cells[a]
glucocorticoid-remediable aldosteronism
adrenal carcinoma

Clinical features

hypertension
muscle weakness (occasionally paralysis)
latent tetany and paraesthesiae
polydipsia, polyuria and nocturia

[a]These conditions account for most cases.

Box 10.5 **Conditions associated with secondary aldosteronism**

Common

congestive cardiac failure
cirrhosis of liver with ascites
nephrotic syndrome

Less common

renal artery stenosis
sodium-losing nephritis
Bartter and Gitelman syndromes[a]
renin-secreting tumours

[a]Bartter and Gitelman syndromes are rare, inherited disorders of renal sodium reabsorption. Sodium loss stimulates aldosterone secretion and leads to hypokalaemia. In Gitelman syndrome, there is also hypercalciuria and hypomagnesaemia.

Box 10.6 **Drugs that potentially interfere with the plasma aldosterone:renin ratio**

Drugs that potentially cause false-positive aldosterone:renin ratio

β-adrenergic receptor blockers
methyldopa
clonidine
non-steroidal anti-inflammatory drugs
renin inhibitors (if plasma renin *activity* measured)
oestrogen-containing drugs (if active renin *concentration* measured)

Drugs that potentially cause false-negative aldosterone:renin ratio

diuretics (all classes)
dihydropyridine Ca^{2+}-channel antagonists
angiotensin-converting enzyme inhibitors
angiotensin II receptor blockers
renin inhibitors (if direct renin *concentration* measured)

activity of the renin–aldosterone axis is affected by several drugs (Box 10.6). Spironolactone (which is an aldosterone antagonist) must be stopped for at least 6 weeks before testing. Most other antihypertensives (with the exception of doxazosin and other alpha-blockers) and diuretics affect renin or aldosterone, or both. If these drugs cannot safely be discontinued, as a minimum, beta blockers and ACE inhibitors should be stopped for 2 weeks beforehand and calcium channel blockers withheld on the day of the test until after its completion. The advice of a clinical biochemist should be sought concerning the precise effects of individual classes of drug. Hypokalaemia should be corrected, because it reduces aldosterone secretion. The patient should be advised not to restrict salt intake for a few days before the test and asked to attend for blood sampling 2 h after waking in the morning to achieve maximum sensitivity. Note that reference ranges for both renin and aldosterone depend on whether the patient is recumbent or ambulant, although the ratios remain the same. The interpretation of results is indicated in Table 10.4: care is necessary because renin can be measured either as enzyme activity or as protein mass. Therefore, local laboratory thresholds should be used for interpretation, taking into account analytical method and units. This is a sensitive test that can detect early disease when aldosterone secretion is only slightly increased, but sufficiently to suppress renin production (Case history 10.4 and 10.5). If the ratio is equivocal, the test should be repeated after rigorous exclusion of all potentially interfering drugs if any of these were not withdrawn. If there is still diagnostic uncertainty a **confirmatory diagnostic test**, most commonly a saline suppression test, is required. This involves the infusion of 2 L of 0.9% saline over a period of 4 h. Sodium loading increases the amount of sodium reaching the distal renal tubules and should inhibit aldosterone secretion: if plasma aldosterone concentration remains >140 pmol/L, the diagnosis is confirmed. Caution is required, particularly in the elderly, because of a small risk of provoking cardiac failure. A more elaborate procedure, regarded by some as the definitive investigation, involves a combination of sodium loading and the administration of fludrocortisone over a period of 4 days. There is a risk of provoking profound hypokalaemia, and potassium replacement may be required. However, this test requires admission to hospital, whereas the saline infusion test can be done as an outpatient; it is contraindicated in the elderly and, like the saline suppression test, may provoke heart failure.

Table 10.4 Screening for Conn syndrome using the plasma aldosterone:renin ratio

Ratio (renin activity in pmol/mL/h)[a]	Ratio (renin mass in mU/L)[a]	Interpretation	Action
<800	<80	diagnosis excluded	seek other causes
800–2000	80–200	diagnosis possible	repeat after excluding all potentially interfering drugs
>2000	>200	diagnosis very likely	confirmatory tests

[a]Note that ranges and thresholds are analytical method, unit and laboratory specific. Aldosterone is measured in pmol/L.

Case history 10.4

History

An apparently healthy 27-year-old woman underwent a medical examination as part of her employer's private medical insurance.

Examination

She was found to have a blood pressure of 158/106 mmHg, confirmed by two repeat measurements. Physical examination was otherwise unremarkable.

Results

The only abnormality on standard biochemical testing was a serum potassium concentration of 3.3 mmol/L. Her eGFR was >90 mL/min/1.73 m². A further blood sample was taken:

Plasma: aldosterone   980 pmol/L (100–800 upright)

renin activity   72 mU/L (5.4–60 upright)

aldosterone:renin ratio   14 (<80)

Summary

Normal aldosterone:renin ratio.

Interpretation

Primary aldosteronism excluded.

Discussion

Although essential hypertension is common, it is prudent always to exclude treatable causes of hypertension in young people, and in hypertension that is resistant to treatment, associated with unusual symptoms or other features suggestive of a specific cause (see Chapter 17). In this patient, both the aldosterone concentration and the renin activity are high, indicating that the increase in aldosterone is secondary to increased renin production. Renal Doppler ultrasound studies indicated a minor degree of unilateral renal artery stenosis; this was confirmed by magnetic resonance angiography. The patient's hypertension proved easy to control with medication. The majority of patients with renal artery stenosis do not develop progressive kidney disease and do not require angioplasty; coexisting essential hypertension may exaggerate the effect of minor degrees of stenosis on the development of hypertension.

Identification of the **cause** of Conn syndrome after a positive diagnostic test result is by CT scanning, although this technique may miss small adrenal adenomas or mistakenly identify non-functioning adenomas as the cause. If surgery is a potential treatment option, CT scanning must be followed up with selective adrenal venous sampling to confirm the site of the aldosterone-producing lesion. Glucocorticoid-remediable aldosteronism can be diagnosed using a genetic test.

If Conn syndrome is shown to be due to a tumour, the tumour should be removed surgically. In patients with bilateral adrenal hyperplasia, treatment with spironolactone, a diuretic that antagonizes the action of aldosterone, may be sufficient to control the blood pressure. Spironolactone is also used in patients with tumours while they await surgery. Glucocorticoid-suppressible hyperaldosteronism is treated with dexamethasone.

Congenital adrenal hyperplasia

The term 'congenital adrenal hyperplasia' encompasses a group of **inherited metabolic disorders** of adrenal steroid hormone biosynthesis. Their clinical features depend on the position of the defective enzyme in the synthetic pathway, which determines the pattern of hormones and precursors that is produced (see Fig. 10.2).

21-Hydroxylase deficiency, with an incidence of 1 in 12 000 live births in the UK, accounts for around 95%

Case history 10.5

History

A 35-year-old woman was found to have a blood pressure of 188/112 mmHg by her general practitioner at a routine health check. He prescribed a thiazide diuretic, but one week later she returned to the surgery complaining of severe muscle weakness and constipation. The doctor arranged an urgent consultation at the local hospital where her serum potassium was found to be 2.6 mmol/L. The diuretic was stopped, her blood pressure was controlled with doxazosin (an alpha-blocker) and she was given oral potassium supplements. After 3 weeks, her serum potassium concentration was only 3.0 mmol/L. She then attended the pathology day unit for collection of samples for measurement of renin and aldosterone.

Results

Plasma:	aldosterone	1570 pmol/L (100–800 upright)
	renin activity	<0.5 mU/L (5.4–60 upright)
	aldosterone:renin ratio	>2500 (≥200 Conn syndrome likely)

Summary

Very high aldosterone:renin ratio.

Interpretation

High probability of Conn syndrome.

Discussion

A CT scan of the abdomen showed a small (1.5-cm) mass arising from the left adrenal gland. This was removed surgically. The patient made a rapid recovery after the operation, and repeated checks showed her to be normokalaemic and normotensive.

Giving a diuretic may provoke symptomatic hypokalaemia in mild aldosteronism. The hypokalaemia in this condition is characteristically resistant to potassium supplementation. Ideally, it should be corrected before measurement of aldosterone because hypokalaemia inhibits aldosterone secretion. However, this patient's plasma aldosterone concentration was high even in the face of ongoing hypokalaemia. In primary aldosteronism, the plasma aldosterone:renin ratio is typically at least >1000 (often >2000), as in this patient.

---

of all cases of CAH. It is an autosomal recessive disorder caused by mutation in the *CYP21* gene. The majority of the remaining 5% are due to deficiency of **11β-hydroxylase**. 21 Hydroxylase deficiency is often incomplete, and adequate cortisol synthesis can be maintained by increased secretion of ACTH by the pituitary. It is this that causes hyperplasia of the glands. Because of the metabolic block, the substrate of the enzyme (17-OHP) accumulates and there is increased formation of adrenal androgens (see p. Figs. 10.2 and 10.5).

There are three clinical forms of 21-hydroxylase deficiency CAH. In about one-third of neonates with 21-hydroxylase deficiency, the enzyme deficiency is almost complete: they present shortly after birth with a **life-threatening salt-losing state**, in which cortisol and aldosterone production are insufficient to maintain normal homoeostasis. Female infants affected by the **simple virilizing** form of CAH are born with **ambiguous genitalia** caused by increased androgen formation but are able to synthesize sufficient mineralocorticoids to maintain normal renal salt and water homoeostasis. Boys may present with pseudoprecocious puberty in their second or third year of life but are not virilized at birth. When the enzyme deficiency is only partial, the condition may not present until early adulthood (**non-classic or late-onset CAH**), with hirsutism, amenorrhoea or infertility. The various forms of 21-hydroxylase deficiency reflect the degree to which the

CYP21 mutation present reduces the activity of the enzyme: the manifestations of the condition run true to type within affected families.

Diagnosis is made by demonstrating an elevated concentration of 17-OHP in the plasma at least 2 days after birth (before this time, maternally derived 17-OHP may still be present in the infant's blood). An abnormal result may be followed up with analysis of a full urine steroid profile to confirm the expected accumulation of androgens and by testing for *CYP21* gene mutations. In patients with suspected late-onset CAH, plasma 17-OHP concentrations are sometimes within the reference range but increase after stimulation of the glucocorticoid synthetic pathway with tetracosactide. **Treatment** involves replacement of glucocorticoid (usually as hydrocortisone, but synthetic agents, which have a longer duration of action, are sometimes used in young adults) to suppress ACTH production, and hence the excessive androgen synthesis. Some patients also need mineralocorticoid replacement with fludrocortisone. Treatment is monitored by measurement of plasma 17-OHP, androstenedione, testosterone and renin together with measures of growth.

Partial **11β-hydroxylase deficiency** is also more common than complete deficiency of the enzyme. Increased androgen production causes virilization, which tends to be more severe than in 21-hydroxylase deficiency (but again is not present in males at birth). Hypertension develops, because of the accumulation of 11-deoxycorticosterone, a

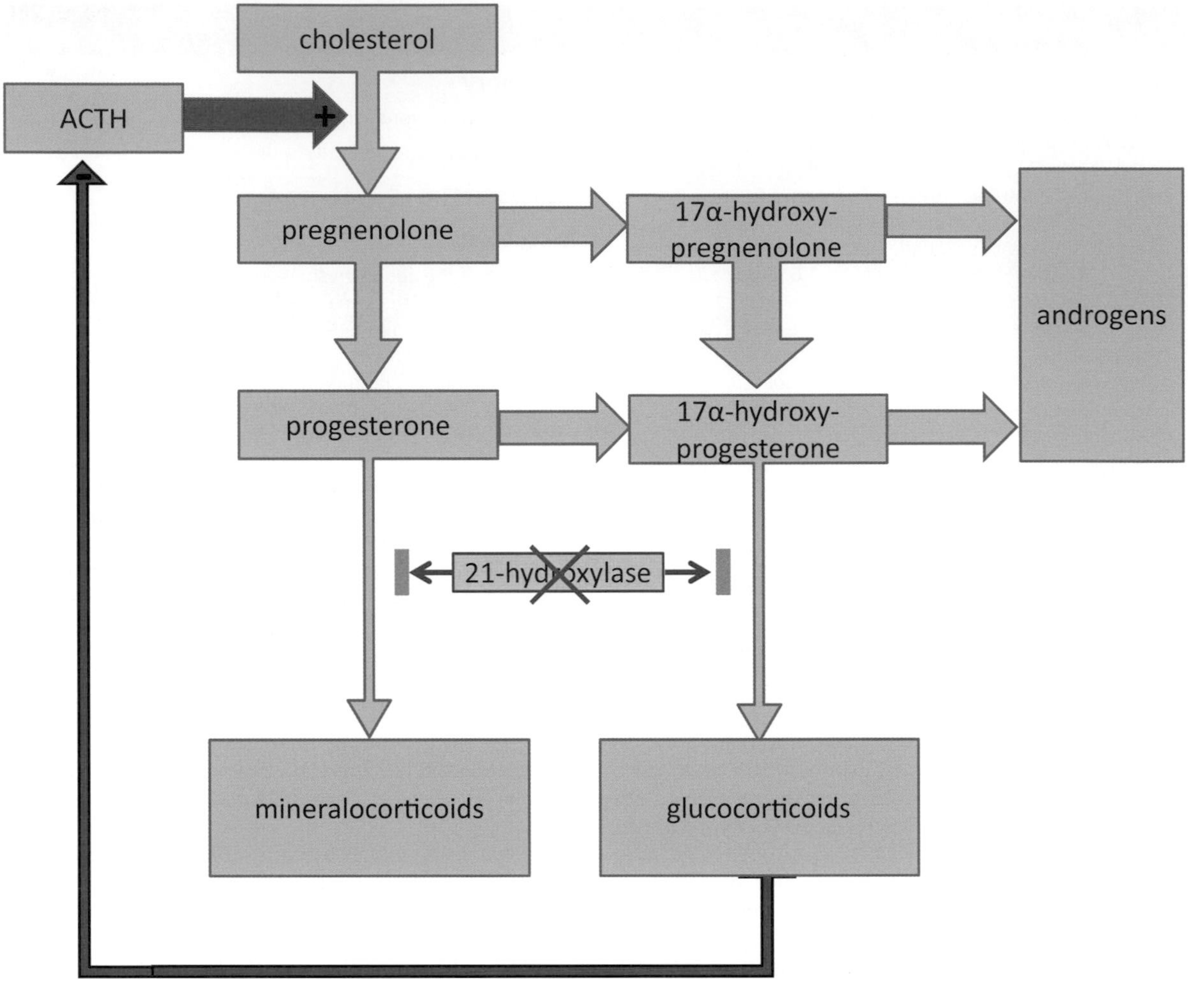

Fig. 10.5 Adrenal steroid synthesis, showing the consequences of 21-hydroxylase deficiency in congenital adrenal hyperplasia (CAH). Decreased cortisol synthesis results in reduced negative feedback to pituitary adrenocorticotrophin (ACTH) production. This in turn stimulates the conversion of cholesterol to pregnenolone and progesterone, leading to increased androgen synthesis. In the salt-losing form of CAH, both cortisol and aldosterone synthesis are insufficient for normal homeostasis, whereas in the simple virilizing form mineralocorticoid synthesis remains sufficient. In late-onset CAH, the enzyme deficiency is only partial and normal mineralocorticoid and glucocorticoid secretion are maintained but patients present in early adulthood with signs of androgen excess.

substrate of the defective enzyme that has mineralocorticoid (salt-retaining) properties. The diagnosis rests on the demonstration of an increased plasma concentration of either 11-deoxycortisol or its urinary metabolite. Treatment is with cortisol alone: although aldosterone secretion is defective, 11-deoxycorticosterone provides adequate mineralocorticoid activity.

Other forms of CAH involving, for example, 17-hydroxylase, corticosterone methyloxidase (thus affecting aldosterone secretion only) and steroid 3β-hydroxydehydrogenase Δ5 isomerase, are rare. Some indication of their consequences, in terms of adrenal steroid metabolism, should be apparent from studying Figs. 10.2 and 10.5 (simplified version).

Disorders of the Adrenal Medulla

The main interest in the adrenal medulla for clinical biochemistry relates to **phaeochromocytomas**. These are tumours that secrete catecholamines, the normal secretory products of the organ, and which are a rare (~0.5% of all cases), but treatable, cause of hypertension. Approximately 10% of phaeochromocytomas are found in extramedullary tissue that shares the same embryological origin (i.e. chromaffin tissue derived from neuroectoderm). Catecholamines can also be produced by tumours of embryologically related tissue, for example, the carotid bodies, and by neuroblastomas, which are rare tumours that occur only in infants and young children and usually present as a rapidly enlarging abdominal mass.

Patients with phaeochromocytomas typically present with **symptoms** such as headache, palpitation, sweating, pallor, tremor and abdominal discomfort. These often occur sporadically. **Hypertension** is common: although this may be episodic, it is usually sustained. Although phaeochromocytomas are rare, they are a potentially curable cause of hypertension, which is a very common condition. Therefore, it is important to have available a simple screening test that identifies patients who are likely to have a phaeochromocytoma and who should be subjected to

more definitive investigation, and eliminates the majority in whom this probability is very low.

The metabolism of catecholamines is outlined in Fig. 10.6. Adrenaline (epinephrine) and noradrenaline (norepinephrine) are metabolized by catechol-O-methyltransferase (COMT) to metadrenaline and normetadrenaline, respectively. They are also converted by the consecutive action of monoamine oxidase and COMT to 4-hydroxy-3-methoxymandelic acid (HMMA), also known as vanillylmandelic acid (VMA).

Approaches to screening and diagnosis vary, and the laboratory should be contacted to ensure that appropriate samples are collected and that drugs that may affect the results of assays are avoided. The simplest **screening test** is measurement of urinary catecholamines or metanephrines (i.e. metadrenaline and normetadrenaline): metanephrines are more sensitive and thus are the preferred test when available. Measurement of plasma metanephrine concentrations has the highest diagnostic sensitivity and specificity, but sample collection and measurement are difficult. Some drugs—for example, methyldopa, α-adrenergic antagonists, paracetamol and labetalol—can cross-react in assays for catecholamines or increase plasma and urine catecholamine concentrations. After diagnosis, the site of the tumour is identified by either CT or MRI scanning. Uptake of ^{131}I-metaiodobenzylguanidine (MIBG) is a useful technique, especially for detecting extraadrenal tumours. Most phaeochromocytomas secrete predominantly noradrenaline; if adrenaline is also secreted, the tumour is more likely to be in the adrenal medulla than extraadrenal (Case history 10.6).

Although phaeochromocytomas are benign in 90% of cases, all tumours should be removed surgically. However, this is a potentially hazardous operation because large quantities of catecholamines may be released into the circulation during the procedure. Full α-adrenergic blockade followed by β-adrenergic blockade should be established before, and maintained during, surgery. Notably, 10% of patients with phaeochromocytomas have multiple tumours. The tumours may be a component of multiple endocrine neoplasia types 2A and 2B (see p. 357), and thus evidence of other relevant endocrine disorders should be sought in affected patients.

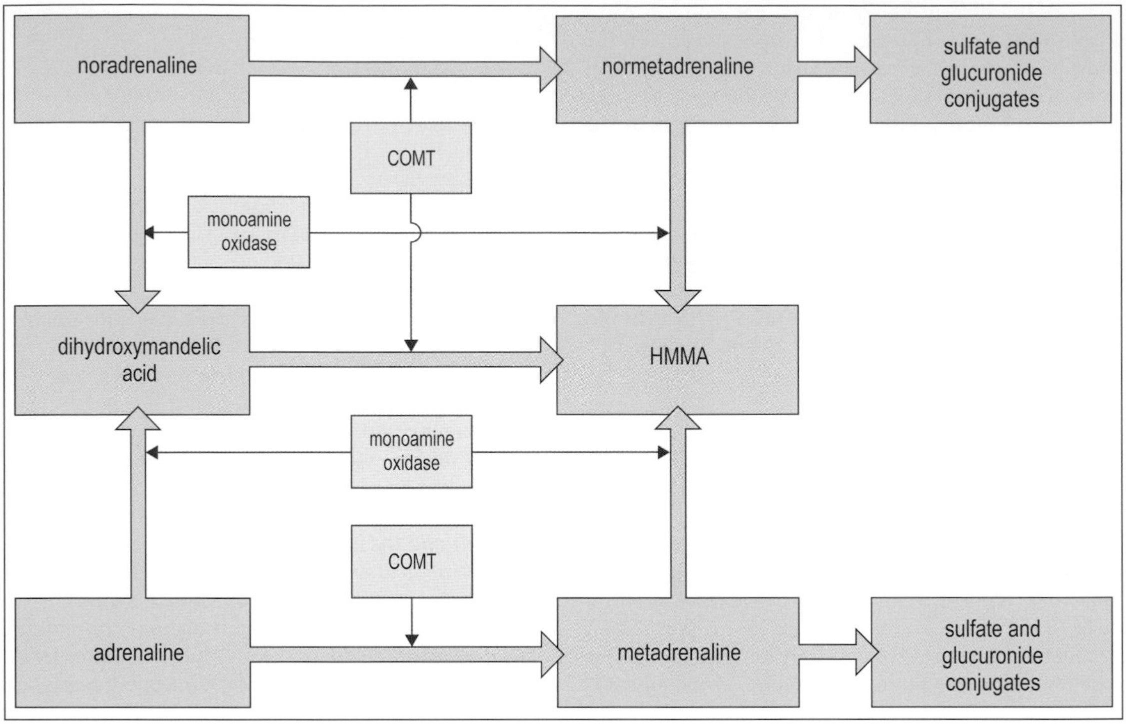

Fig. 10.6 Metabolism of catecholamines. COMT, catechol-*O*-methyltransferase; HMMA, 4-hydroxy-3-methoxymandelic acid.

Case history 10.6

History

A 75-year-old woman presented with anxiety, palpitations and sweating. Her pulse was 80 beats per minute, regular, and her blood pressure was 158/102 mmHg. She had previously been investigated for abdominal pain, for which no cause had been found.

Results

Tests of thyroid function were normal. A 24-h urine collection was made.

Urine: metadrenaline 15.1 µmol/24 h
(<1.3)
normetadrenaline 7.2 µmol/24 h
(<3.0)

Investigations

A CT scan of the abdomen showed a mass arising from the left adrenal gland, and an isotopic scan of the adrenals, using MIBG, showed a single left adrenal mass.

Summary

High urine metanephrine excretion in a patient who has an adrenal mass.

Interpretation

The high metadrenaline excretion suggests that the tumour is of adrenal origin, a location confirmed by the imaging procedures. After 3 days of treatment with phenoxybenzamine and propranolol (α- and β-adrenergic antagonists, respectively), a 5-cm left adrenal phaeochromocytoma was removed by laparoscopic surgery.

The clinical features initially suggested thyrotoxicosis, but the normal thyroid function tests excluded this more common diagnosis.

SUMMARY

- The **adrenal cortex** secretes three classes of steroid hormones: glucocorticoids, mineralocorticoids and androgens.
- The secretion of **cortisol** is controlled by ACTH; ACTH secretion is subject to feedback inhibition by cortisol. Control is also exerted from the higher centres through the hypothalamus. Cortisol secretion shows a diurnal variation, with peak plasma concentrations in the morning and a trough in the late evening. Cortisol is essential to life: it is involved in the response to stress and, with other hormones, regulates many pathways of intermediary metabolism. Its metabolic action is largely catabolic.
- ACTH also stimulates the production and secretion of **adrenal androgens**; these hormones have a role in determining secondary sexual characteristics in the female but do not appear to have a specific role in the male.
- **Aldosterone** is the most important mineralocorticoid; it stimulates sodium reabsorption in the distal tubules of the kidneys in exchange for potassium and hydrogen. It is an important determinant of the ECF volume. Its secretion is controlled by the renin–angiotensin system, in response to changes in blood pressure and blood volume.
- **Adrenal failure** is most frequently due to autoimmune destruction of the glands, although there are many other causes. It can present acutely as a medical emergency with hypoglycaemia and circulatory collapse caused by renal salt wasting. In more chronic cases, lassitude, weight loss and postural hypotension are frequent clinical features, and it should also be considered in patients with otherwise unexplained hyperkalaemia. Diagnosis depends on demonstrating failure of the adrenal to produce cortisol in response to ACTH (tetracosactide or Synacthen test). Pituitary disease can cause secondary adrenal failure by reducing ACTH secretion.
- Overproduction of adrenal cortical hormones can affect predominantly cortisol (producing **Cushing syndrome**) or aldosterone (**Conn syndrome**). Cushing syndrome can also be secondary to excess ACTH production by a pituitary tumour or by a non-endocrine tumour (ectopic ACTH production), or be iatrogenic, due to treatment with corticosteroids or ACTH. Clinical features of Cushing syndrome include characteristic somatic changes, muscle weakness, glucose intolerance, hypokalaemia and hypertension. Patients with Conn syndrome develop hypertension and hypokalaemia. The diagnosis of both of these conditions involves initial screening tests to demonstrate high, non-suppressible concentrations of the hormones and then elucidation of the cause.
- The various forms of Congenital adrenal hyperplasia (**CAH**) are inherited metabolic disorders of adrenal steroid hormone biosynthesis. The clinical features derive from a mixture of underproduction of either cortisol or aldosterone, or both, and increased production of androgens. The most common type is steroid 21-hydroxylase deficiency.
- The **adrenal medulla** produces catecholamines but is not essential to life. There appear to be no clinical sequelae of decreased adrenal medullary activity, but tumours of the glands (neuroblastomas and phaeochromocytomas) can produce excessive quantities of catecholamines. These cause hypertension and other clinical features related to increased sympathetic activity.

Chapter 11

The thyroid gland

Introduction

The thyroid gland secretes three hormones: **thyroxine** (T4) and **triiodothyronine** (T3), both of which are iodinated derivatives of tyrosine (Fig. 11.1), and calcitonin, a polypeptide hormone. T4 and T3 are produced by the follicular cells, but calcitonin is secreted by the C cells, which are of separate embryological origin. Calcitonin is functionally unrelated to the other thyroid hormones. It has a minor role in calcium homoeostasis, and disorders of its secretion are rare (see Chapter 14). Thyroid disorders in which there is either oversecretion or undersecretion of T4 and T3 are, however, common.

T4 synthesis and release are stimulated by the pituitary trophic hormone, **thyroid-stimulating hormone** (TSH). The secretion of TSH is controlled by negative feedback by the thyroid hormones (see p. 157), which modulate the response of the pituitary to the hypothalamic hormone, **thyrotrophin-releasing hormone** (TRH; Fig. 11.2). This feedback is mediated primarily by T3 produced by the action of iodothyronine deiodinase on T4 in the thyrotroph cells of the anterior pituitary. Glucocorticoids, dopamine and somatostatin inhibit TSH secretion. The physiological significance of this is not known, but it may be relevant to the disturbances of thyroid hormones that can occur in non-thyroidal illness (see p. 201). The feedback mechanisms result in the maintenance of steady plasma concentrations of thyroid hormones.

The **major product of the thyroid gland** is T4. Ten times less T3 is produced (the proportion may be greater in thyroid disease), most (~80%) T3 being derived from T4 by deiodination in peripheral tissues, particularly the liver, kidneys and muscle, catalysed by selenium-containing iodothyronine deiodinases. T3 is three to four times more potent than T4. In tissues, most of the effect of T4 results from this conversion to T3, so that T4 itself is essentially

a prohormone. Deiodination can also produce reverse triiodothyronine (rT3; see Fig. 11.1), which is physiologically inactive. It is produced instead of T3 in starvation and many non-thyroidal illnesses, and the formation of either the active or inactive metabolite of T4 appears to play an important part in the control of energy metabolism.

Thyroid Hormones

Actions

Thyroid hormones are essential for **normal growth and development** and have many **effects on metabolic processes**. They act by entering cells and binding to specific receptors in the nuclei, which in turn bind to hormone response elements in DNA. This stimulates the synthesis of messenger RNA and hence polypeptides, including hormones and enzymes. Among the latter are key enzymes involved in energy metabolism, including cytochrome oxidase. Their most obvious overall effect on metabolism is to **stimulate the basal metabolic rate**, oxygen consumption and heat production, through actions that include stimulating Na^+,K^+-ATPases involved in ion transport and increasing the availability of energy substrates. Overall, the effect of thyroid hormones is to increase net catabolism: weight loss and muscle wasting are typical features of excessive secretion of thyroid hormones. Thyroid hormones also increase the sensitivity of the cardiovascular and nervous systems to catecholamines, the former leading to increases in heart rate and cardiac output, and the latter to increased arousal.

Synthesis

Thyroid hormone synthesis involves a number of specific enzyme-catalysed reactions, beginning with the uptake of

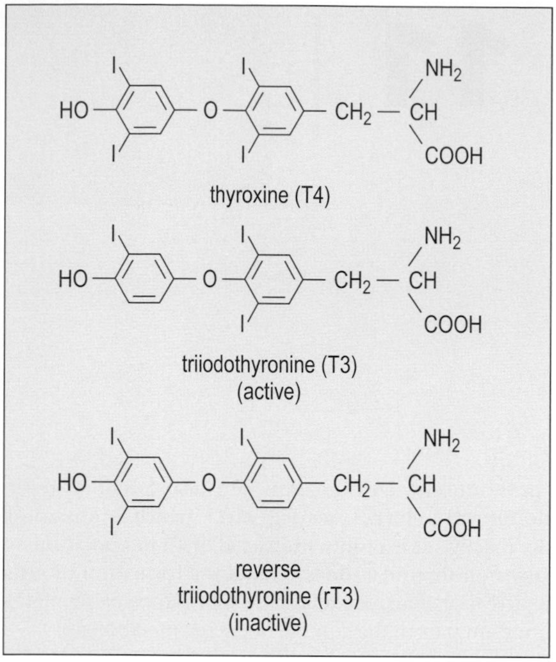

Fig. 11.1 Chemical structure of the thyroid hormones, T4 and T3, and the inactive metabolite of T4, rT3.

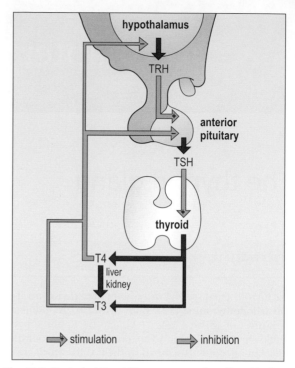

Fig. 11.2 Control of thyroid hormone secretion. Thyroid-stimulating hormone (TSH) is released from the pituitary in response to the hypothalamic hormone, thyrotrophin-releasing hormone (TRH), and stimulates the synthesis and release of thyroid hormones. TSH release is inhibited by thyroid hormones, which decrease the sensitivity of the pituitary to TRH. They may also inhibit TRH release by the hypothalamus.

iodide by the gland and culminating in the iodination of tyrosine residues in the protein thyroglobulin (Fig. 11.3); these reactions are all stimulated by TSH. Rare, congenital forms of hypothyroidism caused by inherited deficiencies of each of the various enzymes concerned have been described.

Thyroglobulin is stored within the thyroid gland in colloid follicles. These are accumulations of thyroglobulin-containing colloid surrounded by thyroid follicular cells. Release of thyroid hormones (stimulated by TSH) involves pinocytosis of colloid by follicular cells and fusion with lysosomes to form phagocytic vacuoles (see Fig. 11.3). After proteolysis, thyroid hormones are released into the bloodstream. Proteolysis also results in the liberation of monoiodotyrosines (MITs) and diiodotyrosines (DITs); these are usually degraded within thyroid follicular cells and their iodine is retained and re-utilized. A small amount of thyroglobulin also reaches the bloodstream.

Thyroid hormones in blood

The **normal plasma concentrations of T4 and T3** are 60–150 and 1.0–2.9 nmol/L, respectively. **Both hormones are extensively protein bound:** some 99.98% of T4 and 99.66% of T3 are bound, principally to a specific thyroxine-binding globulin (TBG) and, to a lesser extent, to prealbumin and albumin. Only the free, non-protein-bound, thyroid hormones are physiologically active. Although the total T4 concentration is normally 50 times that of T3, the different extents to which these hormones are bound to protein mean that the free T4 (fT4) concentration is only 2 to 3 times that of free T3 (fT3). Typical reference ranges are 12–22 pmol/L for fT4 and 3.9–6.7 pmol/L for fT3, but this varies depending on the assay method used.

The precise physiological function of TBG is unknown; individuals who have a genetically determined deficiency of the protein show no clinical abnormality. TBG is approximately one-third saturated at normal concentrations of thyroid hormones. It has, however, been suggested that it provides a buffer that maintains the free hormone concentrations constant in the face of any tendency to change. Protein binding also reduces the amount of thyroid hormones that would otherwise be lost by glomerular filtration and subsequent renal excretion.

Total (free + bound) thyroid hormone concentrations in plasma are dependent not only on thyroid function but also on the concentrations of binding proteins. If these

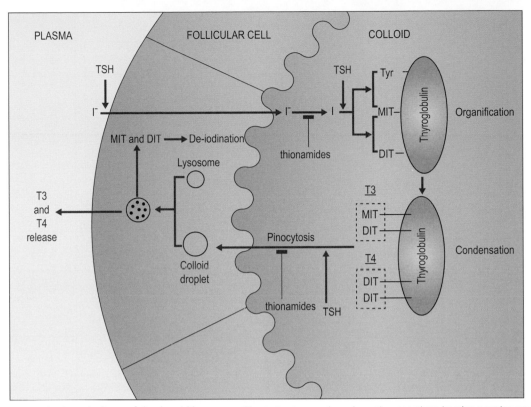

Fig. 11.3 Biosynthesis and release of the thyroid hormones. The iodination and condensation reactions involve tyrosine residues that are an integral part of the thyroglobulin polypeptide. The thyroid hormones remain protein bound until they are released from the cell. Iodide is actively absorbed through the thyroid cells into the colloid of the thyroid follicle, where it is oxidized to iodine and immediately incorporated into tyrosine (Tyr) residues to form monoiodotyrosine (MIT) and diiodotyrosine (DIT). These undergo coupling to form T3 and T4. Antithyroid thionamide drugs, such as carbimazole, act by inhibiting the oxidation of iodide and the coupling reaction. Before secretion of thyroid hormones, colloid droplets are taken up into follicular cells by pinocytosis and undergo lysosomal proteolysis. T3 and T4 are released and MIT and DIT are degraded, with recycling of their iodine content. TSH, thyroid-stimulating hormone.

were to increase (Fig. 11.4), the temporary decline in free hormone concentration caused by increased protein binding would stimulate TSH release, and this would restore the free hormone concentrations to normal: if binding protein concentrations were to fall, the reverse would occur. In either situation, there would be a change in the concentrations of total hormones, but the free hormone concentrations would remain normal.

Changes in the concentrations of the binding proteins occur in many circumstances (Box 11.1), causing changes in total hormone concentrations, but not necessarily in those of the free (physiologically available) hormones. Furthermore, certain drugs—for example, salicylates and phenytoin—displace thyroid hormones from their binding proteins, thus reducing total, but not free, hormone concentrations once a new steady state is attained.

Only small amounts of T4 and T3 are excreted by the kidneys because of the extensive protein binding. The major route of thyroid hormone degradation is by deiodination and metabolism in tissues, but they are also conjugated in the liver and excreted in bile.

Tests of Thyroid Function

Laboratory tests of thyroid function are required to assist in the diagnosis and monitoring of thyroid disease. Most laboratories offer a standard 'profile' of thyroid function tests (e.g. TSH alone or TSH and fT4) and perform additional tests only if these results are equivocal or the clinical circumstances require it.

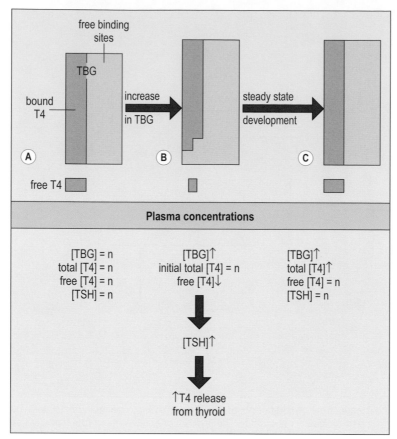

Fig. 11.4 Effect of an increase in thyroxine-binding globulin (TBG) concentration on plasma thyroxine (T4) concentration. **A,** In the initial steady state, TBG is one-third saturated with T4. **B,** TBG concentration increases, causing more T4 to be bound, thus reducing the free T4 concentration. This stimulates thyroid-stimulating hormone (TSH) secretion, which leads to an increase in the release of T4 from the thyroid. **C,** T4 becomes redistributed between the bound and the free states, leading to a new steady state with the same free T4 concentration but an increased total T4.

Box 11.1 **Causes of abnormal plasma thyroxine-binding globulin concentrations**

Increase

genetic
pregnancy
oestrogens, including oestrogen-containing oral contraceptives

Decrease

genetic
protein-losing states, e.g. nephrotic syndrome
malnutrition
malabsorption
acromegaly
Cushing syndrome
corticosteroids (high dose)
severe illness
androgens

Free thyroxine and triiodothyronine

Since total thyroxine and triiodothyronine concentrations depend on binding protein concentration as well as thyroid activity, assays for free thyroid hormones have been developed. The measurement of free hormone concentrations poses technical problems because the binding of free hormones in an immunoassay will disturb the equilibrium between bound and free hormone and cause release of hormone from binding proteins. However, various techniques have been developed to overcome this, and free thyroid hormone assays are now sufficiently reliable for most clinical purposes. However, with gross abnormalities of binding protein concentrations, the results of measurements of free hormones may still be misleading.

In **pregnancy**, fT4 concentrations may rise slightly, early in the first trimester, probably as a result of the weak thyroid-stimulating properties of chorionic gonadotrophin, but then fall in the second and third trimesters. Measured values should be compared with trimester-specific (and method-specific) reference ranges.

Free T3 concentrations can be normal in hypothyroidism (especially in mild cases), and its measurement is of no value in the diagnosis of this condition. Free T3 is, however, a sensitive test for hyperthyroidism. In hyperthyroid patients, both fT4 and fT3 are usually elevated (fT3 to a proportionately greater extent), but there are exceptions to this. In a small number of patients with hyperthyroidism, the fT3 concentration is elevated but fT4 is not (although it is usually high–normal), a condition called 'T3-toxicosis'. Occasionally, fT4 is elevated but not fT3. This is usually due to concomitant non-thyroidal illness resulting in decreased conversion of T4 to T3, and the fT3 concentration increases when this illness resolves. The same pattern is observed in patients with treated hypothyroidism if the dose of T4 is too high (the body protects itself from the adverse effect of over-replacement by decreasing conversion of T4 to T3), although most laboratories do not routinely measure fT3 in such patients.

Thyroid-stimulating hormone

Because the release of TSH from the pituitary is controlled through negative feedback by thyroid hormones, measurements of TSH can be used as an index of thyroid function provided that pituitary function is normal.

If primary thyroid disease is suspected and the plasma TSH concentration is normal, it can be safely inferred that the patient is euthyroid. In overt **primary hypothyroidism, TSH concentrations are greatly increased**, often to >10 times the upper reference limit. Smaller increases are seen in borderline (or subclinical) cases. TSH is a more sensitive marker of early or borderline thyroid dysfunction than is T4: TSH concentrations rise above the reference range before those of T4 fall below it. TSH can also increase transiently during recovery from non-thyroidal illness (see later). **Plasma TSH concentrations are suppressed to very low values in hyperthyroidism**, but low concentrations can also occur in individuals with subclinical hyperthyroidism and in euthyroid patients with non-thyroidal illness ('the sick euthyroid syndrome', see p. 201). Indeed, in hospital patients, a low plasma TSH concentration is more often due to non-thyroidal illness than to hyperthyroidism, whereas a slightly elevated concentration is as frequently due to recovery from such illness as to mild or incipient hypothyroidism.

Clinical biochemistry laboratories undertake large numbers of tests of thyroid function. To simplify their procedures, and to reduce unnecessary cost, many adopt the approach of measuring TSH as a first-line test of thyroid function, adding other tests as required, for example, if the concentration of TSH is found to be outside the euthyroid reference range or if there is a strong suspicion that thyroid dysfunction is secondary to pituitary disease (although this

is far less common than primary thyroid dysfunction). A combination of tests may also be required to assess patients being treated for thyroid disease, particularly in the early stages, because TSH takes typically around 6 weeks to reach a new steady state after a change in the plasma concentration of thyroid hormones.

TSH is a peptide hormone that has the same α-subunit as luteinizing hormone (LH), follicle-stimulating hormone (FSH) and human chorionic gonadotrophin (hCG). Measurement of plasma α-subunit concentration is helpful in the diagnosis of rare TSH-secreting pituitary tumours.

Notably, immunometric assays (such as are used for TSH) are subject to interference by naturally occurring heterophilic antibodies against the monoclonal antibodies used in the assay; such interference occurs only infrequently but can create either high or low results. Some assays also suffer from interference if patients are taking high doses of the vitamin biotin (see p. 208).

Rarely, antibodies cause a proportion of TSH molecules to aggregate to form macro-TSH (a similar phenomenon involving prolactin is described on p. 158). Macro-TSH is not physiologically active; patients have normal plasma T3 and T4 concentrations and are clinically euthyroid because non-complexed TSH concentration is normal. Macro-TSH is, however, detected to a varying degree by most TSH immunoassays.

Typical results of thyroid function tests in various conditions are shown in Table 11.1.

Thyrotrophin-releasing hormone test

In the TRH test, plasma TSH is measured immediately before and 20 and 60 min after giving the patient 200 µg TRH intravenously (i.v.) (Fig. 11.5). The normal response is an increase in TSH concentration of 5–30 mIU/L at 20 min, with reversion towards the basal value at 60 min.

This test is mainly used in the investigation of patients with pituitary or hypothalamic disease, to assess the capacity of the pituitary to secrete TSH. TSH secretion is rarely completely lost in pituitary disease, and thus the TSH response to TRH is more usually decreased than absent. In hypothalamic disease, the response is characteristically (although not invariably) delayed, with the plasma TSH concentration at 60 min exceeding that at 20 min. The TRH test may also be of value in the diagnosis of TSH-secreting tumours, in which the response is usually flat, and thyroid hormone resistance, in which it is normal or exaggerated (see Case history 11.3).

Other tests for thyroid disease

Thyroid scintigraphy is in common use for the identification of thyroid lesions. In this technique, a dose of an isotope, usually [99mTc]-pertechnetate, is given and its distribution within the thyroid is determined using a

Table 11.1 Results of thyroid function tests in various conditions

		PLASMA fT4		
		High	**Normal**	**Low**
Plasma **TSH**	**High**	TSH-secreting tumour (rare) (fT3 ↑; TSH may be high–normal)	subclinical/borderline hypothyroidism	hypothyroidism (primary) recovery from sick euthyroid state
	Normal	euthyroid with T4 autoantibodies (uncommon) thyroid hormone resistance	euthyroid	sick euthyroid (fT3 ↓) hypopituitarism (other pituitary hormones ↓)
	Low	hyperthyroidism (fT3 ↑)	T3 thyrotoxicosis (fT3 ↑) early in treatment of hyperthyroidism subclinical hyperthyroidism (fT3 N/↑)	hypopituitarism (other pituitary hormones ↓) sick euthyroid (severe) (fT3 ↓)

fT3, free triiodothyronine; T4, thyroxine; TSH, thyroid-stimulating hormone.

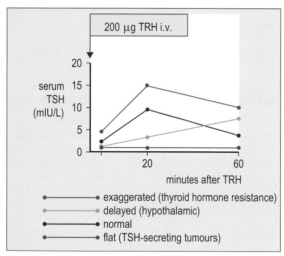

Fig. 11.5 Thyrotrophin-releasing hormone (TRH) test: 200 µg is given i.v. and serum thyroid-stimulating hormone (TSH) is measured at 0, 20 and 60 min. Typical responses are shown.

gamma camera. Scintigraphy allows the identification of 'hot' (active) or 'cold' (inactive and potentially malignant) nodules in patients with lumps in the thyroid. It can also distinguish between Graves disease (uniformly increased uptake), multinodular goitre (patchy uptake) or an adenoma (single 'hot' spot) in patients with thyrotoxicosis, and detect aberrant or ectopic thyroid tissue.

Various **autoantibodies to thyroid-related antigens** may be detectable in the plasma of patients with thyroid disease. Graves disease is caused by **TSH receptor antibodies** that bind to and stimulate TSH receptors. Assays for these antibodies are not yet universally available, but their measurement may be particularly valuable in the diagnosis of Graves disease in the absence of the characteristic eye signs, in the prediction of relapse after a course of antithyroid drugs and in determining the risk of fetal or neonatal thyrotoxicosis in pregnant women with current or previously treated Graves disease. **Thyroid peroxidase antibodies** (formerly called 'thyroid microsomal antibodies') are present in the blood of almost all patients with autoimmune thyroiditis (particularly Hashimoto disease and primary atrophic hypothyroidism). They are also frequently present in Graves disease. Their presence predicts risk of progression from subclinical to frank hypothyroidism (see pp. 205–206). They are, however, also detectable in the plasma of ~20% of people with normal thyroid function. **Antithyroglobulin antibodies** are present in many patients with destruction of the thyroid gland of any cause. They are not pathogenic and have no diagnostic value but may cause abnormal results in assays for plasma thyroglobulin, which is a tumour marker used for monitoring patients treated for thyroid cancer (see p. 361). Autoantibodies to thyroid hormones can occasionally cause abnormal assay results, but these are usually so bizarre that, in practice, they are rarely a cause of diagnostic confusion.

Other biochemical disturbances, not involving the thyroid hormones, occur in thyroid disease but are of no value diagnostically; examples are hypercalcaemia, hyperphosphataemia and an elevated plasma sex hormone-binding

Case history 11.1

History

Knowing that thyroid disease is common in the elderly, a junior doctor requested thyroid function tests on an elderly woman admitted to hospital with severe cellulitis of the leg secondary to an infected ingrowing toenail.

Results (see Appendix for reference ranges)

Serum:		
	TSH	0.1 mIU/L
	fT4	8.0 pmol/L
	fT3	2.0 pmol/L

Summary

TSH, fT4 and fT3 are all low.

Interpretation

The low TSH, fT4 and fT3 results might at first glance suggest thyroid failure secondary to hypopituitarism. However, a TSH this low would be unusual except in severe hypopituitarism. These results are more likely to be due to the 'sick euthyroid syndrome'.

Discussion

A random serum cortisol concentration was 950 nmol/L, indicating normal response of the hypothalamo–pituitary–adrenal axis to stress, and effectively ruling out hypopituitarism as a cause for these results. The infection was treated successfully and thyroid function tests were repeated before discharge: serum TSH concentration was 3.6 mIU/L, fT4 12 pmol/L and fT3 4.7 pmol/L. Unless there is a high probability that a patient's presenting illness is a result of thyroid disease, thyroid function testing should not be performed during acute illness.

Case history 11.2

History

A 24-year-old physiotherapist consulted her general practitioner because excessive moistness of her skin was causing embarrassment at work. She was also concerned that her eyes seemed to have become more prominent and that she had lost weight, although her appetite was unchanged.

Examination

Her pulse was 102/min at rest and that she had a slightly enlarged thyroid gland.

Results

Serum:		
	TSH	<0.01 mIU/L
	fT4	34 pmol/L
	fT3	12 pmol/L

Summary

Undetectable TSH with high fT4 and fT3.

Interpretation

The high fT3 and fT4 concentrations with very low TSH are diagnostic of thyrotoxicosis.

A ^{99m}Tc isotope scan of the thyroid showed an enlarged gland, with uniformly increased uptake. Autoantibodies to thyroid peroxidase were present in the serum at high concentration.

Discussion

This patient's clinical features and scan appearance are typical of thyrotoxicosis due to Graves disease (Box 11.2). Milder cases, particularly in the elderly, may be less obvious and may initially suggest an anxiety state. Measurement of thyroid peroxidase autoantibodies was not necessary to establish the diagnosis in this instance, but when ocular manifestations are absent, measurement of TSH receptor antibodies may be helpful. Some clinical features are specific to Graves disease and can have a course independent of the hyperthyroidism. Patients may present with the ocular manifestations of Graves disease (ophthalmic Graves disease) yet be clinically euthyroid. However, the TSH is usually suppressed even though fT3 may not be elevated, and such patients eventually become biochemically and clinically thyrotoxic. The combination of a low TSH with a normal (usually high–normal) fT3 ('subclinical' or 'borderline' hyperthyroidism) can occur early in the course of Graves disease and other conditions that cause thyrotoxicosis.

globulin (SHBG) concentration in some patients with hyperthyroidism, and hypercholesterolaemia, hyponatraemia and elevated plasma creatine kinase activity in hypothyroidism.

Problems in the interpretation of thyroid function tests

As indicated earlier, no biochemical test of thyroid function can be guaranteed to be reliable in patients with **non-thyroidal illness**. Abnormal results may occur in patients with infections, malignancy, myocardial infarction, following surgery, etc. who do not have thyroid disease. In general, thyroid function tests should not be performed on such patients unless there is a strong suspicion that they have thyroid disease.

Typically, during the acute phase of an illness, fT3 concentration and, less often, fT4 concentration is decreased. TSH is usually normal but may be undetectable in severely ill patients. During recovery, TSH may rise transiently into the hypothyroid range as thyroid hormone concentrations return to normal. In chronic illness, for example chronic kidney disease, free hormone concentrations are typically

---

Case history 11.3

History

Shortly before her final examinations, a medical student experienced sleep disturbance, tachycardia with palpitations and noticed that her hands were warm and sweaty. Her doctor thought it most likely that her symptoms were due to anxiety but arranged a blood sample for thyroid function tests.

Results

Serum:

	TSH	5.2 mIU/L
	fT4	34 pmol/L
	fT3	12.9 pmol/L

Summary

High fT4 and fT3 with slightly raised TSH.

Interpretation

This is an unusual combination of results. The high thyroid hormone results are compatible with hyperthyroidism, but the high TSH excludes primary thyroid disease as a cause. Possible explanations include interference with the hormone immunoassays by heterophilic antibodies (antibodies in a patient's plasma that bind to the antibodies used in the assay), a TSH-secreting pituitary tumour (a rare cause of hyperthyroidism) or thyroid hormone resistance (an inherited disorder in which there is an abnormality of thyroid hormone receptor function but patients are clinically euthyroid).

Discussion

Repeating the measurements using a different assay (using different antibodies) produced essentially the same results, making assay interference very unlikely. A TRH test (see p. 199) was performed. There was a normal TSH response to TRH: with TSHomas, there is typically no response. The plasma concentration of TSH α-subunit was normal: elevated concentrations are usual in patients with TSHomas. It was concluded that the patient had thyroid hormone resistance; this was supported when similar thyroid function test results were demonstrated in her sister and confirmed with a genetic test. Patients with thyroid hormone resistance are usually clinically euthyroid and do not usually require treatment, although some present with symptoms of hyperthyroidism. They frequently undergo repeated investigation before the diagnosis is made.

---

decreased (to an extent that may reflect the severity of the underlying disease); TSH is usually normal but occasionally is decreased.

The occurrence of abnormalities of thyroid function tests in patients with non-thyroidal illness has been termed the 'sick euthyroid syndrome'. Causes include decreased peripheral conversion of T4 to T3; changes in the concentration of binding proteins (to an extent that may reveal technical limitations in the ability of free hormone assays to provide a true measurement of free hormone concentrations); increased plasma concentrations of free fatty acids, which displace thyroid hormones from their binding sites, and non-thyroidal influences on the hypothalamo–pituitary–thyroid axis, for example, by cortisol, which can inhibit TSH secretion.

Many drugs can influence the results of tests of thyroid function. Some examples are given in Table 11.2. Amiodarone is particularly noteworthy. This iodine-containing antiarrhythmic can either increase or decrease thyroid hormone synthesis and may occasionally cause clinical thyroid disease, more often hypothyroidism in iodine-sufficient areas and hyperthyroidism in iodine-deficient areas.

In the rare condition **familial dysalbuminaemic hyperthyroxinaemia**, mutations in the gene for albumin increase its affinity for T4 by approximately 60-fold. Because protein-bound T4 is not physiologically active, this affects plasma total but not fT4 concentrations. However, the high-affinity albumin also binds the T4 'tracer' reagent used in fT4 assays, so its presence causes spuriously high fT4 results with many assays.

Like other immunoassays, thyroid hormone assays are occasionally susceptible to interference from antibodies to animal immunoglobulins that are present in the plasma of a small proportion of healthy people (see p. 208).

Disorders of the Thyroid

The metabolic manifestations of thyroid disease relate to either excessive or inadequate production of thyroid hormones (hyperthyroidism and hypothyroidism, respectively). The clinical syndrome that results from hyperthyroidism is thyrotoxicosis. The term **'myxoedema'** is often used to describe the entire clinical syndrome of hypothyroidism, but strictly refers specifically to the dryness of the skin, coarsening of the features and subcutaneous swelling characteristic of severe hypothyroidism. Patients with thyroid disease may present with a thyroid swelling or goitre. Investigation may reveal hypothyroidism or (more frequently) hyperthyroidism, but there may be no functional abnormality. A goitre can be the presenting feature of thyroid cancer.

Table 11.2 Effects of drugs on thyroid function

Drug	Effect
corticosteroids, dopaminergic drugs	inhibit TSH secretion
lithium[a], iodine, carbimazole, thiouracils	inhibit T3 and T4 secretion
oestrogens, tamoxifen, methadone, heroin	increase TBG[b]
corticosteroids, androgens	decrease TBG[b]
salicylates, phenytoin	compete with T4 for binding by TBG[b]
β-antagonists, amiodarone[c]	inhibit conversion of T4 to T3
cholestyramine, aluminium hydroxide, sucralfate, ferrous sulphate, calcium salts	impair absorption of thyroxine
phenytoin, carbamazepine	increase hepatic metabolism of T4 (so patients on replacement may need an increased dose)

[a]Regular monitoring (6- to 12-monthly) of thyroid hormone concentration is mandatory for patients treated with lithium.
[b]No effect on free hormone concentrations.
[c]Amiodarone is an iodine-containing drug. In addition to its effect on T4 metabolism, it sometimes precipitates hypothyroidism or hyperthyroidism: patients with high thyroid autoantibody concentrations are at increased risk.
T3, triiodothyronine; T4, thyroxine; TBG, thyroxine-binding globulin; TSH, thyroid-stimulating hormone.

Box 11.2 Causes and clinical features of hyperthyroidism.

Causes

Graves disease[a]
toxic multinodular goitre[a]
solitary toxic adenoma[a]
thyroiditis
exogenous iodine and iodine-containing drugs, e.g. amiodarone
excessive T4 or T3 ingestion
ectopic thyroid tissue, e.g. struma ovarii, functioning metastatic thyroid cancer
hCG dependent: choriocarcinoma
TSH dependent: pituitary tumour

Clinical features

weight loss (but normal or increased appetite)[b]
sweating, heat intolerance[b]
fatigue[b]
palpitation[b]: sinus tachycardia or atrial fibrillation
angina, heart failure (high output)
agitation, tremor[b]
warm, moist skin[b]
generalized muscle weakness, proximal myopathy
diarrhoea
oligomenorrhoea, infertility
goitre
ophthalmopathy, lid retraction, lid lag[c]

[a]These account for >90% of cases.
[b]Indicates the most common features.
[c]Eye disease is a feature of Graves disease only.
hCG, human chorionic gonadotrophin; T3, triiodothyronine; T4, thyroxine; TSH, thyroid-stimulating hormone.

Hyperthyroidism

The major causes and clinical features of hyperthyroidism are shown in Box 11.2. Primary hyperthyroidism is far more common than secondary hyperthyroidism (TSH-dependent or hCG-dependent). The commonest single cause is **Graves disease**, an autoimmune disease characterized by the presence of thyroid-stimulating antibodies in the blood. These autoantibodies bind to TSH receptors in the thyroid and stimulate them in the same way as TSH, through activation of adenylate cyclase and the formation of cyclic adenosine monophosphate, resulting in overactivity of the gland. Thyrotoxicosis can also occur as a result of release of preformed thyroid hormones from a damaged gland (e.g. in thyroiditis) and from excessive intake of thyroid hormones.

The laboratory **diagnosis** of primary hyperthyroidism depends on the demonstration of a high plasma concentration of fT3 (and usually fT4) with a very low (usually undetectable) TSH. These tests are also used to monitor the response to treatment and for long-term follow-up. The concentrations of fT3 and fT4 fall as patients become euthyroid, but some time may elapse before normal pituitary responsiveness to thyroid hormones is regained and there is an increase in TSH into the normal range. Thus, although a normal TSH concentration indicates that a patient is euthyroid, a low value is not on its own indicative of persisting hyperthyroidism.

There are three options for the **treatment** of thyrotoxicosis: antithyroid drugs, radioactive iodine and surgery (subtotal thyroidectomy). Treatment with β-adrenergic blocking drugs may provide temporary symptomatic relief but has no effect on the underlying disease process.

Rarely, patients with thyrotoxicosis present with, or develop, thyroid storm. The diagnosis is initially made on clinical grounds and it is one of the rare instances when

> Thyroid storm (thyrotoxic crisis) is a rare but potentially life-threatening medical emergency. It may occur after infection in those with long-standing thyrotoxicosis. Other triggers include thyroid manipulation (e.g. surgery or trauma), administration of radioiodine or iodine contrast media, childbirth, myocardial infarction and diabetic ketoacidosis. Clinical features include tachycardia, fever, atrial fibrillation, heart failure, fever, diarrhoea, vomiting, dehydration, jaundice, agitation, delirium and coma.

the laboratory should be asked to measure thyroid function tests urgently. Inorganic iodine solution (e.g. Lugol iodine) may be administered to block thyroid hormone secretion in patients with thyroid storm and is also used for the same purpose before thyroidectomy.

Unless they have a very large goitre, in the UK it is usual to treat younger patients with Graves disease with **antithyroid drugs**. These suppress thyroid hormone synthesis, although not the release of preformed hormone, and thus there is usually a delay before any response is seen. Although one of the most frequently used drugs, carbimazole, is immunosuppressive, it is uncertain whether it has a significant effect on the underlying pathogenic process. **Radioactive iodine** (^{131}I) therapy is more commonly used as first-line treatment in the USA, but in other countries is used if antithyroid drug therapy is not appropriate or if patients relapse following a course of drug treatment: it is contraindicated in pregnancy.

Antithyroid drugs are given in high doses initially, but once the patient has become euthyroid, a decrease in dosage is often possible (titration regimen). An alternative approach is to continue with a high dose of the chosen drug and give T4 at a replacement dose, for example, 150 μg/day (block and replacement regimen).

Untreated Graves disease has a natural history of remission and relapse. Some patients (30–40%) have only a single episode of hyperthyroidism. It is usual to give antithyroid drugs for a period of 18 months to 2 years. Thyroid status is monitored during this time and thereafter. If the patient relapses, a further course of drug treatment or another mode of treatment is indicated.

Long-term follow-up of patients treated for Graves disease is essential. Patients treated with antithyroid drugs may relapse, occasionally after many years; conversely, most ultimately become hypothyroid. Recurrences of the disease also occur in patients treated surgically or with radioactive iodine. Up to 35% of patients treated surgically, and the majority of patients treated with radioactive iodine, will eventually become hypothyroid, sometimes as long as 10 years or more after treatment. Hypothyroidism that develops within 6 months of either surgery or radioactive iodine treatment may be temporary, but abnormalities

of thyroid function tests, in particular a slightly raised TSH but with normal plasma fT4 and fT3 concentrations, may persist although the patient remains clinically euthyroid. This is illustrated in Fig. 11.6.

The pathogenic thyroid-stimulating autoantibody in Graves disease is an IgG immunoglobulin. In a pregnant woman with Graves disease, the immunoglobulin can cross the placenta and may cause **fetal or neonatal hyperthyroidism**, even if the mother is euthyroid. Measurement of maternal TSH receptor antibody concentration is recommended in women who have either current or previous Graves disease. Early involvement of an endocrinologist in the management of such women is appropriate. Fetal growth and heart rate should be monitored closely if the TSH receptor antibody concentration is high. Neonatal hyperthyroidism is a transient phenomenon because the maternal immunoglobulins are gradually cleared from the neonatal circulation, but treatment may be required in the short term.

Transient biochemical (but usually asymptomatic) hyperthyroidism occurs in up to 5% of women after pregnancy. The changes are usually maximal at 1–3 months after delivery and are often succeeded by symptomatic hypothyroidism (which sometimes persists) at 4–6 months.

The typical ophthalmopathy of Graves disease can present before a patient becomes thyrotoxic and may persist even after successful treatment of the thyrotoxicosis. Specific intervention is occasionally required; for example, to prevent or manage corneal ulceration or visual loss.

Hypothyroidism

There are many causes of primary hypothyroidism (Box 11.3), but hypothyroidism can also occur secondarily to decreased trophic stimulation both in hypopituitarism and in hypothalamic disease. It is, however, uncommon for patients with pituitary failure to present with clinical features of hypothyroidism alone. The commonest cause of hypothyroidism in developed countries is autoimmune destruction of the gland due to **Hashimoto thyroiditis**. Iodine deficiency is a major cause of hypothyroidism in developing countries, particularly in mountainous areas, although its incidence has been reduced by supplementation programmes. Affected individuals usually have a goitre as a result of the increased secretion of TSH. The increased drive to the thyroid may be sufficient to prevent the development of frank hypothyroidism in borderline deficiency. Among drugs that can cause hypothyroidism, lithium is particularly important; regular checks of thyroid function are mandatory in patients treated with lithium.

The clinical manifestations of hypothyroidism (see Box 11.3) are variable and may result in the patient being referred to almost any medical specialty. Clinical

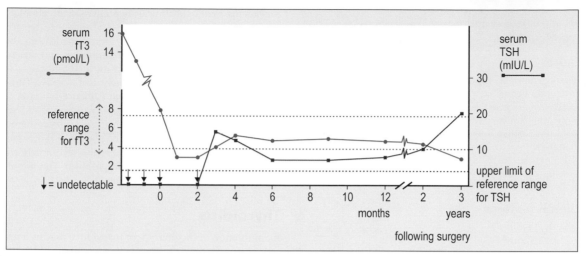

Fig. 11.6 Changes in serum free triiodothyronine (fT3) and thyroid-stimulating hormone (TSH) concentrations after partial thyroidectomy for Graves disease. The patient was rendered euthyroid with antithyroid drugs before surgery. Initially, TSH secretion remained suppressed but eventually rose in response to the low fT3. Normal thyroid hormone secretion by the remaining thyroid tissue was maintained by increased TSH stimulation, but eventually the patient became hypothyroid, as shown by the increased TSH. Hypothyroidism can also develop in patients treated with antithyroid drugs or radioiodine.

diagnosis is confirmed by the finding of a high plasma TSH concentration (unless the condition is secondary to hypopituitarism) and low fT4 concentration. Measurement of fT3 is of no value in the diagnosis of hypothyroidism (see p. 199).

Hypothyroidism is treated by replacement of thyroid hormones, usually T4 (levothyroxine). It is usual to start with a small dose (e.g. 50 µg/day) and increase this at 4- to 6-week intervals on the basis of the results of thyroid function tests. In elderly patients and patients with ischaemic heart disease, a lower starting dose (e.g. 25 µg) should be used, there is a risk that the increase in metabolic rate and demand for oxygen prompted by hormone replacement may precipitate angina or myocardial infarction. T3 has a more rapid onset of action and is preferable in the initial treatment of patients in myxoedema coma (see later).

Thyroid hormone replacement can be monitored by measuring plasma TSH and, if this is abnormal, fT4 concentrations (fT3 if the patient is being treated with T3). Ideally, the replacement dosage should be sufficient to maintain TSH within the reference range. Too high a concentration indicates inadequate replacement; a suppressed TSH suggests excessive replacement and a risk of causing atrial fibrillation and, possibly, osteoporosis. In patients treated with T4, plasma fT4 concentrations associated with a clinically euthyroid state are generally somewhat higher than the normal euthyroid range, because there is no contribution to endogenous hormone activity by secreted T3. If the dosage is changed, the results of thyroid function tests will not reach a new steady state for several weeks. Thyroid

hormones should not be measured until at least 6 weeks have elapsed. The expected fall in TSH concentration lags behind the increase in that of fT4 when treatment is started, and if the TSH has been suppressed because of overreplacement, months may elapse before normal thyrotrophic responsiveness to T4 is regained. Occasional patients experience ongoing symptoms of hypothyroidism during treatment with T4 at a dose sufficient to normalize TSH, and appear to require additional replacement with T3.

Adherence to, and the adequacy of, treatment should be checked annually by measurements of TSH and, if this is abnormal, fT4. Usually, non-adherent patients who begin to take their tablets regularly only a few days before a blood test will be revealed by their having a raised TSH but a normal or even elevated fT4.

Occasionally, patients with hypothyroidism present as an emergency, with stupor and hypothermia. This **myxoedema coma** has a high mortality. Immediate treatment is usually with both T4 and T3, since the latter has a more rapid onset of action. The patient must also be treated with a glucocorticoid, at least until coexistent adrenal insufficiency has been ruled out. Appropriate measures must also be taken to treat any infection, heart failure or electrolyte imbalance and to restore body temperature to normal.

Subclinical hypothyroidism

It is not unusual to find patients whose plasma TSH concentration is elevated but have a free T4 concentration within the reference range. This may be associated

Box 11.3 Causes and clinical features of hypothyroidism

Causes

idiopathic atrophic hypothyroidism[a]
Hashimoto thyroiditis[a]
postsurgery, radioactive iodine, antithyroid drugs (e.g. carbimazole)[a]
drugs (e.g. lithium, amiodarone)[a]
congenital
dyshormonogenic
secondary (pituitary or hypothalamic disease) iodine deficiency

Clinical features

lethargy, tiredness[b]
cold intolerance[b]
goitre[b]
constipation[b]
carpal tunnel syndrome[b]
weight gain[b]
slow relaxation of muscles and tendon reflexes[b]
hypercholesterolaemia[b]
bradycardia[b]
hoarse voice
dryness and coarsening of skin and hair
many others, including:
  anaemia, typically macrocytic, non-megaloblastic but pernicious in 10% of cases
  dementia, psychosis
  angina
  pericardial and/or pleural effusion
  muscle stiffness
  infertility, menorrhagia, galactorrhoea

[a]These account for >90% of cases.

[b]Indicates the most common features.
Children with hypothyroidism may present with growth failure, delayed pubertal development or a deterioration in academic performance.

with a history of treated hyperthyroidism but can occur *de novo*. In the absence of clinical features of hypothyroidism, this is termed 'subclinical' or 'borderline' hypothyroidism. Some patients with subclinical hypothyroidism are in a stable, compensated state in which the thyroid continues to produce adequate amounts of thyroid hormone under trophic stimulation from a higher than normal plasma concentration of TSH. In other patients, although plasma thyroid hormone concentrations are within the population reference range, they are lower than 'normal' for that patient, and the patient may experience mild symptoms of hypothyroidism. A third group of patients are in progression to full hypothyroidism.

Patients with subclinical hypothyroidism should be treated if they are symptomatic. UK guidance regarding asymptomatic patients currently recommends measurement of thyroid peroxisomal autoantibodies and review, if the biochemical abnormality persists, at yearly intervals if antibody positive but at 3-year intervals if negative. Particularly in the elderly, however, recent evidence indicates that the risk of progression to overt hypothyroidism after 5 years in asymptomatic patients is low. Treatment is recommended even in asymptomatic patients if the plasma TSH concentration rises to >10 mIU/L. Treatment is also recommended in all patients with subclinical hypothyroidism who are pregnant or planning to become pregnant.

Thyroiditis

Inflammation of the thyroid, or thyroiditis, may be a result of infection (usually viral) or autoimmune disease. In viral thyroiditis associated with coxsackie, mumps and adenovirus, the inflammation results in a release of preformed colloid and there is an increase in the concentration of thyroid hormones in the blood. Patients may become transiently, and usually only mildly, thyrotoxic. This phase persists for up to 6 weeks and is followed by a similar period in which thyroid hormone output may be decreased, although not sufficiently to cause symptoms. Thereafter, normal function is regained.

Hashimoto thyroiditis is a chronic autoimmune disorder associated with high titres of autoantibodies causing hypothyroidism. Patients often develop a goitre and may have other organ-specific autoimmune diseases. Occasionally, transient hyperthyroidism may occur early in the course of the disease because of, as in viral thyroiditis, increased release of preformed colloid.

Thyroid hormone resistance

Thyroid hormone resistance is a rare autosomal dominant inherited disorder (prevalence ~1/50,000) that results from a genetic mutation that reduces the affinity of the nuclear receptor for T3. Patients are clinically euthyroid because of compensatory increases in plasma thyroid hormone concentrations driven by a small increase in TSH secretion. This combination of raised free thyroid hormone and TSH concentrations is also seen in patients with rare TSH-secreting pituitary adenomas, but in contrast, the latter are clinically thyrotoxic (see Case history 11.3).

Goitre and thyroid cancer

Goitre, or enlargement of the thyroid, can occur in patients with hyperthyroidism (e.g. in Graves disease, toxic multinodular goitre or a thyroid adenoma), hypothyroidism (e.g. in Hashimoto disease or iodine

---

Case history 11.4

History

A senior civil servant was persuaded to seek medical advice because of his increasingly bizarre behaviour. He had slowed down mentally, become indecisive and had given up his daily game of squash, claiming that he no longer had the energy to play. Whereas in the past he had annoyed his colleagues by opening windows even on cold days, he now no longer objected to them remaining closed. His general practitioner suspected hypothyroidism and elicited a history of recent constipation.

Examination

His skin appeared sallow and his hair was coarse and lacked lustre. Bradycardia was present, and when the peripheral reflexes were tested, slow quadriceps relaxation was noted. There was no goitre.

Results

Serum:		
	TSH	>100 mIU/L
	fT4	3.9 pmol/L

Summary

Very high TSH with low fT4.

Interpretation

The clinical diagnosis of hypothyroidism is confirmed by the very high serum TSH concentration.

Discussion

The very high TSH concentration reflects the lack of negative feedback from circulating thyroid hormones. Measurement of fT4 is strictly not necessary for diagnosis, although, as discussed on p. 199, some laboratories routinely measure TSH and fT4 on all samples submitted for thyroid function tests, and most others add fT4 as a second-line confirmatory test when an abnormal TSH result is obtained.

Case history 11.5

History

A 55-year-old businesswoman underwent the medical screening programme provided by her company. Various tests were performed, including assessment of thyroid function.

Results

Serum:		
	TSH	8.0 mIU/L
	fT4	12.5 pmol/L

Summary

Slightly high TSH, fT4 towards the bottom of the reference range.

Interpretation

Serum TSH concentration is slightly elevated, and fT4, although within the reference range, is near the lower end, compatible with subclinical, or borderline, hypothyroidism.

Discussion

Patients with subclinical hypothyroidism are at increased risk of progression to full hypothyroidism in future. Some laboratories automatically measure thyroid peroxisomal antibodies when subclinical hypothyroidism is detected, because the risk of progression is higher if antibody concentration is increased. Sufficient function of the failing thyroid may be maintained by increased secretion of TSH in the early stages. Measurement of fT4 concentration may not be of practical help in management since it is usually not known whether it has fallen significantly in comparison to previous normal values for that patient.

This patient was not initially started on T4 replacement, but 6 months later she had begun to feel increasingly tired and her serum TSH concentration had increased to 19 mIU/L, with a fT4 of 9 pmol/L. Replacement was then started, and 3 months later she commented that she felt 'better than for many years'. Because the clinical features of hypothyroidism can be so non-specific, patients may only recognize that they were present after they improve in response to thyroid replacement therapy.

---

deficiency) and in euthyroid individuals with benign or malignant tumours of the gland. Physiological enlargement of the thyroid may occur during adolescence and pregnancy, unaccompanied by any change in function, but thyroid function tests should be performed even in apparently euthyroid patients presenting with a goitre, because the results may provide a clue to the cause.

Immunoassay interference

Between 2% and 5% of people have antibodies in their plasma that can bind animal immunoglobulins. These so-called heterophilic antibodies are of no clinical significance but have the potential to bind the animal antibodies used in immunoassays, resulting in falsely high (or, more rarely, falsely low) assay results. Manufacturers have adapted their assays to minimize this effect, but it is still sometimes of clinically significant magnitude. In many UK laboratories, abnormal immunoassay results are reviewed by a clinical biochemist before issue to check that they are consistent with previous findings, with other tests in a profile (e.g. fT3 with fT4 and TSH) and with the clinical details provided with the request. The requestor himself or herself should, however, also be aware of this possibility, and is often best placed to identify it if otherwise inexplicable results are obtained. Heterophilic antibody interference sometimes comes to light when there is an unexpected step change in results after the laboratory changes to a new assay.

The laboratory may investigate the presence of heterophilic antibody interference in three ways. First, for most assays, the effect of the interfering antibody can be reduced by diluting the sample (this cannot be done with fT3 and fT4 assays because it disturbs the equilibrium between bound and free hormone). Second, the heterophilic antibody can be neutralized by adding 'blocking antibodies'. Third, the sample can be analyzed by a different method, using reagent antibodies from a different animal species. This process inevitably delays the issuing of a final result, and sometimes it is concluded that the hormone in question cannot reliably be measured. Most laboratories keep records of patients with heterophilic antibodies, but the medical record should also flag this information and clinicians should, if possible, adopt alternative investigative strategies (e.g. monitor fT4 rather than TSH) if repeat testing is necessary.

A rarer type of immunoassay interference results from the presence in the patient's plasma of an antibody to the analyte being tested. For example, some patients with thyroid cancer develop thyroglobulin antibodies, which compete with the antibodies used in the thyroglobulin immunoassay. Most laboratories screen for the presence of antithyroglobulin antibodies and may suppress or provide a caution with the thyroglobulin result if they are present at high concentration.

More recently, immunoassay interference caused when patients take high doses of the vitamin biotin has been identified. This occurs because biotin is a key component of some immunoassay reagents. Clinicians should be aware of this and avoid drawing blood samples from patients who take high dose biotin until at least eight hours after the last dose.

Biochemical tests have no part to play in the diagnosis of **thyroid cancer**, with the exception of calcitonin-secreting medullary carcinoma (see p. 360), but they do have a role in monitoring the efficacy of treatment by total thyroidectomy or ablative doses of radioactive iodine. **Thyroglobulin** is detectable in plasma if there is persistent thyroid activity, because small amounts are released into the plasma together with thyroid hormones. Treatment of thyroid cancers (other than medullary cell) is usually followed by prescription of T4 at supraphysiological doses to suppress TSH secretion, and thus reduce the trophic stimulus to any residual thyroid tissue. The dose of T4 should be adjusted to maintain plasma TSH at very low (or undetectable) concentrations rather than within the reference range in these patients.

Screening for thyroid disease

Congenital hypothyroidism (usually caused by thyroid agenesis or dysgenesis) is sufficiently serious and common (~1/4000 live births in the UK but considerably higher in some other countries) for it to be appropriate to screen for the condition. Untreated, affected children have severe learning disabilities, growth impairment and poor motor skills (a syndrome formerly described as cretinism). Treatment by replacement of T4 is simple and effective, but this must be started as soon after birth as a reliable diagnosis can be made. In the UK, the screening method involves measurement of TSH in a capillary blood sample collected onto a Guthrie card (see p. 382). Screening is delayed until 6–8 days of age to avoid the normal physiological neonatal surge in TSH secretion. Screening for phenylketonuria and some other inherited conditions is performed at the same time.

Hypothyroidism and hyperthyroidism are both common in the elderly (more so the former), with a combined prevalence rate of ~5%. Both the conditions may present insidiously and atypically, so thyroid function testing is often indicated in patients with non-specific symptoms. However, general screening is not appropriate, in part because of the increased prevalence of non-thyroidal illness that might influence the results of thyroid function tests in this patient group.

SUMMARY

- The thyroid gland secretes two iodine-containing hormones, **thyroxine (T4)** and **triiodothyronine (T3).** More T4 is secreted than T3. Some T4 is metabolized to T3 in peripheral tissues; T3 is the more active hormone. The synthesis and secretion of thyroid hormones is stimulated by the pituitary hormone thyroid-stimulating hormone (TSH). The release of TSH is in turn controlled by thyrotrophin-releasing hormone (TRH) from the hypothalamus. T4 and T3 exert negative feedback inhibition on TSH release.

- Thyroid hormones are **essential for normal growth and development**, and **also control basal metabolic rate** and stimulate many metabolic processes.

- T4 and T3 are extensively **protein bound in the blood** (T4 to an even greater extent than T3), to thyroxine-binding globulin, albumin and prealbumin, the free, physiologically active fractions being <1% of the total. Clinical biochemistry laboratories therefore measure free rather than total hormone concentrations, because these are not affected by changes in the concentration of binding proteins, unless extreme.

- Thyroid status is best assessed biochemically by measurement of **plasma TSH and free T4 (fT4) concentrations**, with **free T3 (fT3)** being measured in addition if hyperthyroidism is suspected. Typically, **in primary hypothyroidism, fT4 concentration is low and TSH is high; in hyperthyroidism, TSH is very low and fT3 is high, as usually is fT4.**

- Drug treatment and non-thyroidal disease frequently cause the results of thyroid function tests to be abnormal in patients who do not have thyroid disease.

- Patients with thyroid disease may present as a result of overactivity of the gland (**hyperthyroidism**, causing thyrotoxicosis) or underactivity (**hypothyroidism**, causing myxoedema). Both conditions have **widespread systemic effects.** Patients in either category may have enlargement of the gland (**goitre**), but patients with goitres can be euthyroid. Both hyperthyroidism and hypothyroidism are commonly the result of autoimmune disease, although there are many other causes. The measurement of specific autoantibodies can provide useful diagnostic information in thyroid disease. Options for the treatment of hyperthyroidism include antithyroid drugs, radioactive iodine and surgery; patients with hypothyroidism require hormone replacement.

- The thyroid also secretes **calcitonin**, a polypeptide hormone with a minor role in calcium homoeostasis.

Chapter | **12** |

The gonads

Introduction

Androgens and testicular function

The testes are responsible for the synthesis of the male sex hormones (androgens) and the production of spermatozoa. The most important androgen, both in terms of potency and the amount secreted, is testosterone. Other testicular androgens include androstenedione and dehydroepiandrosterone (DHEA). These weaker androgens are also secreted by the adrenal glands, but adrenal androgen secretion does not appear to be physiologically important in the male. In the female, however, it contributes to the development of certain secondary sexual characteristics, in particular the growth of pubic and axillary hair. The pathological consequences of increased adrenal androgen secretion are discussed in Chapter 10 and on p. 218.

Testosterone is a powerful anabolic hormone. It is essential both for the **development of secondary sexual characteristics** in the male and for **spermatogenesis**. It is secreted by the Leydig cells of the testes under the influence of luteinizing hormone (LH). Spermatogenesis is also dependent on the function of the Sertoli cells of the testicular seminiferous tubules. These cells are follicle-stimulating hormone (FSH) dependent; they secrete inhibin, which inhibits FSH secretion, and androgen-binding protein, the function of which is probably to increase the concentration of androgens within the seminiferous tubules.

Testosterone concentrations in the plasma are very low before puberty, but then rise rapidly to reach normal adult values. A slight decline in concentration may be seen in the elderly.

In the circulation, ~97% of testosterone is protein bound, principally to sex hormone-binding globulin (SHBG) and to a lesser extent to albumin. The free fraction is readily available to tissues; albumin binds testosterone more loosely than SHBG, and albumin-bound testosterone may be in part available. Free testosterone is considered a better indicator of effective androgen availability than total testosterone, but its measurement is technically difficult. A free androgen index, the ratio of testosterone/SHBG concentrations, is sometimes useful when testing for possible hyperandrogenism in females. Bioavailable testosterone, comprising the free fraction and that loosely bound to albumin, can be estimated from testosterone, SHBG and albumin concentrations using the Vermeulen equation (available on-line at www.issam.ch), and it is of value when investigating possible hypogonadism in men when the total testosterone concentration is close to the lower end of the reference range. Both approaches provide relatively imprecise estimates and are rarely necessary if total testosterone concentrations are unequivocally normal or abnormal.

The biological activity of testosterone is mainly due to dihydrotestosterone (DHT). This is formed from testosterone in target tissues in a reaction catalysed by the enzyme 5α-reductase. In a rare condition in which there is deficiency of this enzyme, DHT cannot be formed; male internal genitalia develop normally (Wolffian duct development in the fetus is testosterone dependent), but masculinization, which requires DHT, is incomplete. In states of androgen insensitivity, defects of the receptors for either testosterone or DHT, or both, can cause a spectrum of clinical abnormalities ranging from gynaecomastia to disorders of sex development.

Testosterone is also present in females, at much lower concentrations, with about one third being derived from the ovaries and the remainder from the metabolism of adrenal androgens.

Specific assays are readily available for testosterone, SHBG and the individual adrenal androgens.

Oestrogens and ovarian function

The cyclical control of ovarian function during the reproductive years is discussed in Chapter 9. The principal ovarian hormone is **oestradiol**, but some oestrone is also produced by the ovaries. Oestrogens are also secreted by the corpus luteum and the placenta.

Oestrogens are responsible for the development of many **female secondary sexual characteristics**. They also stimulate the **growth of ovarian follicles** and the proliferation of uterine endometrium during the first part of the menstrual cycle. They have important effects on cervical mucus and vaginal epithelium, and on other functions associated with reproduction.

Plasma concentrations of oestrogens are low before puberty. During puberty, oestrogen synthesis increases and cyclical changes in concentration occur thereafter until menopause, unless pregnancy occurs. After menopause, the sole source of oestrogens is from the metabolism of adrenal androgens; plasma concentrations fall to very low values. In the plasma, oestrogens are transported bound to protein, 60% to albumin and the remainder to SHBG. Only 2–3% remains unbound. Oestrogens stimulate the synthesis of SHBG and also that of other transport proteins, notably thyroxine-binding globulin (TBG) and transcortin, and thus increase total thyroxine and total cortisol concentrations in the plasma.

Slowly rising or sustained high concentrations of oestrogens, together with progesterone, inhibit pituitary gonadotrophin secretion by negative feedback, but the rapid rise in oestrogen concentration that occurs before ovulation stimulates LH secretion (positive feedback).

Oestradiol is present in low concentrations in the plasma of normal men. Approximately one-third is secreted by the testes, the remainder being derived from the metabolism of testosterone in the liver and in adipose tissue.

Progesterone

Progesterone is an important intermediate in steroid hormone biosynthesis but is secreted in appreciable quantities only by the corpus luteum and the placenta. Its concentration in plasma rises during the second half of the menstrual cycle, but then falls if conception does not take place. In the plasma, it is extensively bound to albumin and transcortin: only 1–2% is free. Progesterone has many important effects on the uterus, including preparation of the endometrium for implantation of the conceptus, and also on the cervix, vagina and breasts. It is pyrogenic and mediates the increase in basal body temperature that occurs with ovulation. Measurement of plasma progesterone concentration is of value in the investigation of infertility in women (see p. 219).

Sex hormone-binding globulin

SHBG binds both testosterone and oestradiol in the plasma, although it has greater affinity for testosterone.

> **Box 12.1 Factors that affect sex-hormone binding globulin concentration**
>
> **Increase**
> oestrogens
> hyperthyroidism
> liver cirrhosis
> anorexia
>
> **Decrease**
> androgens
> hypothyroidism
> glucocorticoids
> obesity, particularly in women

The plasma concentration of SHBG in men is about half that in women. Factors that affect SHBG concentration (Box 12.1) alter the ratio of free testosterone to free oestradiol. If SHBG concentration decreases, the ratio of free testosterone to free oestradiol increases, although there is an absolute increase in the free concentrations of both hormones. If SHBG concentration increases, the ratio decreases. Thus, in either sex, the effect of an increase in SHBG is to increase oestrogen-dependent effects, whereas a decrease in SHBG increases androgen-dependent effects (Fig. 12.1).

Disorders of Male Gonadal Function

Delayed puberty and hypogonadism in males

It is uncommon for a boy to enter puberty before the age of 9 years. Precocious puberty is discussed in Chapter 22. Boys who have not entered puberty by the age of 14 years are considered to have **delayed puberty**. They often present earlier than this, more often with short stature (a result of the delayed pubertal growth spurt) than with concern about gonadal development. Delayed puberty can be constitutional (i.e. idiopathic, often associated with a family history), related to chronic illness (e.g. coeliac disease, cystic fibrosis) or a consequence of hypogonadism. Delayed puberty should be investigated to diagnose any pathological disorder: constitutional delayed puberty is essentially a diagnosis of exclusion.

The term **hypogonadism** implies defective spermatogenesis or testosterone production, or both. It can be primary (i.e. caused by testicular disease) or occur secondarily to pituitary or hypothalamic disease. **Primary hypogonadism** is sometimes referred to as 'hypergonadotrophic hypogonadism' (decreased feedback causes increased

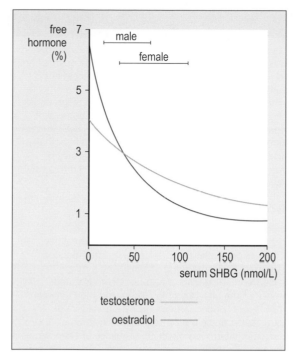

Fig. 12.1 Effect of a change in serum sex hormone-binding globulin (SHBG) concentration on free oestradiol and testosterone concentrations. A decrease in SHBG increases free testosterone concentration more than free oestradiol, and thus is androgenic; an increase in the concentration of SHBG is anti-androgenic. The normal ranges of SHBG in males and females are shown.

Box 12.2 Some causes of male hypogonadism

Primary (serum testosterone ↓; FSH and LH ↑)

congenital
    testicular agenesis
    Klinefelter syndrome (47XXY)
    5α-reductase[a] and other enzyme defects
    untreated cryptorchidism
    haemochromatosis[b]
acquired
    bilateral orchitis (mumps)
    bilateral testicular torsion
    irradiation
    cytotoxic drugs
    bilateral varicocele

Secondary (serum testosterone ↓; FSH and LH normal or ↓)

pituitary disorders
    tumours (especially if causing hyperprolactinaemia)
    panhypopituitarism
hypothalamic disorders
    Kallmann syndrome

FSH, follicle-stimulating hormone; LH, luteinizing hormone.
[a]Testosterone normal but low dihydrotestosterone.
[b]Iron can deposit in either the testicles or the pituitary leading to primary or secondary hypogonadism in haemochromatosis.

---

gonadotrophin secretion) and **secondary hypogonadism** as 'hypogonadotrophic hypogonadism' (the hypogonadism is a consequence of decreased gonadotrophin secretion because of either pituitary or hypothalamic disease). Some of the causes are indicated in Box 12.2. Primary hypogonadism can be caused by defective seminiferous tubule function alone, defective Leydig cell function alone or both. The former leads to infertility through decreased production of spermatozoa, but masculinization is usually normal. Defective Leydig cell function, in contrast, results in a failure of testosterone-dependent functions, including spermatogenesis. The effects of decreased testosterone secretion depend on age at the time of onset of the disorder. Secondary sexual characteristics are in part preserved if secretion is lost after puberty.

The basic **biochemical characteristics** that distinguish between primary and secondary hypogonadism are not always clear-cut. The plasma concentration of testosterone shows a circadian rhythm. It falls during the course of the day and in response to food intake, so the usual recommendation if the result is low is to repeat the test after an overnight fast at 9:00 a.m. Also, since the secretion of gonadotrophins and testosterone is pulsatile, measurements should be made on more than one occasion, particularly if results are borderline.

The use of provocative tests of the hypothalamo–pituitary–gonadal axis in hypogonadism is discussed in Case history 12.1.

Although biochemical tests are important in establishing that a patient has primary, rather than secondary, gonadal failure, they are less useful in distinguishing between the various causes of primary hypogonadism. In general, seminiferous tubule defects are associated with raised plasma FSH concentrations; Leydig cell defects are associated with raised plasma LH concentrations. Human chorionic gonadotrophin (hCG), which has an action similar to LH, can be used to test Leydig cell function (Box 12.3). Semen analysis will provide an indication of seminiferous tubule function, and testicular biopsy is valuable in patients with low sperm counts if the cause is not obvious clinically. Careful clinical examination is essential in all patients with gonadal failure.

Testosterone production sometimes declines after the age of 50 years, even in healthy men, and this trend is more marked in those who have type 2 diabetes. It is usually a result of primary testicular dysfunction, and it is accompanied by a rise in LH as a result of reduced feedback

Case history 12.1

History

A 20-year-old man presented with impotence.

Examination

He had a eunuchoid appearance, i.e. there was only sparse pubic and axillary hair, the genitalia were infantile, muscular development was poor and his span exceeded his height with a sole to pubic symphysis distance greater than symphysis to crown.

Results (see Appendix for reference ranges)

Serum:	testosterone	3.0 nmol/L
	LH	0.8 IU/L
	FSH	0.9 IU/L

Gonadotrophin-releasing hormone (GnRH) test (100 µg GnRH i.v.):

Time (min)	FSH (IU/L)	LH (IU/L)
0	0.7	0.9
20	1.1	1.3
60	1.3	1.8

Summary

Low testosterone with low LH and FSH concentrations, within the prepubertal range. Subnormal and delayed response to GnRH.

Interpretation

The low testosterone and gonadotrophin concentrations in this case suggest a lesion at the level of either the pituitary or hypothalamus. Boys with constitutional delayed puberty occasionally do not enter puberty until 16–18 years of age and have a similar pattern of results, but this patient is clearly hypogonadal. GnRH stimulation tests the function of the hypothalamo–pituitary axis. A normal response is at least a doubling of LH and FSH concentrations, with a peak at 20 min. The test is also sometimes used in an attempt to distinguish between pituitary and hypothalamic causes of hypogonadism; a delayed response may be observed in the latter, but it does not reliably differentiate between them.

Discussion

Patients with pituitary lesions may have clinical or biochemical evidence of other pituitary abnormalities (none was present in this case). He was later found to be anosmic (lacking a sense of smell) and a magnetic resonance imaging scan of his brain demonstrated absence of the olfactory bulbs. The association between anosmia and hypogonadotrophic hypogonadism of hypothalamic origin is called 'Kallmann syndrome'. The eunuchoid habitus is a direct consequence of testosterone deficiency. Testosterone promotes epiphyseal fusion, and when its secretion is inadequate, there is continued growth of long bones, which become disproportionate to the axial skeleton. Had the FSH and LH concentrations been elevated in this patient, and with nothing in the history to suggest acquired testicular failure, the next investigation would have been karyotyping, to investigate for possible Klinefelter syndrome.

Box 12.3 A protocol for the human chorionic gonadotrophin test

Procedure	Results
day 0: 9:00 a.m.; take blood for testosterone; give 5000 U hCG i.m.	normal response: plasma testosterone concentration increases to more than upper limit of reference range
day 4: 9:00 a.m.; take blood for testosterone	primary testicular failure: little or no response
	secondary testicular failure: response may be normal

hCG, human chorionic gonadotrophin.

inhibition. Some authorities recommend testosterone replacement therapy in men who experience symptoms and signs of androgen deficiency such as reduced libido, erectile dysfunction, fatigue and depressed mood if plasma testosterone concentrations are low in a fasting sample taken between 8:00 a.m. and 10:00 a.m. (when they are normally at their highest).

The **treatment** of hypogonadism in males should be directed towards the underlying cause wherever possible. Testosterone is given in testosterone deficiency syndromes, but if fertility is required, treatment must be with gonadotrophin replacement or, in hypothalamic disorders, pulsatile gonadotrophin-releasing hormone (GnRH) administration. Even in constitutional delayed puberty, a course of testosterone can be beneficial, giving a 'kick-start' to puberty, which often continues naturally thereafter. Testosterone replacement should aim to maintain plasma concentrations in the reference range for as long as possible between doses. The actual targets vary with the preparation and apply only once steady state has been reached (after a minimum of four treatments). With implants or injected long-acting testosterone, the concentrations should be measured before the next dose is due, with a target range of 10–15 nmol/L; with transdermal patches or gel, 4–6 h after application, with a target range of 15–20 nmol/L. Because prostate cancer is testosterone-dependent, testosterone replacement must not be given to men with a history of prostate or breast cancer and is generally avoided in men aged >65 years or who have a plasma prostate-specific antigen (PSA) concentration of >4 ng/mL (see p. 361). Replacement treatment increases the haematocrit and therefore may increase risk of thrombotic disease. PSA and haematocrit must be monitored at yearly intervals for the duration of treatment.

Gynaecomastia

Breast development in males is usually related to a disturbance of the balance of oestrogens to androgens. It may occur physiologically in neonates as a result of exposure to maternal oestrogens. During puberty, ~50% of healthy boys develop gynaecomastia because of temporarily increased secretion of oestrogens relative to androgens. In both instances, the gynaecomastia resolves spontaneously. Mild gynaecomastia may also occur in the elderly, as a result of a decrease in testosterone secretion.

Gynaecomastia occurring at other times should be regarded as pathological. The principal causes are shown in Box 12.4. Testicular germ cell tumours sometimes secrete hCG, which stimulates oestrogen production, thereby causing gynaecomastia. Drugs are responsible in 10–20% of patients. The cause may be obvious from either the history or clinical examination. Investigations that may help to establish the cause include measurement of plasma testosterone, oestradiol, gonadotrophins, hCG, SHBG and prolactin, and tests of kidney, liver, thyroid, adrenal and pituitary function. Karyotyping is required to diagnose Klinefelter syndrome, in which an additional X chromosome is present (47XXY). Magnetic resonance imaging of the brain and ultrasound of the testes are required especially if initial biochemistry investigations suggest pituitary disease or a germ cell tumour.

Disorders of Female Gonadal Function

Delayed puberty and hypogonadism in females

Few girls enter puberty before about 8 years of age. Precocious puberty is discussed in Chapter 22. The great majority of girls will have entered puberty by about 13 years of age. Girls with **delayed puberty** usually present because of absence of breast development or amenorrhoea (see later). Girls with no breast development by the age of 13 years or with primary amenorrhoea after the age of 15 years require

---

Box 12.4 Some causes of gynaecomastia

Physiological

neonatal
pubertal
old age

Pathological

increased oestrogens
    chronic liver disease[a], chronic kidney disease, Cushing syndrome, hyperthyroidism[a], testicular tumours (hCG secreting)
decreased androgens
    Klinefelter syndrome
androgen insensitivity
    androgen receptor defect (androgen insensitivity syndrome)
    refeeding after starvation (LH secretion increased)
prolactinoma

Pharmacological

antiandrogens (e.g. flutamide, finasteride)
gonadorelin (GnRH) analogues (e.g. goserelin, buserelin; reduce LH secretion)
anabolic steroids (suppress testosterone)
spironolactone (antiandrogenic)
digoxin (oestrogen agonist)
oestrogens
antiretrovirals (mechanism unknown)
cytotoxics (testicular damage)
antipsychotics (mechanism unknown)

[a]Increased sex hormone-binding globulin (SHBG) may contribute in these conditions through reducing free testosterone concentrations.

GnRH, gonadotrophin-releasing hormone; hCG, human chorionic gonadotrophin; LH, luteinizing hormone

---

further investigation. As in boys, constitutional delayed puberty is essentially a diagnosis of exclusion. The pathological causes (Box 12.5) can be divided into hypogonadism (hypergonadotrophic, i.e. primary ovarian failure, and hypogonadotrophic, i.e. secondary to pituitary or hypothalamic disease) or chronic disease (e.g. coeliac disease, chronic kidney disease).

The principles of **treatment** of female hypogonadism are similar to those in males: low doses of oral oestrogens are used initially to promote feminization, then sequential oestrogen and progestogen to induce menstruation. Treatment with gonadotrophins or GnRH is required to stimulate ovulation.

Amenorrhoea and oligomenorrhoea

Amenorrhoea can be primary (menstruation has never occurred) or secondary. Oligomenorrhoea is sparse or infrequent menstruation; it can be because of less severe forms of some of the causes of amenorrhoea. Primary amenorrhoea can occur as part of the syndrome of female hypogonadism but can also be present in normally feminized women.

The commonest cause of amenorrhoea in women of childbearing age is **pregnancy**, and this possibility, however unlikely, must be investigated using a urine pregnancy test (which detects hCG) before other investigations are undertaken.

Pregnancy apart, amenorrhoea in normally feminized women is most frequently due to a hormonal disturbance that results in a failure of ovulation. Causes include:

- disordered hypothalamo-pituitary function, related to weight loss (30–35% of patients in most series) or hyperprolactinaemia (10–12%), but idiopathic in some 10% of patients
- ovarian dysfunction (e.g. autoimmune premature ovarian failure) (10–12%)
- increased androgen production (particularly polycystic ovary syndrome [PCOS] and late-onset congenital adrenal hyperplasia [CAH]) (30–35%).

Weight loss can lead to a decrease in the frequency of the pulsatility of GnRH secretion, and thus decreased secretion of LH and FSH. Amenorrhoea is a near-universal occurrence in patients with anorexia nervosa and is common in women with a body mass index (BMI) <19 kg/m^2 or after rapid loss of >10% of body weight. Regular menstruation returns if weight is regained.

Severe stress and intensive exercise regimens, such as are adopted by elite athletes, ballet dancers and gymnasts, can also lead to amenorrhoea, probably for complex neuroendocrinological reasons in addition to any effect of decreased body weight.

Amenorrhoea caused by excessive androgen secretion is often associated with hirsutism or even virilism. These conditions are discussed in the next section.

Uterine dysfunction is an uncommon cause of amenorrhoea. It can be excluded, if necessary, by the progestogen challenge test. If medroxyprogesterone acetate is given orally (10 mg daily for 5 days), the occurrence of vaginal bleeding 5–7 days later signifies that the uterus was adequately oestrogenized. If bleeding does not occur, the test is repeated, after priming with oestrogen (ethinyloestradiol 50 µg daily for 21 days, with progestogen on the last 5 days). Absence of bleeding indicates uterine disease. If bleeding occurs, oestrogen deficiency is present.

The **diagnosis** of hormonal causes of amenorrhoea requires basal measurements of plasma FSH, LH and prolactin concentrations. A high FSH concentration is indicative of ovarian failure (and is more sensitive in this respect than LH). If LH, but not FSH, is elevated, the most likely diagnosis is PCOS; plasma testosterone and SHBG concentrations should be measured and pelvic ultrasonography performed (see p. 218). If LH and FSH concentrations are normal or low, a pituitary or hypothalamic disorder should be sought using imaging studies and dynamic testing of the hypothalamo–pituitary axis in a manner similar to that described for male hypogonadism. As in males, however, the results of such tests do not always distinguish between pituitary and hypothalamic disorders.

The **management** of amenorrhoea depends on the cause and whether fertility is required. In hyperprolactinaemia (see Chapter 9), the treatment is directed to the underlying cause wherever possible (e.g. withdrawal of drugs, treatment of hypothyroidism).

In ovarian, pituitary or hypothalamic disease, when fertility is not required, cyclical oestrogen and (if the patient has a uterus) progestogen replacement is given. In established ovarian failure, pregnancy is usually only possible using donated ova.

If fertility is required in patients with pituitary dysfunction, treatment is with pulsatile GnRH or human FSH and LH; hCG is used to mimic the midcycle LH peak and stimulate ovulation. Careful monitoring of plasma oestradiol concentrations is necessary to detect hyperstimulation, which carries a risk of multiple pregnancy and the development of ovarian cysts.

Patients with hypothalamic disease may respond to clomifene. This substance blocks oestradiol receptors in the hypothalamus and stimulates GnRH (and thus LH and FSH) secretion. Non-responders are treated with gonadotrophins or pulsatile GnRH. Clomifene is also useful in inducing ovulation in patients with PCOS. When it has not been possible to distinguish between hypothalamic and pituitary disease, a failure to respond to pulsatile GnRH suggests that amenorrhoea is due to pituitary dysfunction.

A simple protocol for the investigation of endocrine causes of amenorrhoea is given in Fig. 12.2.

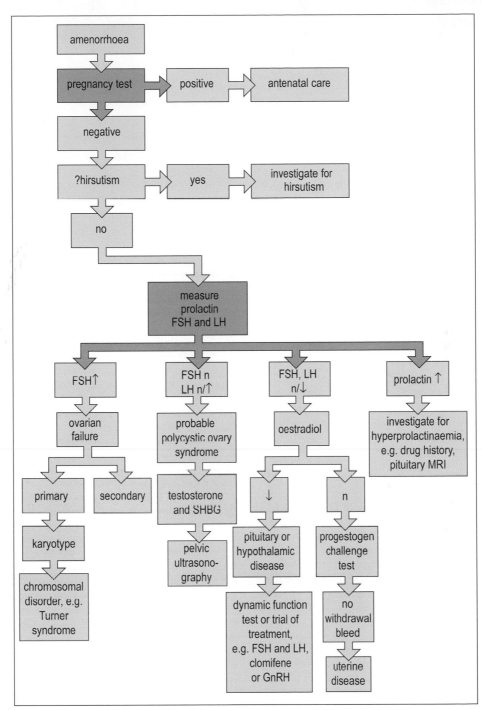

Fig. 12.2 Protocol for the investigation of amenorrhoea; dynamic function tests (gonadotrophin-releasing hormone (GnRH), clomifene) may distinguish between hypothalamic and pituitary causes, although in practice this may only become clear when treatment aimed at restoring fertility is instituted. FSH, follicle-stimulating hormone; LH, luteinizing hormone; MRI, magnetic resonance imaging; SHBG, sex hormone-binding globulin.

The climacteric

During the climacteric, **progressive ovarian failure** causes a decline in ovarian oestrogen secretion and eventually menstruation ceases: **menopause** is defined as occurring 12 months after the last menstrual period. The only oestrogen produced after menopause is the small amount derived from metabolism of adrenal androstenedione in adipose tissue. Plasma FSH concentrations become greatly elevated. Measurement of FSH is sometimes useful in women who are experiencing symptoms of possible menopause before the age of 45 but is not necessary in older women. Plasma LH concentrations are also elevated but to a lesser extent, and measurement of LH or oestradiol is of no value in the diagnosis of menopause. **Metabolic changes** that occur after menopause include decreases in plasma high-density lipoprotein and increases in plasma low-density lipoprotein and urate concentrations. Oestrogen deficiency is a major factor contributing to the development of postmenopausal osteoporosis.

Hormone replacement treatment (HRT) can be effective in controlling the acute symptoms of menopause and is of proven benefit in preventing postmenopausal osteoporosis, although it increases the risk of venous thromboembolism and stroke, and long-term use carries a small increase in the risk of breast cancer. Oestrogen can be given alone in women who have had a hysterectomy, but cyclical progestogen also must be given to women who have not, to prevent endometrial hyperplasia and possible malignant transformation. Biochemical monitoring of HRT is not required routinely.

Hirsutism and virilism

Hirsutism is an increase in body hair in an androgen-related distribution. In most instances, menstruation is normal, but it may be accompanied by menstrual irregularity. Virilisation (e.g. clitoromegaly, male-pattern hair loss) indicates more severe hyperandrogenism, often due to androgen-secreting tumours. There is considerable racial variation in the amount of body hair in women, and what may be regarded as normal in some races may be thought excessive by others.

The clinical features of hirsutism and virilism result from excessive exposure of tissues to androgens. This may be because of increased androgen secretion, a low plasma concentration of SHBG, which increases the free testosterone fraction, or both. In some patients, there appears to be an increased sensitivity to androgens. The causes of hirsutism and virilism are indicated in Box 12.6.

The commonest cause of hirsutism (>75% of patients) is **PCOS**, a condition of hyperandrogenisation and chronic anovulation in the absence of specific underlying adrenal

---

> **Box 12.6 Causes of hirsutism and virilization**
>
> **Idiopathic**
>
> **Ovarian**
> polycystic ovary syndrome
> androgen-secreting tumours
> postmenopausal
>
> **Adrenal**
> congenital adrenal hyperplasia
> Cushing syndrome
> androgen-secreting tumours
>
> **Iatrogenic**
> androgens
> progestogens
>
> Idiopathic causes and polycystic ovarian syndrome account for most cases.

---

or pituitary disease. Its diagnosis requires at least two of the following three features to be present:

- polycystic ovaries (demonstrated by ultrasound)
- chronic anovulation or oligomenorrhoea
- clinical or biochemical evidence of androgen excess.

The condition shows considerable variation in its expression: many women previously classified as having 'idiopathic hirsutism' have a mild form of PCOS. The precise aetiology is uncertain; both genetic and environmental factors appear to be involved.

The ovaries are the source of the excess androgens in PCOS, although the cause of the excessive secretion remains unclear. Plasma LH concentration is often elevated, but although this finding is relatively specific, it is insensitive, in that many patients who otherwise satisfy the diagnostic criteria for the condition have normal concentrations. Plasma testosterone concentration is moderately increased (see later). Plasma oestradiol concentrations are usually in the normal midfollicular range.

Many patients with PCOS are overweight and have insulin resistance with hyperinsulinaemia. This increases ovarian androgen production and suppresses SHBG synthesis, thereby further increasing plasma free androgen concentrations. There is a strong association with other features of the **metabolic syndrome** (see p. 152), including dyslipidaemia and hypertension, which are recognized risk factors for cardiovascular disease. Some current guidelines recommend screening for diabetes and assessment of cardiovascular risk every 3–5 years in women who have PCOS.

The **management** of PCOS depends on the severity of the condition and individual circumstances. The combined oral contraceptive pill is recommended (unless otherwise contraindicated) as first-line treatment for the menstrual abnormalities and hirsutism that are associated with hyperandrogenism. Oestrogens increase plasma SHBG concentrations and are therefore antiandrogenic (see Fig. 12.1). Weight loss has beneficial effects on both reproductive and metabolic dysfunction because it reduces insulin resistance. Metformin is recommended for women who have impaired glucose tolerance or type 2 diabetes mellitus and is sometimes used in overweight or obese women without these features who do not respond adequately to oestrogens or are unable to lose weight. The antioestrogen drug clomifene is a useful treatment for anovulatory infertility that does not respond to weight loss.

The appropriate **investigation** of hirsutism depends on the clinical context, although if menstruation is normal, no endocrine abnormality may be found. Measurement of LH, FSH, testosterone and SHBG is desirable in all patients. A normal plasma total testosterone concentration does not rule out hyperandrogenism, so the free androgen index (see p. 211) should be calculated. Testosterone concentrations are rarely >5.0 nmol/L in PCOS or late-onset CAH (see p. 188). Concentrations >5.0 nmol/L are more likely to be associated with virilization and are strongly suggestive of an androgen-secreting tumour, which may be in an adrenal gland or an ovary. Testosterone immunoassays are susceptible to analytical interference from other steroids, so it is sometimes necessary to confirm a high result using a more specific mass spectrometry method.

The presence of other clinical features (e.g. of Cushing syndrome) in a hirsute patient may suggest a specific diagnosis and thus appropriate further investigations. In patients with severe hirsutism, or if menstrual disturbance or virilism is present, adrenal androgens and 17-hydroxyprogesterone (17-OHP) should be measured. A diagnosis of late-onset CAH is supported by the finding of an elevated concentration of 17-OHP, which increases to more than twice the upper limit of normal 60 min after an injection of synthetic adrenocorticotrophic hormone (ACTH, tetracosactide or Synacthen, 250 µg intramuscularly [i.m.] or intravenously [i.v.]). High concentrations of 17-OHP, DHEA sulphate and androstenedione are found in patients with adrenal tumours, but 17-OHP does not increase significantly in response to ACTH.

Infertility

Infertility is a common clinical problem, leading approximately one in six couples in the UK to seek professional advice. Investigation is usually considered appropriate when a couple has been unable to conceive after 12 months of trying, assuming frequent unprotected intercourse. It can be **primary** (conception has never occurred) or **secondary**, and caused by problems that affect either the male or the female partner. Ovulatory failure, most frequently caused by hyperprolactinaemia or hypothalamo-pituitary dysfunction, is responsible in ~20% of infertility cases, and

---

Case history 12.2

History

A young woman consulted her doctor because she was embarrassed by excessive body hair. Her periods had always been irregular and light, and she had begun her current menstrual period 3 days ago.

Examination

She was moderately obese, and had hirsutism involving her upper lip, lower abdomen and thighs.

Results

Serum:		
	testosterone	1.6 nmol/L
	SHBG	25 nmol/L
	LH	14.2 IU/L
	FSH	3.8 IU/L

Ultrasound examination of the ovaries: multiple cysts present, bilaterally.

Summary

Testosterone at the high end of the reference range. Low SHBG, high LH.

Interpretation

Although the serum testosterone concentration is within the reference range, the SHBG concentration is low, so the free (bioavailable) testosterone concentration is likely to be raised. The calculated free androgen index (100 × testosterone/SHBG, reference range 0–4) is high at 6.4%. A high LH concentration in relation to that of FSH is another characteristic, although not diagnostic, feature of PCOS.

Discussion

This patient has all three diagnostic features of PCOS: polycystic ovaries (demonstrated by ultrasound), oligomenorrhoea and evidence of androgen excess. The clinical features of this condition include hirsutism, acne, menstrual disturbances and obesity, but there is considerable variation in their prevalence and severity. Neither are the typical hormonal changes always present. The pathogenesis of the condition is uncertain. The normal ovaries synthesize androgens (principally testosterone and androstenedione), but their secretion is increased in PCOS. Conversion of androgens to oestrogens in liver and adipose tissue is thought to inhibit secretion of FSH (preventing ovulation) and stimulate that of LH (further stimulating androgen secretion).

---

defective sperm production is responsible in ~25%. Endocrine causes of infertility are rare in males.

The **investigation** of infertility requires a thorough clinical and laboratory assessment of both partners. Anatomical causes—for example, damage to the Fallopian tubes—are

Case history 12.3

History

A couple in their late 20s was infertile in spite of regular intercourse over a 2-year period. Each partner had a child by a previous marriage. The woman's periods had recently become irregular, the last occurring 2 months ago. A semen sample contained a normal count of motile sperm. The woman was on steroid replacement treatment for adrenal failure, which had been diagnosed in her late teens.

Results

Serum:

	prolactin	300 mIU/L
	LH	10.7 IU/L
	FSH	28.2 IU/L

Summary

High FSH with LH concentration at the high end of the reference range and normal prolactin.

Interpretation

The elevated FSH concentration (caused by decreased negative feedback by oestrogens) indicates incipient ovarian failure. FSH is a more sensitive test for this than LH, although, in established ovarian failure (after menopause), the plasma concentrations of LH and FSH are usually both very high. Hyperprolactinaemia, an alternative cause of menstrual disturbance and infertility, has been ruled out.

Discussion

This is secondary infertility. The adrenal failure in the woman had been shown to be caused by autoimmune disease, and there is a recognized association between autoimmune adrenal and ovarian failure (Schmidt syndrome). Two months later she had not had a period, and the plasma concentrations of LH and FSH were less than the lower limit of the assay. On the same sample hCG was measured and its concentration was found to be high, indicating that she was pregnant. LH and FSH production is subject to negative feedback inhibition from oestradiol and inhibin during pregnancy. Ovarian failure develops gradually and occasional ovulation may still occur in the early stages, as in this patient.

relatively common. Semen must be examined to ensure that adequate numbers of normal sperm are present. If menstruation is regular, ovulation is probably occurring. Detection of the rise in basal body temperature that follows ovulation is a useful indicator of this. More reliably, the concentration of **progesterone** (secreted by the corpus luteum) in plasma increases after ovulation. Values >30 nmol/L, 7 days before the next period is due, indicate that ovulation has occurred. Lower values do not exclude ovulation but suggest

poor function of the corpus luteum and are associated with reduced probability of conception. A concentration <10 nmol/L is highly suggestive of an anovulatory cycle: up to 30% of cycles are anovulatory even in women who have normal fertility, so progesterone measurement may have to be repeated during several cycles if initial results are low.

The plasma concentration of **anti-Müllerian hormone** (AMH), a hormone secreted by developing ovarian follicles, is sometimes used as a test for ovarian reserve, especially in women who have a family history of early menopause or in whom there is other concern about premature ovarian failure. In those being considered for assisted conception, very low plasma AMH concentrations help to identify those who will not respond to ovarian stimulation and high concentrations those who may be at risk of hyperstimulation.

If cycles are anovulatory but regular, treatment with clomifene may restore fertility. If not, or if there is oligorrhoea or amenorrhoea, measurements of prolactin and gonadotrophins may indicate a diagnosis (see amenorrhoea, p. 215). Defective sperm production should be investigated by measurements of testosterone and gonadotrophins and, if necessary, by testicular biopsy. The postcoital test, previously used to determine the presence of motile sperm, is now considered unreliable.

Assisted pregnancy

Numerous treatments for infertility are available, ranging from stimulation of ovulation with clomifene or gonadotrophins to *in vitro* fertilization and embryo transfer. Close cooperation between the laboratory and clinical teams is essential to maximize the chance of success and to reduce the risk of complications during treatment to induce ovulation. Monitoring of plasma oestradiol concentration is used together with transvaginal ultrasound to determine whether follicles have developed to an appropriate stage for induction of ovulation and to prevent the onset of the potentially fatal ovarian hyperstimulation syndrome.

Pregnancy

Many physiological and metabolic changes take place in the body during pregnancy. These include changes in the concentrations of hormones directly related to pregnancy and resulting secondary metabolic changes.

Specific hormonal changes
Human chorionic gonadotrophin

Fertilization of the ovum prevents regression of the corpus luteum. Instead, the corpus luteum enlarges, stimulated by the glycoprotein hormone hCG produced by the trophoblast (the developing placenta). This hormone can be detected in maternal blood 7–9 days after conception and may be detectable in urine 1–2 days later. Its detection in the urine provides a highly sensitive and specific test for the diagnosis of pregnancy. The secretion of hCG begins to fall by 10–12 weeks, although it remains detectable in the urine throughout pregnancy. Some tumours can produce hCG; its use as a tumour marker is discussed in Chapter 20.

Quantitative measurement of plasma hCG is valuable in the diagnosis of suspected **ectopic pregnancy**: if the concentration is >1000 IU/L but an intrauterine sac cannot be visualized on transvaginal ultrasound, ectopic pregnancy is likely. In addition, plasma hCG concentrations double every 2 days in normal pregnancy, but the rate in ectopic pregnancy is usually less.

Oestrogens

The stimulated corpus luteum secretes large amounts of oestrogens and progesterone, but after 6 weeks the placenta becomes the major source of these hormones. There is a massive increase in the production of oestriol during pregnancy, but production of oestrone and oestradiol increases also. Oestriol is synthesized in the placenta from androgens

secreted by the fetal adrenal glands. High plasma oestrogen concentrations, and increased inhibin production, result in suppression of LH and FSH synthesis by the pituitary.

Secondary metabolic changes

Many of the metabolic changes that occur in pregnancy are discussed elsewhere in this book. They are summarized in Table 12.1.

Maternal monitoring

Patients with medical conditions may require close monitoring immediately before, and during, pregnancy. For example, strict control of **diabetes mellitus** is vital, for both maternal and fetal health. Women should self-monitor their capillary blood glucose concentration and adjust diet and insulin regimens to maintain near-normal concentrations both before and during pregnancy. Pregnancy can adversely affect maternal glucose homoeostasis: insulin requirements in patients with type 1 diabetes may increase during pregnancy; patients with type 2 diabetes are usually treated with insulin. Some women develop diabetes during pregnancy (gestational diabetes, see p. 235). Risk factors for gestational diabetes include:

Table 12.1 Metabolic changes that occur during pregnancy and the use of oral contraceptives

Change	Cause	Pregnancy	Oral contraceptive use
↓ urea	↑ GFR; ↑ plasma volume	*	
↓ albumin	↑ plasma volume	*	
↓ total protein	↑ plasma volume	*	
↓ TSH	↑ hCG	*see legend*	
↑ cortisol	↑ transcortin	*	*
↑ copper	↑ caeruloplasmin	*	*
glycosuria	↓ renal threshold	*	
↓ glucose tolerance (but normal fasting concentrations)	insulin resistance	*	
↑ triglyceride (VLDL)	↑ oestrogens	*	*
↑ LDL-cholesterol	↑ oestrogens; ↑ progesterone	*	variable
↑ HDL-cholesterol		*see legend*	variable
↑ alkaline phosphatase	placental isoenzyme	*	

Thyroid stimulating hormone (TSH) concentrations fall in early pregnancy because of increased thyroid hormone production in response to human chorionic gonadotrophin (hCG) but subsequently rise again. High-density lipoprotein (HDL)–cholesterol concentrations increase slightly in early pregnancy but then stabilize or even decline to non-pregnant values. The effects of oral contraceptives on lipids are hormone and dose dependent (see p. 222).
GFR, glomerular filtration rate; LDL, low-density lipoprotein; TBG, thyroxine-binding globulin; VLDL, very low-density lipoprotein.

- BMI >30 kg/m^2
- previous large baby
- gestational diabetes during previous pregnancy
- a first-degree relative with diabetes.

Women who are at high risk of gestational diabetes should be offered an oral glucose tolerance test at 24–28 weeks' gestation (16–18 weeks in those with previous gestational diabetes). Screening using urinalysis for glucose is no longer recommended because many pregnant women have glycosuria because of the lower renal threshold for glucose during pregnancy. Treatment for gestational diabetes is usually stopped shortly after giving birth, but fasting plasma glucose concentration should be checked at about 6 weeks after delivery because of the high risk of developing type 2 diabetes in the future. This condition is discussed further in Chapter 13.

Urine should be tested for **proteinuria** (and blood pressure measured) at all clinic attendances. The presence of proteinuria may be an early sign of **pregnancy-induced hypertension**. This condition, also known as preeclampsia, is peculiar to pregnancy. It is characterized by hypertension, proteinuria and oedema. If left untreated, it can lead to severe hypertension and acute kidney injury.

Liver disease that occurs during pregnancy is discussed on p. 121. The placenta produces variable, but sometimes large, amounts of alkaline phosphatase. The resulting increase in plasma alkaline phosphatase activity is of no clinical significance but creates the potential for misinterpretation of liver enzyme results. The presence of placental alkaline phosphatase could be confirmed by isoenzyme analysis, although this is rarely necessary.

In patients with **hypothyroidism**, the replacement dose of thyroxine usually needs to be increased early in pregnancy and should be adjusted to keep the plasma thyroid-stimulating hormone (TSH) concentration within the lower half of the reference range to ensure an adequate supply of thyroxine to both mother and fetus.

Fetal monitoring

The antenatal diagnosis of inherited metabolic disease, chromosomal disorders such as Down syndrome and neural tube defects is considered in Chapter 19.

Fetal blood can be obtained antenatally by **cordocentesis**, the aspiration of fetal blood from the umbilical cord under ultrasound control. Analysis of fetal blood for blood gases, hydrogen ion concentration and lactate can aid in the assessment of fetal well-being when non-invasive studies (e.g. ultrasonic determination of umbilical artery blood flow) suggest that the fetus is at risk.

Fetal fibronectin is a protein that is involved in attaching the fetal sac to the uterine lining. It is normally present in cervico-vaginal secretions up to 22 weeks of gestation, but then disappears until the end of the third trimester. Detection of fetal fibronectin in these secretions during weeks 22–34 in high-risk pregnancies may indicate the possibility of a preterm delivery, although the test is more useful if it is negative, when it is a reliable indicator that preterm delivery will not occur in the next 2 weeks.

During labour, once the cervix is sufficiently dilated, **fetal blood hydrogen ion concentration** can be measured in capillary samples obtained from the scalp. A concentration >60 nmol/L (pH <7.22) suggests potentially dangerous

---

Metabolic and cardiovascular effects of oral contraceptives

Oral contraceptives contain either a combination of an oestrogen and a progestogen or a progestogen alone. In addition to suppressing ovulation, these contraceptives have a number of metabolic effects similar to some of those that occur in normal pregnancy (see Table 12.1). There has been considerable interest in the effects of oral contraceptives on plasma lipid concentrations, and hence on cardiovascular risk. The precise effects depend on the agents used and the dose of oestrogen. Combined oral contraceptives containing low-strength oestrogen tend to slightly increase plasma low-density lipoprotein and reduce high-density lipoprotein (HDL) concentrations, whereas those that contain higher doses of oestrogens have the opposite effect. Combined contraceptives containing relatively androgenic progestogens—for example, gestodene, desogestrel, norgestimate and levonorgestrel—have a greater HDL-lowering effect. These agents are safe for use in younger women but should be used with caution or avoided, because of increased cardiovascular risk, in older women and those with additional risk factors such as smoking or poorly controlled hypertension. There is a slightly increased risk of venous thromboembolic disease, but the absolute risk is very low, and lower than that associated with pregnancy. There is no increase in cardiovascular or thromboembolic disease associated with progestogen-only contraception.

---

lactic acidosis as a result of fetal hypoxaemia. A continuous, direct measurement of fetal P_{O_2} can be made using a transcutaneous oxygen electrode.

SUMMARY

- The principal female sex hormone, or **oestrogen**, is **oestradiol**, secreted by the ovaries. The principal male sex hormone, or **androgen**, is **testosterone**, secreted by the testes.
- The secretion of both these hormones is stimulated by pituitary **luteinizing hormone (LH).** Spermatogenesis and the maturation of ovarian follicles are dependent on testosterone and oestradiol, respectively, and pituitary **follicle-stimulating hormone (FSH).** The secretion of LH and FSH is in turn controlled by gonadotrophin-releasing hormone, released from the hypothalamus, and subject to feedback control by the gonadal hormones. Androgens are also produced by the adrenal glands, and in males, there is some production of oestrogens by metabolism from androgens.
- Both testosterone and oestradiol are transported in the plasma bound to **sex hormone-binding globulin (SHBG)**, with only about 3% of each hormone being in free solution. Because of the greater avidity of testosterone for SHBG, factors that increase the concentration of SHBG tend to increase oestrogen-dependent effects, whereas those that decrease it increase androgen-dependent effects.
- The secretion of testosterone in men is generally maintained throughout life, with a gradual decline in some after the age of 50 years. In women, oestrogen secretion declines sharply in the months leading up to **menopause.**
- Both male and female **hypogonadism** can be either primary or secondary to pituitary or hypothalamic dysfunction. Measurement of the appropriate gonadal hormone and the gonadotrophins, often after attempted stimulation of their secretion, will usually indicate the correct diagnosis and permit rational treatment.
- Hormone measurements are also valuable in the investigation of **gynaecomastia** in men and **virilism** in women. The commonest feature of excessive androgenisation in women is **hirsutism**, which is most frequently due to **polycystic ovary syndrome (PCOS)**: other features of this condition include menstrual irregularity, infertility and the metabolic syndrome. **Congenital adrenal hyperplasia (CAH)** can present for the first time in young adults, causing hirsutism, menstrual irregularity and infertility. However, the presence of severe hirsutism and virilism should suggest the possibility of an **androgen-secreting tumour** of the adrenal glands or ovaries.
- The laboratory investigation of **infertility** also depends heavily on hormone measurements, although many non-endocrine factors must also be considered. A prime consideration is to establish whether ovulation is taking place: this can be inferred from finding an increase in plasma progesterone concentration during the luteal phase (on day 21 of a 28-day menstrual cycle).
- **Pregnancy** can be diagnosed by the detection of human chorionic gonadotrophin (hCG) in the urine. Pregnancy causes a number of physiological changes in biochemical variables, including an increase in the plasma concentrations of hormone-binding proteins. Women with pre-existing diabetes or hypertension and those who develop these conditions during pregnancy require close monitoring to avoid complications for both the mother and the fetus.

Chapter | 13 |

Disorders of carbohydrate metabolism

Introduction

Glucose is a major energy substrate. It typically provides more than half the total energy obtained from a 'western' diet and is the only utilizable source of energy for some tissues, for example, erythrocytes and, in the short term, the central nervous system. Many tissues are capable of oxidizing glucose completely to carbon dioxide; others metabolize it only as far as lactate, which can be converted back into glucose, principally in the liver and also in the kidneys, by gluconeogenesis. Even in tissues capable of completely oxidizing glucose, lactate is produced if insufficient oxygen is available (anaerobic metabolism, see p. 74). The body's **sources of glucose are dietary carbohydrate** and endogenous production by **glycogenolysis** (release of glucose stored as glycogen) and **gluconeogenesis** (glucose synthesis from, for example, lactate, glycerol and most amino acids). Glycogen is stored in the liver and skeletal muscle, but only the former contributes to plasma glucose.

Plasma glucose concentration depends on the relative rates of influx of glucose into the circulation and of its utilization. Its concentration is normally subject to rigorous control, rarely falling below 2.5 mmol/L at any time or rising above 8.0 mmol/L in healthy subjects after a meal or above 5.0 mmol/L after an overnight fast. After a meal, glucose is stored as glycogen, which is mobilized during fasting. Plasma glucose concentration usually falls to pre-meal concentrations within 4 h of a meal, but then continues to fall somewhat as fasting continues and hepatic glycogen stores are used up until, after about 24 h, adaptive changes lead to the attainment of a new steady state. After ~72 h, plasma glucose concentration stabilizes and can then remain constant for many days. The principal source of glucose becomes gluconeogenesis, from amino acids and glycerol, whereas ketones, derived from fat, become the major energy substrate (see p. 226).

The integration of these various processes, and thus the control of plasma glucose concentration, is achieved through the concerted action of various hormones: these are insulin (the actions of which tend to lower plasma glucose concentration) and the 'counterregulatory' hormones, namely glucagon, cortisol, catecholamines and growth hormone, which have the opposite effect. Their effects are summarized in Table 13.1.

The two **most important hormones in glucose homoeostasis** are **insulin** and **glucagon**. Insulin is a 51–amino acid polypeptide, secreted by the β-cells of the pancreatic islets of Langerhans in response to a rise in plasma glucose concentration. It is synthesized as a prohormone, proinsulin. This molecule undergoes cleavage before secretion to form insulin and C-peptide (Fig. 13.1). **Insulin secretion** is also stimulated by gut hormones collectively known as incretins, particularly glucagon-like peptide-1 (GLP-1) and glucose-dependent insulinotropic peptide (GIP, formerly known as gastric inhibitory polypeptide). Incretin release is stimulated by food, so that insulin secretion begins to increase before plasma glucose concentration.

Insulin promotes the removal of glucose from the blood through stimulating the relocation of insulin-sensitive GLUT-4 glucose transporters from the cytoplasm to cell membranes, particularly in adipose tissue and skeletal muscle. Insulin also stimulates glucose uptake in the liver, but by a different mechanism: it induces the enzyme glucokinase, which phosphorylates glucose to form glucose 6-phosphate, a substrate for glycogen synthesis. This process maintains a low intracellular glucose concentration, and thus a concentration gradient that facilitates glucose uptake.

Insulin stimulates glycogen synthesis (and inhibits glycogenolysis) through interaction with an exquisitely coordinated control mechanism that is central to the regulation of plasma glucose concentration. In summary, binding of insulin to its receptor leads to activation of phosphoprotein phosphatase, which dephosphorylates both glycogen synthase (thereby activating it and promoting glycogen synthesis) and

Table 13.1 **Hormones involved in glucose homoeostasis**

Hormone	Principal actions		Site of action
insulin	increases	cellular glucose uptake	M, A
		glycogen synthesis	L, M
		protein synthesis	*L, M*
		fatty acid and triglyceride synthesis	*L, A*
	decreases	gluconeogenesis	L
		glycogenolysis	L, M
		ketogenesis	*L*
		lipolysis	*A*
		proteolysis	*M*
glucagon	increases	glycogenolysis	L
		gluconeogenesis	L
		ketogenesis	*L*
		lipolysis	*A*
adrenaline (epinephrine)	increases	glycogenolysis	L, M
		lipolysis	*A*
growth hormone	increases	glycogenolysis	L
		lipolysis	*A*
cortisol	increases	gluconeogenesis	L
		glycogen synthesis	L
		proteolysis	*M*
	decreases	tissue glucose utilization	L, M, A

Letters indicate sites of action: A, adipose tissue; L, liver; M, skeletal muscle. Normal type indicates actions that directly affect glucose; other effects are shown in italics.

phosphorylase kinase (rendering it inactive, and thus preventing the activation of glycogen phosphorylase, the key enzyme of glycogenolysis). As a result of these actions, in the fasting state, when insulin secretion is inhibited, hepatic glycogenolysis is stimulated and glucose is liberated into the blood.

Insulin also exerts control over glycolysis and gluconeogenesis, stimulating the former and reciprocally inhibiting the latter, by stimulating the expression of phosphofructokinase, pyruvate kinase and the synthesis of its key allosteric activator, fructose 2,6-bisphosphate (Fig. 13.2). Insulin is also important in the control of fat metabolism: it stimulates lipogenesis and inhibits lipolysis. Another aspect of its anabolic function is stimulation of amino acid uptake and protein synthesis. It also stimulates the cellular influx of the predominantly intracellular ions potassium, magnesium and phosphate. Both insulin and incretins have a paracrine effect in the pancreas, reducing the secretion of glucagon by α-cells.

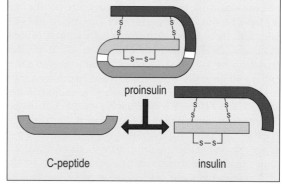

Fig. 13.1 Biosynthesis of insulin. The cleavage of proinsulin produces insulin, consisting of two polypeptide chains linked by disulphide bridges, and C-peptide.

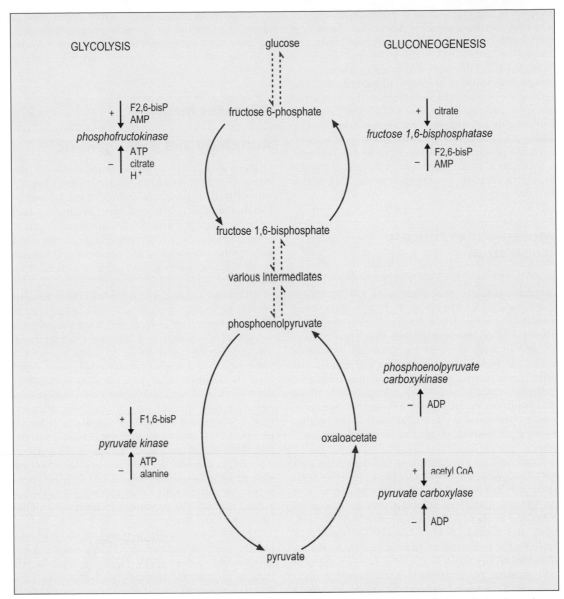

Fig. 13.2 Reciprocal control of glycolysis and gluconeogenesis in the liver. Insulin (released in the fed state) stimulates the expression of phosphofructokinase, pyruvate kinase and the synthesis of its key allosteric activator, fructose 2,6-bisphosphate (F2,6-bisP): glycolysis is promoted and gluconeogenesis is inhibited. Glucagon (released in the fasting state) inhibits expression of these enzymes and stimulates the synthesis of phosphoenolpyruvate carboxykinase and fructose 1,6-bisphosphatase: gluconeogenesis is stimulated and glycolysis is inhibited. The names of enzymes are given in italics. Plus signs (+) indicate substances that activate enzymes; minus signs (−) indicate substances that inhibit enzymes. ADP, adenosine diphosphate; AMP, adenosine monophosphate; ATP, adenosine triphosphate; CoA, coenzyme A.

Glucagon is a 29–amino acid polypeptide secreted by the α-cells of the pancreatic islets; its secretion is decreased by a rise in the plasma glucose concentration. In general, its actions oppose those of insulin: it stimulates hepatic (although not muscle) glycogenolysis through activation of glycogen phosphorylase, gluconeogenesis, lipolysis and ketogenesis. The control of ketogenesis is discussed on pp. 239–240. The combined effects of insulin and glucagon are shown diagrammatically in Fig. 13.3.

Disordered glucose homoeostasis can lead to hyperglycaemia (often to a degree diagnostic of diabetes) or hypoglycaemia. It is to these conditions that the bulk of this chapter is devoted.

Measurement of Glucose Concentration

Plasma glucose concentration tends to be 10–15% higher than that of whole blood because a given volume of red cells contains less water than the same volume of plasma. The difference is of little significance at normal concentrations, and in any case most measurement techniques that use whole blood are calibrated to give results that are equivalent to plasma glucose concentration. However, when glucose concentration is changing rapidly, there may be a considerable discrepancy between the results of whole blood and plasma glucose measurements because of delayed equilibration of glucose across the red cell membranes.

Red blood cells *in vitro* continue to utilize glucose, with the result that, unless a blood sample can be analyzed immediately, it is essential to collect it into a tube that contains sodium fluoride to inhibit glycolysis. Potassium oxalate is used as an anticoagulant in such 'fluoride–oxalate' tubes, and plasma obtained from this blood is thus unsuitable for the measurement of potassium and calcium concentrations (see p. 14).

Blood glucose concentrations are frequently measured on capillary blood samples obtained by 'finger prick' using glucose-sensitive reagent strips and a hand-held blood glucose meter. These instruments are generally robust and produce reliable results provided that users adhere to the simple instructions for their use. They are widely used both by healthcare professionals and by patients, and their use is essential in the management of many patients with diabetes, especially to permit appropriate adjustment in insulin dose or to confirm hypoglycaemia. Their use is discussed further on p. 236; however, they should not be relied on for the diagnosis of diabetes, for which formal laboratory measurement is necessary.

Continuous monitoring of extracellular fluid glucose concentration (which mirrors plasma glucose) using an implanted subcutaneous glucose sensor is also now possible and used by a small number of patients (see p. 236).

Diabetes Mellitus

Aetiology and pathogenesis

Diabetes mellitus (DM) is a **systemic metabolic disorder** characterized by a tendency towards **chronic hyperglycaemia with disturbances in carbohydrate, fat and protein metabolism** that arise from a defect in insulin secretion or action, or both. It is defined clinically from plasma glucose concentrations above which patients are at increased risk of retinopathy, nephropathy and neuropathy. It is a common condition, with a prevalence rate of ~8% in the developed world.

Diabetes can occur secondarily to other diseases (e.g. chronic pancreatitis), after pancreatic surgery and in conditions where there is increased secretion of hormones antagonistic to insulin (e.g. Cushing syndrome and acromegaly). Secondary diabetes is, however, uncommon. There are two main types of primary diabetes. In **type 1 DM**, there is destruction of pancreatic cells, leading to a decrease in, and eventually cessation of, insulin secretion. Approximately 10% of all patients with diabetes have type 1. They have an absolute requirement for insulin. In **type 2 DM**, insulin secretion is defective and delayed, and there is resistance to its actions. Most patients with type 2 DM can initially be successfully treated by diet, with or without antidiabetic drugs, but many eventually require treatment with insulin to achieve adequate glycaemic control. The prevalence of both types of diabetes (although particularly type 2) is increasing.

Type 1 DM usually presents acutely in younger people, with symptoms developing over a period of days or only a few weeks. However, there is evidence that the appearance of symptoms is preceded by a 'prediabetic' period of several months, during which growth failure (in children), a decline in insulin response to glucose and various immunological abnormalities can be detected. **Type 2 DM tends to present more insidiously in middle-aged and elderly adults** (although it is increasingly being diagnosed in obese young people), with symptoms developing over months or even longer. The prevalence rate of type 2 DM is >10% in individuals older than 75 years. Some of the characteristics of type 1 and type 2 DM are shown in Table 13.2.

Approximately 10% of young adult patients present initially with apparent type 2 DM (but often without obesity), but although initially treated successfully with diet or

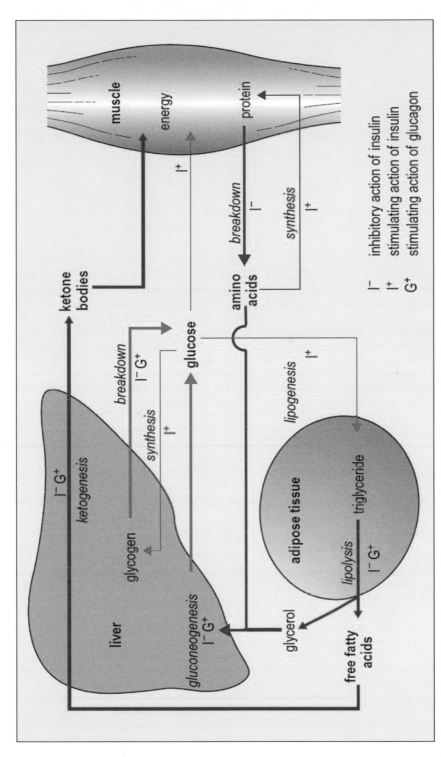

Fig. 13.3 Combined effects of insulin and glucagon on substrate flows between liver, adipose tissue and muscle. When the ratio of the concentrations of insulin to glucagon falls (e.g. during starvation), there is increased hepatic glucose and ketone production and decreased tissue glucose utilization. When the ratio is high (e.g. after a meal), glucose is stored as glycogen and converted into fat.

Table 13.2 **Major characteristics of type 1 and type 2 diabetes mellitus**

Feature	Type 1 diabetes	Type 2 diabetes
typical age of onset	children, young adults	middle-aged, elderly
onset	acute	gradual
habitus	lean	often obese
weight loss	usual	infrequent
ketosis prone	usually	usually not
plasma insulin concentration	low or absent	often normal; may be ↑
family history of diabetes	less common	common
HLA association	DR3, DR4; DQ2, DQ8	none
HLA, human leukocyte antigen.		

antidiabetic drugs, subsequently progress quite rapidly to an absolute requirement for insulin. This group is termed **latent autoimmune diabetes of adulthood**, as patients have the same plasma autoantibodies that are associated with type 1 DM.

A small group of patients develop **maturity onset diabetes of the young** (MODY) as a result of inheritance of a mutation in a single gene that plays a major role in glucose homoeostasis. As these are autosomal dominant disorders, they cluster within families. A diagnosis of MODY should be considered in patients who develop apparent type 2 DM at a relatively young age and have a very strong family history of diabetes. Six types of MODY have been described, each caused by a different mutation. The commonest mutation is in the glucokinase gene (MODY type 2). Glucokinase is the rate-limiting enzyme of glucose metabolism in pancreatic β-cells and, by acting as a 'glucose sensor', is key to the regulation of pancreatic insulin secretion.

Type 1 diabetes mellitus

Type 1 DM is an autoimmune disease. There is a familial incidence, although to a lesser extent than with type 2 DM, and there is a strong association with certain histocompatibility antigens, for example, HLA DR3 and DR4, DQ2 and DQ8. An individual's HLA antigens are genetically determined, but it is clear that type 1 DM is a genetically heterogeneous disorder (the concordance rate in monozygotic twins is only ~40%). Environmental factors are also important, and there is considerable circumstantial evidence that viral antigens (e.g. coxsackie B) may initiate the autoimmune process in some genetically susceptible individuals. Proteins in cow's milk have also been implicated. The incidence shows considerable geographic variation, being particularly high in the Scandinavian countries but low in much of South America. The reason for this variation is unknown.

The pancreatic islets of patients newly diagnosed with type 1 DM show characteristic histological features of autoimmune disease. Islet cell antibodies (ICAs) are frequently present in the plasma (and may be detectable long before the condition presents clinically), together with antibodies to insulin, glutamic acid decarboxylase (GAD) and other proteins, which, like ICAs, are sensitive indicators of risk of progression to diabetes in the apparently healthy members of patients' families (see p. 235).

It is thought that β-cell destruction, via apoptosis, is initiated by activated T-lymphocytes directed against antigens on the cell surface, possibly viral antigens or other antigens that normally are either not expressed or are immunologically tolerated. Clinically overt type 1 DM is a late stage of a process of gradual destruction of islet cells. There is much interest in the possibility of modifying this process, to prevent or retard the development of the disease in susceptible individuals, although clinical trials have thus far had only limited success.

Type 2 diabetes mellitus

Type 2 DM is a heterogeneous disorder. In most cases, insulin resistance is the primary defect. The β-cells compensate by increasing insulin secretion, which may initially maintain normal or near-normal plasma glucose concentrations. Over time, however, insulin secretion becomes inadequate and hyperglycaemia develops, as a consequence both of β-cell failure and worsening insulin resistance. It is thought that hyperglycaemia itself directly contributes to insulin resistance and β-cell dysfunction (glucotoxicity), as does the hyperlipidaemia that is frequently present in diabetes (lipotoxicity). Decreased secretion of incretins has been observed in patients with type 2 DM, but it is unclear whether this is a contributory cause.

Type 2 DM shows a **strong familial incidence**. The concordance rate in monozygotic (identical) twins is >90%, and the risk of an individual developing diabetes is >50% if both parents have the condition. Inheritance is polygenic; >70 genetic loci have been identified that commonly carry polymorphisms (variants) that are each individually associated with a small increase in the risk of diabetes. In contrast, patients with the rarer condition MODY possess a single genetic mutation that has a major effect on glucose homoeostasis.

Environmental factors are also important. Many patients with type 2 DM are obese, particularly tending to have visceral (intra-abdominal) obesity, which is known to cause insulin resistance, and have other features of the 'metabolic syndrome' (see p. 152). Reduced physical activity also causes insulin resistance, and various drugs, including corticosteroids and other immunosuppressants, protease inhibitors, thiazides in high doses, some 'atypical' antipsychotics and β-adrenergic antagonists, are diabetogenic.

The **interaction between genetic and environmental factors** in the pathogenesis of type 2 DM is exemplified by the high prevalence of the condition in certain ethnic groups (e.g. Pacific Islanders) following the adoption of a sedentary westernized lifestyle, with ready access to an assured food supply, in contrast with their aboriginal state. The suggestion is that their genotype evolved to maximize the storage of ingested energy as fat, to provide protection against famine, but that a continuous food supply leads to obesity and insulin intolerance (the 'thrifty genotype' hypothesis). There is also a 'thrifty phenotype' hypothesis, based on the observation that low birthweight is associated with an increased risk of later development of type 2 DM, the putative mechanism being β-cell dysfunction induced by fetal malnutrition.

Type 2 DM is a progressive condition. Although there is evidence that it can be prevented in susceptible individuals by diet and exercise, by the time it presents clinically, it will often have been present for several years. Aggressive treatment may slow its progression, but the tendency is for continuing loss of β-cell function and increasing insulin deficiency. It is of interest that bariatric surgery leads to remission of type 2 DM in up to 90% of patients, often within days of the procedure and before any weight loss has occurred. The mechanism of this phenomenon is unknown: a change in the secretion of incretins is one possibility.

Pathophysiology and clinical features

There are two aspects to the clinical manifestations of DM: those related directly to the metabolic disturbance and those related to the long-term complications of the condition.

The **hyperglycaemia** of diabetes is mainly a result of increased production of glucose by the liver and, to a lesser extent, of decreased removal of glucose from the blood. In the kidneys, filtered glucose is normally completely reabsorbed in the proximal tubules, but at plasma glucose concentrations greater than ~10 mmol/L (the renal threshold) reabsorption becomes saturated and glucose appears in the urine. There is some variation in the threshold between individuals. It is higher in the elderly and lower during pregnancy. Glycosuria results in an osmotic diuresis, increasing water excretion and raising the plasma osmolality, which in turn stimulates the thirst centre. Osmotic diuresis and thirst cause the classic symptoms of polyuria and polydipsia. Other causes of these symptoms include diabetes insipidus, hypercalcaemia, chronic hypokalaemia, and chronic kidney disease (CKD). Polyuria also follows excessive water intake for any reason.

Untreated, the metabolic disturbances may become profound, with the development of life-threatening ketoacidosis (see p. 237) or hyperosmolar hyperglycaemia (see p. 241).

The **long-term complications of diabetes** fall into two groups: **microvascular complications** (i.e. nephropathy, neuropathy and retinopathy) and **macrovascular disease** caused by atherosclerosis. These occur in both type 1 and type 2 DM. The prevalence of all these complications increases with the duration of the disease. The risk of microvascular complications is clearly greater if glycaemic control is poor, but other factors are undoubtedly involved: some patients never develop these complications, even after many years of having diabetes; others develop them rapidly, even with seemingly good control. The development of microvascular disease appears to be directly related to hyperglycaemia, whereas that of macrovascular disease is more closely related to insulin resistance. The results of long-term prospective studies indicate that improved glycaemic control significantly reduces the risk of microvascular complications in both type 1 and type 2 DM. For macrovascular disease, there is evidence of benefit over the long term in type 1 DM, but the evidence is contradictory and controversial in type 2 DM, even though the risk of macrovascular disease is greater in this type of diabetes.

The common pathological feature in microvascular disease is narrowing of the lumens of small blood vessels, and this appears to be directly related to prolonged exposure to high glucose concentrations. The processes involved are complex and still not fully understood; two appear to be particularly important. One is increased formation of sorbitol (an alcohol derived from glucose) by the action of the enzyme aldose reductase, leading to accumulation of sorbitol in cells. This can cause osmotic damage, alter the redox state and reduce cellular myoinositol concentrations. The other relates to the formation of advanced glycation end products. Glucose can react with amino groups in proteins to form glycated plasma and tissue proteins (glycated haemoglobin [HbA_{1c}; see p. 232] is one example). These can undergo cross-linking and accumulate in vessel walls and tissues, leading to structural and functional damage. Other mechanisms of tissue damage may include the generation of free radicals and activation of tissue injury responses secondary to intracellular hyperglycaemia.

The increased predisposition to atherosclerosis in patients with diabetes is also multifactorial. The abnormalities of lipids that occur as a direct result of diabetes (see p. 245) and glycation of lipoproteins leading to altered function are particularly important. Other factors that are implicated include endothelial dysfunction and increased oxidative stress.

The long-term complications of diabetes are a significant source of morbidity and mortality. Their diagnosis, with the exception of nephropathy, is largely clinical, although measurement of plasma lipids is important in assessment of the risk of macrovascular disease. In contrast, the management of the acute metabolic disturbances seen in diabetes requires intensive biochemical monitoring.

Diagnosis

The diagnosis of diabetes depends on the demonstration of hyperglycaemia, using values defined by the World Health Organization (WHO). In a patient with classic symptoms and signs of thirst and polyuria, **a random venous plasma glucose concentration ≥11.1 mmol/L is diagnostic of diabetes; so, too, is a fasting venous plasma glucose concentration ≥7.0 mmol/L**. Most patients presenting with type 1 DM, and some with type 2 DM clearly exceed these diagnostic limits and require no further tests to establish a diagnosis. In the absence of symptoms, these limits must be exceeded on more than one occasion for the diagnosis to be made. Even in symptomatic patients, diabetes is unlikely if a random venous plasma glucose concentration

is ≤5.5 mmol/L. The interpretation of plasma glucose concentrations in the diagnosis of diabetes and glucose intolerance is outlined in Table 13.3.

Individuals who have fasting plasma glucose concentrations that are elevated but not in the diabetic range have **impaired fasting glycaemia** (IFG). The lower threshold for IFG defined by the WHO and used in the UK and much of the rest of the world is 6.1 mmol/L, although the American Diabetes Association (ADA) recommends a value of 5.6 mmol/L. The WHO recommends that patients found to have IFG should undergo an **oral glucose tolerance test** (OGTT, see later) to determine whether they have impaired glucose tolerance (IGT) or diabetes. However, many clinicians treat IFG simply as a state of intermediate glucose intolerance, and the ADA does not endorse the use of the OGTT in this group.

Chronic hyperglycaemia can also be diagnosed using measurements of **glycated haemoglobin (HbA$_{1c}$)**, which is a marker of average plasma glucose concentration over many weeks. Haemoglobin undergoes glycation *in vivo* at a rate proportional to the plasma glucose concentration; the reaction proceeds through a reversible stage but, once the major stable product (HbA$_{1c}$) is formed, it persists in that state for the lifetime of the red cell. HbA$_{1c}$ therefore provides a 'time-weighted' average of plasma glucose concentrations over the previous 2–3 months. More recent glucose concentrations contribute to a greater extent to this average than more historical ones (50% of the HbA$_{1c}$ concentration is accounted for by the average plasma glucose concentration during the last 30 days). HbA$_{1c}$ concentration is expressed as a proportion of total haemoglobin. In the UK and many other countries worldwide, it is reported as mmol/mol haemoglobin, although in some countries it is reported as percentage (%).

Table 13.3 **Diagnostic plasma glucose concentrations (mmol/L)**		
Diagnosis	**Sample**	**Venous plasma**
normal	fasting	<6.1
impaired fasting glycaemia	fasting and (*if measured*)[a] 2 h post-glucose	6.1–6.9 <7.8
impaired glucose tolerance	fasting and 2 h post-glucose	<7.0 7.8–11.0
diabetes mellitus	fasting or 2 h post-glucose	≥7.0 ≥11.1

[a]If an oral glucose tolerance test (OGTT) is performed in a patient with impaired fasting glycaemia (IFG) and the 2 h post-glucose load plasma glucose concentration is 7.8–11.0 mmol/L, a diagnosis of impaired glucose tolerance replaces that of IFG. If a patient is asymptomatic, two results in the diabetic range are required to establish a diagnosis of diabetes mellitus. Note that different diagnostic values are used in pregnancy (see Table 13.4) and the terms 'impaired fasting glycaemia' and 'impaired glucose tolerance' are not used.

Since HbA$_{1c}$ is a marker of long-term glycaemic status, it is a convenient and valid diagnostic test for type 2 DM, which is characterized by slowly developing chronic hyperglycaemia. However, it is not a valid diagnostic test for type 1 DM, in which hyperglycaemia develops rapidly and is therefore unlikely to have been constant over the preceding 2–3 months. HbA$_{1c}$ is also widely used in the monitoring of patients with all types of diabetes (see p. 236).

Since HbA$_{1c}$ reflects average plasma glucose during the life span of the red cells, caution with interpretation is required in patients with decreased red cell life spans, for example because of haemolytic anaemia, or increased life spans, for example in iron deficiency. Abnormal haemoglobins, for example HbS, prevent or interfere with the measurement of HbA$_{1c}$ or cause false results in certain analytical methods. If the abnormal haemoglobin also results in haemolysis, the HbA$_{1c}$ result will in any case underestimate the average plasma glucose concentration because of reduced red cell life spans.

An HbA$_{1c}$ concentration ≥48 mmol/mol is diagnostic of diabetes, provided that the conditions for use described above and in Fig. 13.4 are met. If symptoms of hyperglycaemia are not present and the HbA$_{1c}$ is ≥48 mmol/mol, the test should be repeated to confirm the initial result: although HbA$_{1c}$ concentration varies very little from day to day, a second confirmatory test is important to avoid the risk of making an incorrect lifelong diagnosis as a result, for example, of sample mislabelling or analytical error.

HbA$_{1c}$ concentrations in the range 42–47 mmol/mol signify an intermediate state of hyperglycaemia sometimes called impaired glycaemia or prediabetes. Such patients are at increased risk of developing diabetes in the future, so the test should be repeated in 1 year.

The OGTT assesses the capacity for postprandial metabolism of glucose under controlled conditions. The protocol for the OGTT is given below. In the majority of patients suspected of having diabetes, however, the simple diagnostic thresholds using either plasma glucose or HbA$_{1c}$ measurements as indicated earlier will establish the diagnosis, and formal glucose tolerance testing is unnecessary. The use of the OGTT is now largely limited to the investigation of possible gestational diabetes, but it is also sometimes used in the further investigation of patients who have a fasting plasma glucose concentration in the IFG range (6.1–6.9 mmol/L).

A 2-h OGTT plasma glucose concentration that is below the diagnostic limit for diabetes but greater than normal is diagnostic of **IGT**. This is an intermediate state of hyperglycaemia where plasma glucose concentrations are higher than normal but not so high as to be associated with increased risk of diabetic microvascular disease. IGT is not a

---

The oral glucose tolerance test

The protocol for the OGTT has been very precisely defined by the WHO. Meticulous attention to detail is required to obtain an accurate result.

Patient preparation

The test should not be performed if the patient is febrile or acutely ill, or within 6 weeks of a severe metabolic stress, for example, myocardial infarction or major surgery. At least 3 days of normal diet (carbohydrate intake >150 g/24h) should be allowed before testing. The patient must fast overnight for 8–14 h before the test but may drink water during this time.

The glucose load

The required dose is 75 g anhydrous glucose (children 1.75 g/kg body weight up to a maximum of 75 g) in 250–300 mL water. Partial hydrolysates of starch (e.g. Polycal, or Rapilose) with equivalent carbohydrate content (which are rapidly metabolized to glucose in the intestine) may be used as an alternative; they present a lower osmolar load and thus are less likely to cause nausea. Proprietary glucose drinks are rarely suitable, as most require a volume of >300 mL to deliver the required glucose load.

Procedure

Take blood for the measurement of fasting plasma glucose concentration into a blood tube containing sodium fluoride preservative (to prevent glycolysis).
Administer the glucose load over the course of 5 min.
The patient should rest for the duration of the test and must not smoke.
Take a second blood sample for measurement of glucose after 120 min.

Test interpretation

See Table 13.3

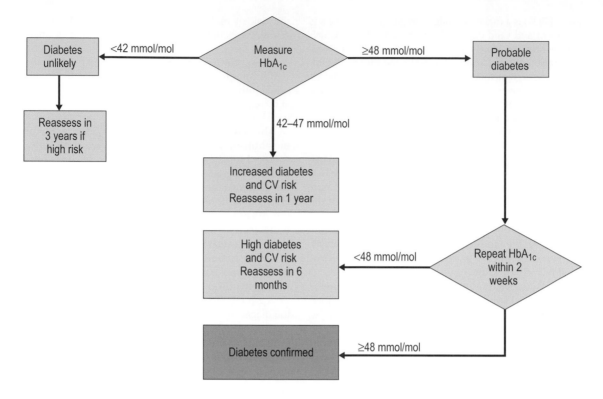

Fig. 13.4 The use of glycated haemoglobin (HbA$_{1c}$) in the diagnosis of diabetes. CV, cardiovascular disease.

HbA$_{1c}$ may be used to diagnose diabetes mellitus in patients with long-standing hyperglycaemia

HbA$_{1c}$ must not be used for diagnosis if hyperglycaemia has developed rapidly, e.g.
- possible type 1 diabetes
- symptomatic children and young adults
- symptoms less than three months
- acutely ill patients
- drugs that may cause rapid rise in glucose e.g. corticosteroids, antipsychotics
- acute pancreatic damage or pancreatic surgery.

HbA$_{1c}$ must not be used for diagnosis in the presence of factors affecting HbA$_{1c}$ formation or measurement. These include:
- iron and vitamin B$_{12}$ deficiency
- haemolytic anaemias
- chronic liver disease
- chronic kidney disease (CKD 4 and 5)
- splenomegaly or splenectomy
- haemoglobinopathies.

HbA$_{1c}$ must not be used to diagnose diabetes in pregnancy

clinical entity in itself. In some patients it is a transitory stage between normal glucose tolerance and diabetes; in others it is a stable state (often associated with obesity). Both IFG and IGT reflect abnormal glucose metabolism and are associated with increased risk of cardiovascular disease and of future development of type 2 DM. Patients should be given dietary and lifestyle advice and followed up regularly.

Notably, measurements of plasma glucose are no exception to the potential for analytical and biological variation to affect results (see Chapter 2). Although precise figures

Table 13.4 The 75g oral glucose tolerance test diagnostic plasma glucose concentrations for gestational diabetes		
	NICE	**IADPSG/WHO**
Fasting	≥5.6 mmol/L	≥5.1 mmol/L *or*
1 h	*or*	≥10.0 mmol/L *or*
2 h	≥7.8 mmol/L	≥8.5 mmol/L

NICE, National Institute for Health and Care Excellence; IADPSG, International Association of Diabetes in Pregnancy Study Groups; WHO, World Health Organization.

are used as cutoffs for diagnosis, the existence of such variation can result in patients being misclassified if their results are close to cutoff values: this is why a confirmatory measurement is required before diabetes is diagnosed in the absence of clinical features. The results of glucose tolerance tests are additionally affected by factors such as the rate of gastric emptying and accurate adherence to the test protocol.

The OGTT is an essential test for the diagnosis of **gestational diabetes** (diabetes with onset during pregnancy, see p. 245). Women who are obese, have close relatives with diabetes, belong to an ethnic group with a high prevalence of diabetes, or who have had a large baby or gestational diabetes in a previous pregnancy are at increased risk. In the UK, a 75 g OGTT is offered to all women at high risk at 24–28 weeks of gestation (earlier if gestational diabetes was diagnosed in a previous pregnancy). Different authorities stipulate different diagnostic criteria; those recommended by the International Association of the Diabetes and Pregnancy Study Groups and by the UK National Institute for Health and Care Excellence are stated in Table 13.4. Women with gestational diabetes may revert to a normal glucose tolerance postpartum. However, they are at increased risk of developing gestational diabetes again in future pregnancies and also of developing type 2 DM.

The type of diabetes is usually apparent from the history and clinical presentation. It is only occasionally necessary to perform specific diagnostic tests. The growth in childhood obesity, however, has resulted in increasing prevalence of type 2 DM in children, a group which almost exclusively developed type 1 DM in previous decades; and some 2% of paediatric diabetes patients have MODY (see p. 230). Establishing the presence of early onset type 2 DM or MODY has implications for treatment and prognosis. The ongoing presence of **C-peptide** in the plasma or urine >3 years after the development of diabetes effectively rules out type 1 DM. Pancreatic **islet cell autoantibodies** (to islet antigen-2 [IA-2], GAD or zinc transporter-8 [ZnT-8]) are present in ~90% of patients with type 1 DM.

Management

The successful management of diabetes requires effective teamwork. Care is frequently shared between a range of healthcare professionals, in both community and hospital settings. The patient plays an active and central role, and effective patient education is of vital importance. Regular follow-up is essential to monitor treatment and to detect early signs of complications, particularly retinopathy, which can in many cases be treated successfully, and nephropathy, as treatment may slow its progression.

The aims of treatment are two fold: to alleviate symptoms and prevent the acute metabolic complications of diabetes, and to prevent long-term complications. In patients with type 2 DM, the first of these objectives is usually attainable with appropriate dietary modification (essentially, substitution of complex for simple carbohydrates, an increase in dietary fibre and restriction of energy intake when necessary) with or without antidiabetic drugs (although insulin is often required later in the course of the condition). Patients with type 1 DM need to adhere to a similar diet but require treatment with insulin from the time of diagnosis.

Since intensive glycaemic control reduces the risk of microvascular complications in diabetes, the goal of treatment should be to maintain plasma glucose concentrations close to the physiological range. In practice, this may be difficult to achieve, as intensification of treatment increases the risk of episodes of hypoglycaemia, particularly in patients treated with insulin or sulfonylurea drugs. Particularly in frail or elderly patients, it may be safer to avoid the risk of hypoglycaemia and maintain a level of glycaemic control that prevents the development of symptomatic acute hyperglycaemia but is less than optimal in terms of reducing the risk of complications long term. Treatment targets should be set and agreed on individually with patients (see p. 236).

It is beyond the scope of this book to discuss treatment strategies in detail. In type 1 DM, the preferred method of treatment is with a 'basal–bolus' regimen of insulin injections, whereby a long-acting insulin is given at night (to mimic the basal insulin secretion that occurs even during fasting) with boluses of short-acting insulin at mealtimes. Such regimens can provide plasma insulin concentrations that closely mimic those seen in individuals without diabetes. They also allow greater flexibility with regard to meals (timing and content) than the traditional twice-daily injections of short- and long-acting insulins. Continuous subcutaneous insulin infusion (insulin pump therapy) is of value in some patients who cannot attain a satisfactory level of glycaemic control with other insulin regimens or if attempts to do so result in severe hypoglycaemia; it is, however, demanding for the patient. 'Closed loop' systems that link a subcutaneous glucose sensor to the insulin pump and thereby adjust or suspend the insulin infusion are now becoming available, but such 'artificial pancreas' systems still require frequent patient attention and intervention.

In patients with type 2 DM, improved control over that achieved with antidiabetic drugs alone can often be achieved by giving a single injection of a long-acting insulin at night, continuing with antidiabetic drugs during the day. However, more intensive insulin regimens, including twice-daily injection of a mixture of short- and long-acting insulins or even the basal–bolus regimen preferred in type 1 DM, may be required for some patients.

Drugs used in the treatment of type 2 DM include: metformin (a biguanide), which suppresses hepatic gluconeogenesis and increases peripheral insulin sensitivity; sulfonylureas, which enhance insulin secretion; pioglitazone (a thiazolidinedione), which activates the peroxisome proliferator-activated receptor γ, thereby enhancing the actions of insulin; and meglitinides, which are rapidly (and short) acting insulin secretagogues. More recently, drugs based on the action of incretins have been developed. These are of two types: incretin enhancers and incretin mimetics. The first group (the gliptins) acts by inhibiting dipeptidyl peptidase 4 (DPP-4), an enzyme responsible for the rapid degradation of GLP-1. The second group (e.g. exenatide and liraglutide) mimics the action of GLP-1 and is resistant to degradation by DPP-4. The newest major class of antidiabetic drugs are the renal tubular sodium–glucose transport protein 2 (SGLT2) inhibitors (e.g. dapagliflozin): by inhibiting renal tubular glucose reabsorption, these lower the renal threshold for glucose and therefore reduce its concentration in the blood.

In both type 1 and type 2 DM, the risk of microvascular complications is reduced by achieving strict glycaemic control, but treatment targets must be appropriate for individual patients and may be more relaxed in patients with multiple comorbidities and relatively short life expectancy, or in frail elderly adults who are at increased risk of harm, such as falls, during episodes of hypoglycaemia.

Macrovascular disease is a major cause of morbidity and mortality, particularly in type 2 DM (but also in type 1 DM). Rigorous management of cardiovascular risk factors including dyslipidaemia and hypertension is of critical importance in reducing the risk of cardiovascular, cerebrovascular and peripheral vascular disease.

Monitoring treatment

The efficacy of treatment in diabetes is monitored clinically, by ensuring that the patient's symptoms are controlled, by measurement of plasma glucose concentration and other objective indicators of glycaemic control (usually HbA$_{1c}$), and monitoring of other biochemical risk factors, principally, plasma lipids and urine albumin.

Capillary blood glucose monitoring using reagent strips and a glucose meter is essential in patients with type 1 DM. This may be done more or less frequently as circumstances require: exercise, illness or a change of diet may alter insulin requirements, and more frequent testing will allow the patient to adjust the dosage accordingly. In type 1 DM, currently recommended targets for treatment in adults in the UK are blood glucose concentrations of 5.0–7.0 mmol/L on waking and 4.0–7.0 mmol/L before meals. Testing after meals is not usually necessary, but if performed, patients should aim to achieve blood glucose concentrations of 5.0–9.0 mmol/L. Self-monitoring of capillary blood glucose is not routinely necessary in patients with type 2 DM unless they are on treatment with insulin or antidiabetic drugs that increase the risk of hypoglycaemia, or if pregnant or planning to become so. **Continuous glucose monitoring** using a portable subcutaneous glucose sensor is now possible, although these are currently expensive and require intensive patient input. This technique is of value in patients with type 1 DM who suffer from hypoglycaemia frequently or without warning, or if hyperglycaemia persists in spite of treatment adjustment based on frequent capillary blood glucose testing.

Urine testing for glucose is no longer recommended in the UK for the monitoring of diabetes. Such testing is only semiquantitative; it is of no value in the detection of hypoglycaemia, and it does not permit achievement of the tight glycaemic control required to minimize long-term complications because glucose is not present in the urine until its concentration in the blood is considerably higher than target values. Urine glucose excretion also depends on the renal threshold for glucose: if this is low (e.g. in pregnancy or renal tubular disorders, p. 245), glucose may be present in the urine at normal plasma glucose concentrations.

The measurement of **HbA$_{1c}$** provides an important means of monitoring glycaemic control over a longer time span (see p. 232). For most patients, especially those on insulin, it is inappropriate to aim for an HbA$_{1c}$ target within the non-diabetic range because this would usually entail an unacceptably high rate of hypoglycaemic episodes. An exception to this is before conception and during pregnancy when normoglycaemia is important to minimize the risk of fetal malformation and health risks to the mother. Treatment targets should be set on an individual basis; current recommendations in the UK are normally to aim to achieve and maintain the HbA$_{1c}$ concentration at ≤48 mmol/mol (≤6.5%) in type 1 diabetes if this can be attained without unacceptably frequent episodes of hypoglycaemia. The general target in type 2 DM is ≤53 mmol/mol (≤7.0%), but the introduction of antidiabetic drug treatment should be considered if HbA$_{1c}$ rises to ≥48 mmol/mol (≥6.5%) on dietary management alone.

Sometimes there is an apparent discrepancy between a patient's capillary blood glucose results and the HbA_{1c} concentration. This is often because the patient is not self-testing at an appropriate range of times (e.g. if readings are only taken before breakfast this will not reveal significant postprandial hyperglycaemia later in the day). Occasionally patients misreport their readings, usually because of fear of having to take more insulin. However, it is always important to consider the possibility of misleading HbA_{1c} results because of abnormal red cell life span or presence of a haemoglobin variant, and to investigate this with appropriate haematological tests. If such a problem is identified, it is possible to monitor glycaemic control by measuring **fructosamine**, which is a collective term for glycated plasma proteins (predominantly glycated albumin). Plasma fructosamine concentration reflects glycaemic control over a much shorter time span than HbA_{1c}, and thus is of less clinical value. Concentrations are misleadingly low when there is increased albumin turnover, for example in patients with albuminuria, and there are no definitive treatment targets. In many patients, clearly documented capillary blood glucose results taken at an appropriate range of times throughout the day are the best option if HbA_{1c} cannot be measured or interpreted.

Other tests of value in monitoring patients with diabetes include screening for microalbuminuria (for incipient diabetic nephropathy) and measurement of plasma creatinine (with estimated glomerular filtration rate [eGFR], to monitor kidney function) and lipids (because of the risk of atherosclerosis). Urine or blood testing for ketones is required in patients with type 1 DM whose diabetes has become poorly controlled because they are at risk of keto acidosis. All of these tests are discussed elsewhere in this chapter.

Notably, both autoimmune thyroid disease (see p. 233) and coeliac disease (see p. 134) have increased prevalence in patients with type 1 DM; guidelines in the UK state that patients with type 1 diabetes should be screened annually for thyroid disease and that children are screened every 3 years for coeliac disease.

Metabolic Complications of Diabetes

Ketoacidosis

Ketoacidosis (diabetic ketoacidosis [DKA]) may be the presenting feature of type 1 DM, or may develop in a patient who omits to take his or her insulin or whose insulin dosage becomes inadequate because of an increased requirement, for example as a result of infection, trauma or any acute illness such as myocardial infarction. Newly diagnosed patients account for 20–25% of cases. It is a rare, although not unknown, occurrence in patients with type 2 DM.

Case history 13.1

History

A 17-year-old man with type 1 DM attended for a routine diabetes review appointment. He reported that he had been in good health during the last 6 months, although he was tired this morning because he had been to a party the night before. He had been taught how to perform capillary blood glucose monitoring but did not do this, because he did not like pricking his finger to obtain blood.

Examination

During the consultation he began to feel slightly sweaty and nauseous so the nurse took a capillary blood glucose measurement as well as sending a venous blood sample to the laboratory for routine HbA_{1c} testing.

Results (see Appendix for reference ranges)

Capillary blood: glucose 18 mmol/L
Venous blood HbA_{1c} 46 mmol/mol (6.4%)

Summary

High capillary blood glucose, but HbA_{1c} result within target for good control.

Interpretation

The capillary blood glucose result rules out hypoglycaemia as a cause for his symptoms. Although his blood glucose concentration is currently too high, the HbA_{1c} result indicates that his long-term control is good.

Discussion

It transpired that he had eaten considerably more than usual the previous evening and had not taken his insulin on the morning of clinic because he had not yet eaten breakfast. Blood glucose is rarely measured at clinic attendances unless patients are suspected of being hypoglycaemic, because random 'one off' results are of little value. Home blood glucose monitoring, especially if samples are taken at a relevant range of times throughout the day (e.g. before meals and before bed) is of much greater use; knowledge of the blood glucose profile is essential if the patient's insulin regimen is to be adjusted effectively.

Pathogenesis

The sequence of events that leads to hyperglycaemia and the consequences of this are illustrated in Figs. 13.3 and 13.5. Insulin deficiency, often combined with increased secretion of glucagon (and other counterregulatory hormones), causes an increase in the glucagon/insulin ratio in the portal blood, which inhibits glycolysis and stimulates gluconeogenesis (see Table 13.1). At the same time, glycogen breakdown is promoted

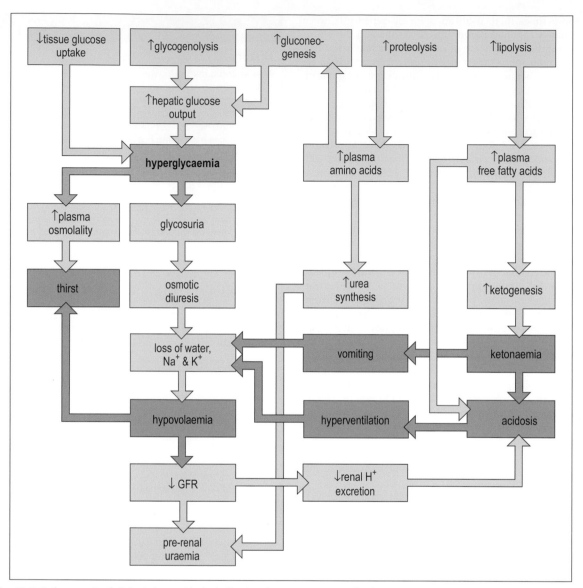

Fig. 13.5 Pathogenesis of diabetic ketoacidosis, indicating the consequences of a decreased insulin/glucagon ratio. Hyperkalaemia is invariably present, in spite of total body potassium depletion, as a result of loss of potassium from the tissues to the extracellular fluid, and, as the glomerular filtration falls, of decreased renal excretion. GFR, glomerular filtration rate.

and glycogen synthesis is inhibited. Decreased peripheral utilization of glucose, resulting from lack of insulin and preferential metabolism of free fatty acids and ketones as energy substrates, contributes to the hyperglycaemia but is less important than the increased rate of glucose production. Increased secretion of catecholamines also contributes to the hyperglycaemia.

Glycosuria causes an osmotic diuresis and hence fluid depletion, which is exacerbated by the hyperventilation and vomiting. The decrease in plasma volume leads to renal hypoperfusion and pre-renal uraemia (acute kidney injury). As the glomerular filtration rate falls, so does the rate of urine production, and the patient, initially polyuric, becomes oliguric. The loss of glucose in the urine affords some protection against the development of severe hyperglycaemia, but this is lost once oliguria develops. Acute kidney injury is a recognized complication of DKA.

Hyperkalaemia is commonly present and is a result of the combined effects of decreased renal excretion and a shift of

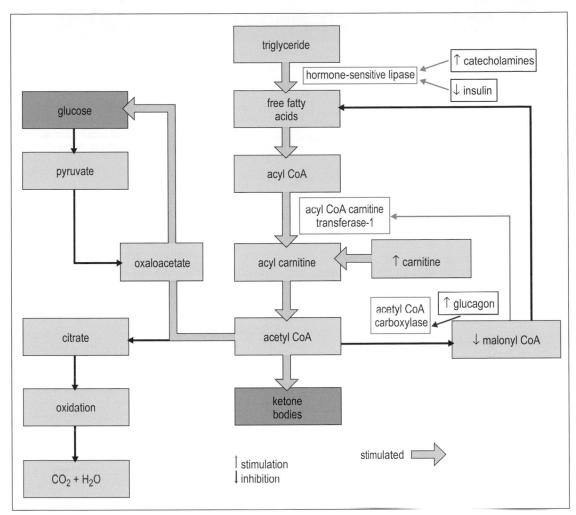

Fig. 13.6 Mechanism of increased ketogenesis in diabetic ketoacidosis. Increased concentrations of catecholamines and decreased concentrations of insulin stimulate hormone-sensitive lipase, promoting lipolysis. Glucagon inhibits the synthesis of malonyl coenzyme A (CoA), an intermediate in fatty acid synthesis (which thus decreases); malonyl CoA is an inhibitor of acyl CoA carnitine transferase, the activity of which thus increases. Increased enzyme activity and substrate supply increase the formation of acyl carnitine, which is required for transport of fatty acids into mitochondria, where ketogenesis takes place. Supplies of oxaloacetate necessary for the oxidation of acetyl CoA in the citric acid cycle are diverted instead to gluconeogenesis.

intracellular potassium into the extracellular fluid (caused by lack of insulin, because insulin promotes cellular potassium uptake, and by acidosis and tissue catabolism). However, in spite of the hyperkalaemia, there is always considerable total body potassium depletion. The plasma sodium concentration is usually decreased because of sodium depletion and the osmotically driven shift of water from the intracellular to the extracellular compartment.

Lack of insulin causes increased lipolysis, with increased release of free fatty acids into the blood from adipose tissue, and decreased lipogenesis. In the liver,

fatty acids normally undergo complete oxidation, and are re-esterified to triglycerides or are converted to acetoacetic and 3-hydroxybutyric acids (ketogenesis). Ketogenesis is promoted in uncontrolled diabetes by the high ratio of glucagon to insulin. The mechanisms involved are shown in Fig. 13.6: increased production of acetyl coenzyme A (CoA) and decreased availability of oxaloacetate necessary for its oxidation are the key abnormalities. Some acetoacetate is spontaneously decarboxylated to acetone. Ketones stimulate the chemoreceptor trigger zone, causing vomiting. Acetoacetic and 3-hydroxybutyric acids are

Case history 13.2

History

An 18-year-old woman consulted her family doctor because of tiredness and weight loss that had come on rapidly during the last 3 weeks. On questioning, she reported feeling thirsty and had noticed that she had been passing more urine than normal. The doctor tested her urine and found glycosuria. He arranged an appointment for her with the hospital diabetes specialist nurse the next day. By then, however, she felt too ill to get out of bed, had started vomiting and had become drowsy. Her mother telephoned the doctor, who arranged for immediate admission to hospital.

Examination

Her blood pressure was 96/60 mmHg with a pulse rate of 112/min and she had cold extremities. She had deep, sighing respiration (Kussmaul respiration) and her breath smelt of acetone.

Results

Serum:	sodium	130 mmol/L
	potassium	5.8 mmol/L
	bicarbonate	5 mmol/L
	urea	18 mmol/L
	creatinine	140 µmol/L
	eGFR	47 mL/min/1.73 m^2
Plasma:	glucose	32 mmol/L
Arterial blood:	hydrogen ion	89 nmol/L (pH 7.05)
	P_{CO_2}	2.0 kPa

Summary

High hydrogen ion concentration with low serum bicarbonate and arterial blood P_{CO_2}. Severe hyperglycaemia.

Raised urea and creatinine, moderate hyperkalaemia and hyponatraemia.

Interpretation

The high plasma glucose concentration, together with the rapid onset of her symptoms, confirm a new diagnosis of type 1 DM. The low bicarbonate and high hydrogen ion concentrations with hyperventilation, and thus a decreased partial pressure of carbon dioxide (P_{CO_2}), indicate a metabolic acidosis with partial respiratory compensation. There is evidence of acute kidney injury (raised urea and creatinine), although eGFR is not a valid estimate of glomerular filtration rate when there has been a rapid loss of kidney function. The disproportionate increase in urea in comparison with creatinine is typical of dehydration compounded by increased urea production caused by increased catabolism of amino acids (see p. 238). The patient has hypotension, tachycardia and cold extremities, suggesting marked extracellular fluid depletion (sodium depletion). The clinical and biochemical features are typical of DKA (Box 13.1).

Discussion

Although this patient is markedly hyperglycaemic, clinically severe DKA can sometimes occur with only a moderate increase in the plasma glucose concentration (10–15 mmol/L). The presence of ketosis should be confirmed by measuring blood 3-hydroxybutyrate concentration with a point-of-care testing meter. The detection of ketonuria using a urine dipstick test is less reliable (see below).

---

the major acids responsible for the acidosis, but free fatty acids and lactic acid also contribute. Notably, in severely ill patients, a shift in redox state promotes conversion of acetoacetate to 3-hydroxybutyrate: this is not detected by conventional urine tests for ketones, so monitoring of ketone concentration during treatment of ketoacidosis is preferably performed by specific measurement of blood 3-hydroxybutyrate concentration, usually using a reagent stick and meter at the bedside.

Management

DKA is a medical emergency. Treatment must be started immediately after the diagnosis has been made, and

patients should be managed in a high-dependency unit. In most cases, with typical clinical features, the diagnosis can be based on a point-of-care glucose measurement, although this must be confirmed by formal laboratory measurement; hydrogen ion concentration (pH) should be measured on a blood gas analyzer to confirm the presence of metabolic acidosis and assess its severity. The **aims of treatment** are to restore kidney function and maintain tissue perfusion by replacement of lost fluid and minerals, and to reverse the metabolic disturbance by providing insulin. Any identifiable precipitating event, such as infection, must also be treated.

Isotonic saline is given intravenously to replace lost fluid. The rate at which it is given will depend on the

Box 13.1 **Clinical and metabolic features of diabetic ketoacidosis**

Clinical

thirst
polyuria (but oliguria late)
dehydration
hypotension, tachycardia and peripheral circulatory failure
ketosis
hyperventilation
vomiting
abdominal pain
drowsiness, coma

Metabolic

hyperglycaemia
glycosuria
metabolic acidosis
ketonaemia and ketonuria
uraemia
hyperkalaemia
hypertriglyceridaemia
haemoconcentration

precise circumstances, but it should usually be given rapidly, at least initially, to restore the extracellular fluid volume to normal. Careful charting of fluid input and output is essential, and physiological monitoring of effective arterial blood volume may be necessary to guide replacement and avoid fluid overload. Catheterization of the bladder may be necessary to assess urine output if the patient is incontinent or anuric. DKA can cause gastric stasis with subsequent risk of aspiration pneumonia, so gastric contents should be aspirated through a nasogastric tube if the patient has a reduced level of consciousness or persistent vomiting.

Potassium supplements are required: insulin causes rapid potassium uptake into cells, with the result that, although patients are usually hyperkalaemic at presentation, hypokalaemia will develop during treatment if potassium is not replaced. Regular monitoring of the plasma potassium concentration is essential, and sufficient potassium should be infused to maintain a plasma potassium concentration of 4.0–5.0 mmol/L.

Treatment with insulin (short acting) is essential; this should be given by constant intravenous infusion, at a rate of 0.1 unit/h per kilogram body weight (typically 6–10 unit/h). The plasma glucose concentration must be monitored frequently: it should ideally fall by 3–5 mmol/L per hour. Over-rapid correction may lead to hypoglycaemia and rebound ketosis driven by counterregulatory hormones. Blood 3-hydroxybutyrate concentration should

fall by ~0.5 mmol/L per hour and venous plasma bicarbonate concentration rise by ~3 mmol/L per hour. When plasma glucose has fallen to 14 mmol/L, the intravenous fluid should be supplemented by 10% dextrose (no more than 2 L in each 24 h) and the insulin infusion continued to maintain euglycaemia and suppress ketogenesis until the metabolic abnormalities have completely resolved. The insulin and dextrose infusions should be continued until it is possible to establish oral food and fluid intake, whereupon a conventional regimen of insulin injections can be introduced. If the patient's insulin regimen includes long-acting insulin, this should not be stopped but should be administered at the usual times and doses throughout.

It is seldom necessary to give **bicarbonate**, except in the severest cases, because restoration of normal renal perfusion allows excretion of the hydrogen ion load and regeneration of bicarbonate, and restoration of normal metabolism reduces the production rate. Intravenous bicarbonate is no longer routinely recommended, because inappropriately rapid correction of an acidosis may impair oxygen delivery to the tissues through an effect on the affinity of haemoglobin for oxygen, increase the rate of hepatic ketogenesis and, paradoxically, increase the cerebrospinal fluid (CSF) hydrogen ion concentration because of delayed equilibration of the bicarbonate between the plasma and the CSF.

The **response to treatment** of a typical patient with DKA is shown in Fig. 13.7. Most patients respond well to the measures described, but fatalities still occur, more frequently in older patients in whom other (e.g. cardiovascular) disease is often present. Cerebral oedema is an occasional complication in young people and is frequently fatal. The deficits present in a patient with ketoacidosis are considerable and may exceed 5 L water and 500 mmol each of sodium and potassium. Considerable depletion of other ions, in particular phosphate, may occur. Plasma phosphate concentration should be measured if skeletal or respiratory muscle weakness develops, and replacement considered if it is low. Other biochemical abnormalities that may be seen include an increase in plasma amylase activity (because of reduced renal excretion), hypertriglyceridaemia and, in severely shocked patients, an increase in aminotransferases (probably related to hypoxic tissue damage).

Hyperosmolar hyperglycaemic state

Not all patients with uncontrolled diabetes develop ketoacidosis. In type 2 DM, severe hyperglycaemia can develop (plasma glucose concentration >50 mmol/L), with extreme dehydration and a very high plasma osmolality, but with no ketosis and minimal acidosis. This complication used to be referred to as 'hyperosmolar non-ketotic hyperglycaemia', but this was misleading

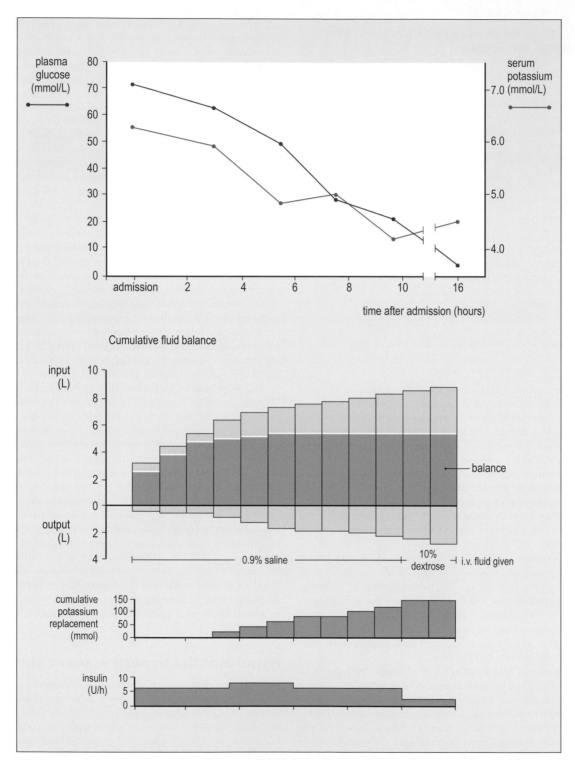

Fig. 13.7 Response to treatment in a patient with severe diabetic ketoacidosis, indicating a fluid deficit of nearly 6 L on admission.

Case history 13.3

History

A 65-year-old widow, who lived alone, was admitted to hospital after her son found her semiconscious at home. She had seemed well when he visited her 1 week previously, although in retrospect he recalled that she had been complaining of thirst and had drunk several glasses of fruit squash that afternoon. She had no significant past medical history.

Examination

She was extremely dehydrated but not ketotic. Her breathing was normal.

Results

Serum:	sodium	149 mmol/L
	potassium	4.7 mmol/L
	bicarbonate	18 mmol/L
	urea	35 mmol/L
	creatinine	180 µmol/L
	eGFR	25 mL/min/1.73 m^2
	total protein	90 g/L
	osmolality	370 mmol/kg
Plasma:	glucose	54 mmol/L

Summary

Very high serum osmolality, and glucose. High urea with relatively lesser increase in creatinine and hypernatraemia. Slightly low bicarbonate.

Interpretation

The very high serum osmolality reflects the severe hyperglycaemia. This has caused an osmotic diuresis, resulting in a decrease in glomerular filtration rate (pre-renal acute kidney injury) with retention of urea and creatinine, and an increase in serum protein concentration caused by the loss of water from the plasma. The serum bicarbonate concentration is a little below normal because of decreased renal hydrogen ion excretion. The raised serum sodium concentration is due to loss of water in excess of sodium as a result of the sustained osmotic diuresis. These results are typical of the hyperosmolar hyperglycaemic state (HSS).

Discussion

The HHS occurs only in type 2 DM, where there is usually sufficient insulin secretion to prevent the excessive lipolysis and oppose the ketogenic action of glucagon essential for the generation of ketoacidosis (possibly because the concentrations of insulin required to do this are lower than those needed to prevent hyperglycaemia). Plasma glucose concentrations are in general higher than in ketoacidosis. Perhaps because vomiting is not a feature, patients do not become acutely ill so quickly. Patients may have a mild metabolic acidosis, largely as a consequence of pre-renal acute kidney injury and lactic acidosis due to reduced tissue perfusion: ketoacidosis should be excluded by measurement of blood 3-hydroxybutyrate concentration using a ketone meter.

because some patients have coexistent mild ketosis. Patients with DKA usually also have increased plasma osmolality, although not to the same extent. Although patients with hyperosmolar hyperglycaemic state (HHS) often appear less severely ill than those with DKA at presentation because of the absence of severe acidosis, the overall mortality rate of this condition is higher, at up to 15%.

Management

Rehydration, to expand the intravascular volume and restore tissue perfusion, is the most important initial priority of treatment. Although these patients have a greatly increased plasma osmolality, fluid replacement should be with isotonic (0.9%) (rather than hypotonic) saline because isotonic saline expands the extravascular compartment more effectively, and it is in any case hypotonic relative to the patient's osmolality. Fluid replacement alone will lower plasma glucose concentrations significantly as a result both of dilution and of increased glucose clearance through the kidney. The latest UK guidelines recommend that **insulin** should be given at presentation only if there is significant ketoacidosis (plasma 3-hydroxybutyrate concentration >1 mmol/L); otherwise it should be delayed until after fluid replacement ceases to cause further reductions in plasma glucose concentrations. A fall in plasma glucose concentration is inevitably associated with a rise in plasma sodium concentration, because of osmotic shift of water into cells: this is a normal compensatory change and it does not usually indicate worsening dehydration. However, it is important to prevent this water shift from occurring too rapidly, to minimize the risk of cerebrovascular complications. Insulin, when indicated, should therefore initially be infused at a slower rate than in DKA, at 0.05 unit/h per kilogram body weight (typically 3–5 unit/h), and the rate of intravenous fluid infusion should be guided by frequent calculation of plasma osmolarity (see p. 38) and monitoring of fluid balance.

Potassium supplements are required, but usually in smaller amounts than in ketoacidosis. Patients with HHS are at high risk of arterial and venous thromboembolism caused by hyperviscosity and should therefore be treated prophylactically with low-molecular-weight heparin throughout the acute illness. In contrast with DKA, continued treatment with insulin may not be required once the acute illness is over; most patients can be managed subsequently with diet and antidiabetic drugs.

Lactic acidosis

Lactic acidosis is an uncommon complication of diabetes. It is occasionally seen in patients treated with metformin, especially if they have CKD and congestive cardiac failure, but it is now more usually associated with severe systemic illness, for example, severe shock and pancreatitis. It is discussed in more detail on p. 62.

Hypoglycaemia in patients with diabetes

Hypoglycaemia can complicate treatment in both type 1 and type 2 DM. It is discussed in more detail on p. 247.

Diabetic nephropathy

Diabetic nephropathy is a major cause of premature death in patients with diabetes, not only directly because of kidney failure but also because of the associated cardiovascular disease. It occurs in about 30% of patients with type 1 DM and 25% of patients with type 2 (more in certain ethnic groups).

The earliest detectable abnormality is **microalbuminuria**. Normal urinary albumin excretion is <20 μg/min (<30 mg/24 h): values between 20 and 200 μg/min (30 and 300 mg/24 h) constitute microalbuminuria. Untreated, microalbuminuria progresses to clinical proteinuria (>200 μg/min: >300 mg/24 h), with the gradually declining glomerular filtration rate and increasing plasma creatinine concentration that characterizes diabetic nephropathy. Hyperlipidaemia and hypertension are frequently present and should be treated appropriately. At the stage of microalbuminuria there is evidence that treatment with angiotensin-converting enzyme inhibitors or angiotensin II receptor antagonists (even in the absence of hypertension) delays progression of proteinuria and CKD. Even in established nephropathy, treatment of hypertension and hyperlipidaemia, as well as dietary protein restriction, may be beneficial. Optimization of glycaemic control is recommended. In addition to being indicative of nephropathy, microalbuminuria is predictive of cardiovascular disease, particularly in type 2 DM. Patients who develop kidney failure (CKD stage 5) require renal replacement therapy.

All patients with diabetes should have their urine albumin excretion measured annually. Microalbuminuria is sometimes detected even at diagnosis in type 2 diabetes (diabetes may have been present but unrecognized for several years) but is rare until 5 years after diagnosis in type 1 DM. **Screening** is done by measuring the albumin:creatinine concentration ratio (ACR), preferably on an early-morning urine sample: this ratio has been shown to correlate well with timed albumin excretion, and measuring it avoids the need to make a timed collection. Precise recommendations vary. In the UK, it is recommended that a raised value (ACR >3.0 mg/mmol) should be followed up by further measurements on two occasions over the succeeding 3–4 months. In the absence of other causes of kidney disease, finding raised ACRs in two of three samples is taken to indicate incipient diabetic nephropathy and should prompt appropriate intervention. Microalbuminuria is undetectable using conventional urine protein reagent strips.

Microalbuminuria is not unique to diabetes. It is a marker of increased endothelial permeability and occurs in any inflammatory state, for example the systemic inflammatory response syndrome; in such conditions, it resolves if improvement in the underlying condition leads to restoration of normal endothelial function.

Lipoprotein metabolism in diabetes mellitus

Insulin has a major role in the control of fat metabolism, and both type 1 and type 2 DM are associated with abnormalities of plasma lipids. In type 1 DM, at presentation, or if glycaemic control deteriorates, marked hypertriglyceridaemia (as a manifestation of an increase in the concentrations of very-low-density lipoprotein [VLDL] and chylomicrons) is often present. This is a result of decreased activity of lipoprotein lipase (which insulin stimulates) and increased activity of hormone-sensitive lipase (which insulin inhibits), leading to increased flux of free fatty acids from adipose tissue that act as a substrate for hepatic triglyceride synthesis. Both these effects are reversed by insulin treatment. Indeed, the degree of hypertriglyceridaemia correlates well with glycaemic control. In well-controlled type 1 DM, low-density lipoprotein (LDL) cholesterol concentrations are unremarkable. High-density lipoprotein (HDL)-cholesterol concentrations are often high although there is evidence that the antiatherogenic properties of HDL (see p. 307) are impaired.

In type 2 DM, hypertriglyceridaemia is also common. Unlike in type 1 DM, it generally persists despite the attainment of adequate glycaemic control. It is a consequence of the combined effects of insulin resistance and relative insulin deficiency, resulting in both increased hepatic synthesis and decreased VLDL catabolism. The VLDL contains increased triglyceride and cholesteryl esters in relation to the amount of apoprotein, and although LDL-cholesterol concentrations are not much increased, the particles tend to be smaller and denser, and are more atherogenic. HDL catabolism is increased, so serum HDL–cholesterol concentrations are often low. In both type 1 and type 2 DM, glycation of apolipoprotein B may enhance the atherogenicity of LDL by reducing its affinity for the LDL receptor, thus leading to increased uptake by macrophage scavenger receptors.

Because of the greatly increased risk of cardiovascular disease, treatment with lipid-lowering drugs should be considered in all patients with diabetes; it is indicated in most patients, especially if other cardiovascular risk factors are present.

Diabetes in Pregnancy

Maternal diabetes increases the risk of congenital malformations and unexplained fetal death. This risk can be greatly reduced by ensuring excellent glycaemic control at conception and during early pregnancy, to which end women with diabetes contemplating pregnancy are offered additional support via special prepregnancy clinics. Maternal hyperglycaemia increases fetal insulin secretion and can cause fetal macrosomia, predisposing to difficult delivery, and neonatal hypoglycaemia. Maintenance of excellent glycaemic control reduces these risks.

Pregnancy reduces glucose tolerance. Women previously treated with insulin often have increased insulin requirements during pregnancy, particularly during the second half. Women normally treated with diet alone or diet and antidiabetic drugs sometimes need treatment with insulin during pregnancy, as do women diagnosed with gestational diabetes (see p. 235), although there is a growing body of evidence that metformin and glibenclamide are safe for use in pregnancy. The rapid reversion of insulin requirements to prepregnancy levels after delivery may precipitate hypoglycaemia, and particularly careful monitoring is required at this time. Patients with gestational diabetes often revert to normal glucose tolerance after delivery (this should be confirmed by measuring fasting plasma glucose concentration about 6 weeks later) but remain at increased risk of developing diabetes in the future.

Glycosuria

Although DM is the commonest cause of glycosuria, it is also seen in patients with a low renal threshold for glucose. This may occur as an isolated and harmless abnormality (renal glycosuria), can develop during pregnancy and is a feature of congenital and acquired generalized disorders of proximal renal tubular function (the Fanconi syndrome, see p. 97).

Glucose in Cerebrospinal Fluid

Glucose concentration in the CSF is frequently measured in patients suspected of having bacterial meningitis because it is usually decreased as a result of bacterial metabolism. If the CSF is frankly purulent, the measurement of CSF glucose provides no useful additional information. The CSF glucose concentration is normally ~65% of the plasma glucose concentration, and CSF glucose should always be interpreted in light of the plasma glucose concentration in a blood sample obtained at the same time. A CSF/plasma glucose ratio ≤0.4 supports a diagnosis of bacterial meningitis.

Hypoglycaemia

Hypoglycaemia is conventionally, although arbitrarily, defined as a plasma glucose concentration <3.0 mmol/L, because symptoms typically begin to develop at around this level, although protective endocrine responses are detectable at higher concentrations. Hypoglycaemia is potentially dangerous: the body's defence mechanisms include both symptoms that may alert the patient and physiological responses that lead to the release of glucose into the circulation. Both are mediated by catecholamines, the latter being augmented by other counterregulatory hormones.

Causes

The causes of hypoglycaemia have been classified in various ways. All are to a greater or lesser extent arbitrary but may provide the basis for a logical approach to investigation. One such is to divide patients into those who appear well from those who are unwell or who are known to have a disease or be on a treatment than can cause to hypoglycaemia. By far the commonest causes are insulin and hypoglycaemic drugs, usually (but not exclusively) in patients with diabetes.

The causes of hypoglycaemia are summarized in Box 13.2. These conditions are discussed further in the following sections.

Clinical features

Glucose is an essential energy substrate for the nervous system, at least in the short term; during starvation, adaptation occurs and ketone bodies can be utilized, but these responses do not develop quickly enough to protect against a rapidly falling plasma glucose concentration. The clinical features of hypoglycaemia are the result of dysfunction of the nervous system (neuroglycopenia) and the effects of catecholamines that are released in response to the stimulus provided by the hypoglycaemia.

The characteristic clinical features of acute hypoglycaemia are summarized in Box 13.2; the features of sympathetic activation typically precede those of neuroglycopenia. The pattern of features, their severity and the plasma glucose concentration at which they occur can vary between individuals. Typical signs and symptoms are more likely to occur if the plasma glucose concentration falls rapidly and if hypoglycaemic episodes are separated by periods of normoglycaemia. These clinical features may become attenuated in insulin-treated patients with diabetes who experience frequent episodes of hypoglycaemia (hypoglycaemia unawareness): this is a result of a lowering of the threshold at which the autonomic nervous system becomes activated. Hypoglycaemia unawareness is usually at least partially reversible with careful adjustment of the insulin regimen and patient education. The clinical features of hypoglycaemia are likely to be enhanced if cerebral blood flow is impaired, whereas they may be attenuated in patients taking β-adrenergic blocking drugs, such as propranolol, and in patients with autonomic nephropathy. In chronic hypoglycaemia, psychiatric manifestations may predominate, and other features may not be present, even with a glucose concentration as low as 1.0 mmol/L.

Diagnosis

There are **two stages in the diagnosis** of hypoglycaemia: **confirmation** of the low plasma glucose concentration and **elucidation of the cause**. Mention has been made of the considerable variation in the plasma glucose concentration at which symptoms of hypoglycaemia begin to appear. In children and young adults, symptoms will usually be present only with a concentration <2.2 mmol/L. Neonates often develop features only when the plasma glucose is <1.5 mmol/L, although brain damage may occur before such low concentrations are reached. The elderly tend to be more sensitive to low plasma glucose concentrations, perhaps because of impaired homoeostatic responses or decreased cerebral perfusion resulting from atheroma, although the condition may go unrecognized if individuals are prone to episodes of dizziness (e.g. because of postural hypotension) or confusion. Although glucose meters can be used to support clinical suspicion of hypoglycaemia, they are insufficiently accurate at low plasma glucose concentrations to provide a definitive diagnosis and formal laboratory measurements should be used. Blood must be collected into a container containing fluoride preservative, to inhibit glycolysis.

Box 13.2 Major causes and clinical features of hypoglycaemia in adults

Causes	Clinical features
Unwell or on causative medication	**Acute**
drugs:	due to neuroglycopenia:
insulin	tiredness
sulfonylureas	confusion
alcohol	detachment
critical illness:	lack of concentration
liver, kidney or heart failure	ataxia
sepsis (including malaria)	dizziness
hormone deficiency:	paraesthesiae
ACTH/cortisol	hemiparesis
growth hormone,	convulsions
pituitary hormones	coma
glucagon (in type 1 diabetes)	due to sympathetic stimulation:
non-islet cell tumours	palpitation and tachycardia
inherited metabolic disorders (paediatric/neonatal):	profuse sweating
galactosaemia	facial flushing
hereditary fructose intolerance	tremor
hyperinsulinaemic hypoglycaemia of infancy	anxiety
glycogen storage disease type I	non-specific:
neonatal hypoglycaemia (various forms)	hunger
	weakness
	blurred vision
Seemingly well	**Chronic neuroglycopenia**
endogenous hyperinsulinism:	personality changes
insulinoma	memory loss
functional β-cell disorders	psychosis
non-insulinoma pancreatogenous hypoglycaemia	dementia
after gastric bypass	
insulin autoimmunity	
antibody to insulin or insulin receptor	
surreptitious, or malicious hypoglycaemia	

Chronic neuroglycopenia is seen mainly in patients with insulin-secreting tumours; the features of acute neuroglycopenia are classically seen in patients with diabetes who have taken too much insulin but may occur with other forms of reactive hypoglycaemia.
ACTH, adrenocorticotrophic hormone.

Clinical features can be confirmed as resulting from hypoglycaemia only if they are alleviated by giving glucose either by mouth or parenterally, as appropriate. Those that are caused by acute neuroglycopenia and catecholamine release should resolve immediately, but those attributable to chronic hypoglycaemia often persist. The presence of a low plasma glucose concentration, symptoms of hypoglycaemia and their abolition by giving glucose constitute 'Whipple's triad'.

Investigation of the cause of hypoglycaemia begins with assessment of the clinical presentation and in particular any intercurrent illness. Critical illness will be obvious, and non-islet cell tumours that cause hypoglycaemia are usually large. A review of medication is essential. Hormonal deficiency states must be sought and, where appropriate, excluded. It is no longer considered useful to distinguish formally between fasting and reactive hypoglycaemia, but if symptoms tend to be associated with either fasting or are postprandial, it may be helpful to attempt to provoke them with either a prolonged fast or a mixed meal test (Box 13.3). In both cases, if the onset of hypoglycaemia is confirmed, measurement of plasma insulin and C-peptide concentrations will then help to determine its cause. An algorithm for the investigation of hypoglycaemia is provided as Fig. 13.8.

Box 13.3 Protocols for mixed meal and prolonged diagnostic fast hypoglycaemia provocation tests

Mixed meal test

fast overnight and delay all non-essential medication

give a mixed meal similar to that which has caused symptoms

collect blood samples every 30 min for 6 h

observe and note all symptoms and signs of possible hypoglycaemia

if hypoglycaemia requires treatment, collect blood immediately before administering glucose

measure plasma glucose at all time points

if glucose <3.0 mmol/L, measure:

    insulin

    C-peptide

    proinsulin

Prolonged diagnostic fast test (72 h)

start time is the time of the last meal

minimise non-essential medication

allow calorie-free drinks and encourage activity

measure plasma glucose every 6 h until plasma glucose <3.3 mmol/L, then increase to every hour

observe and note all symptoms and signs of possible hypoglycaemia

if plasma glucose falls to <2.5 mmol/L and the patient is symptomatic, collect samples for:

    insulin

    C-peptide

    proinsulin

    3-hydroxybutyrate

end the fast if hypoglycaemic and symptoms develop, or after 72 h

if urgent treatment of hypoglycaemia is required, obtain samples before carbohydrate administration.

See Fig. 13.8 and below for interpretation of results.

Insulin-induced hypoglycaemia

Most patients with **type 1 DM** experience occasional episodes of hypoglycaemia. Attempts to attain optimum glycaemic control (i.e. as near physiological plasma glucose concentrations as possible) inevitably increase the risk of hypoglycaemia. The secretion of glucagon becomes impaired in established type 1 DM, and the lack of this important counterregulatory hormone impairs the body's natural defences against hypoglycaemia.

Hypoglycaemia is often related to a missed meal or some other factor such as exercise or stress (see Case history 13.5). The diagnosis must rest on the plasma glucose concentration, but if there is any doubt, giving glucose to a confused or unconscious patient is usually safer than waiting until the result is available. Glucagon can also be used to treat hypoglycaemia if the patient has a reduced level of consciousness and so is unable to take glucose by mouth: it causes rapid mobilization of hepatic glycogen (and thus is not effective in starved individuals). Treatment with β-adrenergic blockers can mask the adrenergic symptoms of hypoglycaemia (except sweating) and delay recovery.

Insulinoma

Insulinomas are tumours of the insulin-secreting β-cells of the pancreatic islets. Although uncommon, they are an important cause of hypoglycaemia. Plasma glucose concentration should be measured in any patient who experiences a fit, faint or 'funny turn' to exclude hypoglycaemia as a cause, although many patients with an insulinoma present with behavioural changes rather than with the classic features of acute hypoglycaemia. For this reason, there is often a delay before the diagnosis is considered and appropriate investigations are performed.

Other causes of hypoglycaemia are usually obvious clinically and, with the exception of insulin- and sulfonylurea-induced hypoglycaemia, are associated with low plasma insulin concentrations. The presence of an insulin-secreting tumour can be inferred from the presence of an inappropriately high plasma insulin concentration (>18 pmol/L) at a time when the glucose concentration is low (<3.0 mmol/L). Measurement of plasma proinsulin concentration may also be useful (concentrations >5.0 pmol/L are inappropriate in the presence of hypoglycaemia), although the results obtained vary from assay to assay and thus should be interpreted carefully. C-peptide should also be measured. Although secreted in equimolar amounts with insulin, C-peptide is cleared from the circulation more slowly, so it may be a more reliable marker of endogenous insulin secretion than insulin itself. A concentration >0.2 nmol/L implies continuing endogenous insulin secretion. Inappropriately high insulin with suppressed C-peptide indicates exogenous insulin administration. Measurement of plasma 3-hydroxybutyrate concentration is sometimes recommended. Insulin inhibits lipolysis and hence the production of 3-hydroxybutyrate. High concentrations (>2.7 mmol/L) occur in hypoglycaemia with suppressed insulin secretion (e.g. cortisol deficiency, liver disease). In hyperinsulinaemia and tumour-related hypoglycaemia, 3-hydroxybutyrate concentrations are usually low even when insulin secretion is suppressed if fat stores are severely depleted.

Ideally, blood should be collected for these measurements while the patient is symptomatic. If this cannot

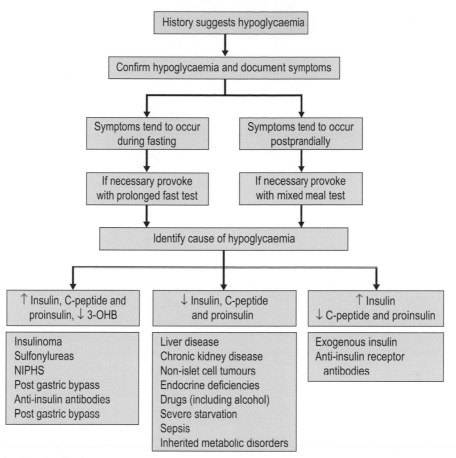

Fig. 13.8 A simple algorithm for the investigation and diagnosis of hypoglycaemia; for definitive investigations, see text. 3-OHB, 3-hydroxybutyrate; NIPHS, non-insulinoma pancreatogenous hypoglycaemia syndrome.

be achieved, or if symptoms of acute hypoglycaemia do not occur, blood samples should be collected after an overnight fast on three consecutive mornings; when this is done, biochemical (although often asymptomatic) hypoglycaemia is demonstrable in 90% of patients with an insulinoma. If hypoglycaemia does not occur under these circumstances, patients suspected of having an insulinoma should undertake a 72-h fast (Box 13.3). Clinical hypoglycaemia develops in almost all patients with an insulinoma during a 72-h fast. Although normal subjects occasionally develop hypoglycaemia during such a fast (women more frequently than men), this is asymptomatic and the plasma insulin concentration is low (usually <18 pmol/L).

Once hyperinsulinism has been demonstrated (and administration of exogenous insulin excluded as a cause of the hypoglycaemia), imaging techniques are used to localize the tumour. The great majority of tumours (~90%) are benign; the treatment of choice is surgical resection, when possible, and the prognosis is good. Diazoxide, a drug that specifically inhibits insulin secretion by β-cells, can be used to prevent hypoglycaemia preoperatively. In some 10% of patients, there are multiple benign or malignant pancreatic tumours and there may be associated adenomas in other endocrine organs (multiple endocrine neoplasia type 1, see p. 357). Diazoxide and somatostatin analogues, such as octreotide, that are less specific inhibitors of gastrointestinal hormone synthesis are valuable in the management of insulinomas when surgical treatment is either not possible or has failed. More recently it has been found that the protein kinase inhibitor everolimus is also an effective treatment.

History

A young man collapsed during a 10-mile charity run. He was conscious but disorientated and his speech was incoherent. The paramedics did a finger prick test, which showed a very low capillary blood glucose concentration, and a venous blood sample was taken and sent to a local laboratory for confirmatory testing. He was given 20 g glucose intravenously and recovered rapidly. He was then able to inform the clinical staff that he was diabetic, treated with insulin; he had injected his normal dose of insulin that morning and eaten his usual breakfast. He was given further carbohydrate by mouth and went home later that evening with a normal blood glucose concentration. The laboratory subsequently reported an initial plasma glucose concentration of 1.6 mmol/L.

Discussion

Exercise increases glucose metabolism and enhances insulin sensitivity. It is important that patients with type 1 DM are aware of this and understand how to reduce their insulin dose or increase their carbohydrate intake accordingly. Patients should always carry sugar and a means of identification to facilitate treatment in an emergency.

Non-pancreatic tumours

Hypoglycaemia can occur in association with non-pancreatic neoplasms, including hepatocellular and adrenal carcinomas, carcinoid tumours and large mesenchymal tumours such as retroperitoneal sarcomas. Patients are usually not ketotic, and except with some carcinoid tumours, plasma insulin concentrations are not increased. It has been suggested that increased glucose uptake by the tumour may be a factor, but this is unlikely ever to be the sole cause. Hepatic glucose output is often reduced, although there is a normal glucogenic response to glucagon. It is probable that most such tumour-related hypoglycaemia is related to the secretion of insulin-like growth factors (IGFs). Plasma IGF-1 concentrations are consistently low in such patients, but IGF-2 (particularly the non-protein-bound form) is often increased, and the IGF-1/IGF-2 ratio decreased. Cytokines such as tumour necrosis factor-α (TNF-α) have also been implicated.

Drug- and alcohol-induced hypoglycaemia

In patients with **type 2 DM**, hypoglycaemia can complicate treatment with sulfonylureas, because they stimulate pancreatic insulin secretion. Some of the sulfonylurea drugs are excreted through the kidneys so patients with CKD are at risk of hypoglycaemia if they do not make appropriate dosage reductions. The treatment of self-poisoning with sulfonylureas (particularly long-acting agents) can be difficult: giving glucose itself stimulates the secretion of insulin and can lead to exacerbation of the hypoglycaemia.

Hypoglycaemia caused by drugs other than those used to treat diabetes is uncommon. Children, but not adults, poisoned with salicylates may develop severe hypoglycaemia. It has also been reported in patients who have taken overdoses of paracetamol, in whom it is probably related to the severe liver damage that this drug can cause. Other drugs reported to cause hypoglycaemia include β-adrenergic blockers, quinidine and pentamidine. Drug-induced hypoglycaemia is treated by administration of glucose (either orally or parenterally) until the effect of the drug has worn off.

Alcohol potentiates insulin- and drug-induced reactive hypoglycaemia. It also increases insulin release in response to an oral glucose load. Alcohol-induced fasting hypoglycaemia is considered in Case history 13.6.

Liver and kidney disease

Although the liver is central to glucose homoeostasis, its functional reserve is so great that hypoglycaemia is a rare feature of liver disease. It may occur, however, with the rapid, massive hepatocellular destruction that can follow poisoning with paracetamol and other toxins. The kidneys are the only organs other than the liver capable of gluconeogenesis; they are also responsible for insulin degradation. These facts may in part explain the severe hypoglycaemia that is occasionally a feature of kidney failure.

Endocrine disease

Deficiency of hormones antagonistic to insulin is a recognized but uncommon cause of hypoglycaemia. **Lack of cortisol** can be caused either by primary adrenal failure or be secondary to panhypopituitarism; hypoglycaemia can be a feature of either condition. Mild hypoglycaemia can occur with isolated **deficiency of adrenocorticotrophic hormone (ACTH) or growth hormone**, but in the latter condition it is rarely symptomatic.

Rather surprisingly, in view of its role in carbohydrate metabolism, decreased secretion of adrenaline (epinephrine) in patients who have undergone bilateral adrenalectomy and who are maintained on corticoid hormone replacement neither causes hypoglycaemia nor interferes with the ability to recover from artificially induced hypoglycaemia.

Sepsis

Hypoglycaemia sometimes develops in patients with septicaemia. It is thought to be a result of the release of

Case history 13.6

History

An elderly man was found to be unrousable one morning by fellow inmates of a derelict house in which they slept. He had been drunk the previous evening and, although this was not uncommon, he had never before been so stuporous in the morning. An ambulance was called and he was admitted to hospital, where he was found to be profoundly hypoglycaemic. He responded rapidly to intravenous glucose and did not then appear inebriated. He refused further treatment and discharged himself later the same day.

Discussion

Alcohol-induced fasting hypoglycaemia is caused mainly by the inhibitory effect of alcohol on gluconeogenesis. However, poor nutrition and liver disease may also contribute. As in this case, hypoglycaemia characteristically develops several hours after alcohol ingestion when hepatic glycogen stores become exhausted. Signs of inebriation may not be present at this time and blood alcohol concentrations can be unremarkable. Although first described, and most commonly seen, in poorly nourished patients with chronic alcoholism, hypoglycaemia can be precipitated by alcohol in healthy subjects whose hepatic glycogen reserves have been depleted by lack of food. It is a particular risk in young children who consume alcohol.

cytokines, which may stimulate insulin secretion or have a direct effect on hepatic glucose production. Impaired kidney function may also be contributory.

Inherited metabolic disease

Hypoglycaemia is an important feature of various inherited metabolic disorders which often present in neonatal and early childhood period (see p. 253). Glycogen storage disease type I is discussed in more detail on p. 337.

Hypoglycaemia after gastrointestinal surgery

Symptoms of hypoglycaemia are common in patients who have undergone gastric surgery involving either a gastrointestinal anastomosis or a pyloroplasty, typically developing 90–150 min after a meal, particularly if it is rich in sugar. There is rapid passage of glucose into the small intestine and release of hormones that stimulate insulin secretion. The insulin response is excessive and hypoglycaemia ensues as glucose absorption from the gut falls off rapidly, rather

than slowly, as it does when gastric emptying is normal. The delivery of an osmotic load to the small intestine also results in rapid influx of fluid, resulting in bloating, nausea and, sometimes, vomiting (dumping syndrome).

Symptoms suggestive of hypoglycaemia after meals may be described by people who have not undergone surgery. Most such people do not, however, demonstrate all three components of Whipple's triad, and so-called idiopathic postprandial hypoglycaemia is no longer widely considered to be a true entity. In patients in whom this is a persistent problem, however, a mixed meal test should be performed to exclude other significant pathology.

Other causes of hypoglycaemia

Sudden cessation of a hypertonic glucose infusion being given as part of a parenteral feeding regimen occasionally precipitates hypoglycaemia; the infusion is often tapered off during the last 2 h of feeding to prevent this. Hypoglycaemia can also occur after dialysis against a glucose-rich dialysate.

Hypoglycaemia has been described as a result of the presence of antibodies that bind to insulin and is thought to be due to the sudden release of insulin from the antibodies. Other patients with antibodies to the insulin receptor have also been described: this usually results in hyperglycaemia due to reduced receptor function, but occasionally the antibodies activate the receptor, causing hypoglycaemia.

Hypoglycaemia in Childhood

Neonatal hypoglycaemia

Hypoglycaemia may occur transiently in apparently healthy babies but is particularly common in those who have respiratory distress, severe infection, brain damage or who are small-for-gestational-age. Premature and small-for-gestational-age babies are particularly at risk of developing neonatal hypoglycaemia because they are born with low hepatic glycogen stores and are more likely to have feeding problems. Extensive physiological changes occur at birth; there is a sudden interruption of the maternal glucose supply, so that glycogenolysis must span the period until feeding becomes established. Babies born to mothers with diabetes may have islet cell hyperplasia, which increases the risk of hypoglycaemia developing in the immediate postnatal period, although this does not persist thereafter. Thresholds for further investigations vary, but they are commonly instigated if the plasma glucose concentration falls to <2.8 mmol/L.

Case history 13.7

History

A woman telephoned for an ambulance when she was unable to rouse her husband one morning; she noticed that his left leg and arm were jerking. In the hospital emergency department, he was found to be pale and sweaty, with a rapid, poor-volume pulse. His plasma glucose concentration was 0.8 mmol/L. He regained consciousness when given a bolus of glucose intravenously, but then became confused and required a continuous glucose infusion for several hours to prevent recurrent hypoglycaemia.

His wife revealed that she had been becoming increasingly worried about her husband. Formerly a man of equable temperament, over the past 6 months he had frequently arrived home in a bad mood, taken little notice of his wife and young child, and sat in sullen silence until his evening meal. After eating, he would behave quite normally, apparently with no recollection of his previous behaviour. On the two mornings immediately before admission, she had found him sitting up in bed, apparently conscious but staring vacantly at the wall and not speaking; after she managed to get him to drink a cup of sweet tea, he had rapidly recovered.

A presumptive diagnosis of insulinoma was made, and this was confirmed by the finding of a serum insulin concentration of 480 pmol/L at a time when he was hypoglycaemic. The C-peptide concentration was also high. He had hepatomegaly, and his serum alkaline phosphatase activity was raised. A magnetic resonance imaging scan showed numerous small lesions in the liver; at laparotomy, the liver was found to have extensive tumour deposits, shown on histological examination to be characteristic of an insulinoma. A single small tumour was present in the pancreas. No surgical treatment was possible; he initially responded well to cytotoxic drugs but relapsed and died 6 months later.

Discussion

This case illustrates the sometimes bizarre symptomatology of patients with insulinomas, who may be chronically hypoglycaemic. The diagnosis in this patient was clear from the results of blood tests taken at the time of admission. However, many patients require several blood tests after overnight fasting to secure the diagnosis. The majority of insulinomas (~90%) are benign, unlike the tumour in this case.

Hypoglycaemia in infancy

Any of the conditions discussed previously can cause hypoglycaemia in infancy. A variety of other conditions that may cause hypoglycaemia at this time (see Box 13.4) are discussed later. The inherited metabolic diseases associated with hypoglycaemia are particularly likely to present during the first few weeks of life.

Beyond the neonatal period, energy stores are usually sufficient to prevent hypoglycaemia during fasting unless there is a defect in homoeostatic mechanisms (e.g. as a result of endocrine disease). In some children, however, starvation—often in the setting of an intercurrent illness—can lead to hypoglycaemia. Insulin secretion is suppressed and ketosis is present. Such children are often thin and sometimes have a history of being small-for-gestational-age. The hypoglycaemia is thought to be a result of impaired mobilization of glucogenic precursors (particularly alanine), but no specific defect has been described and there is no defining test for this condition, often called 'idiopathic ketotic hypoglycaemia'. Affected children usually lose the tendency towards hypoglycaemia by the age of 5 years.

Hyperinsulinism can cause persistent neonatal hypoglycaemia. There is often overgrowth of pancreatic ducts and islet cells. This rare condition was formerly known as 'nesidioblastosis' but is now referred to as 'hyperinsulinaemic

Box 13.4 Causes of hypoglycaemia in childhood

Transient neonatal hypoglycaemia

Hyperinsulinaemia

islet cell hyperplasia
insulinoma

Inherited metabolic disorders, including:

glycogen storage diseases
galactosaemia
hereditary fructose intolerance
fatty acid β-oxidation defects

Other causes

prematurity
small-for-dates
endocrine disorders
starvation
drugs
idiopathic ketotic hypoglycaemia

hypoglycaemia of infancy'. Many cases have been demonstrated to be the result of genetic mutations, for example, in the genes for the sulfonylurea receptor (an adenosine triphosphate [ATP]-dependent potassium channel in the plasma membrane of islet cells), glucokinase or glutamate dehydrogenase. In infants with glutamate dehydrogenase deficiency, a high protein intake can precipitate the hypoglycaemia, which probably explains what was formerly called 'leucine-induced hypoglycaemia'. The diagnosis is made on the basis of persistent hypoglycaemia without ketosis (i.e. low plasma 3-hydroxybutyrate concentration) together with an inappropriately high plasma insulin concentration and ongoing high glucose requirements. No tumour is demonstrable. Hyperinsulinaemic hypoglycaemia of infancy may remit spontaneously in adolescence and should be treated medically (with diazoxide or octreotide): subtotal pancreatectomy may be required, but only if medical treatment fails to control the symptoms.

Other inherited metabolic diseases associated with hypoglycaemia include galactosaemia, certain glycogen storage diseases, defects of the β-oxidation of fatty acids, hereditary fructose intolerance (Case history 13.8) and some organic acidaemias and amino acidopathies. Some of these are discussed in Chapter 19.

Case history 13.8

History

A healthy, 2-month-old female infant, who had previously been breast-fed, vomited when given supplementary feeds of sweetened cow's milk. She reacted similarly when given fruit juice, and sometimes became quiet and sleepy after such a feed. Her mother experimented with various feeds and learned to avoid those that made her child ill. The child grew up with an aversion to sweet foodstuffs and fruit. Her brother, born 3 years later, had a similar history.

Later, when both became medical students, they wondered if their aversion was due to hereditary fructose intolerance. Fructose tolerance tests induced hypoglycaemia, vomiting and hypophosphataemia, which is a characteristic metabolic feature of this condition.

Discussion

If the link between a child's illness and dietary fructose (and sucrose) is not made, there may be serious long-term consequences, for example, failure to thrive, cirrhosis and renal tubular dysfunction. If fructose is avoided and irreversible liver or kidney damage has not occurred, patients with hereditary fructose intolerance remain symptom free. The cause of the intolerance is a lack of the B isoenzyme of fructose 1-phosphate aldolase, which catalyses the conversion of fructose 1-phosphate and fructose 1,6-bisphosphate to trioses.

When fructose is ingested, it is converted to fructose 1-phosphate by fructokinase. In the absence of the B isoenzyme of aldolase, there is insufficient enzyme activity to metabolize fructose 1-phosphate, which accumulates. The A and C isoenzymes normally account for only 15% of the total catalytic activity, although this is sufficient for the metabolism of fructose 1,6-biphosphate, which therefore does not accumulate in this condition.

The clinical manifestations stem from the accumulation of fructose 1-phosphate, which inhibits glucose synthesis, and the depletion of ATP and phosphate as fructose is phosphorylated but not further metabolized. The fructose tolerance test is unpleasant for the patient and potentially dangerous; definitive diagnosis by identification of the causative mutation in the aldolase B gene is now the preferred diagnostic approach.

SUMMARY

- **In health,** homoeostatic mechanisms ensure the maintenance of plasma glucose concentrations within a narrow range, whether an individual is fed or fasting.
- **DM** is a condition characterized by **hyperglycaemia to a degree that is associated with increased risk of microvascular disease** and is due to a relative or absolute deficiency of insulin. It can occur secondarily to other pancreatic disease such as chronic pancreatitis, but the majority of cases are idiopathic. **Type 1** typically affects younger patients. It is an autoimmune disease and usually has an acute onset. **Type 2** typically affects middle-aged and elderly people (although it is increasingly being diagnosed in obese young people) and has a more gradual onset. Genetic and environmental factors are important in its pathogenesis. The prevalence of both types of diabetes, but particularly of type 2, is increasing. Less common types include **latent autoimmune diabetes of adulthood** and **MODY.**
- **Hyperglycaemia** leads to glycosuria and causes an osmotic diuresis, producing the classic clinical features of polyuria and thirst. If inadequately treated, patients with type 1 DM may develop **DKA.** In this condition, hyperglycaemia, together with increased lipolysis, proteolysis and ketogenesis, leads to severe dehydration, mineral loss, pre-renal acute kidney injury and a profound metabolic acidosis. Patients with type 2 DM appear to have sufficient insulin secretion to prevent the excessive lipolysis and ketogenesis that are the hallmarks of ketoacidosis. Instead, inadequate treatment may lead to the development of very severe hyperglycaemia and dehydration, producing a

continued

SUMMARY—cont'd

HHS. Both DKA and HHS are medical emergencies; their management involves provision of fluid and insulin, with general supportive measures and treatment of any specific pre-existing or complicating factors.

- In the longer term, patients with diabetes are at risk of developing **microvascular complications** (retinopathy, neuropathy and nephropathy) and **atherosclerosis.** The presence of **microalbuminuria** may indicate early (and potentially treatable) nephropathy and is also a risk factor for cardiovascular disease. Diabetes is associated with various perturbations of lipid metabolism that predispose to atherosclerosis.

- The **treatment** of diabetes is aimed at relieving symptoms and preventing both short- and long-term complications. Treatment with insulin and antidiabetic drugs that may provoke hypoglycaemia should be monitored by measurements of **capillary blood glucose** concentration made by patients themselves. Measurements of **glycated haemoglobin (HbA$_{1c}$)** provide a valuable index of glycaemic control over a period of several weeks and are of value in the monitoring of all patients with diabetes.

- The **causes of hypoglycaemia** can be divided into two groups according to whether the condition occurs in those who are apparently well or in those who are unwell or with a condition or treatment known to provoke hypoglycaemia. Causes of **hypoglycaemia** in seemingly well patients include insulin-secreting tumours **(insulinomas)** and certain other tumours producing insulin-like substances. Except in patients with insulinomas, clinical features caused by hypoglycaemia are rarely the only feature of any of these conditions. The diagnosis of an insulinoma depends on the finding of inappropriately high insulin (and C-peptide and proinsulin) concentrations in the blood at a time when the patient is hypoglycaemic. This is often demonstrable after an overnight fast, supplemented, if necessary, by exercise.

- Hypoglycaemia can be caused by drugs (including some antidiabetic drugs), insulin and alcohol. Causes associated with illness include pituitary and adrenal failure, severe liver disease and glycogen storage diseases, notably type I (glucose 6-phosphatase deficiency).

- Hypoglycaemia is particularly common in **neonates** who are small for gestational age, and is a risk in babies born to diabetic mothers. It is also a feature of several inherited metabolic diseases.

- Acutely, hypoglycaemia causes **clinical features related to increased activity of the sympathetic nervous system and decreased substrate supply to the central nervous system.** These usually respond rapidly to the administration of glucose. Patients who are chronically hypoglycaemic, for example because of an insulinoma, often present with behavioural disturbance or frank psychosis, and the acute manifestations of hypoglycaemia may be absent.

Chapter 14

Calcium, phosphate and magnesium

Introduction

Calcium is the most abundant mineral in the human body. The average adult body contains ~25 000 mmol (1 kg), of which 99% is bound in the skeleton. The total calcium content of the extracellular fluid (ECF) is only 22.5 mmol, of which about 9 mmol is in the plasma (Fig. 14.1). Bone is not metabolically inert. Most of the calcium in bone is stable, but ~500 mmol/24 h moves between bone and the ECF to support calcium homoeostasis. Approximately 7.5 mmol/24 h moves between the stable pool and the ECF in the course of bone remodelling (see later). In the kidneys, ionized calcium is filtered by the glomeruli (240 mmol/24 h). Most of this is reabsorbed in the tubules, and normal renal calcium excretion is 2.5–7.5 mmol/24 h in men (2.5–6.25 in women). Obligatory renal calcium excretion is ~2.5 mmol/24 h. Because of faecal loss, the minimum dietary requirement is ~12.5 mmol/24 h (although it is higher during growth, pregnancy and lactation). Gastrointestinal secretions contain calcium, some of which is reabsorbed together with dietary calcium. Because calcium in the ECF pool is effectively exchanged through the kidneys, gut and bone about 33 times every 24 h, a small change in any of these fluxes can have a profound effect on ECF, and hence plasma, calcium concentration.

Calcium has many important functions in the body (Table 14.1). Its effect on neuromuscular activity is of particular importance in the symptomatology of hypocalcaemia and hypercalcaemia, as described later in this chapter.

Bone

Bone consists of osteoid, a collagenous organic matrix, on which is deposited complex inorganic hydrated calcium salts known as **hydroxyapatites**. These have the general formula:

$$Ca_{10}(PO_4)_6(OH)_2$$

Even when growth has ceased, bone remains biologically active. Continuous turnover ('remodelling') occurs with bone resorption (mediated by osteoclasts) being followed by new bone formation (mediated by osteoblasts) (see Fig. 15.1). At any one time, up to 10% of bone mass in adults is subject to remodelling. This process is controlled and coordinated by hormones, growth factors and cytokines. **Bone formation** requires osteoid synthesis and adequate calcium and phosphate for the laying down of hydroxyapatite. Alkaline phosphatase, secreted by osteoblasts, is essential to the process, probably acting by releasing phosphate from pyrophosphate. Bone provides an important reservoir of calcium, phosphate and, to a lesser extent, magnesium and sodium.

Plasma Calcium

In the plasma, calcium is present in three forms (Fig. 14.2): bound to protein (mainly albumin), complexed with citrate and phosphate, and as free ions. Only the latter form is physiologically active, and it is the concentration of ionized calcium that is maintained by homoeostatic mechanisms.

In alkalosis, hydrogen ions dissociate from albumin, and calcium binding to albumin increases. There is also an increase in calcium complex formation. As a result, the concentration of free, ionized calcium falls, and this may be sufficient to produce clinical symptoms and signs of hypocalcaemia, although total plasma calcium concentration is unchanged. In an acute acidosis, the reverse effect is observed: that is, the ionized calcium concentration is increased.

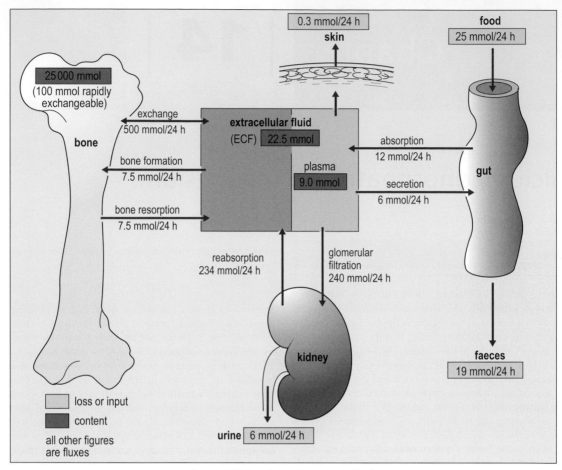

Fig. 14.1 Daily calcium fluxes in the body.

Table 14.1 **Functions of calcium**	
Function	**Example**
structural	bone teeth
neuromuscular	control of excitability release of neurotransmitters initiation of muscle contraction
enzymic	cofactor for coagulation factors
signalling	intracellular second messenger

Changes in plasma albumin concentration will affect total calcium concentration independently of the ionized calcium concentration, leading to possible misinterpretation of results in both hypoproteinaemic and hyperproteinaemic states. Various formulae have been devised to indicate the total calcium concentration to be expected if the albumin concentration were normal. One widely used formula is given in Box 14.1, but such estimates of **'adjusted' calcium** concentration should be interpreted with caution, especially when blood hydrogen ion concentration is abnormal. In this situation, a direct measurement of ionized calcium may be helpful (see p. 271).

A common cause of apparent hyperproteinaemia, and hence hypercalcaemia, is venous stasis during blood sampling, which causes increased efflux of fluid from the vascular to the interstitial compartment. This must be avoided when determinations of plasma calcium are to be made. Ideally, a tourniquet should not be used or, if required, should be applied for the minimum possible time before blood is drawn. Although globulins bind calcium to a lesser extent than albumin, the increase in

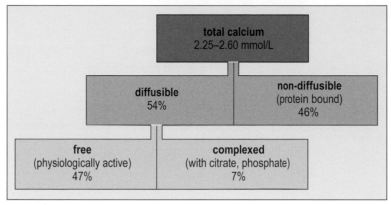

Fig. 14.2 Distribution of calcium in human plasma. Some 80% of the amount bound to protein is bound to albumin, and the remainder to γ-globulins.

γ-globulin in patients with myeloma can be great enough to increase the total plasma calcium concentration. In myeloma, however, there is frequently an increased ionized calcium concentration because of the secretion of calcium-mobilizing substances by the tumour cells (see pp. 292–295).

Calcium-Regulating Hormones

Calcium concentration in the ECF is normally maintained within narrow limits by a control system involving two hormones: **parathyroid hormone** (PTH) and **calcitriol** (1,25-dihydroxycholecalciferol). These hormones also control the inorganic phosphate concentration of the ECF. Calcitonin has only a minor role in calcium homoeostasis.

Parathyroid hormone

PTH is a single-chain polypeptide, comprising 84 amino acids; as with many peptide hormones, it is synthesized as a larger precursor, pre-pro-PTH (115 amino acids). Before secretion, 2 amino acid sequences are lost; the removal of a 25–amino acid chain produces pro-PTH, a further 6 amino acids being removed to form PTH itself (Fig. 14.3). The pre- and pro-sequences are thought to be involved in the intracellular transport of the hormone. The biological activity of PTH resides in the N-terminal 1–34 amino acid sequence of the hormone. PTH is secreted by the parathyroid glands in response to a fall in plasma ionized calcium concentration, and secretion is inhibited by hypercalcaemia. These effects are mediated by the calcium-sensing receptor (CaSR). Calcitriol (see later) inhibits PTH synthesis. PTH acts on bone and the kidneys, tending to increase the plasma concentration of calcium and reduce that of phosphate (Table 14.2).

PTH mobilizes calcium from bone: this action is biphasic, a rapid phase involving existing cells (probably osteocytes) and a longer-term response dependent on the proliferation of osteoclasts. In the kidneys, it increases the fraction of the filtered calcium that is reabsorbed. However, because increased resorption of bone increases the amount of calcium that is filtered, there may be **hypercalciuria** despite the increased reabsorption. PTH promotes **phosphaturia** and mild acidosis by decreasing the reabsorption of filtered phosphate and bicarbonate in the proximal tubules. Also, in the kidneys, PTH stimulates the formation of calcitriol (Fig. 14.4), the calcium-regulating hormone derived from vitamin D.

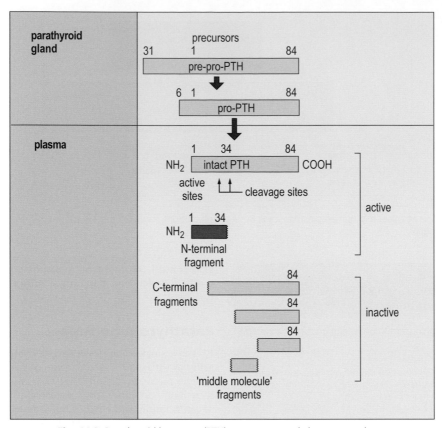

Fig. 14.3 Parathyroid hormone (PTH): precursors and cleavage products.

Table 14.2 **Actions of parathyroid hormone (PTH)**

Target organ	Action	Effect
Bone	rapid release of calcium	↑ plasma $[Ca^{2+}]$
	↑ osteoclastic resorption	
	↑ production of FGF23	↓ plasma $[PO_4^{2-}]$
Kidney	↑ calcium reabsorption	↑ plasma $[Ca^{2+}]$
	↓ phosphate reabsorption	↓ plasma $[PO_4^{2-}]$
	↑ 1α-hydroxylation of 25-hydroxycholecalciferol	↑ calcium and phosphate absorption from gut
	↓ bicarbonate reabsorption	acidosis
FGF23, fibroblast growth factor 23.		

Despite the importance of PTH in the control of phosphate excretion, changes in phosphate concentration do not directly affect secretion of the hormone. Mild hypomagnesaemia stimulates PTH secretion, but more severe hypomagnesaemia reduces it, because the secretion of PTH is magnesium dependent.

Intact PTH has a half-life in the blood of only 3–4 min. It is rapidly metabolized in the liver and kidneys, undergoing

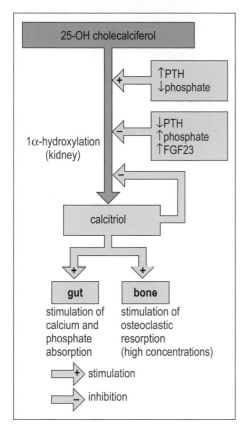

Fig. 14.4 Calcitriol (1,25-dihydroxycholecalciferol): principal actions and control of renal synthesis. These actions increase the extracellular concentrations of calcium and phosphate. Other hormones, including growth hormone, prolactin and oestrogens, have a longer-term stimulatory effect on calcitriol synthesis. FGF23, fibroblast growth factor 23; 25-OH cholecalciferol, 25-hydroxycholecalciferol; PTH, parathyroid hormone.

(1α-hydroxylation). Hydroxylation in the liver is not subject to feedback control, but that in the kidneys is closely regulated (see Fig. 14.4). When the 1α-hydroxylation of 25-hydroxycholecalciferol is inhibited, there is an increase in 24-hydroxylation. The product of this reaction, 24,25-dihydroxycholecalciferol, has no known physiological function. Both this metabolite and calcitriol undergo further metabolism in the kidneys to physiologically inactive products.

The principal actions of calcitriol are indicated in Fig. 14.4. In the gut, it stimulates absorption of dietary calcium and phosphate; this process involves the synthesis of a calcium-binding protein (calbindin D) in enterocytes. This protein is one of a widely distributed group of calcium-binding proteins that are present in many tissues. In bone, calcitriol promotes mineralization largely indirectly, through its role in the maintenance of ECF calcium and phosphate concentrations. The binding of calcitriol to osteoblasts increases the production of alkaline phosphatase and of a calcium-binding protein, **osteocalcin**, the plasma concentrations of which correlate with bone formation rate. At high concentrations, calcitriol stimulates osteoclastic bone resorption, which releases calcium and phosphate into the ECF. In the kidneys, calcitriol inhibits its own synthesis. It may have a small stimulatory effect on calcium reabsorption, acting permissively with PTH.

Many other tissues have receptors for calcitriol, suggesting that it has roles in addition to regulating bone metabolism (see p. 142). It has been shown to influence cellular differentiation in normal and malignant tissues; it also stimulates the production of several cytokines, suggesting that it has a role in immunomodulation.

Calcitonin

Calcitonin, a peptide hormone produced by the C cells of the thyroid, is secreted when plasma calcium concentration rises and also in response to certain gut hormones. It can be shown experimentally to inhibit osteoclast activity, and thus bone resorption, but its physiological role is uncertain. Subjects who have had a total thyroidectomy do not develop a clinical syndrome that can be attributed to calcitonin deficiency. Also, calcium homoeostasis is normal in patients with medullary carcinoma of the thyroid, a tumour that secretes large quantities of calcitonin (although intermittent calcitonin injections can be used as a short-term treatment for hypercalcaemia). The plasma concentrations of both calcitonin and calcitriol are elevated during pregnancy and lactation; during these events calcitonin may block the action of calcitriol on bone and permit increased calcium uptake from the gut to satisfy increased requirements without loss of mineral from bone.

cleavage in the region of amino acids 33–37 and elsewhere. As a result, various fragments of the hormone, as well as the intact hormone, are present in the blood; these include an N-terminal fragment, with a similar half-life to that of the intact hormone, a C-terminal fragment (half-life 2–3 h) and others (see Fig. 14.3). Immunometric assays for 'intact PTH' may detect an inactive fragment missing only the N-terminal six amino acids (PTH 7–84) in addition to intact (1–84) PTH. Assays that measure only PTH 1–84 ('bioactive PTH') have been introduced, although they offer little advantage in the management of patients.

Calcitriol

This hormone is derived from vitamin D by successive hydroxylation in the liver (25-hydroxylation) and kidneys

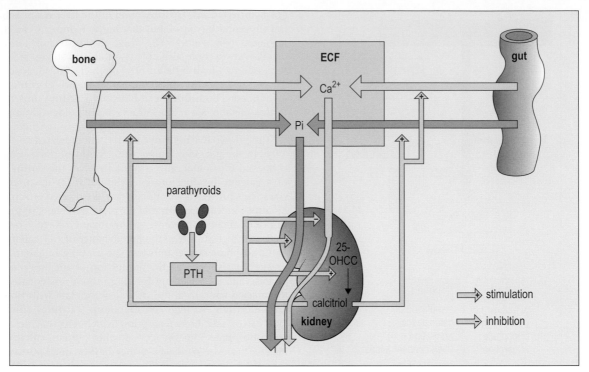

Fig. 14.5 Homoeostatic responses to hypocalcaemia. Hypocalcaemia stimulates the release of parathyroid hormone (PTH), which in turn stimulates calcitriol synthesis. These hormones act together to restore plasma calcium concentration to normal, independently of phosphate concentration. ECF, extracellular fluid; 25-OHCC, 25-hydroxycholecalciferol; Pi, phosphate.

Calcitonin has been detected in many other sites, including the gut and the central nervous system, where it may act as a neurotransmitter. Calcitonin gene-related peptide is produced in neural tissue as a result of alternative splicing of the calcitonin gene. It is a potent vasodilator and is thought to play a role in the sensory pathways for painful stimuli.

Fibroblast growth factor 23

Fibroblast growth factor 23 (FGF23) is a protein produced by osteocytes in response to high circulating concentrations of calcitriol and phosphate. PTH also increases transcription of FGF23. Although it does not affect plasma calcium directly, FGF23 increases loss of phosphate through the kidneys by inhibiting the sodium–phosphate cotransporter and inhibits renal 1α-hydroxylase, thus decreasing circulating concentrations of both phosphate and calcitriol. Mutations in the gene for FGF23 are associated with abnormalities of plasma phosphate concentration (see Chapter 15). Some rare tumours secrete FGF23, causing profound hypophosphataemia and osteomalacia. Measurement of FGF23 can be helpful in patients with severe unexplained hypophosphataemia.

Calcium and Phosphate Homoeostasis

The response of the body to a fall in plasma calcium concentration, provided that this is not due to disordered homoeostasis in the first instance, is illustrated in Fig. 14.5. Hypocalcaemia stimulates the secretion of PTH, which in turn increases the production of calcitriol. There is an increase in the uptake of both calcium and phosphate from the gut, and in their release from bone. The increased concentration of calcitriol stimulates production of FGF23, which together with PTH, increases phosphaturia, so the excess phosphate is excreted. The fractional reabsorption of calcium by the kidneys is increased by PTH, some of the mobilized calcium is retained and the plasma calcium concentration tends to rise towards normal.

Hypophosphataemia (Fig. 14.6) stimulates calcitriol secretion and inhibits FGF23 secretion but has no effect on PTH release. Calcium and phosphate absorption from the gut are stimulated and the resulting tendency for calcitriol

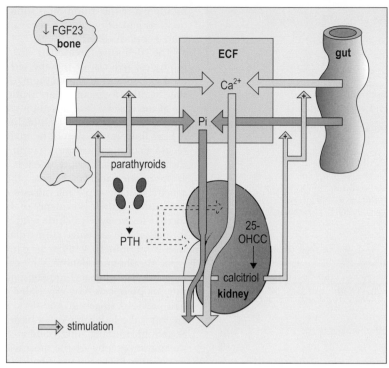

Fig. 14.6 Homoeostatic responses in hypophosphataemia. In the absence of parathyroid hormone (PTH) (secretion is not affected by phosphate), an increase in calcitriol production caused by stimulation of 1α-hydroxylase tends to increase the plasma phosphate independently of calcium concentration. Suppression of fibroblast growth factor 23 (FGF23) release from bone by hypophosphataemia also contributes to maintaining plasma phosphate concentration by allowing the renal tubules to reabsorb more phosphate. ECF, extracellular fluid; 25-OHCC, 25-hydroxycholecalciferol; Pi, phosphate.

to increase the plasma calcium concentration inhibits PTH secretion, with the result that the excess calcium absorbed from the gut is excreted in the urine. The net outcome is the restoration of the phosphate concentration towards normal, independently of that of calcium.

Disorders of Calcium, Phosphate and Magnesium Metabolism

Hypercalcaemia

The causes of hypercalcaemia are listed in Box 14.2. Two conditions account for up to 90% of cases: primary hyperparathyroidism and malignancy. It may be discovered during the investigation of an illness known to cause hypercalcaemia or during the investigation of clinical features suggestive of hypercalcaemia (see Box 14.2). However, it is often clinically silent and discovered incidentally when calcium concentration is measured for other reasons.

Malignant disease

Malignant disease is a common cause of hypercalcaemia, particularly in patients in hospital. There may or may not be obvious metastases in bone. Patients with hypercalcaemia and malignant disease are usually symptomatic, because of the malignancy, the hypercalcaemia or both. Non-metastatic hypercalcaemia is discussed on p. 352; with most solid tumours, it is due to the secretion by the tumour of PTH-related peptide (PTHrP). This peptide has partial N-terminal amino acid sequence homology with PTH. It acts as a growth factor in the fetus but is not detectable in significant amounts in adults except during lactation. It is secreted in breast milk, where it may regulate transfer of calcium from breast tissue. In patients with metastases in bone, there is often no relationship between the extent of metastasis and the severity of the hypercalcaemia, suggesting that humoral factors may be involved in the pathogenesis of hypercalcaemia in malignant disease regardless of whether osseous metastases are present (see p. 352). Other humoral factors that have been implicated include transforming growth factors, prostaglandins and, particularly

Box 14.2 **Causes and clinical features of hypercalcaemia**

Causes

Common

malignant disease, with or without metastasis to bone
primary hyperparathyroidism

Less common

thyrotoxicosis
vitamin D intoxication
thiazide diuretics
sarcoidosis
familial hypocalciuric hypercalcaemia
renal transplantation (tertiary hyperparathyroidism)

Uncommon

milk–alkali syndrome
lithium treatment
tuberculosis
immobilization (especially in Paget disease)
acute adrenal failure
inherited disorders
diuretic phase of acute kidney injury

Clinical features

muscle weakness, tiredness, lassitude, weight loss and
    thirst
mental changes (impaired concentration, drowsiness,
    personality changes, coma)
anorexia, nausea, vomiting and constipation
abdominal pain (rarely peptic ulceration and pancreatitis)
polyuria, dehydration and renal impairment
kidney stones and nephrocalcinosis (mainly associated
    with primary hyperparathyroidism)
short QT interval on ECG
cardiac arrhythmias and hypertension
corneal calcification and vascular calcification
there may also be features of the underlying disorder,
    such as bone pain in malignant disease and
    hyperparathyroidism
mild hypercalcaemia is often asymptomatic

in haematological malignancies, osteoclast-activating cytokines (see Case history 16.1).

Primary hyperparathyroidism

The prevalence of primary hyperparathyroidism is of the order of 1 case per 1000 persons. It can occur at any age but is most common in postmenopausal women (see Case history 14.1). It is usually due to a **parathyroid adenoma**, less often to diffuse hyperplasia of the glands, and only rarely to parathyroid carcinoma. Adenomas may be

multiple and the condition is sometimes familial; it may occur as part of one of the syndromes of multiple endocrine neoplasia (see Box 20.2).

The definitive **treatment** for hyperparathyroidism is surgical removal of the affected glands. Patients with mild (<2.85 mmol/L) asymptomatic hypercalcaemia may stay healthy for many years without an operation but are at increased risk of development of osteoporosis and renal impairment, and should be reassessed regularly. A high fluid intake should be maintained to discourage renal calculus formation. Vitamin D should be given if the patient is deficient. Surgery is recommended for all symptomatic patients (see Box 14.2) and also for asymptomatic patients if plasma calcium concentrations exceed 2.85 mmol/L, there is evidence of decreased bone density, there is severe hypercalciuria with increased risk of stone formation, the estimated glomerular filtration rate (eGFR) is <60 mL/min/1.73 m^2 or in patients younger than 50 years. Parathyroid adenomas are usually small and rarely palpable. **Imaging techniques** may help to localize the tumour preoperatively, especially in patients who have had previous surgery to the neck, in whom the normal anatomical relationships may have been distorted. ^{99m}Tc-Sestamibi scanning, ultrasound and high-definition computed tomography are the most widely used localization techniques. PTH has a short half-life in plasma, and intraoperative measurements of the hormone can be helpful in confirming successful resection of a tumour (because this leads to a rapid fall in concentration).

Secondary and tertiary hyperparathyroidism

Plasma PTH concentrations are also raised in many patients with **chronic kidney disease (CKD)** and with **vitamin D deficiency**. Both these conditions are associated with decreased synthesis of calcitriol, which causes hypocalcaemia, and the increase in PTH secretion is an appropriate physiological response. This is termed **secondary hyperparathyroidism**. The increase in PTH may not normalize the plasma calcium. In the absence of adequate calcitriol, there is resistance to the calcium-mobilizing effect of PTH on bone. Occasionally, patients with established kidney failure become hypercalcaemic, caused by the development of autonomous PTH secretion, presumably as a result of the prolonged hypocalcaemic stimulus. Such hypercalcaemia may manifest for the first time in a patient given a renal transplant who becomes able to metabolize vitamin D normally. This is termed **tertiary hyperparathyroidism**.

PTH is, in part, metabolized and excreted by the kidneys. Increased plasma concentrations of PTH in CKD reflect impairment of these processes, as well as increased secretion. Much of the excess consists of C-terminal fragments, which are inactive in calcium homoeostasis and are not detected in modern PTH assays. Measurement of PTH is

Case history 14.1

History

A 51-year-old woman was investigated after two episodes of ureteric colic, shown to be caused by calcium-containing calculi. She also complained of constipation, although she previously had normal bowel movements, but was otherwise well.

Examination

No abnormality was found.

Results (see Appendix for reference ranges)

Serum:	adjusted calcium	2.95 mmol/L
	phosphate	0.70 mmol/L
	bicarbonate	19 mmol/L
	creatinine, albumin and alkaline phosphatase	within reference range
Plasma:	PTH	18 pmol/L
24-h urine:	calcium	10.8 mmol (2.5–7.5)

Summary

Hypercalcaemia with hypercalciuria, low phosphate and bicarbonate and raised PTH

Interpretation

The high concentrations of both calcium and PTH suggest a diagnosis of hyperparathyroidism. The low concentrations of phosphate and bicarbonate are consistent with the diagnosis, as is hypercalciuria.

Discussion

Hyperparathyroidism can present in many ways (see Box 14.2), including renal or ureteric colic due to calculi that are a result of hypercalciuria. Only about 10% of patients have clinical evidence of bone disease at presentation, although biochemical and radiological evidence is present in >20%. Many patients with hyperparathyroidism have no or few symptoms and are detected as a result of biochemical screening. Indeed, hyperparathyroidism is by far the most common cause of asymptomatic hypercalcaemia.

The plasma calcium concentration is nearly always raised. Exceptions to this occur if there is concomitant kidney disease, vitamin D deficiency or hypothyroidism; occasionally the calcium is raised only intermittently. The phosphaturic action of PTH causes hypophosphataemia, but this is not invariable; the plasma phosphate concentration may be normal or raised, particularly if there is kidney damage. Plasma alkaline phosphatase activity is raised in only 20–30% of patients. Hypercalciuria is a reflection of the hypercalcaemia and should be assessed together with other risk factors for the development of urinary tract stones when considering parathyroidectomy. A low urine calcium excretion in a patient with hypercalcaemia is suggestive of familial hypocalciuric hypercalcaemia (FHH, see p. 264).

The plasma PTH concentration is usually elevated but may be high–normal. Measurements of PTH should be interpreted in relation to the plasma calcium concentration. If calcium is elevated by any mechanism that does not involve PTH, parathyroid activity is suppressed; PTH will be undetectable in plasma or present only at a low concentration.

---

essential to the monitoring of patients with CKD, especially if being treated with calcitriol or the other 1α-hydroxylated derivative of vitamin D, alfacalcidol.

Other causes of hypercalcaemia

Malignancy and hyperparathyroidism account for the majority of cases of hypercalcaemia, but other conditions can be responsible. It is sometimes seen in patients with **thyrotoxicosis**, although thyroid hormones have no specific role in calcium homoeostasis, the hypercalcaemia being caused by the increased osteoclastic activity that may be present in this condition. Coincidental thyrotoxicosis may provoke symptomatic hypercalcaemia in a patient with mild, subclinical hyperparathyroidism. Thyrotoxicosis can also cause osteoporosis (see p. 276).

Excessive intake of vitamin D itself is a rare cause of hypercalcaemia, but the 1α-hydroxylated derivatives (calcitriol, alfacalcidol) are extremely potent and may cause hypercalcaemia. Plasma calcium concentration should be monitored regularly in patients treated with these agents.

In the **milk–alkali syndrome**, hypercalcaemia is associated with the ingestion of milk and antacids for the control of dyspeptic symptoms. The ingestion of alkali is important in the pathogenesis of the hypercalcaemia: it increases the renal reabsorption of filtered calcium, but the precise mechanism is unknown. This syndrome is uncommon, and becoming more so since the introduction of drugs that inhibit gastric acid secretion for the treatment and prevention of peptic ulceration. It should also be remembered that dyspepsia itself may be a feature of hyperparathyroidism, because calcium stimulates gastrin release. Occasionally, patients with parathyroid adenomas may have associated gastrin-secreting tumours (multiple endocrine neoplasia type 1, see p. 357).

Thiazide diuretics sometimes cause mild hypercalcaemia because they increase the reabsorption of calcium by the renal tubules. Chronic **lithium therapy** can cause increased PTH secretion and is an occasional cause of hypercalcaemia.

Approximately 10% of patients with **sarcoidosis** develop hypercalcaemia (see Case history 14.2), as a result of 1α-hydroxylation of 25-hydroxycholecalciferol by macrophages in the sarcoid granulomas, a process that is not regulated by PTH but is dependent on the circulating concentration of the substrate. Hypercalcaemia can also complicate **other granulomatous disorders** (e.g. tuberculosis) for a similar reason.

Hypercalcaemia is a rare feature of **acute adrenal failure**, possibly related to the sudden fall in cortisol concentration and plasma volume contraction.

During a period of **immobilization**, there is a decreased stimulus to bone formation, and continued resorption (a part of normal bone turnover) results in hypercalciuria. Hypercalcaemia is usually only seen in immobilized patients if there is pre-existing increased bone turnover, as occurs during puberty and in patients with Paget disease.

Familial hypocalciuric hypercalcaemia (FHH), also known as 'benign familial hypercalcaemia', is a rare autosomal dominant syndrome. It is most often a result of mutation in the *CaSR* gene, which leads to an increase in the parathyroids' set point for calcium. Hypercalcaemia is present throughout life and is usually asymptomatic. Hypophosphataemia is sometimes present; PTH concentrations are usually normal but may be slightly elevated. The condition is benign but may be misdiagnosed as primary hyperparathyroidism, leading to inappropriate surgery. The key to diagnosis is demonstrating relative hypocalciuria for the degree of hypercalcaemia (the ratio of calcium clearance to creatinine clearance is typically <0.01 in FHH; it is usually >0.02 in primary hyperparathyroidism), or confirming hypercalcaemia in other family members. No treatment is required, but patients should be made aware of their diagnosis to prevent further unnecessary investigations for hypercalcaemia.

Although infants and children can also develop hypercalcaemia from any of the disorders mentioned earlier, they are more likely than adults to have an underlying genetic cause. Severe neonatal hyperparathyroidism causes life-threatening hypercalcaemia in newborns who have inherited two inactivating mutations of the *CaSR* gene. Williams–Beuren syndrome is caused by a microdeletion on chromosome 7 and is associated with characteristic elfin facies, supravalvular aortic stenosis and hypercalcaemia (which usually resolves by the age of 4 years).

Investigation

The way in which hypercalcaemia is investigated is dependent on the clinical setting. In hospitalized patients, malignancy is much commoner than hyperparathyroidism; the reverse is true in asymptomatic individuals with hypercalcaemia. In any patient, clinical features of the causative disorder may be present. The plasma phosphate concentration is of limited diagnostic value: although low in most uncomplicated cases of primary hyperparathyroidism, it can also be decreased in hypercalcaemia caused by malignancy, and can be raised in either condition if there is renal impairment. Plasma alkaline phosphatase activity can be elevated in either condition, although it is more frequently so in malignant disease.

Measurement of PTH, using an assay for the intact hormone, is essential. Even if there is clear evidence of malignant disease or some other cause of hypercalcaemia, hyperparathyroidism is sufficiently common for there to be a real possibility of it being present coincidentally. The measurement of urinary calcium/creatinine clearance ratio will help to differentiate FHH from other causes. Serum protein electrophoresis and measurement of light chains in urine and serum are required if multiple myeloma is suspected (see pp. 285 and 293).

Radiographic examination may occasionally reveal the characteristic subperiosteal bone reabsorption and bone cysts of hyperparathyroidism, but these are only present in a minority of patients. A primary lung tumour or bone metastases will usually be revealed by imaging techniques, but other tumours may not be so easily detected.

If hyperparathyroidism and malignancy are excluded, reassessment of the history, both for drugs and features of other conditions associated with hypercalcaemia, should prompt appropriate further investigations.

Management

When possible, the underlying cause should be treated, but the hypercalcaemia itself may require treatment in the short term. Dehydrated patients should be rehydrated with **intravenous saline**. Once this has been achieved, an intravenous infusion of a **bisphosphonate** can be given to lower the calcium. If hypercalcaemia does not respond to a bisphosphonate, **calcitonin** or high-dose **corticosteroids** may be effective, at least in the short term. Life-threatening resistant hypercalcaemia may require treatment by dialysis or, exceptionally, emergency parathyroidectomy.

Calcimimetic drugs (e.g. cinacalcet) are agonists for the calcium receptors in the parathyroid glands, suppressing PTH secretion and lowering plasma calcium in PTH-dependent hypercalcaemia. They are particularly useful in patients with mild to moderate hyperparathyroidism when surgery is not advisable.

> If a patient is found to have severe hypercalcaemia (adjusted serum calcium concentration >3.4 mmol/L) or has severe symptoms of hypercalcaemia, they should be admitted to hospital for urgent investigation and treatment.

Case history 14.2

History

A 38-year-old man developed thirst and polyuria while on holiday in Spain. He had no other symptoms. He consulted his family doctor when he returned to the UK. He had never smoked and had previously been well, apart from some joint pain and large painful nodules that disappeared to leave bruising on his legs several months before. He was admitted to hospital.

Examination

He appeared dehydrated.

Investigations

A chest x-ray showed some increased hilar shadowing but was otherwise normal.

Results

Serum:	adjusted calcium	3.24 mmol/L
	phosphate	1.20 mmol/L
	alkaline phosphatase	90 U/L
	urea	10.0 mmol/L
	creatinine	150 µmol/L
	eGFR	50 mL/min/1.73 m²
Plasma:	glucose	4.8 mmol/L
	PTH	<1 pmol/L

He was started on a saline infusion. Despite a good diuresis, the serum calcium remained elevated. He was then given prednisolone 30 mg daily, and a week later the serum calcium was 2.80 mmol/L. He was subsequently found to have raised serum angiotensin-converting enzyme (ACE) activity.

Summary

Marked hypercalcaemia with suppressed PTH; reduced kidney function consistent with dehydration.

Interpretation

The suppressed PTH implies that the raised calcium concentration is not due to hyperparathyroidism. The normal glucose concentration excludes diabetes mellitus as the cause of thirst and polyuria. In view of the decreased GFR, the normal serum phosphate is not helpful. The raised ACE activity is suggestive but not diagnostic of sarcoidosis.

Discussion

The patient presented with acute, symptomatic hypercalcaemia. The diagnosis could be hyperparathyroidism, an occult malignancy or some other condition. PTH is undetectable, implying suppression of the parathyroid glands by hypercalcaemia, rather than autonomous PTH secretion. The response to prednisolone also militates against hyperparathyroidism. The hypercalcaemia of malignancy responds unpredictably to steroids. The clue to the diagnosis is provided by the chest x-ray, the serum ACE activity and the previous history of probable erythema nodosum, which are suggestive of sarcoidosis. The hypercalcaemia in this condition is characteristically sensitive to steroids, which suppress the activity of the 1α-hydroxylase enzyme in macrophages. It is often more severe in summer, because of increased synthesis of vitamin D by the action of ultraviolet light on the skin.

Hypocalcaemia

The causes of hypocalcaemia are listed in Box 14.3. Deficiency or impaired metabolism of vitamin D, CKD, hypoparathyroidism and hypomagnesaemia account for the majority of cases. The importance of interpreting a low plasma calcium concentration in relation to the albumin concentration has already been stressed. The clinical features relate to increased neural and muscular excitability (see Box 14.3). Chvostek sign (contraction of facial muscles on tapping facial nerve) and Trousseau sign (carpal spasm when sphygmomanometer cuff applied to upper arm is inflated to midway between systolic and diastolic blood pressures for 3 min) may be positive before other signs are present (latent tetany). Mild hypocalcaemia may be asymptomatic; in severe cases, the condition can be life-threatening.

Vitamin D deficiency

Vitamin D deficiency, which causes **osteomalacia** in adults and **rickets** in children, is discussed in Chapter 15. Deficiency may be caused by inadequate endogenous synthesis or dietary supply of vitamin D, or malabsorption. Whatever the cause, the effect is to decrease the amount of 25-hydroxycholecalciferol available for calcitriol synthesis, leading to decreased absorption of calcium and phosphate from the gut (see Case history 7.2). Although the 1α-hydroxylation of 25-hydroxycholecalciferol is stimulated in hypocalcaemia, with severe deficiency of the vitamin, lack of the substrate will prevent sufficient calcitriol being formed.

Vitamin D deficiency is a cause of secondary hyperparathyroidism. This further lowers the plasma phosphate concentration, and patients with vitamin D

Box 14.3 Causes and clinical features of hypocalcaemia

Causes

Artefactual (blood collected into EDTA tube)

Associated with low PTH concentration
  hypoparathyroidism
  hypomagnesaemia
  hungry bone syndrome (see p. 267)
  inherited disorders

Associated with high PTH concentration
vitamin D deficiency:
  dietary
  malabsorption
  inadequate exposure to ultraviolet light
disordered vitamin D metabolism:
  chronic kidney disease
  anticonvulsant treatment
  1α-hydroxylase deficiency
  vitamin D resistance

pseudohypoparathyroidism
acute pancreatitis
hyperphosphataemia
massive transfusion with citrated blood
acute rhabdomyolysis

Clinical features

behavioural disturbance and stupor
numbness and paraesthesiae
muscle cramps and spasms (tetany)
laryngeal stridor
convulsions
cataracts (chronic hypocalcaemia)
basal ganglia calcification (chronic hypocalcaemia)
papilloedema
Trousseau sign positive
Chvostek sign positive
prolonged QT interval on ECG

Additional features in patients with vitamin D deficiency include myopathy and bone pain.
ECG, electrocardiography; PTH, parathyroid hormone.

---

deficiency often have hypophosphataemia. As deficiency becomes more severe, plasma alkaline phosphatase activity increases and hypocalcaemia may develop. The plasma concentration of 25-hydroxycholecalciferol is low.

Impaired vitamin D metabolism

The formation of calcitriol requires the successive hydroxylation of vitamin D in the liver and kidneys. Kidney disease as a cause of hypocalcaemia is discussed later.

Hypocalcaemia and bone disease are occasionally seen in **patients with epilepsy** treated with phenobarbital or phenytoin. Both drugs are inducers of hepatic microsomal hydroxylating enzymes and are thought to alter the metabolism of vitamin D in the liver. They probably also directly inhibit intestinal calcium absorption. In some forms of **chronic liver disease**, particularly primary biliary cirrhosis, hypocalcaemia and a metabolic bone disease with some features of osteomalacia develop. Mechanisms include malabsorption of vitamin D, decreased 25-hydroxylation and decreased synthesis of vitamin D-binding protein.

Inherited disorders of vitamin D metabolism are discussed on pp. 98 and 274.

Kidney disease

Hypocalcaemia is common in patients with established kidney failure (see Case history 5.3) but is rarely symptomatic. It is often associated with a complex metabolic bone disease known as 'chronic kidney disease–mineral and

Box 14.4 Some causes of hypoparathyroidism

Genetic

DiGeorge syndrome
pseudohypoparathyroidism (high PTH)

Acquired

autoimmune (may be part of polyglandular autoimmune syndrome)
surgery (thyroidectomy)
radiotherapy
haemochromatosis
infiltrative conditions
idiopathic
hypomagnesaemia (reversible)

---

bone disorder' (formerly known as renal osteodystrophy). This condition is discussed in Chapter 5.

Hypoparathyroidism

The causes of hypoparathyroidism are listed in Box 14.4. The commonest is thyroid surgery, after which it may be transient or permanent see Case history 14.3. The congenital form may be associated with thymic aplasia and immune deficiency, the DiGeorge syndrome.

Pseudohypoparathyroidism superficially resembles hypoparathyroidism, but plasma concentrations of PTH are elevated because of resistance to the hormone. It is

Case history 14.3

History

A 56-year-old woman was admitted to hospital for cataract extraction. She was in good health apart from her failing vision. She had undergone thyroidectomy for a multinodular goitre 20 years earlier.

Examination

Both Chvostek and Trousseau signs (see Box 14.3) were positive.

Results

Serum:	adjusted calcium	1.60 mmol/L
	phosphate	2.53 mmol/L
	creatinine	72 µmol/L
	eGFR	81 mL/min/1.73 m^2
	alkaline phosphatase	76 U/L
Plasma:	PTH	<1 pmol/L

Summary

Asymptomatic severe hypocalcaemia and hyperphosphataemia with normal kidney function and low PTH.

Interpretation

The combination of hypocalcaemia, hyperphosphataemia, normal alkaline phosphatase and low PTH is typical of hypoparathyroidism. In most other conditions causing hypocalcaemia (apart from hypomagnesaemia), PTH secretion is increased.

Discussion

Chronic hypocalcaemia from hypoparathyroidism (in this case probably caused by surgical damage to the parathyroid glands) is often asymptomatic and may go undetected for many years. Cataracts are a recognized complication. Patients should be monitored long term after major thyroid or other neck surgery because hypocalcaemia can develop many years later.

found in a group of hereditary disorders caused by molecular defects in the gene *GNAS1*, which encodes the α-subunit of a stimulatory G-protein. The clinical manifestations vary depending on whether the defect is inherited from the mother or the father (an example of genetic imprinting). Patients often have characteristic skeletal abnormalities, including a rounded face, short stature, shortening of the fourth and fifth metacarpals and metatarsals, and a tendency for exostoses to form. They may have learning difficulties. In **pseudopseudohypoparathyroidism** (paternal inheritance of a *GNAS1* defect), similar skeletal abnormalities are present, but the plasma concentrations of calcium

and PTH are normal. These conditions are rare and genetic testing is recommended to confirm the diagnosis.

Other causes of hypocalcaemia

Hungry bone syndrome is a term used to describe the hypocalcaemia (often severe and symptomatic) that can follow the treatment of conditions in which hypercalcaemia has been associated with increased bone resorption. It is particularly prevalent after the surgical treatment of primary hyperparathyroidism and thyrotoxicosis. Removal of the stimulus to bone resorption results in rapid uptake of calcium by bone, leading to hypocalcaemia. With parathyroid adenomas and in hypercalcaemic thyrotoxicosis, prolonged suppression of normal PTH production may contribute to the hypocalcaemia. Hungry bone syndrome should be anticipated and should be preventable by the provision of vitamin D and calcium before and after surgery; this is also the treatment if the condition does occur.

Because magnesium is required for both PTH secretion and its action on target tissues, **severe magnesium deficiency** can cause hypocalcaemia or render patients insensitive to the treatment of hypocalcaemia with vitamin D or calcium, or both. The pathophysiology of hypocalcaemia in **acute pancreatitis** is discussed in Chapter 7.

Management

Patients with symptomatic hypocalcaemia are usually treated with intravenous calcium gluconate, at least until their symptoms are controlled. Any coexisting magnesium deficiency must also be corrected. Persistent hypocalcaemia is usually treated with calcium supplements, vitamin D or both, according to the cause. Because PTH is required for the stimulation of the second hydroxylation step in calcitriol synthesis in the kidneys, patients who lack PTH or have kidney failure require treatment with 1α-hydroxylated derivatives of vitamin D.

Hyperphosphataemia

By far the most common cause of hyperphosphataemia is **renal insufficiency**; other causes are listed in Box 14.5. Transient hyperphosphataemia in milk-fed infants may be secondary to inappropriate constituents of feeds, but excessive intake is an uncommon cause in adults, occurring only if excessive phosphate is given intravenously, for example

Severe (adjusted calcium concentration <1.9 mmol/L) or symptomatic hypocalcaemia is a medical emergency requiring admission to hospital and often requiring intravenous administration of calcium gluconate.

Box 14.5 **Some causes of hyperphosphataemia**

chronic kidney disease
hypoparathyroidism, pseudohypoparathyroidism
acromegaly
excessive phosphate intake/administration
vitamin D intoxication
catabolic states, e.g. tumour lysis syndrome
artefactual (*in vitro*): delayed separation or haemolysis of
blood sample

Box 14.6 **Some causes of hypophosphataemia**

Redistribution

diabetic ketoacidosis (recovery phase)
enteral/parenteral nutrition with inadequate phosphate
(particularly in malnourished patients); intravenous
glucose therapy
respiratory alkalosis

Renal loss

primary hyperparathyroidism
renal tubular disease
diuretics
hypophosphataemic rickets
tumour-associated osteomalacia ($\uparrow$ FGF23)

Decreased intake/absorption

dietary
malabsorption
vomiting
phosphate binding agents, such as magnesium and
calcium salts (rare)
vitamin D deficiency
ethanol withdrawal[a]

[a]Ethanol withdrawal can also cause inappropriate phosphaturia.
FGF23, fibroblast growth factor 23.

during parenteral feeding. Increased **tissue catabolism**, for example in the treatment of malignant disease (particularly haematological malignancy), can cause hyperphosphataemia as part of the tumour lysis syndrome (see p. 354). Tissue catabolism is also one of its causes in diabetic ketoacidosis, but in these patients renal impairment is often also present.

Hyperphosphataemia is potentially important clinically because it results in inhibition of the 1α-hydroxylation of 25-hydroxycholecalciferol in the kidneys; phosphate may also combine with calcium, resulting in metastatic calcium deposits in the tissues and hypocalcaemia.

Management

Management should be directed at the underlying cause, but in practice, the most effective treatment is to give phosphate binders (often calcium salts) by mouth to reduce absorption from the gut. In patients with CKD, a low phosphate diet is also recommended.

Hypophosphataemia

Hypophosphataemia is a common biochemical finding. When mild, it is probably of little consequence, but severe hypophosphataemia (<0.3 mmol/L) can have important consequences on the function of all cells, particularly muscle cells (causing muscle weakness or even rhabdomyolysis), red and white blood cells, and platelets, by limiting the formation of essential phosphate-containing compounds such as adenosine triphosphate (ATP) and 2,3-diphosphoglycerate. Chronic hypophosphataemia is a cause of rickets and osteomalacia.

Hypophosphataemia can be caused by decreased intestinal absorption, increased renal excretion or redistribution from extracellular to intracellular fluid. Specific causes are given in Box 14.6. Although hyperphosphataemia is usual in diabetic ketoacidosis, hypophosphataemia is seen during the recovery phase when there is increased uptake of phosphate into depleted tissues in response to treatment with insulin. This is also the mechanism of hypophosphataemia seen in patients with malnutrition

who are given a high-energy intake (refeeding syndrome) either enterally or parenterally (see Case history 8.3). Hypophosphataemia is common during alcohol withdrawal and is multifactorial. The causes include decreased intake, renal loss, alkalosis and refeeding. Respiratory alkalosis can cause hypophosphataemia by stimulating phosphofructokinase and the formation of phosphorylated glycolytic intermediates.

Several rare inherited disorders can cause hypophosphataemia by increasing the urinary loss of phosphate. This may be part of the renal Fanconi syndrome in which there is generalized failure of reabsorption of many substances in the proximal renal tubules. It can also be a specific failure of phosphate absorption, as occurs in autosomal dominant and X-linked forms of hypophosphataemic rickets (see p. 98).

Management

Hypophosphataemia should be anticipated, and prevented, in conditions where it may occur. It is treated by the administration of phosphate, either enterally or parenterally as appropriate, but intravenous phosphate should not be given to a patient who is hypercalcaemic or oliguric.

Plasma phosphate concentration
Plasma phosphate concentrations vary throughout the 24-h period, particularly in response to carbohydrate intake, when a surge in insulin causes phosphate to move into cells. When monitoring patients, the least variable results are obtained on fasting morning blood samples.

Magnesium

Magnesium is the fourth most abundant cation in the body. The adult human body contains approximately 1000 mmol, with about half in bone and the remainder distributed equally between muscle and other soft tissues. Only 11–17 mmol is found in the ECF, the plasma concentration being 0.7–1.0 mmol/L. The normal daily intake of magnesium (10–12 mmol) is greater than is necessary to maintain magnesium balance (~8 mmol/24 h) and the excess is excreted through the kidneys.

Urinary magnesium excretion is increased by ECF volume expansion, hypercalcaemia and hypermagnesaemia, and decreased in the opposite of these states. There is no one specific homoeostatic mechanism for magnesium. Various hormones, including PTH and aldosterone, affect the renal handling of magnesium; the effects of aldosterone are probably secondary to changes in ECF volume, but PTH, which increases the tubular reabsorption of filtered magnesium, appears to act directly.

Magnesium acts as a cofactor for some 300 enzymes, including those involved in protein synthesis, glycolysis and the transmembrane transport of ions. A magnesium–ATP complex is the substrate for many ATP-requiring enzymes. Magnesium is important in the maintenance of the structure of ribosomes, nucleic acids and some proteins. It interacts with calcium in several ways and affects the permeability and electrical properties of cell membranes such that extracellular magnesium depletion causes hyperexcitability.

Hypermagnesaemia

Significant hypermagnesaemia is uncommon. Cardiac conduction is affected at concentrations of 2.5–5.0 mmol/L; very high concentrations (>7.5 mmol/L) cause respiratory paralysis and cardiac arrest. Such extreme hypermagnesaemia may rarely be seen in established kidney failure. Hypermagnesaemia (3–4 mmol/L) may be induced deliberately in the intensive care setting to reduce bronchospasm in severe asthma or to reduce the risk of fitting in severe pre-eclampsia.

Intravenous calcium may give short-term protection against the adverse effects of hypermagnesaemia, but in established kidney failure, dialysis may be necessary.

Box 14.7 **Causes and clinical features of hypomagnesaemia**
Causes
malabsorption, malnutrition and fistulae
refeeding syndrome
alcoholism (chronic alcoholism and ethanol withdrawal)
cirrhosis
diuretic therapy (especially loop diuretics)
proton pump inhibitors
renal tubular disorders (in advanced kidney disease, hypermagnesaemia is usual)
chronic mineralocorticoid excess
drug toxicity, e.g.:
amphotericin
aminoglycosides
cisplatin
ciclosporin
Gitelman syndrome
Clinical features
tetany (with normal or decreased calcium)
agitation, delirium
ataxia, tremor, choreiform movements and convulsions
muscle weakness, cardiac arrhythmias

Hypomagnesaemia

Hypomagnesaemia usually indicates magnesium deficiency. Surveys have shown that it may be present in up to 10% of hospitalized patients; it occurs more frequently than hypermagnesaemia. The causes and clinical features are summarized in Box 14.7. A proportion of circulating magnesium is bound to albumin, although to a lesser extent than calcium. Severe hypoalbuminaemia may therefore be associated with a low plasma magnesium concentration, which is physiologically appropriate. Hypocalcaemia, caused by decreased PTH secretion, is a clinically important consequence of hypomagnesaemia (Case history 14.4). Hypophosphataemia and hypokalaemia may also be present, but all these abnormalities usually respond to magnesium supplementation. Plasma magnesium concentration should always be measured in patients with hypocalcaemia, or clinical features suggestive of hypocalcaemia, when these do not respond to calcium supplementation (see Case history 14.5), and also in patients with refractory hypokalaemia. Other indications for its measurement include parenteral nutrition, chronic diarrhoea and other conditions listed in Box 14.7.

Mild magnesium deficiency is treated by oral supplementation, although this may induce diarrhoea and further magnesium loss. In severe deficiency, and with malabsorption, magnesium is given by slow intravenous infusion.

Case history 14.4

History

An elderly woman presented with weight loss and malabsorption caused by amyloidosis of the small intestine. She was known to have osteomalacia and had been hypocalcaemic. She was given parenteral nutritional support, but despite what was considered to be adequate calcium and vitamin D supplementation, she remained hypocalcaemic.

Results

Serum:	magnesium	0.35 mmol/L
	adjusted calcium	1.94 mmol/L
Plasma:	PTH	1.1 pmol/L

Summary

Profound hypomagnesaemia and hypocalcaemia with suppressed PTH.

Interpretation

The low calcium and PTH concentrations suggest hypoparathyroidism, with hypomagnesaemia being the likely cause.

Discussion

Patients with malabsorption may develop magnesium deficiency and although this patient's parenteral feeds contained magnesium, there was presumably an insufficient amount to correct her deficit. Magnesium is required for the release of PTH, so long-standing hypomagnesaemia can cause functional hypoparathyroidism. When she was given additional magnesium supplements, her serum calcium concentration rapidly returned to normal.

Case history 14.5

History

A young man presented with a short history of severe diarrhoea, abdominal pain, weight loss and rectal bleeding. He had had several previous episodes of diarrhoea and abdominal pain, but these had been much milder and he had not sought medical advice. He also complained of cramps in his arms and legs.

Examination

Both Chvostek and Trousseau signs (see Box 14.3) were positive, indicating latent tetany.

Investigation

A rectal biopsy indicated Crohn disease.

Results

Serum:	sodium	142 mmol/L
	potassium	3.1 mmol/L
	urea	5.4 mmol/L
	creatinine	96 μmol/L
	eGFR	>90 mL/min/1.73 m^2
	adjusted calcium	2.42 mmol/L
	phosphate	0.9 mmol/L
	magnesium	0.38 mmol/L

Summary

Low serum potassium with very low magnesium; normal calcium and phosphate.

Interpretation

Low calcium concentration is excluded as the cause of his latent tetany, which is explained by the severe hypomagnesaemia.

Discussion

Magnesium was measured because of latent tetany in the presence of normal calcium concentration. Intestinal mucous is rich in magnesium and potassium and patients with diarrhoea can have large losses from the gut as well as decreased absorption from food. He was given oral potassium and parenteral magnesium replacement (not oral, in view of his diarrhoea) and the cramps resolved.

When symptoms of hypocalcaemia occur in a patient whose serum calcium concentration is normal, hypomagnesaemia should be considered as a cause. Low concentrations of magnesium are often found in association with low concentrations of calcium, phosphate and potassium, but hypomagnesaemia can occur in isolation.

Ionized calcium

The most frequently used methods in laboratories for determining plasma calcium concentration measure **total calcium**, although **ionized calcium** can be measured using an ion-selective electrode (usually part of a blood gas analyzer). Because normally ~50% of plasma calcium is in the ionized form, calcium concentrations measured by point-of-care instruments are about half those reported by routine laboratory methods. Accurate measurements of ionized calcium require the exclusion of air from the sample to avoid changes in binding of calcium to albumin in response to changes in hydrogen ion concentration (pH); this is difficult other than for point-of-care testing. Fortunately, measurements of total calcium are satisfactory for most clinical purposes. One undoubted advantage of ionized calcium measurements over conventional measurements of total calcium is the speed with which results are available. They may thus be useful to monitor calcium in circumstances when rapid changes in concentration can occur, for example, during exchange blood transfusion or during surgery with extracorporeal bypass (the citrate used to anticoagulate blood products complexes with calcium). They can also be useful in patients with alkalosis or acidosis when the change in calcium binding to albumin cannot be assessed by measuring total calcium concentrations.

SUMMARY

- **Calcium** has many functions in the body in addition to its **structural role** in bones and teeth. It is essential for **muscle contraction**, affects the **excitability of nerves**, is a **second messenger**, involved in the action of several hormones, and is required for **blood coagulation.**
- About half the calcium in the plasma is **bound to protein**; it is the unbound fraction that is physiologically active and whose concentration is closely regulated.
- Two hormones have a central role in calcium homoeostasis. The main action of **calcitriol**, the hormone derived from vitamin D by successive hydroxylations in the liver and kidneys, is to stimulate calcium (and phosphate) uptake from the gut. **Parathyroid hormone (PTH)**, secreted in response to a fall in plasma ionized calcium concentration, stimulates calcitriol formation, stimulates calcium resorption from bone and reabsorption by the renal tubules, and has a powerful phosphaturic action. These two hormones, along with **fibroblast growth factor 23**, also regulate extracellular phosphate concentration. **Calcitonin** has only a minor role in calcium homoeostasis.
- The common causes of **hypercalcaemia** are **primary hyperparathyroidism**, caused by parathyroid adenomas or hyperplasia, and **malignant disease** (including myeloma), with or without metastasis to bone. Less common causes include sarcoidosis, thyrotoxicosis and overdosage with vitamin D or its derivatives. Mild hypercalcaemia is often asymptomatic; when more severe, clinical features may include bone and abdominal pain, kidney stones, polyuria, thirst and behavioural disturbances.
- **Hypocalcaemia** causes hyperexcitability of nerve and muscle, leading to muscle spasm (tetany) and, in severe cases, to convulsions. Causes include **vitamin D deficiency** and **hypoparathyroidism.** Vitamin D deficiency may be either dietary in origin, often exacerbated by little exposure to sunlight (and hence reduced endogenous synthesis), or caused by malabsorption.
- **Hyperphosphataemia** is particularly associated with renal impairment; it inhibits vitamin D metabolism and can cause hypocalcaemia. Severe **hypophosphataemia**, such as can occur with inadequate phosphate provision during intravenous feeding, has potentially harmful effects on many body tissues, particularly blood cells and skeletal muscle.
- **Magnesium** is an essential cofactor for many enzymes. Its concentration in the extracellular fluid is controlled primarily through regulation of its urinary excretion. **Hypomagnesaemia** can cause clinical features similar to those of hypocalcaemia, and indeed can cause hypocalcaemia, because the secretion of PTH is magnesium dependent. Deficiency of magnesium can occur with prolonged diarrhoea and malabsorption. **Hypermagnesaemia** is common in kidney failure, but it is usually mild and appears to be tolerated well by the body; increased magnesium concentrations rarely cause obvious clinical disturbances.

Chapter | 15 |

Bones and joints

Introduction

Disorders of the bones and joints are very common, with an increasing prevalence related to an ageing population, obesity and vitamin D insufficiency in many developed countries. Although the commonest of these disorders, osteoarthritis, is not associated with biochemical abnormalities, clinical biochemistry laboratories play an important role in the diagnosis and monitoring of many of the other bone and joint disorders.

Bone has **three important functions**: it provides **structural support** to the body; it houses the **haemopoietic bone marrow**; and it is **metabolically active**, being essential for calcium and phosphate homoeostasis (see Chapter 14). Bone consists of a proteinaceous matrix, 90% of which is formed by type I collagen fibres, the remainder being glycoprotein and proteoglycan ground substance. This provides the support for the mineral component, which consists of spindle-shaped crystals of hydroxyapatite, a complex hydrated calcium phosphate. Bone has **two structurally distinct** components: dense **cortical bone** (the major form) and spongy trabecular bone, which is more metabolically active and supports the bone marrow.

Mature bone undergoes constant **remodelling**, a process that involves ~10% of the skeleton at any one time. It takes place within multicellular bone remodelling units on bone surfaces and involves the **resorption** of small volumes of bone by osteoclasts (which subsequently undergo apoptosis) and their **replacement** by osteoid generated by osteoblasts (Fig. 15.1), which rapidly becomes mineralized to form mature bone. Alkaline phosphatase (ALP) promotes bone mineralization by breaking down pyrophosphate (an inhibitor of mineralization) to phosphate (which is required for the process). Some of the osteoblasts become trapped in the new bone and are transformed into osteocytes. The whole process is coordinated by numerous hormones, growth factors and cytokines, including osteoprotegerin (OPG, which decreases osteoclastic activity) and receptor activator of nuclear factor-κB ligand (RANKL, which increases it), such that **under normal circumstances the rates of resorption and bone formation are matched**. Many of the systemic factors that alter bone resorption, such as parathyroid hormone (PTH) and calcitriol, act by altering the balance of RANKL and OPG production.

Synovial joints are found throughout the skeleton wherever a range of movement is required between bones. The typical synovial joint is a closed space, lubricated by a small amount of synovial fluid, which is an ultrafiltrate of plasma with additional secreted components (e.g. hyaluronate) that modify the viscoelastic properties of the fluid. The bone ends that move against each other are covered with articular cartilage composed of proteoglycans and collagen; this cartilage has a dual role of providing a smooth, low-friction surface and acting as a shock absorber during movement. The whole joint is enclosed by a tough capsule which is lined by the synovial membrane. Synovial membrane cells secrete synovial fluid and phagocytose joint debris.

Metabolic Bone Diseases

Metabolic bone diseases are a result of a disruption of the normally orderly process of bone remodelling. The corresponding changes in plasma calcium and phosphate concentrations and ALP activity (a marker of osteoblastic activity) are summarized in Table 15.1.

Rickets and osteomalacia

These conditions are characterized by **defective mineralization of osteoid** and are summarized in Table 15.2.

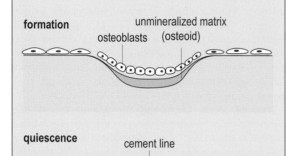

quiescence bone lining cells mineralized bone

resorption

osteoclasts

formation unmineralized matrix

osteoblasts (osteoid)

quiescence

cement line

Fig. 15.1 Cycle of a bone remodelling unit. Quiescent bone surfaces are covered by osteoblast-related bone lining cells. Remodelling begins with the replacement of these cells by osteoclast precursor cells from blood, perhaps in response to cytokines released from areas of microdamage. These cells differentiate into osteoclasts, which excavate resorption pits. When resorption is complete, the osteoclasts undergo apoptosis and are replaced by osteoblasts, which lay down new osteoid. This becomes mineralized, and a new quiescent phase begins. The whole process takes 6–12 months.

Rickets occurs in infancy and childhood (while bones are growing); osteomalacia is its adult equivalent. Defective mineralization is most frequently due to an inadequate supply of calcium, usually because of **deficiency of vitamin D** (see Chapter 8). Such 'calciopenic' rickets and osteomalacia can also be caused by impaired production of calcitriol or resistance to its actions. These are features of two rare, inherited conditions: in

vitamin D–dependent rickets type I, there is deficiency of renal 1α-hydroxylase; in type II, there is resistance to the actions of calcitriol secondary to a receptor defect. Inheritance in both cases is autosomal recessive. Impaired production of calcitriol also occurs in chronic kidney disease (CKD) and contributes to the pathogenesis of CKD–mineral and bone disorder (CKD–MBD), in which features of osteomalacia are usually present. Osteomalacia has also been reported in individuals being treated with anticonvulsants who are living in institutions, probably as a combined result of vitamin D deficiency and altered hepatic metabolism of the vitamin.

Defective bone mineralization can also be caused by an **inadequate supply of phosphate**. The cause is usually a renal tubular phosphate leak, such as occurs in the renal Fanconi syndrome, in proximal renal tubular acidosis and, as an isolated phenomenon, in inherited hypophosphataemic ('vitamin D–resistant') rickets (see pp. 97–98). Many of these disorders result in increased activity of fibroblast growth factor 23 (FGF23), an important stimulator of renal phosphate loss (see p. 260 and Table 15.2). Measurements of plasma FGF23 concentration and tubular reabsorption of phosphate can be helpful in the diagnosis of tumour-induced osteomalacia and in some of the genetic disorders. Hypophosphatasia is a rare, inherited disorder that causes bone features that resemble rickets, in which there is a deficiency of ALP.

The clinical features of rickets and osteomalacia include bone pain and tenderness, and (particularly in rickets) skeletal deformities. Proximal muscle weakness is frequently present; about 50% of patients with privational disease have hypocalcaemia, which is occasionally severe enough to be symptomatic, but in the rest, calcium concentration is maintained just within the reference interval by secondary hyperparathyroidism (increased secretion of PTH in response to falling calcium concentration). Osteomalacia can coexist with osteoporosis.

Both rickets and osteomalacia give rise to characteristic radiological appearances, although these may not always be apparent in osteomalacia, and bone biopsy is sometimes required to confirm the diagnosis. Treatment is with vitamin D or one of its hydroxylated derivatives, together with supplements of calcium or phosphate as appropriate. Biochemical monitoring is through measurement of plasma calcium, phosphate, ALP and PTH, all of which should normalize, although there is often a flare in ALP activity during the first few weeks of treatment. Monitoring of plasma 25-hydroxycholecalciferol or calcitriol concentration is indicated for some of the rare inherited diseases but is not routinely required for privational disease, unless there are concerns about the adequacy of intestinal absorption of vitamin D.

Table 15.1 **Biochemical changes in plasma in metabolic bone disease**

Condition	Calcium	Phosphate	Alkaline phosphatase	Other
osteoporosis	N	N	N	—
osteomalacia	↓ or N	↓	↑ (↑↑[a])	—
Paget disease	N (↑[b])	N	↑↑↑	—
chronic kidney disease–mineral and bone disorder	↓ or N	↑	↑	↑ creatinine
primary hyperparathyroidism	↑	N or ↓	N or ↑	PTH inappropriately high
secondary tumour deposits	N or ↑	↓, N or ↑	↑	—

[a]During early phase of recovery.
[b]During immobilization.
N, normal; PTH, parathyroid hormone.

Table 15.2 **Some causes of osteomalacia and rickets**

Cause	Mechanism
Calciopenic	
nutritional calcium and/or vitamin D deficiency	may be dietary or secondary to malabsorption
lack of sunlight	cholecalciferol is produced in skin exposed to ultraviolet light
anticonvulsants	accelerated clearance of 25-hydroxycholecalciferol
chronic kidney disease	multifactorial (see p. 92)
vitamin D–dependent rickets type I	deficiency of renal 1α-hydroxylase
vitamin D–dependent rickets type II	calcitriol receptor defect
Phosphopenic	

isolated phosphate loss
  X-linked dominant
  autosomal dominant
  X-linked recessive
  autosomal recessive
  tumour associated (oncogenic osteomalacia)
	PHEX mutation causing increased production of FGF23
	FGF23 activating mutation
	Dent disease, associated with hypercalciuria
	various mutations causing increased FGF23 activity
	mesenchymal cell tumours producing FGF23

generalized renal tubular disorders (Fanconi syndrome)
  cystinosis, Wilson disease, tyrosinaemia type 1
  proximal renal tubular acidosis
  autoimmune disorders (e.g. Sjögren syndrome)
  drugs (e.g. cisplatin, amphotericin)
  heavy metal toxicity
	failure of reabsorption of many components of the glomerular filtrate, including phosphate, uric acid, amino acids, glucose, and low molecular weight proteins; the individual disorders are discussed in relevant chapters

PHEX is a phosphate regulating gene on the X chromosome which encodes a protein that controls fibroblast growth factor 23 (FGF23; see p. 260) production. Inactivation of *PHEX* increases FGF23 production, thereby stimulating renal phosphate loss.

Osteoporosis

Osteoporosis is characterized by **reduced bone mass and abnormalities of bone microarchitecture**, which render it more fragile and susceptible to fracture. It is defined as a bone mineral density >2.5 standard deviations below the mean for young adults or by the occurrence of a low-impact (or fragility) fracture (e.g. vertebral or neck of femur). The lifetime risk of fracture because of osteoporosis is about 40% in women and 20% in men; such fractures are a considerable source of morbidity and mortality.

It is now standard practice to assess clinical risk factors (with or without measurements of bone mineral density) in algorithms that estimate future fracture risk for an individual (e.g. QFracture or the WHO-sponsored FRAX tool).

The two greatest risk factors for the development of osteoporosis are **ageing** and **postmenopausal oestrogen deficiency**. Peak bone mass plateaus at about age 30 years and begins to decline from age 40 years at a rate of ~1% of mass per year. This bone loss is a result of the decrease in osteoblastic activity in relation to osteoclastic activity that occurs with ageing. It involves both trabecular and cortical bone, is particularly associated with femoral neck fractures, and affects men and women. Postmenopausal osteoporosis results from accelerated bone loss in the first five years after menopause and primarily affects trabecular bone. It typically leads to compression fractures of the vertebral bodies, leading to deformity and loss of height. The other type of fracture particularly associated with osteoporosis is Colles fracture of the distal radius, which is also more common in women. Osteoporosis can develop at a much earlier age in people with other risk factors (Box 15.1).

The **radiological diagnosis** of osteoporosis is based on measurements of bone density, for example, by dual-energy x-ray absorptiometry (DEXA).

Plasma calcium and phosphate concentrations are normal in uncomplicated osteoporosis; so, too, is ALP activity (unless a fracture has occurred or osteomalacia is also present). Several biochemical **markers of bone turnover** are available for the assessment of both bone resorption and bone formation. Markers of bone resorption include various substances derived from collagen, for example, pyridinium cross-links of collagen (deoxypyridinoline and pyridinoline, both measured in urine) and cross-linking telopeptides of type I collagen (e.g. C-telopeptide of collagen cross-links [CTX], measured in serum). Markers of bone formation include plasma osteocalcin, bone-specific ALP and procollagen type I terminal peptides (N-terminal [P1NP] and C-terminal). Although no one substance in either class has yet been shown conclusively to be superior to any other, the International Osteoporosis Foundation has endorsed the use of CTX and P1NP in clinical trials of osteoporosis treatments. Their value in guiding clinical practice has yet to be fully established, but suppression of markers of resorption during treatment—for example, with bisphosphonates—becomes maximal sooner (approximately 3 months) than changes in bone density can reliably be detected (up to 2 years); furthermore, failure to respond is suggestive of non-adherence to treatment. There is also evidence that changes in the concentrations of these markers correlate more closely with the reduction in risk of fracture than changes in bone mineral density. The place of bone turnover markers is therefore predominantly in monitoring treatment rather than identification of patients at risk of developing osteoporosis, for which DEXA scanning and risk scores are preferred.

> ### Box 15.1 Risk factors for osteoporotic fractures
>
> ageing
> postmenopausal oestrogen deficiency
> low body mass index
> previous osteoporotic fracture
> parental history of hip fracture
> rheumatoid arthritis
> endocrine:
>   premature ovarian failure/hypogonadism
>   thyrotoxicosis
>   Cushing syndrome
>   diabetes mellitus
> drugs:
>   glucocorticoids
>   prolonged heparin treatment
>   androgen deprivation therapy
> ethanol
> smoking
> immobilization
> weightlessness
> malabsorption/malnutrition

Prevention and management

Osteoporosis is associated with high morbidity and mortality. Valuable preventive measures include moderate regular weight-bearing exercise and an adequate dietary calcium intake (including during growth) to optimize peak bone mass, and reduction of alcohol intake and cessation of smoking to reduce the rate of bone loss.

In patients with established osteoporosis, it is important to identify and manage appropriately risk factors for falls (e.g. postural hypotension). Vitamin D deficiency should be corrected with cholecalciferol. Calcium supplements appear to increase cardiovascular risk, so increasing dietary calcium intake may be preferable.

Bisphosphonates are analogues of inorganic pyrophosphate that inhibit bone resorption and are regarded as the drug treatment of choice. They can be given intravenously if oral preparations cause gastrointestinal side effects. **Denosumab**, a monoclonal antibody against RANKL, may be used when bisphosphonates are not tolerated. **Raloxifene** (a selective oestrogen receptor modulator) reduces the risk of vertebral (but not other) fractures and appears to reduce the risk of breast cancer. Treatment with a recombinant fragment of PTH (**teriparatide**) entails daily subcutaneous injections. **Calcitriol** inhibits bone resorption but care must be taken to avoid hypercalcaemia and hypercalciuria. Hormone replacement treatment (HRT) is now mostly reserved for younger women with early menopause. Testosterone is effective in hypogonadal men but increases the risk of prostate cancer in those with normal testicular function.

> Patients who require long-term treatment with glucocorticoids are at increased risk of fragility fractures and should be considered for bone protective treatment according to local guidelines. **!**

All such drug treatment requires monitoring of bone mineral density and fracture risk to determine duration of therapy.

Paget disease of bone

Paget disease of bone is a condition of unknown aetiology (although there is some evidence that paramyxovirus infection in genetically predisposed individuals is responsible). Its incidence and severity have been decreasing in the UK. It is **characterized by increased osteoclastic activity**, which engenders increased osteoblastic activity, and thus new bone formation. The new bone that is formed is abnormal and laid down in a disorganized fashion. As a result, **bones become thickened, deformed and painful**. The most frequently affected bones are those of the pelvis, spine and skull, and the femora.

Paget disease is a disease of the elderly (see Case history 15.1). It is frequently asymptomatic: only about 5% of patients have symptoms, of which the most frequent (80%) is pain. Other features include deformity, pathological fracture, compression of adjacent tissues (e.g. the auditory nerves, causing deafness) and a steal syndrome in which the increased vascularity of the abnormal bone diverts blood flow away from adjacent tissues, causing ischaemia. Osteosarcoma is a serious but rare (<1%) complication.

Plasma ALP activity is increased, often markedly, and reflects disease activity; plasma calcium and phosphate concentrations are usually normal, although hypercalcaemia may develop if a patient with Paget disease is immobilized. It is relatively common to find an unexpectedly increased serum ALP activity in elderly subjects; if serum calcium and phosphate concentrations and liver function tests are normal, Paget disease is the most frequent cause.

The treatment of Paget disease involves the use of analgesics and, in more severe cases, bisphosphonates to reduce osteoclastic activity. Response to treatment can be monitored by measurements of serum ALP activity and P1NP, both of which should decline within a few weeks.

Chronic kidney disease–mineral and bone disorder

Patients with CKD develop a complex bone disease, primarily as a result of disturbance of the PTH–calcitriol axis. This condition is discussed in detail in Chapter 5.

Case history 15.1

History

An elderly man complained of severe pain in his pelvis and thighs and was diagnosed from radiological evidence as having Paget disease of bone. The serum ALP was 750 U/L. He was treated with oral bisphosphonates and made a good clinical recovery, although when his medication was stopped his thighs became painful again.

Results

His serum ALP activities are shown in Fig. 15.2.

Discussion

The primary defect in Paget disease is an increase in osteoclastic activity, but this causes increased osteoblastic activity, reflected by high serum ALP activities. Serial measurements can be used, as in this patient, to monitor the disease and its response to treatment.

Hyperparathyroid bone disease

Clinical evidence of bone involvement used to be a common feature of **primary hyperparathyroidism** (see Chapter 14), but most patients with hyperparathyroidism are now identified when hypercalcaemia is found incidentally. They are usually asymptomatic and have no abnormal physical signs or radiographic findings. Plasma ALP activity is normal unless there is significant bone involvement.

The characteristic features of hyperparathyroid bone disease include bone pain and evidence of localized areas of bone resorption on radiography, for example, subperiosteal bone resorption, small, widespread lucencies in the skull ('pepper-pot skull') and bone cysts ('brown tumours', composed of osteoclasts and fibrous tissue). These features are due to increased osteoclastic activity, and any increase in plasma ALP is due to an associated increase in osteoblastic activity.

Other metabolic bone diseases

Osteogenesis imperfecta (brittle bone disease) is a group of disorders characterized by extreme fragility of bone; in 90% of cases, it is due to one of several genetically determined abnormalities of collagen synthesis. It typically presents in children with fractures and bone deformities, and must be distinguished from fractures caused by non-accidental injury. Most affected children have characteristically blue sclerae. There are no simple biochemical investigations to aid in its diagnosis. Management involves the use of bisphosphonates, physiotherapy and other measures to protect bones against fracture. **Osteopetrosis** is caused by a variety of genetic disorders affecting the number or

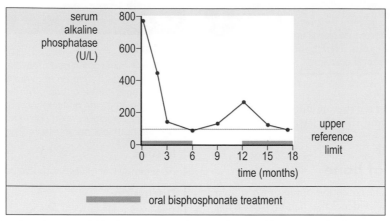

Fig. 15.2 Serum alkaline phosphatase activities in a patient with Paget disease of bone. Periods of treatment with oral bisphosphonates are indicated. After a good response to the first period of treatment, the serum alkaline phosphatase began to rise, indicating recrudescence of the disease; a good response was again achieved when treatment was restarted.

function of osteoclasts, thereby interfering with normal bone resorption. Most patients present in infancy with poor growth and blindness or deafness caused by cranial nerve entrapment. The bone marrow space is occluded by excess bone with resulting failure of haematopoiesis. Some forms can be cured by bone marrow transplantation, which provides healthy osteoclast precursors.

Articular Disease

Joints can be affected by a wide variety of diseases, both specifically and as part of multisystem disease. **Osteoarthritis, rheumatoid arthritis** and other inflammatory arthritides are a major source of pain and disability. For most, the role of the biochemistry laboratory in management is limited: one example is the measurement of C-reactive protein (see p. 289) to monitor inflammatory conditions. For one group, however, biochemical tests are important in both diagnosis and management: these are the crystalline arthritides, in particular, gout.

Measurement of **autoantibodies** plays an important role in the diagnosis of rheumatoid arthritis and other inflammatory arthritides. Plasma concentrations of rheumatoid factor (RhF) are raised in the majority of patients with rheumatoid disease, although a small number of apparently healthy people also have raised concentrations. RhF is an antibody (usually immunoglobulin M, the type detected by most assays for RhF), directed against the Fc portion of the IgG molecule. Anticyclic citrullinated peptide (CCP) antibodies are also frequently present in the plasma. Their detection appears to be more sensitive for diagnosis, and high titres are associated with a greater risk

of developing joint damage. Anti-CCP antibodies may be detectable several years before rheumatoid disease becomes apparent clinically. Approximately 30% of patients with rheumatoid arthritis are also positive for antinuclear antibodies, but these are particularly associated with **systemic lupus erythematosus** (SLE). Both these conditions (particularly SLE) can affect many tissues other than joints.

Laboratory investigations are required for monitoring treatment of rheumatoid arthritis when disease-modifying drugs (e.g. methotrexate) or 'biologics' (monoclonal antibodies) are used. The former can cause liver damage and bone marrow toxicity, and the latter can induce antibody formation which reduces the efficacy of treatment (see pp. 366 and 370).

Gout and hyperuricaemia
Introduction

Clinical gout is the result of the **deposition of crystals of monosodium urate** in the cartilage, synovium and synovial fluid of joints as a consequence of hyperuricaemia. It is the commonest inflammatory joint disease in men older than 40 years. **Uric acid** is the end product of purine metabolism in humans. At physiological pH, uric acid is 98% ionized and is therefore present mainly as the urate ion. In the extracellular fluid (ECF), where sodium is the major cation, uric acid effectively exists as a solution of its sodium salt, monosodium urate. This salt has low solubility, and the ECF becomes saturated at concentrations a little greater than those that normally prevail. In patients with hyperuricaemia, there is thus a tendency for crystals of monosodium urate to form. In addition to acute arthropathy, other manifestations of gout include kidney stones (which may lead to CKD) and tophi (accretions of sodium urate in soft tissues). A sudden increase in urate production, typically seen as a consequence of treatment of haematological malignancy (tumour lysis syndrome, see p. 354), can lead to widespread crystallization in the renal tubules, causing obstruction and acute kidney injury (acute **urate nephropathy**). This is usually avoidable by giving allopurinol (see later); but if it does occur, it can be treated with rasburicase, a recombinant fungus-derived uricase (see lightbulb p. 283).

Uric acid metabolism

Purine nucleotides are essential components of nucleic acids: they are intimately involved in energy transformation and phosphorylation reactions, and act as intracellular messengers. There are three sources of purines in humans: the diet, degradation of endogenous nucleotides and *de novo* synthesis (Fig. 15.3). As purines are metabolized to uric acid, the body urate pool (and hence plasma concentration) depends on the relative rates of both urate formation from these sources and urate excretion. Urate is excreted by both the kidneys and the gut, with renal excretion accounting for approximately two-thirds of the total. Urate secreted into the gut is metabolized to carbon dioxide and ammonia by bacterial action (uricolysis).

Urate handling by the kidney is complex (Fig. 15.4). It is filtered at the glomeruli and almost totally reabsorbed in the proximal convoluted tubules; distally, both secretion and reabsorption occur. Normal urate clearance is about 10% of the filtered load. In healthy subjects, urate excretion increases if the filtered load is increased. In CKD, the plasma concentration rises only when the glomerular filtration rate declines to less than ~20 mL/min.

Dietary purines account for about 30% of excreted urate. The introduction of a purine-free diet typically reduces plasma urate concentrations by only 10–20%.

The **metabolic pathways** involved in uric acid synthesis are shown in Fig. 15.5. *De novo* synthesis leads to the formation of inosine monophosphate (IMP), which can be converted to the nucleotides adenosine monophosphate (AMP) and guanosine monophosphate (GMP). Nucleotide degradation involves the formation of the corresponding nucleosides (inosine, adenosine and guanosine); these are then metabolized to purines. The purine derived from IMP is hypoxanthine, which is converted by the enzyme xanthine oxidase first to xanthine and then to uric acid. Guanine can be metabolized to xanthine (and so to uric acid) directly, but adenine cannot. However, AMP can be converted to IMP by the enzyme AMP deaminase and, at the nucleoside level, adenosine can be converted to inosine. Thus, surplus GMP and AMP can be converted to uric acid and excreted.

However, the excretion of uric acid represents the waste of a metabolic investment, because purine synthesis

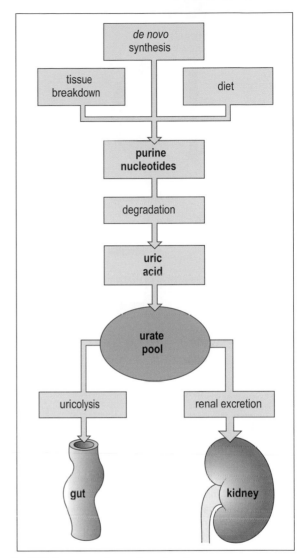

Fig 15.3 Sources and excretion of urate.

requires considerable energy expenditure. Pathways exist whereby purines can be salvaged and converted back to their parent nucleotides. For guanine and hypoxanthine, this is accomplished by the enzyme hypoxanthine–guanine phosphoribosyl transferase (HGPRT), and for adenine by adenine phosphoribosyl transferase (APRT).

Plasma urate concentrations are, in general, higher in men than in women. Marked increases occur at puberty in males (there is a lesser increase in females at this time) and perimenopausally in women (Fig. 15.6). Urate concentrations tend to be higher in people living in the developed world and in those who are obese. There is considerable

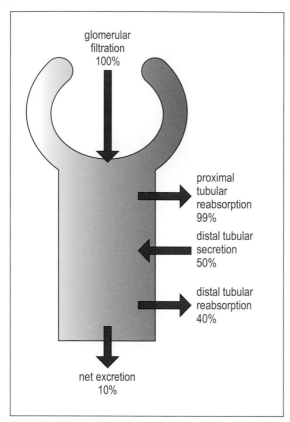

glomerular
filtration
100%

proximal
tubular
reabsorption
99%

distal tubular
secretion
50%

distal tubular
reabsorption
40%

net excretion
10%

Fig. 15.4 Urate excretion in the kidneys.

genetically determined variation in plasma urate concentrations between different ethnic groups, with particularly high concentrations, for example, in Polynesian and Maori people.

In adult men in the UK, the upper limit of the reference range is usually taken as 430 μmol/L (360 μmol/L in women). In an aqueous solution of pH 7.4 ([H$^+$] 40 nmol/L), at 37°C, and with an ionic strength similar to that of plasma, the solubility of monosodium urate is 570 μmol/L; in plasma, the presence of protein appears to reduce this somewhat.

Hyperuricaemia

Hyperuricaemia may occur because of increased formation of uric acid, decreased excretion or a combination of both. Some causes of increased formation are given in Box 15.2.

When hyperuricaemia is due to decreased excretion, it is renal excretion that is usually affected. Indeed, in hyperuricaemia, the total amount of urate removed by uricolysis in the gut is increased. Reference to Fig. 15.4 will show that decreased renal urate excretion could result from decreases in filtration or tubular secretion. Plasma urate concentration rises late in CKD, but many factors can affect tubular function and thereby cause hyperuricaemia at an earlier stage: the more important of these are given in Box 15.2. Excessive ethanol intake probably increases adenine nucleotide degradation (and some alcoholic beverages contain high concentrations of purines), but any increase in lactate production caused by ethanol may also impair urate excretion.

Gout

Acute gout is characterized by **severe joint pain of rapid onset associated with swelling and redness** (see Case history 15.2). The risk of gout increases exponentially with increasing plasma urate concentrations and thus with age. The risk is increased 50-fold once plasma concentrations exceed 540 μmol/L. This is true for both men and women, although women are less likely to develop such high concentrations. However, although hyperuricaemia is a prerequisite for the development of gout, gout by no means always complicates hyperuricaemia. Indeed, some 85% of people with hyperuricaemia remain asymptomatic throughout life.

Gout can be precipitated by a sudden change (either increase or decrease) in urate concentration. When urate concentration has fallen rapidly in a hyperuricaemic individual (e.g. as a result of a change in diet, decrease in alcohol consumption or treatment with a hypouricaemic drug), the plasma urate concentration may not be elevated when the patient presents with gout. The solubility of monosodium urate declines steeply with decreasing temperature and this may, to some extent, explain the tendency for the more peripheral joints, which have lower intraarticular temperatures, to be more frequently affected.

Monosodium urate crystals forming in joints are engulfed by neutrophil leukocytes and damage the lysosomal membranes of these cells, thus causing cellular disruption. The generation of superoxide free radicals and release of lysosomal enzymes into the joint precipitates an acute inflammatory reaction. The release of interleukins (particularly IL-1β) and other inflammatory mediators from monocytes and tissue macrophages also provides an inflammatory stimulus.

Gout is customarily defined as **primary** (idiopathic) or **secondary** (when a condition known to cause hyperuricaemia is present). However, gout is uncommon when hyperuricaemia develops secondarily to other conditions. The tendency for hyperuricaemia and gout to be familial has led to investigation for a causal inherited metabolic defect. Although there are a few rare conditions in which such a defect does lead to hyperuricaemia, none has been found in the great majority of patients with primary gout. Some 90% of patients appear to excrete urate at a rate inappropriately

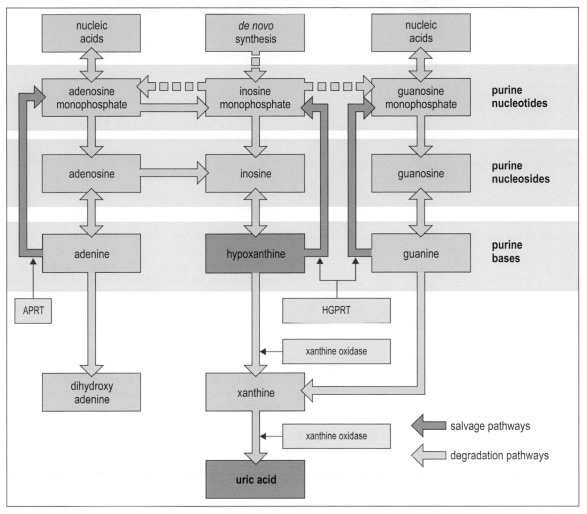

Fig. 15.5 Simplified diagram of the pathways of purine nucleotide metabolism and uric acid synthesis in humans. APRT, adenine phosphoribosyl transferase; HGPRT, hypoxanthine–guanine phosphoribosyl transferase.

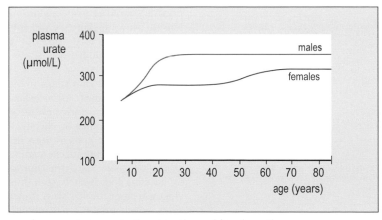

Fig. 15.6 Variation in mean plasma urate concentrations in males and females with age.

low for the plasma concentration, whereas about 10% have excessive urate production. Clearly defined inherited disorders (see later) are responsible for fewer than 1% of cases. Dietary factors and ethanol ingestion exacerbate hyperuricaemia in about 50% of patients, but although their amelioration may reduce plasma urate concentrations somewhat, these usually remain elevated. Gout is rare in women before menopause, but the incidence increases markedly thereafter.

Patients with gout frequently have hyperlipidaemia (particularly hypertriglyceridaemia) and often other features of the metabolic syndrome (p. 309). Hyperuricaemia is associated with the resistance to insulin that is characteristic of this syndrome. However, although the syndrome itself is an important risk factor for cardiovascular disease, it is uncertain whether this is the case with hyperuricaemia alone.

Diagnosis. The **diagnosis of gout is primarily clinical** but is supported by the demonstration of **hyperuricaemia** and can be confirmed by the presence of tophi or of mono-sodium urate crystals in the synovial fluid. These crystals are typically needle shaped, 2 to 10 μm long, and are seen within neutrophils. They show strong negative birefringence when viewed under polarized light.

The differential diagnosis includes other crystalline arthropathies and septic arthritis. Septic arthritis can coexist with gout, and blood and joint fluid should be cultured if there is systemic toxicity. Leucocytosis and an increase in the plasma concentrations of inflammatory markers occur in both conditions.

Management. **Non-steroidal anti-inflammatory drugs** are the usual first-line treatment for acute gout (although not aspirin, which causes urate retention in usual doses). **Colchicine** is also effective but is less well tolerated. Steroids (intraarticular or systemic) are sometimes required.

None of these agents affects the hyperuricaemia. This can be treated by dietary measures, avoidance of alcohol and, if possible, of relevant drugs (especially diuretics). Urate-lowering drugs, of which the most widely used is allopurinol, are used for long-term treatment when there have been recurrent acute attacks of gout, when there are kidney stones with hyperuricaemia, especially if there is kidney damage, and in tophaceous gout. **Allopurinol** is an inhibitor of xanthine oxidase and thus inhibits the synthesis of urate from xanthine. It decreases plasma urate concentration and urinary urate excretion; urinary xanthine excretion is increased, but xanthine is more water soluble than urate. The aim should be to lower the plasma urate concentration to <300 μmol/L. **Febuxostat** is an effective alternative for patients who cannot tolerate allopurinol.

Starting treatment with hypouricaemic drugs may precipitate an acute attack of gout, and most guidelines recommend avoiding them during, or for several weeks after, an acute episode. Colchicine is effective for prophylaxis if recurrent acute attacks occur or attacks occur during treatment. Patients with **asymptomatic hyperuricaemia** should be given dietary and lifestyle advice, but drug treatment is rarely indicated; features of the metabolic syndrome, if present, should be treated appropriately. In treating hypertension, thiazide diuretics and some other drugs (see Box 15.2) should be used with care because they can cause renal urate retention.

Natural history. Four stages in the natural history of gout have been described. *Asymptomatic hyperuricaemia* can be present for years before an *acute attack* is precipitated by, for example, trauma or dietary indiscretion. Symptom-free periods of months or years follow ('*intercritical gout*'), punctuated by acute attacks leading, if untreated, to *chronic tophaceous gout*. Since the introduction of allopurinol, tophaceous gout is rarely seen. It tends to occur mainly in elderly women treated with diuretics (in particular, thiazides, which inhibit renal tubular secretion of urate) for

---

Box 15.2 Causes of hyperuricaemia

Increased urate formation	Decreased renal urate excretion
Primary	**Primary**
increased purine synthesis:	idiopathic
idiopathic	
inherited metabolic	**Secondary**
disease	chronic kidney disease
	increased renal reabsorption/
Secondary	decreased secretion:
excessive dietary purine	thiazide diuretics
intake	loop diuretics (e.g.
disordered ATP	furosemide)
metabolism:	beta blockers
ethanol	salicylates (low doses)[a]
tissue hypoxia	angiotensin-converting
increased nucleic acid	enzyme inhibitors
turnover:	some angiotensin II
malignant disease	receptor blockers (not
psoriasis	losartan)
cytotoxic drugs	organic acids (e.g. lactic
	acid, hence ethanol)
	lead

[a]Note that salicylates reduce urate excretion at low doses only; at high doses (>4 g/24 h) aspirin is uricosuric because it blocks the tubular reabsorption of urate.
ATP, adenosine triphosphate.

many years rather than as a sequel to recurrent attacks of acute gout.

Rare causes of hyperuricaemia

There are a number of rare, inherited metabolic diseases associated with hyperuricaemia and gout (Table 15.3). In all of them, hyperuricaemia results from increased uric acid synthesis.

Hypouricaemia

Hypouricaemia is uncommon and, in itself, clinically inconsequential. It may be caused by either decreased urate synthesis or increased excretion, and thus is seen in congenital xanthine oxidase deficiency (xanthinuria), severe liver disease and renal tubular disorders such as the Fanconi syndrome. It can also result from excessive medication with allopurinol and the use of uricosuric drugs such as probenecid.

Case history 15.2

History

An obese 55-year-old businessman was awoken from sleep by excruciating pain in his left first metatarsophalangeal joint. He was unable to put his foot to the floor. One year previously he had had an episode of renal colic but had declared himself too busy to be investigated in connection with this.

Examination

The affected joint was hot, swollen, red and extremely tender.

Results (see Appendix for reference ranges)

Serum: urate   780 μmol/L

Summary

Very high urate concentration, well above the solubility limit for sodium urate.

Discussion

This is the classic presentation of gout. The onset is often sudden, nocturnal and monoarticular. In 70% of patients, the metatarsophalangeal joint of the great toe is the first to be affected. The classic signs of inflammation were present and hyperuricaemia was confirmed. In this patient, the previous episode of renal colic may well have been caused by a urate kidney stone. Gout is more common in men than in women and is associated with obesity, hypertriglyceridaemia, hypertension, diabetes and excessive alcohol intake.

Other crystalline arthropathies

Gout is not the only crystalline arthropathy. The deposition of **calcium pyrophosphate** in joints may mimic gout clinically (**pseudogout**). It can also cause a chronic arthropathy that mimics and overlaps with osteoarthritis. Calcium pyrophosphate crystals may be demonstrable in synovial fluid. They are characteristically rhomboid or rod shaped and show weak positive birefringence when viewed under polarized light.

Effect of rasburicase on serum urate measurement

Laboratory methods for the measurement of serum urate produce falsely low results in patients who are taking the drug rasburicase to prevent acute hyperuricaemia during cytotoxic cancer chemotherapy (see p. 354). This is due to the urate oxidase activity of the drug; it continues to metabolize urate *in vitro* (i.e. in the specimen container). Monitoring of plasma urate concentration is rarely necessary after rasburicase treatment has been started, but if it is, the sample must be transported to the laboratory on ice and assayed as quickly as possible.

Table 15.3 Some inherited metabolic diseases associated with hyperuricaemia

Enzyme abnormality	Consequence
hypoxanthine–guanine phosphoribosyl transferase deficiency (Lesch–Nyhan syndrome and less severe variants)	decreased activity of salvage pathway decreases purine reutilization, and thus increases uric acid synthesis
glucose 6-phosphatase deficiency (glycogen storage disease type I)	increased metabolism of glucose 6-phosphate through pentose phosphate pathway increases formation of ribose 5-phosphate, a substrate for purine nucleotide synthesis hyperlactataemia decreases uric acid secretion in renal tubules
phosphoribosyl pyrophosphate synthetase (PRPP synthetase) variant (with increased activity)	PRPP is a substrate for purine nucleotide synthesis and also activates the rate-limiting enzyme

Other disorders include adenosine monophosphate deaminase deficiency and hereditary fructose intolerance.

Chondrocalcinosis (calcium deposition in articular cartilage) may also be present. Calcium pyrophosphate arthropathy is predominantly a disease of the elderly. The condition may be familial, but most cases occur in association with hyperparathyroidism, haemochromatosis or other metabolic disorders.

Hydroxyapatite crystals can occur in joints. This is often asymptomatic but can occasionally cause an acute synovitis clinically resembling gout. Rarely, other crystals occur in joints, for example, calcium oxalate in patients with type 1 hyperoxaluria.

SUMMARY

- The **metabolic bone diseases** include osteoporosis, osteomalacia, Paget disease, hyperparathyroid bone disease and chronic kidney disease–mineral and bone disorder. Characteristic biochemical changes in plasma occur in all of them, with the exception of osteoporosis.
- **Osteomalacia** is usually due to deficiency or abnormal metabolism of vitamin D but may also be seen in phosphate wasting disorders; **rickets** is its childhood equivalent. In **osteoporosis**, a decrease in osteoid and mineral reduces the strength of bone and predisposes it to fracture. It is a major cause of morbidity and mortality in the elderly, particularly in women. **Paget disease** is also primarily a condition of the elderly; increased osteoclastic activity and abnormal new bone formation cause bone pain and, in severe cases, deformity.

- **Gout** is an arthropathy caused by the precipitation of monosodium urate crystals in synovial joints. This occurs when plasma urate concentrations are elevated. Secondary causes of **hyperuricaemia** include kidney disease, thiazide diuretics, increased cell turnover and a high intake of purine-rich foods. Gout and hyperuricaemia show a strong familial incidence. Some rare inherited defects in purine metabolism that cause hyperuricaemia have been described, but in the majority of patients there is no such defect, and hyperuricaemia is thought to be due to decreased renal urate excretion. Gout usually presents as an acute arthritis but can lead to chronic joint disease, and crystals of monosodium urate can be deposited in tissues and in the renal tubules, causing an obstructive uropathy.

Chapter | **16** |

Plasma proteins and enzymes

Introduction

Proteins are present in all body fluids, but it is the proteins of the blood plasma that are examined most frequently for diagnostic purposes. More than 100 individual proteins have a physiological function in the plasma. Their principal functions, with relevant examples, are indicated in Table 16.1. Quantitatively, the single most important protein is **albumin**. With the exception of fibrinogen, the other proteins are known collectively as **globulins**. Changes in the concentrations of individual proteins occur in many conditions, and their measurement can provide useful diagnostic information.

Some plasma proteins are **enzymes** (e.g. renin, coagulation factors). In addition to these, many primarily intracellular enzymes are detectable in plasma as a result of their loss from cells during normal cell turnover. The measurement of such enzymes provides a sensitive (although often relatively non-specific) indicator of **tissue damage**. Most of these enzymes are described in chapters that describe conditions in which their measurement is of particular value, but some general principles of the use of enzyme measurements are discussed in this chapter.

Measurement of Plasma Proteins

Total plasma protein

In very general terms, variations in plasma protein concentrations can be caused by changes in any of three factors: the rate of protein **synthesis**, the rate of **removal** and the **volume of distribution**.

The concentration of proteins in plasma is affected by **posture**: an increase in concentration of 10–20% occurs within 30 min of becoming upright after a period of recumbency. Also, if a **tourniquet** is applied before venipuncture, a significant rise in protein concentration can occur within a few minutes. In both cases, the change in protein concentration is caused by increased diffusion of fluid from the vascular into the interstitial compartment. These effects must be borne in mind when blood is being drawn for the determination of protein concentration.

Only changes in the more abundant plasma proteins (i.e. albumin or immunoglobulins) will have a significant effect on the total protein concentration. Except when patients have been given blood or proteins intravenously, a rapid increase in total plasma protein concentration is always due to a decrease in the volume of distribution (in effect, to dehydration). A rapid decrease is often the result of an increase in plasma volume. Thus, changes in plasma protein concentration can provide a valuable aid to the assessment of a patient's **state of hydration**.

The total protein concentration of plasma can also fall rapidly if capillary permeability increases, because protein will diffuse out into the interstitial space. This can be seen, for example, in patients with **sepsis** or **the systemic inflammatory response syndrome**. Causes of increased and decreased total plasma protein concentration are summarized in Table 16.2.

Capillary zone electrophoresis of proteins

Capillary zone electrophoresis is commonly used for the detection of **paraproteins** (monoclonal proteins produced by tumours of B-lymphocyte origin, particularly myeloma). The technique separates the proteins into distinct regions (**albumin, α_1- and α_2-globulins, β_1- and β_2-globulins and γ-globulins)** and is performed on serum rather than plasma, because the clotting of plasma to form serum removes fibrinogen. The latter produces a large peak in the β_2 region that can complicate interpretation of the

Table 16.1 Functions of plasma proteins

Function	Example
transport	thyroxine-binding globulin (thyroid hormones) apolipoproteins (cholesterol, triglyceride) transferrin (iron)
humoral immunity	immunoglobulins
maintenance of oncotic pressure	all proteins, particularly albumin
enzymes	renin coagulation factors complement proteins
protease inhibitors	α_1-antitrypsin
buffering	all proteins

Table 16.2 Causes of changes in total plasma protein concentration

Increase	
hypergammaglobulinaemia, paraproteinaemia	↑ protein synthesis
artefactual	haemoconcentration caused by stasis of blood during venepuncture
dehydration	↓ volume of distribution
Decrease	
malnutrition and malabsorption liver disease humoral immunodeficiency	↓ protein synthesis
overhydration increased capillary permeability	↑ volume of distribution
protein-losing states catabolic states	↑ excretion/catabolism

Table 16.3 Principal plasma proteins

Class	Protein	Approximate mean serum concentration (g/L)
	prealbumin	0.25
	albumin	40
α_1-globulin	α_1-antitrypsin α_1-acid glycoprotein	2.9 1.0
α_2-globulin	haptoglobin α_2-macroglobulin caeruloplasmin	2.0 2.6 0.35
β_1-globulin	transferrin low-density lipoprotein	3.0 1.0
β_2-globulin	complement components (C3)	1.0
γ-globulins	IgG IgA IgM IgD IgE	14.0 3.5 1.5 0.03 trace

Many other important proteins are present in only very low concentrations, for example, thyroxine-binding globulin, transcortin and vitamin D-binding globulin.

scan. Plasma proteins are often still classified into groups according to their electrophoretic mobility (Table 16.3), although this classification has no relevance in relation to their function, with the exception that most of the normal immunoglobulins migrate (and are still often referred to) as γ-globulins.

Fig. 16.1 shows diagrammatically the appearance of normal serum (see Fig. 16.1A) and serum containing a paraprotein (see Fig. 16.1B) after capillary zone electrophoresis. Note that in Fig. 16.1B, there is a decrease in normal immunoglobulins, as characteristically occurs in patients with paraproteinaemia caused by myeloma (see p. 292). Paraproteins typically migrate in the γ region but (especially the IgA class) may migrate towards the β region. Fig. 16.1C shows a polyclonal increase in immunoglobulins (as may occur in some autoimmune diseases and chronic infections).

Some laboratories still use agarose gel electrophoresis to separate proteins, including paraproteins, into distinct bands, but this is a less precise technique.

Specific Plasma Proteins

Albumin

Albumin, the most abundant plasma protein, makes the major contribution (~80%) to the oncotic pressure of plasma. Oncotic (or colloid osmotic) pressure is the osmotic pressure due to the presence of proteins and is an important determinant of the distribution of extracellular

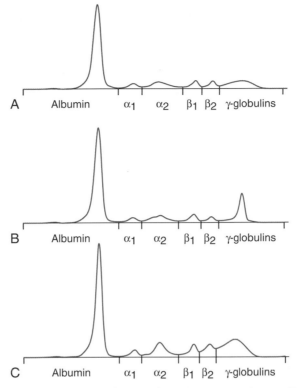

Fig. 16.1 Some typical findings on capillary zone electrophoresis of proteins. **A,** Normal serum. **B,** Sharp peak in the γ region representing a paraprotein, with reduction in the surrounding γ-globulins indicating immune paresis. **C,** Polyclonal increase in γ-globulins.

fluid (ECF) between the intravascular and extravascular compartments.

In **hypoalbuminaemic** states, the decreased plasma oncotic pressure disturbs the equilibrium between plasma and interstitial fluid, with the result that there is a decrease in the movement of the interstitial fluid back into the blood at the venular end of the capillaries (Fig. 16.2). The accumulation of interstitial fluid is seen clinically as **oedema**. The relative decrease in plasma volume results in a fall in renal blood flow. This stimulates the secretion of renin, and hence of aldosterone, through the formation of angiotensin (secondary aldosteronism, see p. 187). This results in **sodium retention**, and thus an increase in ECF volume, which exacerbates the oedema.

There are many possible causes of hypoalbuminaemia (Box 16.1), a combination of which may be implicated in individual cases. For example, in a patient with malabsorption caused by Crohn disease, a low albumin concentration may reflect both **decreased synthesis** (decreased supply of amino acids because of malabsorption) and

increased loss (directly into the gut from ulcerated mucosa).

Hyperalbuminaemia can be either an artefact, usually as a result of venous stasis during blood collection, or a result of dehydration. Albumin synthesis is increased in some pathological states as a response to protein loss, but this never causes hyperalbuminaemia.

Measurements of albumin concentration are frequently used in relation to the assessment of patients who have **malnutrition**. This topic is discussed in detail in Chapter 8, but it should be noted that, because of its relatively long half-life (~20 days), plasma albumin concentration is not a useful marker of the response to nutritional support in the short term (<10 days).

Low concentrations of albumin are characteristic of chronic liver disease, being caused by both decreased synthesis and an increase in the volume of distribution as a result of fluid retention and the formation of ascites. Because of its relatively long half-life in the plasma, albumin concentration is usually normal in acute hepatitis.

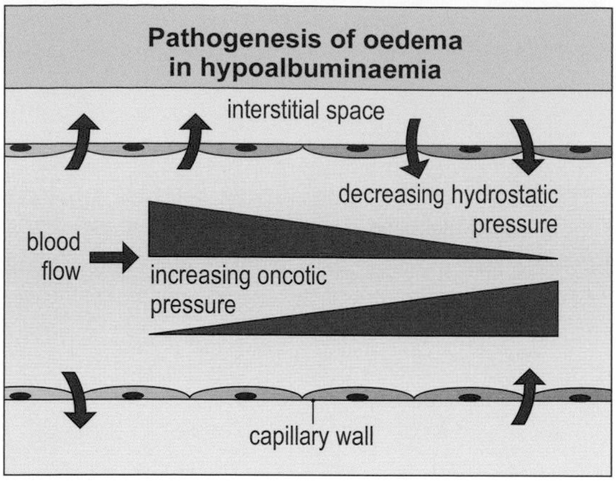

Pathogenesis of oedema in hypoalbuminaemia

interstitial space

decreasing hydrostatic pressure

blood flow

increasing oncotic pressure

capillary wall

Fig. 16.2 Pathogenesis of oedema in hypoalbuminaemia. The normal balance of hydrostatic and oncotic pressures is such that there is net movement of fluid out of the capillaries at their arteriolar ends and net movement in at their venular ends (indicated here by arrows). Oedema can thus be caused by an increase in capillary hydrostatic pressure, a decrease in plasma oncotic pressure or an increase in capillary permeability.

Box 16.1 Causes of hypoalbuminaemia

Decreased synthesis

malnutrition
malabsorption
liver disease

Increased volume of distribution

overhydration
increased capillary permeability
  septicaemia
  hypoxia

Increased excretion/degradation

nephrotic syndrome
protein-losing enteropathies
burns
haemorrhage
catabolic states
  severe sepsis
  fever
  trauma
  malignant disease

Albumin is a high-capacity, low-affinity **transport protein** for many substances, such as thyroid hormones, calcium and fatty acids. The influence of low plasma albumin concentration on measurements of thyroid hormones and calcium is considered on pp. 196 and 256, respectively. Albumin binds unconjugated bilirubin, and hypoalbuminaemia increases the risk of kernicterus in infants with unconjugated hyperbilirubinaemia (see p. 383). Salicylates, which displace bilirubin from albumin, can have a similar effect.

Many drugs are bound to albumin in the blood, and a decrease in albumin concentration can have important pharmacokinetic consequences. Phenytoin, for example, is highly protein bound, so a decrease in plasma albumin, will increase the concentration of free drug, and thus the risk of toxicity, if the dose of phenytoin is not reduced. Some laboratories provide phenytoin concentration values adjusted for serum albumin.

A number of molecular variants of albumin exist. In **bisalbuminaemia**, the variant protein has a slightly different electrophoretic mobility from normal albumin, and a pair of albumin peaks is seen on electrophoresis: there are no clinical consequences. **Analbuminaemia** is a rare, inherited condition in which the plasma albumin concentration is <1 g/L. People with this condition tend to suffer episodic mild oedema, but are otherwise well.

α₁-Antitrypsin

α_1-Antitrypsin, an α_1-globulin produced by the liver, is a naturally occurring inhibitor of proteases. Inherited deficiencies of α_1-antitrypsin synthesis can cause **emphysema**, occurring at a younger age (third and fourth decades of life) than is usual for this condition, and **neonatal hepatitis**, which can progress to cirrhosis.

Homozygotes for the normal protein are termed Pi (protease inhibitor) MM. More than 70 alleles of the gene have been described. α_1-Antitrypsin deficiency is most frequently due to homozygosity for the Z allele (PiZZ), with this genotype having a frequency of about 1 in 3000 in the UK. In affected individuals, plasma α_1-antitrypsin concentration is reduced to 10–15% of normal. The defect is due to a single amino acid substitution, which causes the protein to form aggregates that cannot be secreted from the liver and, as a result, cause liver damage. The development of emphysema is due to a lack of natural inhibition of the enzyme neutrophil elastase, which results in destructive changes in the lung. Not all PiZZ homozygotes develop liver or lung disease, but the manifestations tend to be similar within families. The risk of development of emphysema is greatly increased by smoking: cigarette smoke oxidizes a thiol group at the active site of α_1-antitrypsin, decreasing the inhibitory activity of what small amounts of the protein are present.

PiMZ heterozygotes have plasma α_1-antitrypsin concentrations that are about 60% of normal; there is probably only a very slightly increased tendency for these individuals to develop lung disease compared with normal PiMM homozygotes. Although homozygotes for the relatively common S allele have markedly reduced α_1-antitrypsin activity, they rarely present clinically. PiSZ heterozygotes, however, have increased susceptibility to lung disease, albeit not to the same extent as those with PiZZ.

Accurate phenotyping and genotyping are required for the screening of an affected individual's family members. Isoelectric focusing is a technique that allows identification of individual protein variants; allele-specific oligonucleotides can be used to determine the genotype. α_1-Antitrypsin is an **acute phase protein** (see later). Its concentration increases in acute inflammatory states, and this may be sufficient to bring a genetically determined low concentration of the protein, for example, in a PiMZ heterozygote, into the reference range. However, even with an acute phase response, the α_1-antitrypsin concentration in PiZZ homozygotes never rises to >50% of the lower reference limit.

Haptoglobin

Haptoglobin is an α_2-globulin. Its function is to **bind free haemoglobin** released into the plasma during intravascular haemolysis. The haemoglobin–haptoglobin complexes formed are removed by the reticuloendothelial system, thereby conserving iron, and the concentration of haptoglobin falls correspondingly. Thus, a low plasma haptoglobin concentration can be indicative of **intravascular haemolysis**. However, low concentrations due to decreased synthesis are seen in chronic liver disease, metastatic disease and severe sepsis.

Haptoglobin is an acute phase protein and its concentration also increases in hypoalbuminaemic states such as the nephrotic syndrome. It demonstrates considerable genetic polymorphism: the molecule consists of pairs of two types of subunit, α and β, and although the β-chain is constant, there are three alleles for the α-chain. These different proteins appear to be functionally similar.

α_2-Macroglobulin

α_2-Macroglobulin is a high molecular mass protein (820 kDa) that constitutes approximately one-third of the α_2-globulins. Hepatic synthesis of the protein increases in the nephrotic syndrome and, because it is too large to be filtered even through a damaged glomerular basement membrane, plasma concentrations rise. Like α_1-antitrypsin, α_2-macroglobulin is an inhibitor of proteases, although it has a broader spectrum of activity.

Caeruloplasmin

Caeruloplasmin is a copper-containing protein, which functions as a ferroxidase and superoxide scavenger. Its synthesis and plasma concentration are greatly reduced in **Wilson disease** (p. 118). Its concentration is increased in pregnancy (an oestrogen-related effect). It is an acute phase protein.

Transferrin and ferritin

Transferrin is a β_1-globulin and is the major **iron-transporting protein** in the plasma; normally ~30% saturated with iron, it is characteristically >60% saturated in **haemochromatosis**. Ferritin is the principal iron storage protein, and measurement of its plasma concentration is used as a test for assessing body iron stores. Transferrin and ferritin are discussed in more detail in Chapter 8. The plasma concentration of carbohydrate-deficient transferrin can be used to assess exposure to ethanol (see p. 113), although it is neither a specific nor a sensitive test.

Acute phase proteins and the acute phase response

The term 'acute phase response' encompasses a complex range of physiological changes that occur after trauma and in burns, infection, inflammation and other related conditions. It comprises **haemodynamic changes**, increases in the activity of the **coagulation** and **fibrinolytic** systems, **leucocytosis**, changes in the concentration of many **plasma proteins** and **systemic effects**, particularly **pyrexia**. It is mediated by a host of cytokines, tumour necrosis factor and vasoactive substances.

Increases occur in the plasma concentrations of C-reactive protein (CRP) and procalcitonin (see later), protease inhibitors, caeruloplasmin, α_1-acid glycoprotein, fibrinogen and haptoglobins: these are a result of increased synthesis, mediated primarily by interleukin-6 (IL-6) and other cytokines. At the same time, there are **decreases** in the concentration of albumin, prealbumin and transferrin: these are mainly a result of increased vascular permeability, mediated by prostaglandins, histamine and other vasoactive substances.

CRP is so called because of its property of binding to a polysaccharide (fraction C) from the cell walls of pneumococci. It may have a general function in defence against bacteria and foreign substances. Its concentration can increase 30-fold from a normal value of <5 mg/L during the acute phase response, for which it is a valuable marker, particularly in the context of monitoring patients with inflammatory conditions such as rheumatoid arthritis and Crohn disease. It is both more sensitive and more specific than measurements of the **erythrocyte sedimentation rate** (ESR) and **plasma viscosity** in this respect. The CRP concentration begins to rise at about 6 h after the initiation of an acute phase response and reaches a peak after about 48 h before beginning to fall if the inflammatory stimulus remits. The concentrations of α_1-acid glycoprotein and fibrinogen rise and fall more slowly: peak concentrations occur at about 70 and 90 h, respectively.

A raised CRP concentration is unequivocal evidence of an inflammatory response, but viral infections usually cause only a small rise in CRP, and some autoimmune diseases, for example, systemic lupus erythematosus (SLE) and scleroderma, do not cause any increase.

Procalcitonin is a 116 amino acid protein that is normally produced by neuroendocrine cells in the lungs and intestine and also by the C cells of the thyroid where it undergoes cleavage to produce calcitonin. It is another acute phase protein and its plasma concentration increases to particularly high levels in response to infection owing to increased gene expression in most differentiated cell types. It is not a substitute for CRP as a marker of an acute phase response, but its measurement may provide additional information, because it appears to have greater sensitivity and specificity for bacterial infection than CRP, and it appears to be a better prognostic indicator and particularly helpful in reducing unnecessary antibiotic prescribing.

Other plasma proteins

Measurements of other plasma proteins may provide useful information in particular circumstances. Measurement of **coagulation factors** (e.g. fibrinogen, factor VIII) is usually conducted in haematology laboratories and is essential in the investigation of some bleeding disorders. Measurement of the proteins of the **complement system** is of considerable value in the investigation of some diseases with an immunological basis. The **apolipoproteins** are considered in detail in Chapter 17. The importance of hormone-binding proteins, such as cortisol-binding globulin and sex hormone-binding globulin, is considered in Chapters 10 and 12, respectively. Plasma proteins used in the assessment of **nutritional status** are discussed in Chapter 8. Measurement of the plasma concentration of β_2-**microglobulin** is of value in monitoring patients with myeloma (see p. 294). The measurement of plasma proteins derived from tumours (**tumour markers**) is discussed in Chapter 20.

Immunoglobulins

The immunoglobulins are a group of plasma proteins that function as antibodies, recognizing and binding foreign antigens. This facilitates the destruction of these antigens by the cellular immune system.

Because every immunoglobulin molecule is specific for one antigenic determinant, or epitope, there are vast numbers of different immunoglobulins. All share a similar basic structure (Fig. 16.3), consisting of two identical 'heavy' polypeptide chains and two identical

'light' chains, linked by disulphide bridges. There are five types of **heavy chain** (γ, α, μ, δ, ε) and two types of **light chain** (κ, λ), the immunoglobulin class being determined by the type of heavy chain that the molecule contains (Table 16.4).

The N-terminal amino acid sequences of both the heavy and the light chains show considerable variation between individual immunoglobulin molecules; these form the part of the immunoglobulin molecule responsible for recognition of the antigen (**the antigen binding site**). The amino acid sequence of the rest of the chains varies little within one immunoglobulin class; this constant part of the molecule is concerned with complement activation and interaction with the cellular elements of the immune system. The characteristics and functions of the immunoglobulins are summarized in Table 16.4.

On electrophoresis, immunoglobulins behave mainly as γ-globulins, but IgA and IgM may migrate with the β- or α_2-globulins. Because the normal plasma concentration of IgG is much higher than that of the other immunoglobulins, the γ-globulin peak seen on electrophoresis of normal serum is largely due to IgG.

Pleural fluid and ascites

The protein concentration of pleural fluid or abdominal ascites is occasionally measured to determine whether the sample is a transudate (fluid with a low protein content derived by filtration across capillary endothelium) or an exudate (fluid with a high protein content actively secreted in response to inflammation). A value of 25 or 30 g/L is often taken as the dividing line between the two types of fluid, but this is not a reliable criterion as the protein content of both is very variable. Measurement of lactate dehydrogenase (LDH; see later) is also helpful, because its activity is higher in exudates than in transudates, although values are also influenced by the plasma activity of the enzyme (Box 16.2).

Measurement of pleural fluid pH ([H+]) has been advocated to detect infection if the fluid is not obviously purulent. Although a low pH can also be associated with malignancy and connective tissue disorders, in clinical practice it is most often related to infection, and a pH value <7.2 ([H+] >63 nmol/L) in the absence of systemic acidosis indicates the need for insertion of a drain.

A chylous leak from the thoracic duct may be confirmed by the detection of a high triglyceride concentration in the pleural fluid.

The critical question is more often whether the ascites or pleural fluid is infected or if it is related to the presence of a tumour. This can only be determined by microbiological and cytological examination: protein measurement is of limited value.

Decreases and increases of plasma immunoglobulin concentrations can be either physiological or pathological in origin.

Hypogammaglobulinaemia

Physiological causes

At birth, IgA and IgM concentrations are low and they rise steadily thereafter (Fig. 16.4), although IgA may not reach the normal adult concentration until the end of the first decade of life. IgG is transported across the placenta, mainly during the last trimester of pregnancy, and concentrations are high at birth (except in premature infants). IgG concentration then declines, as maternal IgG is cleared from the body, before rising again as it is slowly replaced by the infant's own IgG.

Physiological hypogammaglobulinaemia is one of the reasons for the susceptibility of infants (especially the premature) to infection.

Pathological causes

Various inherited disorders of immunoglobulin synthesis are known, ranging in severity from **X-linked** agammaglobulinaemia (Bruton disease), in which there is a complete absence of immunoglobulins and affected children develop recurrent bacterial infections, to milder dysgammaglobulinaemias, in which there is a defect or partial defect of only one or two immunoglobulin classes. The commonest of these, **IgA deficiency**, has a prevalence of about 1 in 700 in the UK.

Hypogammaglobulinaemia can also be **acquired**. It commonly occurs in haematological malignancies, such as chronic lymphocytic leukaemia, multiple myeloma and Hodgkin disease. It can be a complication of the use of cytotoxic drugs and is a feature of severe protein-losing states, for example, the nephrotic syndrome. Increased catabolism also contributes to hypogammaglobulinaemia in protein-losing states.

Measurement of the specific class of immunoglobulin is essential for the diagnosis of hypogammaglobulinaemia. Electrophoresis is not sufficient for this purpose because the normal concentrations of the immunoglobulins, with the exception of IgG, are relatively low and the effect of any decrease in the size of the γ-globulin peak is too small to be detectable. IgG deficiency can be inferred if the γ-globulin peak is subnormal, but possible coexistent deficiencies of other immunoglobulins will not be apparent.

Hypergammaglobulinaemia

Physiological causes

Increased concentrations of immunoglobulins are seen in both acute and chronic infections, such as tuberculosis and infection with the human immunodeficiency virus (HIV). Serological investigations, involving the measurement of antibodies against specific antigens (e.g. hepatitis B surface

---

Box 16.2 Light's criteria for differentiation of an exudate and transudate in pleural fluid

Pleural fluid is an exudate if one or more of the following criteria are met:
   pleural fluid protein >0.5 × serum protein concentration
   pleural fluid LDH >0.6 × serum LDH activity
   pleural fluid LDH >2/3 of upper reference limit for serum

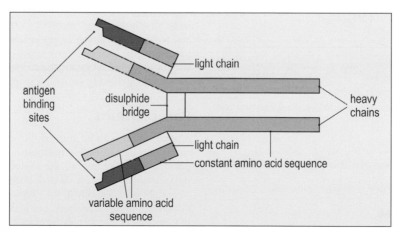

Fig. 16.3 Structure of immunoglobulins. All immunoglobulins have the same basic structure. IgM consists of a pentamer of the basic structure. IgA is secreted as a dimer.

Table 16.4 **Characteristics of the immunoglobulins**

Class	Heavy chain	Mean plasma concentration (g/L)	Molecular mass (kDa)	Function
IgG	γ	14.0	146	the major antibody of secondary immune responses
IgA	α	3.5	160	secreted as a dimer (molecular mass 385 kDa), the major antibody in seromucous secretions, e.g. saliva, intestine, bronchial mucus
IgM	μ	1.5	970	a pentamer, confined to the vascular spaces; the major antibody of the primary immune response
IgD	δ	0.03	184	present on the surface of B-lymphocytes, involved in antigen recognition
IgE	ε	trace	188	present on surface of mast cells and basophils; probable role in immunity to helminths and associated with immediate hypersensitivity reactions

Immunoglobulins of each class contain either κ or γ light chains. In IgA and IgG, slight variations in the structure of the constant regions of the heavy chains create different subclasses.

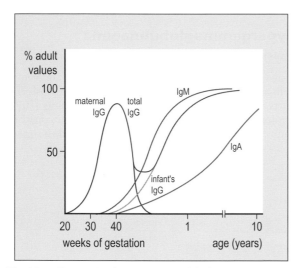

Fig. 16.4 Changes in plasma immunoglobulin concentrations with age.

antigen), are widely used in the diagnosis of infectious diseases.

Pathological causes

Increases in plasma immunoglobulin concentrations are common in **autoimmune diseases**, for example, rheumatoid disease and SLE, and in **chronic liver diseases**, some of which have an autoimmune basis.

The measurement of specific autoantibodies is of great value in the diagnosis of autoimmune disease. Many examples are described elsewhere in this book. Many different immunoglobulins are produced in these conditions and they give rise to a diffuse (polyclonal) increase in the γ-globulin region on electrophoresis (see Fig. 16.1C). Occasionally, several discrete ('oligoclonal') peaks are seen. Measurement of specific antibodies to known allergens may also be helpful in establishing the cause of type 1 hypersensitivity reactions such as urticaria or anaphylactic shock. However, results can be difficult to interpret and testing should only be undertaken if it will alter future management. Detailed discussion of the investigation of allergic reactions is beyond the scope of this book and readers are encouraged to consult textbooks of immunology.

Paraproteins

A paraprotein is an immunoglobulin produced by a single clone of cells of the B-lymphocyte series, most frequently **plasma cells**. Because all the molecules are identical, the paraprotein is seen on electrophoresis of serum as a discrete tight peak, usually in the γ region (see Fig. 16.1B). The peak may migrate elsewhere, particularly if the protein is an IgA or IgM, or if complex formation with another plasma protein has occurred. More than one paraprotein peak can occasionally be seen: this may be because of dimerization, as frequently occurs with IgA paraproteins, or the presence of complexes or fragments of paraproteins in addition to the intact molecule.

If plasma is inadvertently used for capillary zone electrophoresis (see p. 22), the presence of a fibrinogen peak may mimic or mask a paraprotein. Even with serum, a paraprotein may be missed on electrophoresis if, as occasionally happens, it coincides exactly with a normal peak, for example, α_2-globulin.

Paraproteins (usually IgG or IgA) occur most frequently in **multiple myeloma** (disseminated malignant proliferation of plasma cells, see Case history 16.1). They are also seen in the much rarer conditions of **solitary plasmacytoma**, and **Waldenström macroglobulinaemia** (IgM). Paraprotein secretion (usually IgM) occurs less frequently and, to a lesser extent, in **chronic lymphocytic leukaemia** and **B-cell lymphomas**.

Examination of serum is essential for the detection of paraproteins, but the urine can be examined as well. In ~11% of patients with myeloma, the tumour secretes only immunoglobulin light chains. These are of low molecular mass and are rapidly cleared from the plasma and are therefore not detected by routine protein electrophoretic techniques. They are, however, readily detectable in urine; immunoglobulin light chains found in the urine are known as **Bence Jones protein** and are present in some 75% of all cases of myeloma. **Free light chains** can also now be measured directly in serum and testing is recommended in all patients with suspected myeloma to identify those who would be missed using capillary electrophoresis alone because they produce very little abnormal protein (oligosecretory) or produce light chains only. Some guidelines no longer recommend screening urine, as serum analysis of light chains is a more sensitive test

---

Case history 16.1

History

A 70-year-old man presented with back pain and loss of weight. Although a non-smoker, he had had several recent chest infections and was increasingly short of breath on exercise.

Examination

He was anaemic, but there were no other obvious abnormalities.

Investigations

Radiological examination showed punched-out lytic lesions in the lumbar vertebrae, ribs and pelvis.

Results (see Appendix for reference ranges)

Serum:	sodium	130 mmol/L
	urea	15.3 mmol/L
	creatinine	212 µmol/L
	eGFR	26 mL/min/1.73 m^2
	calcium (adjusted)	2.75 mmol/L
	total protein	85 g/L
	albumin	30 g/L
	urate	610 µmol/L
Blood:	ESR	>100 mm/h (ref. range <22)
	haemoglobin	85 g/L
	film	normochromic, normocytic anaemia, rouleux and increased background staining

Summary

Severe anaemia with hypercalcaemia, kidney impairment and very high ESR.

Interpretation

The combination of these laboratory findings and lytic bone lesions is highly suggestive of myeloma. Capillary zone electrophoresis of serum proteins revealed a paraprotein in the γ-globulin region (see Fig. 16.1B); this was shown to be IgG-κ. There was a decrease in the normal γ-globulins. Bence Jones protein was present in the urine and identified as κ in type. Serum free light chain analysis confirmed an excess of the κ class.

Discussion

This is a typical presentation of multiple myeloma. The paraprotein is an IgG in 52% of patients (Table 16.5). Replacement of normal bone marrow by malignant plasma cells frequently results in anaemia and in decreased synthesis of normal immunoglobulins.

The diagnosis rests on the presence of all three of the following: a monoclonal protein in serum or urine, typical radiological appearances or other evidence of end-organ damage and increased numbers of abnormal plasma cells in the bone marrow. Examination of a bone marrow trephine biopsy and aspirate allows phenotyping of the plasma cells by flow cytometry and immunohistochemistry and identification of myeloma-associated genetic changes that give important prognostic information. Free light chains are readily filtered by the glomeruli but are toxic to the renal tubules; acute or chronic kidney injury is therefore a frequent complication when excess light chains are being produced.

Table 16.5 Incidence of paraprotein types

Protein	Incidence (%)
IgG	52
IgA	21
IgD	1.5
IgM (predominantly WM)	12
Bence Jones only	11

Up to 75% of patients have detectable free light chains (Bence Jones protein) in urine. IgE and IgM myelomas occur, but are rare. In about 1% of all cases, no paraprotein can be detected. WM, Wladenström macroglobulinaemia.

Box 16.3 Features of monoclonal gammopathy of undetermined significance (MGUS)

Diagnostic

paraprotein concentration <30 g/L
no clinical features of myeloma (no anaemia or hypercalcaemia, normal kidney function)
no lytic lesions in bone on radiography
<10% plasma cells in bone marrow aspirate
no evidence of other B-cell proliferative disorders

Other features

no suppression of other immunoglobulins
no Bence Jones proteinuria
normal κ/λ light chain ratio
no increase in paraprotein concentration with age

for the identification of abnormal light chain production. Raised serum concentrations of light chains associated with an abnormal ratio of κ to λ chains (normal being 0.26–1.65) confirm monoclonal rather than polyclonal immunoglobulin production. Monitoring of free light chain concentrations following treatment is especially helpful in patients with light chain or oligosecretory myeloma but is increasingly used to assess response in all types of myeloma.

The presence of paraprotein causes red cells to adhere to each other (rouleaux formation) and may be sufficient to cause an increase in the background staining of the blood film. Spurious hyponatraemia can occur in patients with paraproteinaemia, because of replacement of plasma water with protein ('pseudohyponatraemia', see p. 42).

Paraproteins are not always associated with overt malignant disease. **Monoclonal gammopathy of undetermined significance (MGUS)** becomes increasingly common with advancing age (prevalence rate of 5% in people older than 70 years) and is known to confer a significant risk of developing symptomatic myeloma; this necessitates regular follow-up of the patient. Thorough investigation is required to exclude malignancy (Box 16.3).

Kidney disease is the cause of death in approximately one-third of patients with myeloma. It is often multifactorial in origin: contributory factors include obstruction of nephrons by protein, hypercalcaemia, pyelonephritis (because of immune suppression) and renal amyloid (light chain deposits). Hypercalcaemia is common in myeloma; its cause is discussed elsewhere (see p. 261).

Despite the extensive lytic lesions of bone, there is no increase in osteoblastic activity and plasma alkaline phosphatase (ALP) activity is usually normal. The **laboratory findings** in myeloma are summarized in Box 16.4. It should be appreciated that metabolic abnormalities may not be present when the condition is first diagnosed ('asymptomatic myeloma'): they may develop subsequently, and so patients should be monitored periodically for these complications. Serum β_2-microglobulin concentration is a good prognostic indicator in myeloma because it reflects both the activity of the tumour and renal function: an increased concentration (>3.5 mg/L) implies a poorer prognosis. A staging system has been devised based on the serum β_2-microglobulin and albumin concentrations, in which patients with a β_2-microglobulin <3.5 mg/L and albumin >35 g/L are predicted to have the longest median survival time. Other features associated with a poor prognosis include anaemia, kidney disease, hypercalcaemia, hypoalbuminaemia, specific genetic abnormalities and a high paraprotein concentration, which reflects tumour bulk (see p. 360). Myeloma is treated using cytotoxic and immunomodulatory drugs, but the prognosis is variable, with the disease often becoming refractory to treatment. Local radiotherapy may be useful for isolated lesions (including plasmacytomas) and for localized bone pain. Younger patients are now commonly treated with high-dose chemotherapy followed by autologous stem cell transplantation.

Waldenström macroglobulinaemia is also a B-cell tumour. The paraprotein is an IgM, and a hyperviscosity syndrome, causing sludging of red cells in capillaries and predisposing to thrombus formation, is a prominent feature. It is much less common than myeloma.

Rarer still is Franklin (heavy chain) disease, in which the paraprotein produced is an immunoglobulin heavy chain only. This is usually an α-chain, but may also be a γ- or μ-chain. Patients with α-chain disease typically present with malabsorption caused by infiltration of the gut by lymphoma cells.

Some paraproteins precipitate out of solution when cooled to 4 °C and redissolve on warming. These proteins are known as **cryoglobulins** and are associated with Raynaud phenomenon, although the majority of patients with this condition do not have cryoglobulinaemia. Cryoglobulins can also occur in other conditions in which high concentrations of immunoglobulins occur such as connective tissue disorders (e.g. SLE) and chronic viral infections, most notably hepatitis C.

Cytokines

Cytokines are low molecular weight (<80 kDa) peptides secreted by cells involved in inflammation and immunity, which control the activity and growth of these cells. Most of their functions are local, either on nearby cells (**paracrine**) or on the cells that secrete the peptide (**autocrine**), but some have remote (**endocrine**) effects. They show some functional overlap with **peptide growth factors** (GFs), which influence the growth of non-immune cells. The two groups of factors are collectively known as peptide regulatory factors.

There is no unified classification system for cytokines but examples include **interleukins**, which are regulators of inflammation; **interferons**, which have antiviral properties and in general have an inhibitory effect on cell growth; **colony-stimulating factors**, which stimulate the growth of macrophages and white blood cells; **chemokines**, which induce chemotaxis in nearby responsive cells and **tumour necrosis factors**, which stimulate the proliferation of many cells, including cytolytic T cells.

Many cytokines have multiple properties and some cytokine-mediated responses can be brought about by more than one cytokine. Cytokines interact with each other, with the result that the effect of an individual cytokine depends on which other cytokines are present. They are also capable of inducing and inhibiting each other's secretion. More information on these substances can be found in textbooks of immunology.

Cytokines are of considerable importance in the coordination of the immune and inflammatory responses, and in the control of myelopoiesis. Some cytokines are secreted by tumours and can contribute to the effects of those tumours. They can be measured in serum by sensitive and specific assays, although as yet there are few clear clinical indications for doing so in routine practice.

GFs include epidermal GF, platelet-derived GF, transforming GF and the insulin-like GFs. Secretion of the latter by mesenchymal tumours is a cause of tumour-associated hypoglycaemia. GFs are used therapeutically to stimulate haemopoietic cells after bone marrow grafting for haematological malignancies. Cytokine inhibitors are used to treat disorders in which the immune system causes damage to organs, such as rheumatoid arthritis and ulcerative colitis.

Plasma Enzymes

Measurements of the activity of enzymes in serum or plasma are of value in the diagnosis and management of a wide variety of diseases. Most such enzymes are primarily intracellular, being released into the blood when there is damage to cell membranes, but many enzymes, for example, renin, complement factors and coagulation factors, are actively secreted into the blood, where they fulfil their physiological functions. The use of enzyme measurements in tissue for the diagnosis of inherited metabolic diseases is discussed in Chapter 19.

Small amounts of intracellular enzymes are present in the blood as a result of normal cell turnover. When damage to cells occurs, increased amounts of enzymes will be released and their concentrations in the blood will rise.

However, such increases are not always due to tissue damage. Other possible causes include:

- increased cell turnover
- cellular proliferation (e.g. neoplasia)
- increased enzyme synthesis (enzyme induction)
- obstruction to secretion
- decreased clearance (removal).

Little is known about the mechanisms by which enzymes are removed from the circulation. Small molecules, such as amylase, are filtered by the glomeruli, but most enzymes are probably removed by reticuloendothelial cells. Plasma amylase activity rises in acute and chronic kidney disease, but in general, changes in clearance rates are not known to be important as causes of changes in plasma enzyme activities.

Enzyme activity

Enzyme assays usually depend on the measurement of the catalytic activity of the enzyme, rather than the concentration of the enzyme protein itself. Because each enzyme molecule can catalyse the reaction of many molecules of substrate, measurement of activity provides great sensitivity.

Reference ranges for plasma enzymes are dependent on assay conditions and may also vary according to age and sex. It is thus important to be aware of both the reference range used by the laboratory providing the assay and the physiological circumstances when interpreting the results of enzyme assays. Ranges quoted in the Appendix are from a laboratory in the UK and may not necessarily be the same as the reader's ranges.

Disadvantages of enzyme assays

A major disadvantage of the use of enzymes in the diagnosis of tissue damage is their lack of specificity for a particular tissue or cell type. Many enzymes are common to more than one tissue, with the result that an increase in the plasma activity of a particular enzyme could reflect damage to any one of these tissues. This problem may be obviated to some extent in two ways: first, different tissues may contain (and thus release when they are damaged) two or more enzymes in different proportions; thus alanine (ALT) and aspartate aminotransferases (AST) are both present in cardiac and skeletal muscle and hepatocytes, but there is only a little ALT in either type of muscle; second, some enzymes exist in different forms (isoforms), colloquially termed **isoenzymes** (although, strictly, the term 'isoenzyme' refers only to a genetically determined isoform). Individual isoforms are often characteristic of a particular tissue: although they may have similar catalytic activities, they often differ in some other measurable property, such as electrophoretic mobility, heat stability or binding by a specific antibody.

After a single insult to a tissue, the activity of intracellular enzymes in the plasma rises following release from the damaged cells and then falls as the enzymes are cleared. It is thus important to consider the time at which the blood sample is taken in relation to the insult. If taken too soon, there may have been insufficient time for the enzyme to reach the bloodstream, and if too late, it may have been completely cleared. As with all diagnostic techniques, data acquired from measurements of enzymes in plasma must always be assessed in light of whatever clinical and other information is available, and their limitations borne in mind.

Several enzymes can form complexes with other proteins, most often immunoglobulins; they are cleared from the plasma more slowly than the native forms and are referred to as '**macro**' enzymes. The consequence may be a sustained increase in plasma activity, which may cause diagnostic confusion if the possibility is not considered (e.g. macroamylasaemia p. 128). Macro enzymes are rarely of pathological significance, although occasionally they are associated with paraproteins.

In the boxes and figures that follow, typical plasma activities of enzymes in various conditions are given. Higher (or lower) values may of course occur in more (or less) severe cases.

Specific enzymes
Alkaline phosphatase

The enzyme ALP is present in high concentrations in the liver, bone (osteoblasts), placenta and intestinal epithelium. These tissues each contain specific isoenzymes (strictly, isoforms) of ALP. Pathological increases in ALP activity are most frequently seen in **cholestatic liver disease** and in **bone diseases** in which there is an increase in osteoblastic activity (e.g. fractures, Paget disease and osteomalacia).

Some causes of an increase in plasma ALP activity are summarized in Box 16.5. Physiological increases are seen in **pregnancy**, because of the placental isoenzyme, and in **childhood** (when bones are growing), because of the bone isoenzyme. Plasma ALP activity is high at birth but falls rapidly thereafter. However, it remains two to three times the normal adult range, and rises again during the adolescent growth spurt before falling to adult values as bone growth ceases (Fig. 16.5). Plasma ALP activity increases slightly in the elderly, even in the absence of apparent bone or liver disease. Activities of ALP as high as 10 times the upper reference limit (URL) may be seen in severe Paget disease of bone, rickets and osteomalacia, and occasionally in cholestatic liver disease. Lesser increases are, however, more common in these conditions (see Box 16.5). Note that total ALP activity is not increased in uncomplicated osteoporosis.

Plasma ALP is frequently elevated in **malignant disease**: it may be of bony or hepatic origin and associated with the presence of either primary or secondary tumours in these tissues. A number of tumours secrete the placental

Box 16.5 **Some causes of increased plasma alkaline phosphatase activity**

Physiological

pregnancy (last trimester)
childhood

Pathological

often >5 × URL
  Paget disease of bone
  osteomalacia, rickets
  cholestasis (intrahepatic and extrahepatic)
  cirrhosis
usually <5 × URL
  bone tumours (primary and secondary)
  chronic kidney disease–mineral and bone disorder
  primary hyperparathyroidism with bone involvement
  healing fractures
  osteomyelitis
  hepatic space-occupying lesions (tumour, abscess)
  infiltrative liver disease
  hepatitis
  inflammatory bowel disease
  drugs

URL, upper reference limit.

or placental-like (Regan) isoenzymes. The placental isoenzyme is used as a tumour marker in germ cell malignancies.

ALP is frequently measured as part of a biochemical profile and it is not uncommon to find a raised activity in the absence of clinical evidence of bone or liver disease, and in the absence of other biochemical abnormalities. In establishing the cause of such an increase, it is clearly helpful to determine the tissue of origin. This can be done by measuring tissue-specific isoenzymes of ALP using various specialist techniques. A simpler but less reliable alternative is to measure plasma γ-glutamyl transferase. This enzyme is found in the liver but not in bone. Its plasma activity is often (but not always) increased when there is an excess of hepatic ALP in the plasma.

Aminotransferases

Two aminotransferases are used in diagnosis and management: aspartate aminotransferase (AST) and alanine aminotransferase (ALT; the 'T' in the abbreviations stands for 'transaminase'; this term has now been replaced by 'aminotransferase', although the abbreviation has not been changed and indeed the term 'transaminase' remains colloquial). Both enzymes are widely distributed in body tissues, but ALT is present in only small amounts, except in the liver. Even here, there is more than three times as much

AST; in cardiac and skeletal muscle, there is 20 times as much AST as ALT.

Some causes of increased plasma ALT activity are shown in Box 16.6. Very high values, sometimes in excess of 100 × URL, are seen in acute hepatitis. More usually in hepatitis, the peak value is only 10–20 × URL. In myocardial infarction, plasma aminotransferases begin to rise some 12 h after the infarct. AST rises to a much greater extent than ALT, reaching a peak of up to 10 × URL at 24–36 h and then declining over 2–3 days, providing that there is no further cardiac damage. However, AST is not a specific or sensitive enough marker for the diagnosis of myocardial infarction, for which measurement of cardiac troponins should be used.

In most conditions in which transaminases are elevated, there is a proportionately smaller rise in ALT than AST. In hepatitis, however, plasma activities of ALT may exceed those of AST. The use of AST:ALT ratio measurements in liver disease is discussed on p. 113. Aminotransferases are often measured as part of a biochemical profile. It is very uncommon to find values >20 × URL unexpectedly; this is most likely to occur in the prodromal phase of viral hepatitis. Values of up to 3 × URL are sometimes found in patients who have no clinical evidence of tissue damage (see p. 113). Ethanol abuse and non-alcoholic steatohepatitis should be considered as possible causes in such cases, as should the use of many commonly prescribed drugs, such as statins. If there are no other biochemical changes, or any readily apparent cause of the raised value, the test should be repeated after an interval of a few weeks.

γ-Glutamyltransferase

The enzyme γ-glutamyltransferase (γGT) is present in high concentrations in the liver, kidney and pancreas. Measurement of its plasma activity provides a sensitive indicator of **hepatobiliary disease**, although it is of no value in distinguishing *between* cholestatic and hepatocellular disease. In biliary obstruction, plasma γGT activity may increase before that of ALP.

Plasma γGT activity is raised in the absence of liver disease in many patients taking anticonvulsant drugs such as phenytoin and phenobarbital; rifampicin, used in the treatment of tuberculosis, can have a similar effect. This is an example of **enzyme induction**. The increased plasma γGT is not due to cell damage but to an increase in enzyme production within cells, with the result that an increased amount is released during normal cell turnover.

Plasma γGT activity is frequently very high in patients with **alcoholic liver disease**, but it can be elevated in heavy ethanol drinkers, in the absence of other evidence of liver damage, because of enzyme induction. Up to 70% of such people have elevated activities of the enzyme, but it should be appreciated both that similar increases may be seen in other

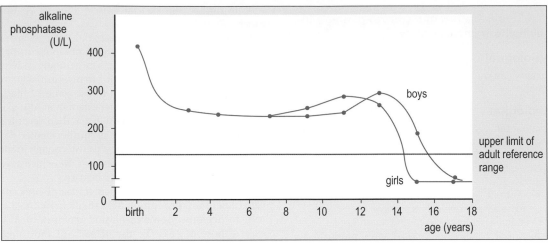

Fig. 16.5 Serum alkaline phosphatase activity as a function of age in childhood. Mean values are shown; the peaks between 10 and 16 years correspond to the pubertal growth spurt, and values of up to three times the upper limit of the adult reference range may be seen at this time.

Box 16.6 **Some causes of an increased plasma alanine aminotransferase activity**

Often >10 × URL

acute hepatitis and liver necrosis
  (values may sometimes exceed 100 × URL)

5–10 × URL

liver hypoxia
cholestasis
chronic hepatitis

Usually <5 × URL

physiological (neonates)
other liver diseases
pancreatitis
myocardial infarction
haemolysis (*in vivo* and *in vitro*)
skeletal muscle disease
following surgery or trauma
drugs, e.g. statins

Plasma aspartate aminotransferase is raised to a similar extent in liver diseases, but to a much greater degree in the other conditions.

URL, upper reference limit.

Lactate dehydrogenase

Increases in plasma LDH activity are seen in a wide variety of conditions, including acute damage to the liver, pancreas, skeletal muscle and kidneys, and also in megaloblastic and haemolytic anaemias. In patients with **lymphoma or testicular cancers**, a high plasma LDH activity indicates a poor prognosis. There is a correlation between enzyme activity and tumour bulk, and thus serial measurements may be useful in following response to treatment.

Plasma activities of LDH increase several hours after myocardial infarction and remain elevated for some days, but measurement is of no practical value in the management of this condition. An increased plasma activity (both from red blood cells and from damaged tissues) occurs in haemolytic crises in sickle cell anaemia, and measurement of LDH may be of value to assess severity.

Creatine kinase

Increases in plasma creatine kinase (CK) activity are usually the result of **skeletal** or **cardiac muscle** damage, although moderate increases can be seen after physical exertion. Some racial groups have higher plasma activities in health (Box 16.8). Measurement of plasma CK activity is used in the investigation of skeletal muscle disease, especially if rhabdomyolysis is suspected, when it is a key decision-making test. It is rarely used now in the investigation of myocardial damage. The diagnostic uses of CK measurements are discussed in Chapter 18.

The enzymatically active CK molecule is a dimer; there are two monomers, M and B. Three isoenzymes, BB, MM and

conditions (Box 16.7) and that a significant number of people who abuse ethanol have a normal γGT activity. Plasma γGT activity can remain elevated for up to 3–4 weeks after abstinence from alcohol, even in the absence of liver damage.

MB, occur. BB is confined mainly to the brain. The CK normally present in plasma is mainly the MM isoenzyme. Even in severe brain damage, the contribution of the BB isoenzyme to plasma activity is minimal. The CK in healthy skeletal muscle is almost entirely MM but in muscle disorders with a high proportion of regenerating fibres, there is an increase in the MB isoenzyme. In cardiac muscle, up to 30% is the MB isoenzyme and in the past, the demonstration that >5% of a total high CK activity was due to the MB isoenzyme, suggested a cardiac origin, unless the patient had a history of chronic muscle disease. The presence of **macro-CK** (see earlier) is relatively common and should be excluded in patients with an unexplained, persistent rise in plasma CK activity.

Amylase and lipase

Amylase is found in the salivary glands and exocrine pancreas, and tissue-specific isoenzymes can be distinguished by means of electrophoresis or the use of inhibitors. It is cleared by the kidneys, and plasma activities increase in patients with chronic kidney disease.

Plasma amylase activity is usually increased, often to 5× or even to >10 × URL, in **acute pancreatitis**. Its use in the diagnosis of patients presenting with an acute abdomen and the other causes of an increase in plasma amylase activity, including **macroamylasaemia**, are discussed in Chapter 7.

Lipase is also found in the exocrine pancreas and the finding of a raised plasma activity is thought to be a more specific and sensitive indicator of pancreatitis than amylase (see Chapter 7).

Cholinesterase

This enzyme is secreted by the liver into the bloodstream, and low plasma activities occur in chronic liver disease. It is, however, rarely measured for this reason. Plasma cholinesterase activity also falls in organophosphate poisoning. Low activities occur physiologically during pregnancy.

Interest in this enzyme derives largely from the fact that it hydrolyses certain anaesthetic drugs including the muscle-relaxant succinylcholine (suxamethonium, scoline). Occasionally, patients are found in whom the effect of this drug, which paralyses respiration, persists for several hours after it has been administered (scoline apnoea). Many of these patients have an abnormal cholinesterase activity caused by inherited mutations of the butyrylcholinesterase (pseudocholinesterase) gene.

Four enzyme variants have been recognized and are characterized on the basis of their activity in the presence of inhibitors: normal, dibucaine-resistant, fluoride-resistant and inactive. Normal homozygotes (genotype $E_1^u E_1^u$) account for 95% of the population, and heterozygotes for dibucaine resistance ($E_1^u E_1^a$) account for 4%. Such individuals do not usually react abnormally to succinylcholine, but homozygotes for dibucaine resistance ($E_1^a E_1^a$) (0.05%) are at risk of developing scoline apnoea, as are patients who produce an inactive enzyme ($E_1^s E_1^s$). Individuals having an adverse reaction to succinylcholine, and their relatives, should be screened to identify those who have an abnormal cholinesterase so that these drugs can be avoided should they need to undergo anaesthesia. Direct genetic testing to identify individual mutations is now available in some laboratories.

Tryptase

Mast cells contain high concentrations of tryptase and histamine, the massive release of which contributes to the symptoms and signs of anaphylactic shock. Measurement of plasma tryptase concentrations is most commonly used in the assessment of suspected anaphylactic reactions. UK guidelines recommend blood sampling as soon as possible after emergency treatment has started and again 1–2 h later. A significant rise confirms the diagnosis, and referral to an allergy specialist is advised. A sustained increase in concentration is found in the rare condition of mastocytosis, in which there is abnormal proliferation of mast cells.

SUMMARY

- The most abundant protein in plasma is **albumin**, which is synthesized in the liver. Through its contribution to the **colloid osmotic pressure**, albumin has an important role in determining the distribution of the ECF between the vascular and extravascular spaces. It is also an important **transport protein** for several hormones, drugs, free fatty acids, unconjugated bilirubin and various ions. Its concentration is, however, affected by so many pathological processes (decreases occur in chronic liver disease, protein-losing states, malabsorption, after trauma and when capillary permeability is increased) that measurements must be interpreted with caution.

- Most of the other plasma proteins are classified as globulins. The **immunoglobulins** are synthesized by plasma cells and constitute the **humoral arm of the immune system.** There are five classes, of which the most abundant are IgG, IgA and IgM. IgM is the main antibody of the primary immune response and is largely confined to the vascular compartment; IgG is involved in the secondary response and is distributed throughout the ECF; IgA is secreted onto mucosal surfaces. An increase in total immunoglobulins is characteristic of chronic inflammatory conditions and autoimmune diseases. Measurement of immunoglobulins is of value in the investigation of immunodeficiency syndromes. Measurement of **specific antibodies** is of value in the investigation of autoimmune and infectious diseases and some allergies.

- **Myeloma** is a malignant tumour of plasma cells, which produce large amounts of identical, monoclonal, immunoglobulin molecules or fragments thereof, known as **paraproteins.** Electrophoresis of serum proteins and measurements of serum free light chain concentrations are used to diagnose myeloma. **Metabolic features** of myeloma include renal impairment, hypercalcaemia and hyperuricaemia. Patients are frequently anaemic and may have an immune paresis. Causes of death include infection and kidney disease.

- **Other plasma proteins** include the coagulation factors, complement components, various transport proteins, for example, thyroxine-binding globulin, transcortin, sex hormone-binding globulin, transferrin and caeruloplasmin. Increases in the concentration of certain proteins occur in association with acute inflammatory reactions. These **acute phase proteins** include α_1-antitrypsin, CRP and haptoglobin. α_1-Antitrypsin is a protease inhibitor; inherited deficiency of the protein can cause neonatal hepatitis, which may progress to cirrhosis, and emphysema in adults, particularly those who smoke. Measurement of CRP is valuable in following the course of conditions characterized by episodes of acute inflammation, such as rheumatoid arthritis and Crohn disease. Haptoglobin binds free haemoglobin and plasma concentrations fall with haemolysis.

- The **cytokines** are a large group of autocrine and paracrine regulatory peptides, which modulate the activity of the immune system and are involved in the coordination of acute inflammation and the immune response.

- The **enzymes** present in the plasma include those that have a physiological function there, for example, renin and the blood clotting factors, and those that have been released from cells as a result of damage or normal cell turnover. Diagnostic enzymology is principally concerned with the latter; the measurement of enzyme activity in the plasma can give useful diagnostic information concerning the site and extent of tissue damage. Examples of such enzymes include **CK**, which is released after damage to skeletal muscle, and the **aminotransferases**, which are widely distributed and are released into the blood in a variety of conditions, including hepatitis and skeletal muscle injury.

- Few enzymes that are measured for diagnostic purposes in plasma are tissue specific, but when the origin of increased plasma activity is not obvious either clinically or for other reasons, measurement of the **isoenzymes** (molecular variants of the enzymes that have similar catalytic activity but a different chemical structure, rendering them distinguishable, for example, immunochemically or by electrophoresis) can often provide this information. Thus, the measurement of ALP isoenzymes will distinguish

SUMMARY—cont'd

between a hepatic, bony or other source for increased plasma activity of this enzyme. Another method to improve specificity involves measuring more than one enzyme, because the concentration of different enzymes, and thus the amount released when cells are damaged, varies between different tissues.

- Many enzymes can form complexes with other proteins, usually immunoglobulins, which are cleared more slowly than the native forms, leading to a sustained rise in plasma activities. These **'macro' enzymes** are rarely of pathological significance but may lead to diagnostic confusion if not recognized.

- Although tending to lack specificity, the measurement of plasma enzyme activity can provide a very sensitive means of detecting tissue damage and can be invaluable in following the course of an illness such as hepatitis or Paget disease of bone, even though the diagnosis may have been established using another technique.

Chapter | 17 |

Lipids, lipoproteins and cardiovascular disease

Introduction

The major lipids present in the plasma are **fatty acids, triglycerides, cholesterol** and **phospholipids**. Other lipid-soluble substances, present in much smaller amounts, include **fat-soluble vitamins** and **steroid hormones** (discussed in Chapters 8 and 10, respectively).

Elevated plasma concentrations of lipids, particularly cholesterol, are causally related to the pathogenesis of **atherosclerosis**, the process responsible for the majority of **cardiovascular disease** (coronary, cerebrovascular and peripheral vascular disease). Cardiovascular disease is the commonest cause of death in the UK; many of these are in people younger than 60 years. Effective management of hypercholesterolaemia and other risk factors is of proven benefit in reducing cardiovascular disease mortality.

Triglycerides, Cholesterol and Phospholipids

Triglycerides are more correctly called 'triacylglycerols', a term not in general use; the more colloquial term is used in this book to avoid confusion. Triglycerides consist of **glycerol** esterified with three **long-chain fatty acids**, such as stearic (18 carbon atoms) or palmitic (16 carbon atoms) acids (see p. 3 and Figs. 1.4 and 1.5). Triglycerides are present in dietary fat and can be synthesized in the liver and adipose tissue to provide a source of stored energy; this can be mobilized when required, for example during starvation. Although the majority of fatty acids in the body are **saturated**, certain **unsaturated** fatty acids are important as precursors of prostaglandins and in the esterification of cholesterol. Triglycerides containing both saturated and unsaturated fatty acids are important components of cell membranes.

Cholesterol is also important in **membrane structure** and is the precursor of **steroid hormones** and **bile acids**. Cholesterol is present in dietary fat and can be synthesized in the liver by a mechanism that is under close metabolic regulation. Cholesterol can be excreted in the **bile either** *per se* or after metabolism to **bile acids**.

Phospholipids are compounds similar to the triglycerides but with one fatty acid residue replaced by phosphate and a nitrogenous base.

Because they are **not water soluble**, lipids are transported in the plasma in association with proteins. Albumin is the principal carrier of free fatty acids (FFAs); the other lipids circulate in complexes known as **lipoproteins**. These consist of a non-polar core of triglycerides and cholesteryl esters surrounded by a surface layer of phospholipids, cholesterol and proteins known as apolipoproteins (Fig. 17.1). The latter are important both structurally and in the metabolism of lipoproteins, as receptor ligands and enzyme activity regulators.

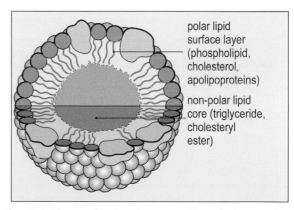

Fig. 17.1 Diagram showing the composition of a lipoprotein particle. A segment has been removed to reveal the non-polar core of cholesteryl esters and triglycerides surrounded by phospholipids and apolipoprotein.

polar lipid surface layer (phospholipid, cholesterol, apolipoproteins)

non-polar lipid core (triglyceride, cholesteryl ester)

Classification of Lipoproteins

Lipoproteins are classified by their densities as demonstrated by their ultracentrifugal separation. Density increases from **chylomicrons** (of lowest density) through lipoproteins of very-low-density (**VLDL**), intermediate-density (**IDL**) and low-density (**LDL**), to high-density lipoprotein (**HDL**) (Table 17.1). Distinct subtypes of HDL and LDL are also recognized; a preponderance of small, dense LDL is associated with increased risk of cardiovascular disease. IDL, normally only present in small amounts, can accumulate in pathological disturbances of lipoprotein metabolism. The approximate lipid and apolipoprotein content of the circulating lipoproteins is illustrated in

Fig. 17.2, but it is important to appreciate that their composition is not static. They are in a dynamic state with continuous exchange of components between the various types. Their principal functions are summarized in Table 17.1 and discussed in the next section.

Lipoprotein(a), or **Lp(a)**, is a lipoprotein of unknown function. It is larger and denser than LDL but has a similar composition, except that it contains in addition one molecule of apolipoprotein(a) (apo(a)) for every molecule of apo B-100. Apo(a) shows considerable homology with plasminogen. The concentration of Lp(a) in the plasma varies 1000-fold between individuals, with significant ethnic differences, and in a skewed distribution with most people having low concentrations. An elevated concentration of Lp(a) appears to be an independent risk factor for coronary

Table 17.1 Classification and characteristics of lipoproteins

Lipoprotein	Density (g/mL)	Mean diameter (nm)	Source	Principal function
chylomicron	<0.95	500	intestine	transport of exogenous triglyceride
VLDL	0.96–1.006	43	liver	transport of endogenous triglyceride
IDL	1.007–1.019	27	catabolism of VLDL	precursor of LDL
LDL	1.02–1.063	22	catabolism of VLDL, via IDL	cholesterol transport
HDL	1.064–1.21	8	liver, intestine; catabolism of chylomicrons and VLDL	reverse cholesterol transport

HDL, high-density lipoprotein; IDL, intermediate-density lipoprotein; LDL, low-density lipoprotein; VLDL, very low-density lipoprotein.

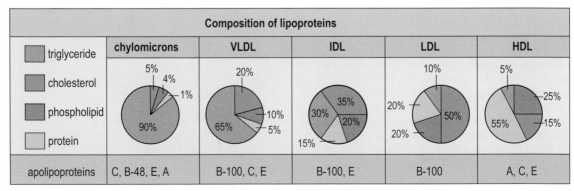

Fig. 17.2 Composition of lipoproteins; although the composition in each class is similar, the particles are heterogeneous, so the percentages given are approximate. Only the principal apolipoproteins are shown. HDL, high-density lipoprotein; IDL, intermediate-density lipoprotein; LDL, low-density lipoprotein; VLDL, very-low-density lipoprotein.

heart disease (CHD). Conventional drug treatments that lower LDL have little effect on Lp(a) concentration. Measurement is not currently recommended for cardiovascular risk screening, but this may change, particularly as specific treatments are developed and evaluated.

Lipoprotein Metabolism

Chylomicrons

Chylomicrons (Fig. 17.3) **are formed from dietary fat** (principally triglycerides, but also cholesterol) in enterocytes; they enter the lymphatics and reach the systemic circulation via the thoracic duct. Chylomicrons are the major transport form of **exogenous (dietary) fat**. Triglycerides constitute about 90% of the lipid. Triglycerides are removed from chylomicrons by

the action of the enzyme **lipoprotein lipase** (LPL), located on the luminal surface of the capillary endothelium of adipose tissue, skeletal and cardiac muscle and lactating breast, with the result that FFAs are delivered to these tissues to be used either as **energy substrates** or, after re-esterification to triglyceride, for **energy storage**. LPL is activated by apo C-II.

Apo A and apo B-48 are synthesized in the gut and are present in newly formed chylomicrons; apo C-II and apo E are transferred to chylomicrons from HDL. As triglycerides are removed from chylomicrons by the action of LPL, these particles become smaller; cholesterol, phospholipids, apo A and apo C-II are released from the surface of the particles and taken up by HDL. Esterified cholesterol is transferred to the chylomicron remnants from HDL, in exchange for triglycerides, by **cholesteryl ester transfer protein**. The **chylomicron remnants**, depleted of triglycerides and enriched in cholesteryl esters, are cleared rapidly from the circulation

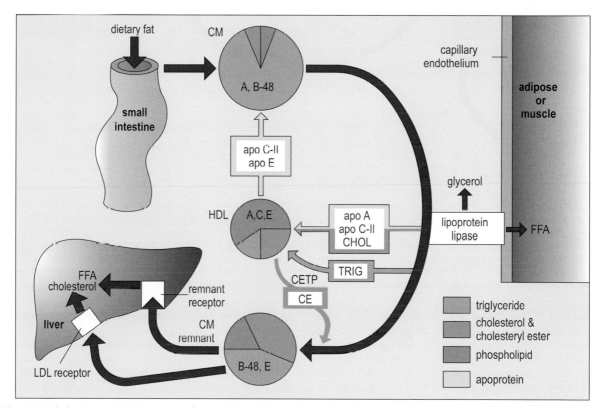

Fig. 17.3 Chylomicrons (CMs) transport dietary triglycerides to tissue where they are removed by the action of lipoprotein lipase. The resulting remnant particles are removed from the bloodstream by the liver. They bind to remnant receptors (which recognize apo E) and low-density lipoprotein (LDL) receptors (which also recognize apo E, but not the truncated form of apo B, B-48) on hepatic cells, are internalized and catabolized. Apo A and B-48 are synthesized in intestinal cells; apo C and apo E are acquired, together with cholesteryl esters (CEs), from high-density lipoprotein (HDL). Apolipoprotein C-II activates lipoprotein lipase. As triglycerides (TRIG) are removed from CMs, apo A, apo C, cholesterol (CHOL) and phospholipids are released from their surfaces and transferred to HDL where the cholesterol is esterified. CEs are transferred back to the remnant particles in exchange for triglycerides by the CE transport protein (CETP). FFA, free fatty acid.

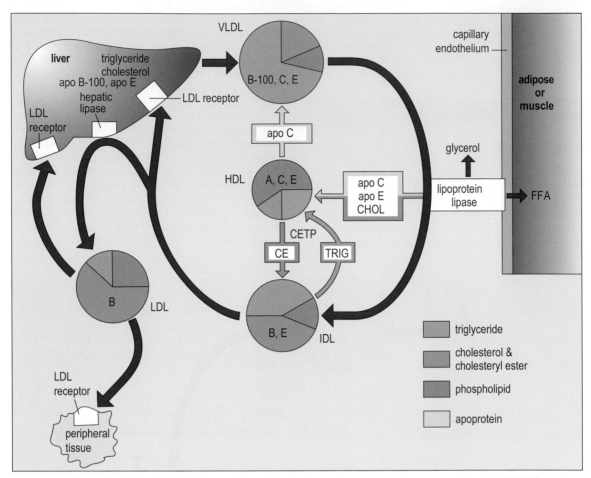

Fig. 17.4 Very-low-density lipoprotein (VLDL) is synthesized in the liver and transport endogenous triglyceride (TRIG) from the liver to other tissues where they are removed by the action of lipoprotein lipase. At the same time, cholesterol (CHOL), phospholipids and apo C and apo E are released and transferred to high-density lipoprotein (HDL). By this process, VLDL is converted to intermediate-density lipoprotein (IDL). CHOL is esterified in HDL, and cholesteryl esters (CEs) are transferred to intermediate-density lipoprotein (IDL) by CE transfer protein (CETP). Some IDL is removed by the liver, but most has more triglyceride removed by hepatic triglyceride lipase and is thereby converted into low-density lipoprotein (LDL). FFA, free fatty acid.

by the liver. This process depends on the recognition of apo E by chylomicron remnant receptors (also known as LDL receptor-related protein) and LDL receptors (see later).

Although their major function is the transport of dietary triglycerides, chylomicrons also transport dietary cholesterol and fat-soluble vitamins to the liver. Under normal circumstances, chylomicrons cannot be detected in plasma in the fasting state (>12 h after a meal).

Very-low-density and intermediate-density lipoproteins

VLDL (Fig. 17.4) **is formed from triglycerides synthesized in the liver either** *de novo* **or by re-esterification of FFAs.** VLDL also contains some cholesterol, apo B, apo C and apo E; the apo E and some of the apo C is transferred from circulating HDL.

VLDL is the principal transport form of **endogenous** triglycerides and initially shares a similar fate to chylomicrons, triglycerides being removed by the action of LPL. As the VLDL particles become smaller, phospholipids, free cholesterol and apolipoproteins are released from their surfaces and taken up by HDL, thus converting the VLDL to denser particles, IDL. Cholesterol that has been transferred to HDL is esterified and the cholesteryl ester is transferred back to IDL by cholesteryl ester transfer protein in exchange for triglyceride. More triglycerides are removed by **hepatic triglyceride lipase**, located on hepatic endothelial cells, and IDLs are thereby converted to LDL, composed mainly of cholesteryl esters, apo B-100 and phospholipid. Some

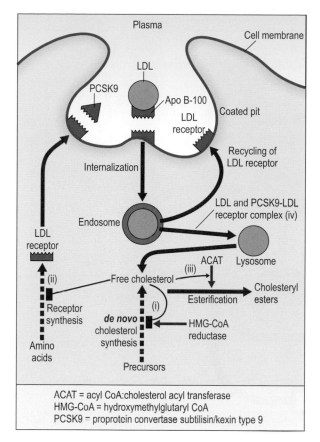

ACAT = acyl CoA:cholesterol acyl transferase
HMG-CoA = hydroxymethylglutaryl CoA
PCSK9 = proprotein convertase subtilisin/kexin type 9

Fig. 17.5 Low-density lipoprotein (LDL) uptake and catabolism. LDL is derived from very-low-density lipoprotein, via intermediate-density lipoprotein. It is removed by the liver and other tissues by a receptor-dependent process involving the recognition of apo B-100 by the LDL receptor. The LDL particles are hydrolysed by lysosomal enzymes, releasing free cholesterol which: (i) inhibits hydroxymethylglutaryl coenzyme A (HMG-CoA) reductase, the rate-limiting step in cholesterol synthesis; (ii) inhibits LDL receptor synthesis; and (iii) stimulates cholesterol esterification by augmenting the activity of the enzyme acyl CoA: cholesterol acyl transferase (ACAT). LDL receptors that have bound circulating proprotein convertase subtilisin/kexin type 9 (PCSK9) are directed to the lysosome (iv) for destruction.

IDL is taken up by the liver via **LDL receptors**. These receptors are capable of binding apo B-100 and apo E (but not apo B-48).

Under normal circumstances, there are very few IDL particles in the circulation because of their rapid removal or conversion to LDL.

Low-density lipoprotein

LDL is the principal carrier of cholesterol, mainly in the form of cholesteryl esters. LDL is formed from VLDL via IDL

(see Fig. 17.4). It can pass through the junctions between capillary endothelial cells and bind to **LDL receptors** on cell membranes that recognize apo B-100, both in the liver and in peripheral tissues. This is followed by internalization and lysosomal degradation with release of free cholesterol (Fig. 17.5). Cholesterol can also be synthesized in these tissues, but the rate-limiting enzyme, hydroxymethylglutaryl coenzyme A reductase (**HMG-CoA reductase**), is inhibited by cholesterol, with the result that, in healthy adults, cholesterol synthesis occurs only in the liver. Free cholesterol also stimulates its own esterification to cholesteryl esters by stimulating the enzyme acyl coenzyme A (CoA): cholesterol acyl transferase.

LDL receptors are saturable and subject to down-regulation by an increase in intracellular cholesterol. LDL receptors are targeted for destruction by the lysosome if bound to proprotein convertase subtilisin/kexin type 9 (PCSK9), which prevents the necessary conformational changes that cause the release of LDL within the endosome and recycling of the receptor to the cell membrane.

Macrophages derived from circulating monocytes can take up LDL via scavenger receptors. This process occurs at normal LDL concentrations but is enhanced when LDL concentrations are increased and by modification (e.g. oxidation) of LDL. Uptake of LDL by macrophages in the arterial wall is an important event in the pathogenesis of atherosclerosis. When macrophages become overloaded with cholesteryl esters, they are converted to **foam cells**, the classic components of atheromatous plaques.

In human neonates, plasma LDL concentrations are much lower than in adults, and cellular cholesterol uptake is probably all receptor mediated and controlled. LDL concentrations increase during childhood and reach adult levels after puberty.

High-density lipoprotein

HDL (Fig. 17.6) is synthesized primarily in the liver and, to a lesser extent, in small intestinal cells, as a precursor ('nascent HDL') comprising phospholipid, cholesterol, apo E and apo A. Uptake of cholesterol is stimulated by ATP-binding cassette protein A1 (ABCA1). Nascent HDL is disc shaped; in the circulation, it acquires apo C and apo A from other lipoproteins and from extrahepatic tissues, assuming a spherical conformation. The free cholesterol is esterified by the enzyme lecithin-cholesterol acyltransferase (LCAT), which is present in nascent HDL and activated by its cofactor, apo A-I. This increases the density of the HDL particles, which are thus converted from HDL3 to HDL2.

Cholesteryl esters are transferred from HDL2 to remnant particles in exchange for triglycerides, this process being mediated by cholesteryl ester transfer protein. Cholesteryl esters are taken up by the liver in chylomicron remnants and IDL and excreted in bile, partly after metabolism to bile acids.

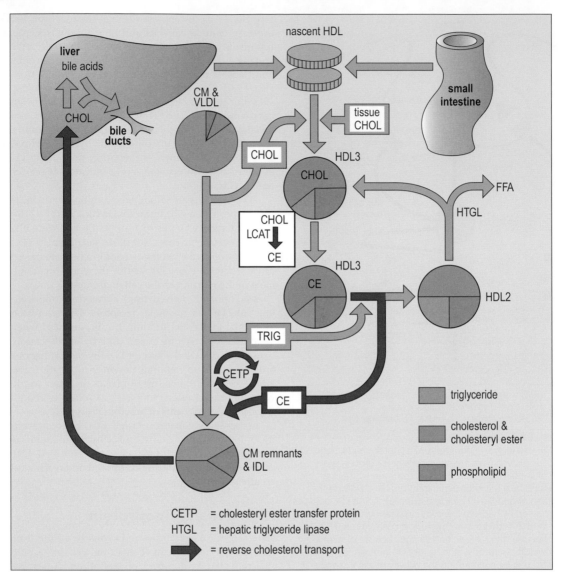

Fig. 17.6 High-density lipoprotein (HDL) metabolism and reverse cholesterol transport. Nascent HDL acquires free cholesterol (CHOL) from extrahepatic cells, chylomicrons (CM) and very-low-density lipoprotein (VLDL), and is thereby converted to HDL3. The cholesterol is esterified by the enzyme lecithin-cholesterol acyltransferase (LCAT), and cholesteryl esters (CEs) are transferred to remnant lipoproteins by CE transport protein (CETP) in exchange for triglyceride. Remnant particles are removed from the circulation by the liver, whence the cholesterol is excreted in bile both *per se* and as bile acids. Much HDL is recycled, although some is probably taken up by the liver and steroidogenic tissues. Apoprotein transfers have been omitted for clarity. FFA, free fatty acid; IDL, intermediate-density lipoprotein.

The triglyceride-enriched HDL2 is converted back to HDL3 by the removal of triglycerides by the enzyme hepatic triglyceride lipase, located on the hepatic capillary endothelium. Some HDL2 is probably removed from the circulation by the liver and steroidogenic tissues, through receptors that recognize apo A-I (scavenger receptor type B1).

Thus, HDL has two important functions: it is a **source of apoproteins** for chylomicrons and VLDL, and it mediates **reverse cholesterol transport**, taking up cholesterol from senescent cells and other lipoproteins and transferring it to remnant particles, which are taken up by the liver. Cholesterol is excreted by the liver in bile, both as free and esterified cholesterol and through metabolism to bile acids. In addition, HDL has anti-inflammatory properties and transports the protein paraoxonase, which is an antioxidant.

Summary

The essential features of lipoprotein metabolism are as follows:

- dietary triglycerides are transported in chylomicrons to tissues where they can be used as an energy source or stored
- endogenous triglycerides, synthesized in the liver, are transported in VLDL and are also available to tissues as an energy source or for storage
- cholesterol synthesized in the liver is transported to tissues in LDL, derived from VLDL; dietary cholesterol reaches the liver in chylomicron remnants
- HDL acquires cholesterol from peripheral cells and other lipoproteins and this is esterified by LCAT. Cholesteryl esters are transferred to remnant particles, which are taken up by the liver, whence the cholesterol is excreted.

Lipid Investigations

Reference ranges and clinical goals

At birth, the plasma cholesterol concentration is very low (total cholesterol <2.6 mmol/L, LDL-cholesterol <1.0 mmol/L). There is a rapid increase in the first year of life: the mean total cholesterol concentration in childhood is ~4.2 mmol/L. In affluent societies in particular, concentrations rise further in early adulthood.

Elevated plasma cholesterol concentrations are a **major risk factor for cardiovascular disease**, because in the majority of people most plasma cholesterol is present in the LDL fraction. The relationships between cholesterol concentration and mortality from CHD is curvilinear (Fig. 17.7). The curve becomes increasingly steep as cholesterol concentration increases: CHD mortality doubles between concentrations of 5.2 and 6.5 mmol/L and quadruples between 5.2 and 7.8 mmol/L. At concentrations <5.2 mmol/L the curve becomes ever shallower, but there is no threshold concentration below which there is no further reduction in CHD mortality. In individuals with other risk factors—for example, **cigarette smoking** (see later)—the curve is moved upwards and is steeper.

Approximately two-thirds of adults in the UK have plasma cholesterol concentrations >5.2 mmol/L and one-quarter have concentrations >6.5 mmol/L. It is, however, inappropriate to define a reference range for plasma

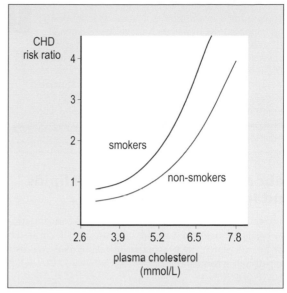

Fig. 17.7 Mortality from coronary heart disease (CHD) and plasma cholesterol concentration. Mortality is expressed as risk relative to that associated with a concentration of 5.2 mmol/L. With additional risk factors (e.g. cigarette smoking), the curve is shifted upwards and is steeper.

cholesterol concentration based on population values, because there is a graduation of cardiovascular risk across the entire range of concentrations found in the general population. Rather, it is preferable to consider an individual person's concentration in terms of its implication for their risk of future cardiovascular events: this will depend on the presence or absence of other cardiovascular risk factors and whether they already have clinical evidence of cardiovascular disease.

In contrast with the association between plasma cholesterol concentration (and, in particular, LDL-cholesterol) and increased risk of cardiovascular disease, there is **an inverse correlation between plasma HDL–cholesterol concentration (when below median values only) and cardiovascular risk**. This is attributed to the observation that **LDL particles** become **smaller, denser and more atherogenic** as the HDL–cholesterol concentration falls. Many physiological factors influence LDL- and HDL-cholesterol, some of which are indicated in Table 17.2.

Hypertriglyceridaemia is also a cardiovascular risk factor, albeit a less important one. Certain triglyceride-rich lipoproteins, particularly IDLs, are directly atherogenic. Hypertriglyceridaemia is also usually associated with the presence of small, dense LDL particles, which are more atherogenic than other LDL subtypes: this pattern is particularly associated with type 2 diabetes mellitus.

> **!**
>
> Triglyceride concentration is linearly associated with an increased risk of pancreatitis: values >10 mmol/L should trigger intervention and patient counselling; specialist advice should be considered for patients with triglycerides >20 mmol/L.
>
> Triglyceride concentrations >1.7 mmol/L associated with low HDL-cholesterol (<1.2 and <1.0 mmol/L in women and men, respectively) is also associated with increased risk of cardiovascular disease; the pattern can be reversed by weight loss.

Laboratory measurement of lipids and lipoproteins

Triglyceride and total and HDL-cholesterol concentrations can easily be measured in the laboratory. LDL-cholesterol can be calculated, in plasma from fasting patients, using the following formula:

$$\text{LDL CHOL} = \text{TOTAL CHOL} - \left(\text{HDL CHOL} + \frac{\text{TRIG}}{2.2} \right)$$

where all quantities are expressed in mmol/L. This formula becomes increasingly inaccurate as triglyceride concentrations increase above normal values, and is invalid if they exceed 4.5 mmol/L. In addition, calculation of LDL-cholesterol concentration is relatively imprecise because it summates the results of three separate laboratory assays, and the testing process is inconvenient to the patient because it requires fasting. Calculation of non-HDL-cholesterol (total cholesterol – HDL-cholesterol) provides an alternative measure of total atherogenic lipoprotein concentration. It has the added advantages that it does not require the patient to fast and uses only two laboratory measurements. Monitoring of plasma non-HDL-cholesterol, rather than LDL-cholesterol concentration, is recommended in current UK guidelines for the management of lipid disorders. Total and HDL-cholesterol concentrations are the lipid parameters used in the estimation of cardiovascular risk.

Although (with the exception of HDL-cholesterol) routine laboratory lipid assays measure the total cholesterol or triglyceride concentration regardless of their lipoprotein distribution, the concentration of individual lipoproteins can be inferred from the results. An increase solely in cholesterol indicates high concentrations of lipoproteins that contain mostly cholesterol, principally LDL (see Fig. 17.2). An increase in both cholesterol and triglycerides suggests an increase in lipoproteins that contain both lipids, that is, VLDL and IDL, assuming that the patient is

fasting and, therefore, that chylomicrons are unlikely to be present.

Lipoproteins can be separated by ultracentrifugation, after which their concentration is measured in terms of their cholesterol content, but this is not a convenient technique for routine use and is primarily a research tool. Lipoproteins can also be separated by electrophoresis, which is occasionally useful to confirm the presence of an atypical 'broad beta' band if increased amounts of IDL are present, as in patients with remnant hyperlipoproteinaemia (see p. 314).

Apolipoprotein analysis is largely of value in the rarer types of primary hyperlipidaemia. Apo E genotyping or phenotyping is necessary to confirm the diagnosis of remnant hyperlipoproteinaemia. Measurement of LPL and apo C-II are required for the diagnosis of the cause of fasting chylomicronaemia (see p. 315). Because each LDL particle contains only one apo B molecule, whereas the cholesterol content of LDL is variable, apo B concentration provides a better measure of LDL particle concentration (but it has not been shown to have greater value than LDL- or non-HDL-cholesterol in CHD risk assessment). Apo B production by the liver is increased in familial combined hyperlipidaemia (see p. 315): a high concentration in patients with the increase in plasma concentrations of both cholesterol and triglycerides that characterizes this condition supports this diagnosis. Apo A-I is present largely in HDL, but its measurement has not been proved to provide additional useful information. High plasma concentrations of Lp(a) indicate additional CHD risk independently of LDL-cholesterol concentration, and measurement may have a role in refining risk-based treatment decisions, although it is not widely used currently (see p. 304).

The **appearance of the plasma** (after separation from blood cells in the laboratory) may provide useful information about the nature of a hyperlipidaemia. In health, in the fasting state, plasma is clear. Following a meal, it often becomes opalescent because of the light-scattering properties of chylomicrons and VLDL. At triglyceride concentrations greater than ~4 mmol/L, the plasma becomes increasingly turbid; with severe hypertriglyceridaemia, it appears milky (lipaemic). If plasma is left undisturbed, chylomicrons float to the surface, leaving a clear layer underneath; VLDL remains in suspension. LDL does not scatter light and, even at high plasma cholesterol concentrations, the plasma remains clear.

Clinical indications for lipid testing

There is conclusive evidence from clinical trials that lowering plasma cholesterol concentrations by any means, not just with HMG-CoA reductase inhibitors

Table 17.2 Some physiological influences on lipoproteins and secondary causes of dyslipidaemia

	HDL cholesterol	LDL cholesterol	Triglycerides
sex	F > M	F = M	F < M
age	slight ↓ in F	↑	↓
exercise	↑	↓	↓
obesity	↓	N	↑
ethanol	↑	N	↑
exogenous oestrogens	↑	↓	↑
diabetes mellitus	↓	N	↑↑
hypothyroidism	N	↑↑	N/↑
nephrotic syndrome	↓	↑↑	↑↑
chronic kidney disease	↓	N/↑	↑
cholestasis[a]	N	↑	N

[a]In cholestasis, much of the hypercholesterolaemia is due to the accumulation of lipoprotein X, an aggregate of free cholesterol, lecithin, albumin and apo C.
F, female; HDL, high-density lipoprotein; LDL, low-density lipoprotein; M, male; N, no significant effect.

Patient preparation for lipid testing

In patients who are not already on lipid-lowering therapy, measurement of lipids is most commonly requested in the context of cardiovascular risk assessment (see later). The lipid tests required are total and HDL-cholesterol, although triglycerides are also included in some guidelines. The concentration of the cholesterol parameters changes little after eating, and postprandial hypertriglyceridaemia is associated with increased cardiovascular risk, hence the patient does need not to fast before the blood sample is taken. A 12-h fast, but with free access to water, is needed only if calculation of LDL–cholesterol concentration is required, because the formula used (see p. 310) assumes that no chylomicrons are present.

When lipid studies are done on a patient who has had a myocardial infarction (MI) or stroke, blood should either be taken **within 24 h** or after an **interval of 3 months**, because the metabolism of lipoproteins is disturbed during the convalescent period, so results may be misleading.

whom there is no evidence of disease). Lowering cholesterol also reduces the risk of ischaemic **stroke**. Lowering cholesterol is not associated with an increase in mortality from other diseases (e.g. cancer). Treatment of hypercholesterolaemia with statins is associated with a slightly increased incidence of type 2 diabetes in those in whom the diagnosis was imminent, but the theoretical increase in mortality is far outweighed by the anticipated reduction in cardiovascular mortality resulting from lowering cholesterol.

It is therefore clear that lipid measurements should be made in all patients known to have cardiovascular disease, in those at increased risk because of the presence of other risk factors (see p. 316) and where the family history suggests an inherited disorder such as familial hypercholesterolaemia (FH; see p. 313). Thus, plasma lipids should be measured in individuals with the following:

- clinical evidence of cardiovascular disease
- a family history of premature CHD (occurring at age <60 years)
- other major cardiovascular risk factors (e.g. diabetes mellitus, hypertension)
- patients with clinical features of hyperlipidaemia (see later)
- patients whose plasma is seen to be lipaemic.

In the absence of these indications, recommendations regarding screening vary from country to country. Current UK

(statins), **reduces mortality** from CHD and decreases overall mortality. This has been demonstrated both in the context of **secondary prevention** (treatment of individuals with pre-existing cardiovascular disease) and **primary prevention** (treatment of individuals in

practice recommended by the National Institute for Health and Care Excellence in 2014 is to commence regular comprehensive cardiovascular risk assessment, including measurement of lipids, in all adults from the age of 40 years onwards.

Disorders of Lipid Metabolism

Several rare inherited metabolic diseases are associated with the accumulation of lipids in tissues, and in others plasma lipoprotein concentrations are reduced. By far the commonest disorders, however, are the hyperlipidaemias, both primary (genetic) and secondary.

Classification

Hyperlipidaemias are classified as either **primary**, comprising a group of genetically determined disorders, or **secondary**, in which the abnormalities are the result of an acquired condition.

Hyperlipidaemias previously were classified using the World Health Organization (WHO) system, based on the work of Fredrickson, according to the pattern of lipoprotein abnormality present. This classification is now largely obsolete and hyperlipidaemias are classified by their metabolic cause (if secondary) or their specific type (if primary).

Secondary hyperlipidaemias

Secondary hyperlipidaemias are common (see Table 17.2 and Case histories 17.1, 17.2 and 17.3): management should initially be directed at the underlying condition. It is always important to exclude secondary causes in the investigation of patients with hyperlipidaemias, even if the presence of a primary disorder is inferred from the family history. Occasionally, such a cause may coexist with a primary hyperlipidaemia and exacerbate its manifestations.

Several **drugs** can also cause or exacerbate hyperlipidaemia, including thiazides (at high dose), beta blockers lacking intrinsic sympathomimetic activity, corticosteroids, immunosuppressants, retinoids and antiretroviral drugs. Oestrogens, especially when given to postmenopausal women, may lower plasma cholesterol concentrations but may cause, or exacerbate, hypertriglyceridaemia. Certain progestogens used in oral contraceptives also have a small adverse effect on plasma lipids (see p. 222).

Case history 17.1

History

A 55-year-old man presented with a history of lethargy, loss of concentration and constipation. He had suffered from angina for 2 years, but this had become less of a problem recently, as he had become much less active.

Examination

He appeared myxoedematous.

Results (see Appendix for reference ranges)

Serum:		
	thyroid-stimulating hormone (TSH)	>100 mIU/L
	cholesterol	12.2 mmol/L
	HDL-cholesterol	1.3 mmol/L
	LDL-cholesterol	10.2 mmol/L
	non-HDL-cholesterol	10.9 mmol/L
	triglycerides	1.5 mmol/L

Summary

Significantly raised TSH with isolated hypercholesterolaemia.

Interpretation

Biochemical and clinical hypothyroidism; hypothyroidism frequently causes hypercholesterolaemia, because of decreased removal of LDL from the circulation. Treatment with thyroxine, starting with a low dose to avoid exacerbation of angina, should return his cholesterol to normal.

Discussion

His serum cholesterol concentration fell to 8.2 mmol/L when euthyroid, with an LDL-cholesterol of 6.4 mmol/L. The persistence of a raised cholesterol concentration despite adequate treatment of the hypothyroidism is suggestive of the presence of an underlying primary hypercholesterolaemia.

In view of his ischaemic heart disease, this man's LDL-cholesterol concentration should be reduced to <1.8 mmol/L (see p. 317). Statin treatment is indicated, but only after becoming biochemically euthyroid: there is theoretically an increased risk of myopathy if statins are given to hypothyroid patients.

Note that hypothyroidism should be treated under close medical supervision in patients with ischaemic heart disease. The increase in metabolic rate increases the body's oxygen requirements and can exacerbate angina or precipitate myocardial infarction.

Primary hyperlipidaemias

Familial hypercholesterolaemia

Familial hypercholesterolaemia (FH) is characterized by high plasma cholesterol concentrations that are present from early childhood and do not depend on the presence of environmental factors (see the following section, Polygenic hypercholesterolaemia). It is inherited as an **autosomal dominant** characteristic, with a prevalence in the population in the UK of about 1 in 250. Huge numbers of different mutations (>90% affecting four genes) have been described worldwide, with the commonest affecting **LDL receptor** function or the structure of **apo B**. In all cases, there is a defect in the uptake and catabolism of LDL, and its plasma concentration is increased. In heterozygotes, total cholesterol is typically in the range 7.5–12 mmol/L (see Case history 17.4). When a diagnosis of FH is made, the patient's first-degree relatives should also be tested because each has a 50% probability of having the same disorder. Identification of the specific genetic mutation is preferable as the phenotype varies considerably between affected family members, limiting the utility of lipid analysis alone, although this can be done. Such 'cascade' testing is of great clinical value because treatment (which is primarily with statin drugs) significantly reduces the risk of developing CHD, especially if the disorder is identified early in life.

Heterozygotes tend to develop coronary artery disease some 20 years earlier than the general population; more than half of those untreated die before the age of 60 years. In the rare **homozygotes** (prevalence ~1/1 000 000), no functional receptors are present. Plasma cholesterol

> !
>
> Familial hypercholesterolaemia is probable when cholesterol concentration is >7.5 mmol/L (LDL-cholesterol >4.9 mmol/L) in adults or >6.7 mmol/L (LDL >4.0 mmol/L) in children, together with **tendon xanthomata** in the individual or close relative, or on DNA evidence of a recognized mutation. 'Possible' FH is suspected in patients who do not meet these definitive criteria but who have the same degree of hypercholesterolaemia together with a family history of premature CHD or hypercholesterolaemia. Tendon xanthomata always and corneal arcus or xanthelasma before the age of 40 years should alert one to the possibility of FH. Corneal arcus and xanthelasmata may occur in the absence of an obvious disturbance of lipid metabolism, although usually only in older people (>60 years of age). Patients with FH require rigorous cardiovascular risk management, invariably requiring lipid-lowering drugs as well as lifestyle modification (see later), initiated ideally before the age of 10 years.

concentrations are usually >15 mmol/L. These individuals develop coronary artery disease in childhood and, if untreated, rarely survive into adult life.

Polygenic hypercholesterolaemia

In FH, the distribution of plasma cholesterol concentrations in relatives of the proband is mostly bimodal, with a clear distinction between heterozygotes and normals. More

---

Case history 17.2

History

A 45-year-old obese barman, with a history of heavy alcohol ingestion, presented with recurrent epigastric pain.

Investigation

Endoscopy revealed a duodenal ulcer; a blood sample was taken for liver function tests.

Results

Serum:		
	cholesterol	7.5 mmol/L
	HDL-cholesterol	1.4 mmol/L
	LDL-cholesterol	N/A (calculation not possible)
	non-HDL-cholesterol	6.1 mmol/L
	triglyceride	8.4 mmol/L

Lipaemia was detected by the laboratory analyser, and on inspection the plasma looked turbid. The duty biochemist therefore requested analysis of a full lipid profile.

Summary

Significant mixed dyslipidaemia.

Interpretation

Ethanol causes hypertriglyceridaemia by increasing triglyceride synthesis, and the insulin resistance seen in obesity has a similar effect. Massive hypertriglyceridaemia (>20 mmol/L) may occur in patients with a high alcohol intake when there is an additional, inherited tendency to hypertriglyceridaemia. Moderate alcohol intake increases HDL-cholesterol concentrations but this is not cardioprotective.

Discussion

It was not possible to estimate the LDL-cholesterol concentration in this sample because the triglyceride concentration was >4.5 mmol/L. Non-HDL-cholesterol could still be calculated: this illustrates one of the advantages of this parameter over LDL-cholesterol.

Case history 17.3

History

An obese 44-year-old woman with type 1 diabetes was found to have a blood glucose concentration of 32 mmol/L at the outpatient clinic and was admitted to hospital. The serum obtained from a subsequent blood sample was seen to be grossly lipaemic.

Results

Serum:		
	cholesterol	53 mmol/L
	triglyceride	150 mmol/L

The sample was inspected after standing overnight and had a creamy, supernatant layer, although the infranatant remained lipaemic.

Summary

Gross mixed dyslipidaemia.

Interpretation

The appearance of the serum indicates the presence of both chylomicrons and VLDL. Hyperlipidaemia can complicate uncontrolled type 1 and type 2 diabetes and is due to a combination of decreased lipoprotein lipase activity and increased hepatic triglyceride synthesis. It may exacerbate a coexisting familial hyperlipidaemia.

Discussion

This patient was treated with an intravenous insulin infusion. Her blood glucose concentration fell rapidly, and she was re-stabilized on an appropriate regimen of subcutaneous insulin injections. After a week, her serum cholesterol and triglycerides were 8.0 and 11 mmol/L, respectively. Thereafter, her diabetes remained well controlled and follow-up lipid analysis showed cholesterol 6.0 mmol/L, HDL-cholesterol 0.6 mmol/L and triglycerides 5.3 mmol/L. Her immediate family had normal serum lipids, and it was concluded that her persistently elevated triglyceride and low HDL were related at least in part to her obesity. She was started on a statin to reduce her CVD risk.

Case history 17.4

History

A 36-year-old man attended an appointment with his general practitioner after his optician noticed that he had bilateral corneal arcus. He was a non-smoker and not overweight. His father had died of a heart attack at the age of 40 years.

Examination

Achilles tendon xanthomata were present. Blood pressure was normal.

Results

Serum:		
	cholesterol	13.2 mmol/L
	HDL-cholesterol	1.3 mmol/L
	LDL-cholesterol	11.4 mmol/L
	non-HDL-cholesterol	10.1 mmol/L
	triglyceride	1.3 mmol/L

Summary

Isolated hypercholesterolaemia with tendon xanthomata and family history of premature cardiovascular disease.

Interpretation

This is the characteristic picture of FH.

Discussion

Tendon xanthomata, although not an invariable finding, are virtually pathognomonic of FH. Their development is age related. They are accumulations of cholesterol, but deep-seated, with the result that the overlying skin has a normal colour (see Red Flag on p. 313).

Remnant hyperlipoproteinaemia

Remnant hyperlipoproteinaemia is also known as **familial dysbetalipoproteinaemia** (see Case history 17.5). Biochemically, it is characterized by the presence of an excess of IDL and chylomicron remnants; chylomicrons are sometimes also present. Total **cholesterol and triglyceride concentrations are elevated**, typically to **approximately equal values**. This condition previously was called 'broad beta disease', because the remnant particles create a broad band on serum lipoprotein electrophoresis. Patients are at increased risk for cerebrovascular, coronary and peripheral artery disease. Remnant hyperlipoproteinaemia is characterized clinically by the presence of fat deposits in the **palmar creases** and by **tuberous xanthomata**; the latter tend to occur over bony prominences and, unlike tendon xanthomata, are reddish. However, neither of these cutaneous stigmata is invariably present. In some patients, eruptive xanthomata occur periodically.

frequently, when the family of an individual with hypercholesterolaemia is studied, a continuous distribution is found, consistent with the plasma cholesterol being influenced by several genes. Multiple single nucleotide polymorphisms have been identified (at least 50).

The significance of this condition again lies in its relationship to the risk of coronary artery disease, and the principles of management are similar to those for FH. In polygenic hypercholesterolaemia, however, dietary treatment alone may sometimes be adequate to lower the cholesterol concentration to acceptable levels and the cardiovascular disease rates are lower than in FH.

Case history 17.5

History

A middle-aged man was referred to a dermatologist because of extensive yellowish papules on his buttocks and elbows.

Examination

The papules were typical of eruptive xanthomata, with erythematous bases. He also had yellow, fatty streaks in the palmar creases and was overweight.

Results

Serum:		
	slightly turbid on inspection	
	cholesterol	8.5 mmol/L
	triglyceride	6.4 mmol/L

Apo E genotyping indicated that the patient was homozygous for the *APOE e2* allele. Thyroid function tests and fasting glucose were within reference limits.

Interpretation

He has a mixed dyslipidaemia with similar increases in cholesterol and triglycerides; this is consistent with remnant hyperlipoproteinaemia.

Discussion

This patient was treated with a low-fat diet and fenofibrate with subsequent introduction of atorvastatin, and after 3 months his serum lipid concentrations had become normal. There was also considerable regression of the xanthomata. When the fenofibrate was stopped, the lipid abnormalities recurred, but resolved again on restarting the drug.

The apo E gene shows **polymorphism**. The commonest apo E phenotype is termed E3/E3. Remnant hyperlipoproteinaemia is associated with the **E2/E2 phenotype**, which can result in impaired IDL uptake by the liver. However, although the phenotype is present in 1 in 100 of the healthy population, remnant hyperlipoproteinaemia is an uncommon disorder (prevalence ~1/10 000), implying that other factors contribute to its expression. Such factors include obesity, alcohol, hypothyroidism and diabetes. Notably, although the variant apoprotein is present from birth, the condition does not appear clinically until adult life. Although the diagnosis can be inferred from the clinical and biochemical findings, it should ideally be confirmed by apo E genotyping.

The significance of apo E polymorphism is not limited to lipid metabolism. Increased frequency of the *e4* allele has been demonstrated in patients with familial Alzheimer disease.

Familial chylomicronaemia

Fasting chylomicronaemia is a feature of two rare hyperlipidaemias, both having an **autosomal recessive** inheritance: in one, there is a deficiency of the enzyme **LPL**, and in the other a deficiency of **apo C-II**, which is required for activation of this enzyme. The result in each case is a failure of chylomicron clearance from the bloodstream. Presentation is usually in childhood, with eruptive xanthomata, recurrent abdominal pain caused by pancreatitis and sometimes hepatosplenomegaly. Lipaemia retinalis may also be present.

Chylomicronaemia may also be seen in other patients with a genetic predisposition to hypertriglyceridaemia when this is exacerbated by obesity, diabetes mellitus, hyperuricaemia or alcohol ingestion; some drugs—for example, thiazides—may also have this effect.

Management involves giving a **very-low-fat diet**, with substitution of some fat by triglycerides based on medium chain fatty acids: these are absorbed directly from the gut into the bloodstream and therefore do not produce chylomicrons. The major complication of the chylomicronaemic syndromes is recurrent pancreatitis, but this is usually prevented if plasma triglyceride concentrations can be maintained at <10 mmol/L. A drug targeting apo-CIII (which inhibits LPL) has recently been developed.

Familial hypertriglyceridaemia

Familial hypertriglyceridaemia, which has a prevalence of approximately 1 in 600, is usually associated with an excess of VLDL in plasma. It is usually not manifest until adulthood. The molecular basis is uncertain (there is increased hepatic synthesis of VLDL). Inheritance appears to be **autosomal dominant**, although a polygenic aetiology is suggested. Triglyceride concentrations are not usually >5 mmol/L, but in severe cases, in which other factors (e.g. obesity and alcohol) are implicated, they can be much higher; chylomicronaemia can occur, and only then are physical signs (e.g. eruptive xanthomata and lipaemia retinalis) usually present.

It is uncertain whether there is an increased risk of CHD in patients with familial hypertriglyceridaemia, although HDL concentration is often reduced; in severe cases, there is a risk of pancreatitis.

Familial combined hyperlipidaemia

Familial combined hyperlipidaemia is due to hepatic overproduction of apo B, leading to increased VLDL secretion and increased production of LDL from VLDL. Either plasma cholesterol or triglyceride, or both, may be elevated;

typically, in affected relatives, one-third have an increase in LDL, one-third have an increase in VLDL and one-third have an excess of both lipoproteins. Cutaneous manifestations of hyperlipidaemia may be present, and in all cases, there is an increased risk of coronary artery disease.

The prevalence is approximately 1 in 200; inheritance is probably autosomal dominant. There are no distinctive clinical features, and the diagnosis is often presumptive, based on the increase in both cholesterol and triglyceride in the absence of tendon xanthomata or a secondary cause of hyperlipidaemia.

Familial hyperalphalipoproteinaemia

In familial hyperalphalipoproteinaemia, there is hypercholesterolaemia due to an increase in only the HDL fraction, which may be present in other members of the family. CHD risk may be decreased, but this is debated. No specific treatment is required. The existence of this condition underlines the need to measure HDL-cholesterol in patients with hypercholesterolaemia. Generally, if total cholesterol is >7 mmol/L, there will always be an increase in LDL, but even then, measurement of HDL-cholesterol is essential in the assessment of CHD risk.

Cardiovascular Risk Management

Risk factors and risk assessment

The major reason for treating hyperlipidaemia is to decrease the risk of cardiovascular disease. In patients with severe hypertriglyceridaemia, treatment may be necessary to reduce the risk of pancreatitis. It cannot be overemphasized that hyperlipidaemia is only one of many risk factors for cardiovascular disease: more than 200 have been identified. The decision to treat a patient with hyperlipidaemia must be based on an adequate assessment of risk: with the exception of patients with very high lipid concentrations and those known to have arterial disease, the decision to prescribe lipid-lowering treatment should not be based on measurements of lipids alone. Some of the more important risk factors are indicated in Table 17.3.

These risk factors tend to be **multiplicative**: in people in the lowest quintile of cholesterol concentrations, hypertension increases cardiovascular risk by approximately 2-fold and cigarette smoking by a factor of ~1.6; a combination of hypertension and smoking increases risk by a factor of ~3.4. Risk attributable to the major cardiovascular risk factors present in an individual patient can be quantified using a risk-prediction model such as the Framingham system or QRISK3 (recommended in the UK because it is based on a large UK epidemiological database). Risk is usually expressed as percentage risk of developing symptomatic cardiovascular disease over the next 10 years. However, lifetime risk calculations are increasing in popularity.

Table 17.3 Risk factors for cardiovascular disease

Modifiable	Not modifiable
hypercholesterolaemia[a]	personal history of cardiovascular disease[a]
hypertension[a]	family history of premature cardiovascular disease[a]
cigarette smoking[a]	male sex[a]
diabetes mellitus[a]	age[a]
hyperfibrinogenaemia[b]	
hyperhomocysteinaemia[b]	
low HDL-cholesterol[b]	
hypertriglyceridaemia[b]	
overweight[b]	
sedentary lifestyle[b]	

[a]Major risk factors, proven benefit from clinical intervention if modifiable.
[b]Potentially modifiable risk factors (although the benefit of doing so is either uncertain or unproven).

Cigarette smoking, hypertension and diabetes are all major risk factors that are susceptible to intervention. A family history of premature vascular disease, age and being male are not susceptible, but may require a more aggressive approach to the management of those factors, including hyperlipidaemia, which are susceptible. It should be appreciated that the single most important risk factor for future symptomatic coronary disease is a history of previous MI or other clinical evidence of cardiovascular disease. This has major implications for treatment (see later).

A number of additional potential biochemical markers of cardiovascular risk have been identified. C-reactive protein and fibrinogen predict future cardiovascular disease, probably because they are markers of inflammation, and treating inflammation is associated with significant reduction of associated cardiovascular risk, but their clinical role is uncertain. The use of Lp(a) measurement is discussed on p. 304. High plasma concentrations of homocysteine occur in the inherited metabolic disease homocystinuria (classically a result of a deficiency of the enzyme cystathionine β-synthase); patients with this disease are at increased risk of premature vascular disease. A lesser degree of hyperhomocysteinaemia is also a cardiovascular risk factor, possibly through promotion of the oxidation of LDL and a direct toxic action on the vascular endothelium. Folate supplementation lowers plasma homocysteine concentration, but has not been shown to prevent vascular disease, and thus routine measurement of homocysteine as a cardiovascular risk factor is not recommended.

Rationale for treatment of hyperlipidaemia

All patients at risk of CHD should be encouraged to make appropriate changes to their diet and lifestyle, particularly increasing physical activity. The diet should be designed to achieve/maintain an ideal body weight, and not more than 30% of energy should be provided by fat, of which not more than one-third should be saturated. The effects of dietary intervention on lipid concentrations are, however, more apparent in clinical trials than in free-living subjects.

Targets for lipid concentrations during treatment reflect those achieved in randomized controlled clinical trials (although recent studies have demonstrated that there is no lower limit of LDL beneath which no further benefit is gained). On this basis, in **secondary prevention** (patients with established CHD, cerebrovascular disease and peripheral vascular disease), current guidelines recommend a target LDL-cholesterol concentration <1.8 mmol/L (equivalent to a non-HDL-cholesterol concentration of 2.5 mmol/L) or a reduction of >40% in non-HDL-cholesterol. The benefits of prescribing **statins** to achieve target concentrations in this context are well established. Such treatment clearly reduces mortality and is cost-effective. It must, of course, be combined with other appropriate intervention, including both adoption of a **healthier lifestyle** (improved diet, increased exercise, cessation of smoking, etc.) and **other drugs** (e.g. aspirin, beta blockers, angiotensin-converting enzyme [ACE] inhibitors and additional antihypertensive medication when required).

In the context of **primary prevention**, however, the situation is less clear-cut. Because the risks for CHD are lower, the benefits of intervention (in terms of the numbers of patients treated in relation to numbers of lives saved) are also lower. Guidelines for the prescription of lipid-lowering drugs in primary prevention are usually set around specific levels of risk. Some guidelines recommend treatment at a cumulative risk of developing cardiovascular disease over 10 years as low as 10%. It cannot, however, be overemphasized that such guidelines are only guidelines: they should not be regarded as prescriptive and are not a substitute for the exercise of clinical judgement in individual patients. Most patients with **diabetes** are at high risk of CHD: some guidelines recommend treatment of almost all patients, whereas others advocate frequent review of 10-year cardiovascular risk. Patients with **chronic kidney disease, major psychiatric disease** and those with **chronic inflammatory diseases** are also at high risk of cardiovascular disease and should be treated accordingly.

In practice, lipid-lowering medication is likely to be indicated in most individuals whose total cholesterol concentration remains >7.8 mmol/L after an adequate trial of dietary modification. It will be indicated at lower concentrations if other risk factors are present. At any given cholesterol concentration, the indication for intervention will be strengthened by the presence of hypertriglyceridaemia or a low HDL-cholesterol concentration.

Hypercholesterolaemia

The drugs of choice for the treatment of hypercholesterolaemia are the **statins**, inhibitors of HMG-CoA reductase, the rate-limiting step in cholesterol synthesis. These decrease intracellular cholesterol concentrations and thus increase LDL receptor expression and decrease plasma LDL. Statins lower triglycerides slightly and tend to increase HDL. They are the only class of lipid-lowering drugs that have been shown to reduce overall mortality. **Ezetimibe** inhibits cholesterol absorption and thereby interrupts its enterohepatic circulation and decreases the delivery of dietary cholesterol to the liver, thus increasing LDL receptor expression. Its action is therefore synergistic with that of the statins, with which it may usefully be used in combination. Monoclonal antibodies to **PCSK9** inhibit LDL receptor recycling and thus increase LDL receptor expression, resulting in further LDL reduction.

Less specific inhibitors of lipid and bile acid uptake, the **bile acid sequestrants**, are less effective and poorly tolerated: their use is declining.

Several new powerful classes of drugs to treat hypercholesterolaemia have recently become available or are in a late stage of development and trial. These include **apo-B antisense oligonucleotides** and **microsomal triglyceride transfer protein inhibitors,** which reduce VLDL synthesis and hence LDL production.

Patients with homozygous FH tend to respond poorly to drugs and are usually treated with repeated **LDL apheresis**, a process that physically removes LDL from the circulation. Microsomal triglyceride transfer protein inhibitors are powerful LDL-lowering agents that sometimes avoid or reduce the need for apheresis.

Hypertriglyceridaemia

Hypertriglyceridaemia may respond well to control of body weight and any coexistent exacerbating factors (e.g. excessive alcohol intake and diabetes). The main classes of drug used for treating hypertriglyceridaemia are the **fibrates** and **fish oils**. Fibrates have various effects on lipid metabolism, but work primarily by stimulating LPL and reducing liver triglyceride synthesis. Fish oils are rich in the ω-3 polyunsaturated fatty acids that decrease VLDL synthesis. Antisense oligonucleotide therapy directed at apo-CIII is licensed only for patients with very severe hypertriglyceridaemia due to familial chylomicronaemia (see p. 315).

High lipoprotein(a)

Lipid apheresis is effective but is undertaken only very rarely. Cholesterol reduction, with statins and consideration of low-dose aspirin therapy, is the mainstay of therapy. Antisense oligonucleotide therapy is under development and should provide useful data on the clinical effectiveness of treatments aimed specifically at Lp(a).

Lipoprotein Deficiency

There are three rare, inherited lipoprotein deficiencies: abetalipoproteinaemia, hypobetalipoproteinaemia and Tangier disease.

Abetalipoproteinaemia

In abetalipoproteinaemia, there is a defect in the synthesis of apo B; chylomicrons, VLDL and LDL are absent from the plasma. Clinically, there is malabsorption of fat, acanthocytosis, retinitis pigmentosa and an ataxic neuropathy.

Hypobetalipoproteinaemia

In hypobetalipoproteinaemia, there is partial deficiency of apo B; chylomicrons, VLDL and LDL are present but in low concentrations. Clinical features vary from no apparent abnormality to fat malabsorption, hepatic steatosis and failure to thrive.

Tangier disease

In Tangier disease, plasma HDL concentrations are reduced; clinically, the condition is characterized by hyperplastic, orange tonsils and the accumulation of cholesteryl esters in other reticuloendothelial tissues. Patients are at increased risk of cardiovascular disease. The condition is due to a loss-of-function mutation in the gene that codes for the protein ABCA1, which normally stimulates the uptake of cholesterol into HDL.

Myocardial Infarction

Some patients with MI have a typical history of crushing central **chest pain**, perhaps radiating to the arm or jaw, associated with **typical electrocardiogram (ECG)** changes of ST segment elevation. This type of MI is at the severe end of the spectrum of **acute coronary syndrome** (ACS), which also includes non-ST elevation MI (NSTEMI) and unstable angina. ACS can also present atypically (without typical chest pain), or be clinically silent, particularly in the elderly. The ECG changes may not always be typical, particularly where there has been previous infarction, or in left bundle branch block. Also, even apparently typical chest pain is not always due to MI.

The measurement, in plasma, of biomarkers released from the myocardium plays a central role in the diagnosis and management of ACS. Indeed, the 2018 universal definition of MI is an acute rise in cardiac biomarkers in a clinical context of symptoms of ischaemia or new ECG changes. The cardiac biomarker with the best diagnostic performance for routine clinical purposes is cardiac troponin (see Case histories 17.6 and 17.7).

Cardiac biomarkers that enable earlier diagnosis continue to be investigated, e.g. myoglobin, heart-type fatty acid binding protein and copeptin. It is likely that no single test will combine adequate sensitivity and specificity, but there may be potential for developing combinations of tests that can be deployed as point-of-care testing.

Biochemical monitoring has an important role in the monitoring of patients with ACS. Plasma lipids should be measured at presentation, as treatment with a high potency statin is almost invariably required. Testing also gives the opportunity to identify genetic dyslipidaemias that require both patient counselling and family screening. Repeat measurement of lipids should be no sooner than 3 months

---

Troponin

Troponin I and **troponin T** are component proteins of the contractile apparatus in muscle cells. Their cardiac-specific isoforms can be measured by immunoassays that do not cross-react with the skeletal isoforms. Although the presence of increased concentrations in plasma indicates **myocardial injury**, this could be due to many causes, for example myocarditis or pulmonary embolism. Therefore, troponin measurement is only clinically indicated if acute coronary syndrome (ACS) is suspected. New high-sensitivity assays enable detection of an acute rise in plasma earlier than 4 h after onset of ACS in many patients, but neither troponin I nor troponin T increases in plasma sufficiently early to inform the use of thrombolysis or primary angioplasty in patients with ST elevation MI. Their greatest use is in distinguishing which patients with ACS have NSTEMI and which have angina: the former group requires specific urgent investigation and treatment because they are at much higher risk of death.

The high-sensitivity troponin assay is useful for acute admission units. If there is no rise in troponin 3 h after the admission test, the patient is likely to have either non-cardiac chest pain or stable angina caused by coronary stenosis (without acute thrombosis). This can facilitate rapid and accurate triage and discharge of patients.

Case history 17.6

History

A recently retired lawyer was admitted to a hospital with chest pain that had developed during the evening after a day spent digging in his garden.

Investigation

There were no specific signs of myocardial infarction on the ECG.

Results

		On admission	3 h
Serum:	high sensitivity troponin T	6 ng/L	8 ng/L

Interpretation

ACS was ruled out by demonstrating no significant increase in serum high sensitivity troponin T.

Discussion

A significant rise would be a troponin concentration increase of >50% after 3 h, although this may vary depending on assay and patient pathway. In the absence of other causes, it was concluded that the chest pain was musculoskeletal in origin, and as the pain subsided rapidly, he was discharged. One of the junior doctors requested measurement of creatine kinase (CK) on the 3-h sample and it was found to be high at 950 U/L. This result, however, is of little clinical value because heavy exercise almost invariably causes an increase in plasma CK activity, which may reach a peak of >10 × the upper reference limit in untrained individuals.

Case history 17.7

History

A general practitioner was called to see a previously fit elderly man in a residential home. The patient had become acutely short of breath 1 h earlier, soon after his breakfast, and developed a cough with frothy white sputum. He also complained of dizziness but denied chest pain.

Examination

He had widespread crepitations throughout his lung fields; his blood pressure was 122/70 mmHg, but had been 152/92 mmHg when checked by the doctor 2 months previously.

He was given a diuretic, with considerable ensuing symptomatic relief. An electrocardiogram (ECG) showed changes consistent with a very recent myocardial infarction. He was admitted to hospital for emergency percutaneous coronary intervention (PCI).

Results

Serum:	high sensitivity troponin T	62 ng/L

Discussion

The breathlessness, cough and crepitations are classic features of left ventricular failure. A likely cause of this, and the fall in blood pressure, was myocardial infarction: chest pain does not always occur, particularly in the elderly. A second troponin measurement would demonstrate the acute rise characteristic of myocardial infarction. However, the typical ECG changes in this case obviated the need for repeat measurement. Patients with a typical clinical presentation and ST segment elevation on ECG should be referred immediately for PCI; measurement of troponin is not required for diagnosis in such circumstances.

later (see p. 311) because the metabolic stress of ACS causes a prolonged fall in plasma cholesterol concentrations.

Cerebrovascular disease and peripheral vascular disease

The approach to risk factor assessment and management in patients with cerebrovascular and peripheral vascular disease is very similar to that for CHD. However, some types of dyslipidaemia, particularly remnant hyperlipoproteinaemia predispose more to peripheral vascular disease than CHD and the relative importance of risk factors is subtly different in the different types of vascular disease. For example, hypertension is more important for cerebrovascular disease, and peripheral vascular disease is classically seen in those with the worst burden of atherosclerotic plaque such as patients who smoke and have diabetes mellitus. Aggressive risk factor modification is required, as for MI, and again the clinician should look for evidence of genetic dyslipidaemias.

Heart Failure

Heart failure has been defined as a failure of the cardiac output to meet the needs of the tissues (excluding situations where this is caused by volume depletion, e.g. haemorrhage). However, it is probably more useful to regard it as a clinical syndrome with a variety of causes. It may present as a **medical emergency** (acute pulmonary oedema) or be **asymptomatic** in the early stages. It is relatively common, with an overall prevalence rate in the UK of about 2%, although this rises to 8% in those older than 65 years. The condition is chronic and progressive, and patients with heart failure have a shortened life expectancy and impaired quality of life. The prognosis can be improved by appropriate treatment, but because the symptoms and signs are non-specific, particularly in the early stages, the diagnosis can only reliably be made by echocardiography.

As discussed in Chapter 3, the heart secretes two natriuretic peptides: atrial natriuretic peptide (ANP) and B-type natriuretic peptide (BNP). ANP is produced mainly in the atria, and BNP (although first isolated from brain) comes mainly from the cardiac ventricles. Release of both is increased in heart failure, although BNP is the better marker of ventricular function and prognosis. It is synthesized as a prohormone, which is cleaved on release from cardiac muscle cells to produce **BNP** itself and an N-terminal fragment of the prohormone called **NT-proBNP** (see Case history 17.8).

Laboratory investigations are also important in the general assessment of patients with heart failure: some examples are given in Table 17.4.

Hypertension

Hypertension is a common condition that affects ~15% of the adult population. Although usually itself asymptomatic, it is an important cause of morbidity and mortality, particularly from stroke and CHD. In ~95% of patients, a specific cause for raised blood pressure cannot be demonstrated. Such hypertension is termed **essential**: its pathogenesis is not clear, although in some 70% of cases at least one other member of the family also has hypertension. Around 5% are **secondary** to other disorders (Box 17.1). Several rare, inherited conditions also cause hypertension, mostly via the aldosterone pathway. They are listed in Table 17.5, not because of their individual importance, but because of the clinicopathological correlations that they demonstrate.

BNP

A normal value of either plasma **BNP (<100 ng/L) or NT-proBNP (<300 ng/L) virtually excludes heart failure** in those presenting with suggestive symptoms, although a raised concentration may occur in other conditions. Their main use is therefore as a 'rule-out' test; patients with normal concentrations should be investigated further for other causes of their symptoms. Natriuretic peptides may also prove useful in monitoring the progression of heart failure, in tailoring its treatment and as prognostic indicators in both heart failure and CHD.

Case history 17.8

History

A 75-year-old man arranged to see his GP because he felt that he was becoming increasingly breathless on exertion. He had a 20-year history of type 2 diabetes, with stage 3 chronic kidney disease caused by diabetic nephropathy.

Results

Serum:	creatinine	156 µmol/L
	eGFR	37 mL/min/1.73m^2
	urea	7.2 mmol/L
	sodium	135 mmol/L
	potassium	3.7 mmol/L
Plasma:	NT-proBNP	480 pg/mL

Summary

Raised creatinine and upper limit urea and a mildly raised NT-proBNP.

Interpretation

UK guidelines on heart failure indicate that plasma NT-proBNP concentrations <400 pg/mL rule out the diagnosis, therefore this patient should be referred for further investigations (such as echocardiography) to determine the cause of his symptoms. The creatinine and urea could be in keeping with the expected chronic kidney disease but result trends should be checked before making this decision.

Discussion

Echocardiography demonstrated an ejection fraction of 57%, which is within the reference range, indicating normal heart function. However, aortic stenosis was identified, explaining his symptom of breathlessness.

Plasma NT-proBNP or BNP measurement is a useful 'rule-out' test, but moderately increased values may be caused by many reasons other than heart failure. Concentrations increase with age and are higher in patients with diabetes and chronic kidney disease, for example.

Table 17.4 Laboratory investigations in patients with heart failure

Investigation	Explanation
full blood count	anaemia is a cause of 'high-output' heart failure
plasma albumin	hypoalbuminaemia is another cause of oedema
plasma creatinine	chronic kidney disease
plasma potassium	diuretic-induced hypokalaemia
thyroid function tests[a]	thyrotoxicosis
plasma ferritin[a]	haemochromatosis
serum and urine electrophoresis[a]	myeloma-related amyloid
endocrine causes of hypertension[a]	see Box 17.1

[a]Investigations appropriate only if indicated clinically.

Box 17.1 Causes of secondary hypertension

coarctation of the aorta
chronic kidney disease
endocrine disease
   Conn syndrome
   Cushing syndrome
   phaeochromocytoma
   hyperparathyroidism[a]
pregnancy-associated hypertension
obesity (and sleep apnoea)

[a]There is an association between hyperparathyroidism and hypertension, but the hypertension often persists after parathyroidectomy.

Biochemical investigations play no part in the diagnosis of essential hypertension, although they are important in assessing possible adverse effects of medication (e.g. diuretic-induced hypokalaemia) and complications of hypertension (particularly chronic kidney disease). They are, however, of value in diagnosing some causes of secondary hypertension, particularly kidney and endocrine disease and the rare inherited causes.

Because it is so common, it is clearly impractical to investigate all patients with hypertension for secondary and other rare causes. All patients should, however, have simple investigations performed (Table 17.6), to look for evidence of kidney damage and as part of overall cardiovascular risk assessment. More complex investigations, particularly to diagnose **Conn syndrome, phaeochromocytoma** or **Cushing syndrome**, should be reserved for patients in whom the simple testing suggests a specific cause (e.g. hypokalaemia in an untreated patient should raise a suspicion of excessive mineralocorticoid secretion), those with clinical features suggestive of an underlying cause and patients with more severe hypertension, particularly if the hypertension is difficult to control with conventional treatment or occurs at a relatively young age.

Table 17.5 Inherited conditions associated with hypertension

Condition	Inheritance	PLASMA Aldo	Renin	Cause	Other features
glucocorticoid-suppressible aldosteronism	AD	N/↓	↓	mutation causes fusing of regulatory sequence of steroid 11β-hydroxylase with coding sequence of aldosterone synthase: aldosterone synthesis is controlled by ACTH rather than angiotensin II	variable hypokalaemic alkalosis ↑ plasma 18-hydroxycortisol
Liddle syndrome	AD	↓	↓	activating mutation in distal tubular sodium transporter leads to sodium retention and ↑ ECF volume	variable hypokalaemic alkalosis
syndrome of apparent mineralocorticoid excess	AR	↓	↓	11β-hydroxysteroid dehydrogenase deficiency, causing decreased metabolism of cortisol to cortisone: allows cortisol to exert mineralocorticoid effect	hypokalaemic alkalosis
Gordon syndrome (pseudohypoaldosteronism type II)	AD	↓	↓	mutation leading to distal renal tubular chloride reabsorption leads to sodium retention and ↑ ECF volume	hyperkalaemia, renal tubular acidosis; responds to salt restriction and thiazides
steroid 11β-hydroxylase deficiency	AR	↓	↓	↑ plasma 11-deoxycorticosterone, which has mineralocorticoid activity	hypokalaemic alkalosis virilization
steroid 17α-hydroxylase deficiency	AR	↓	↓	↑ plasma 11-deoxycorticosterone, which has mineralocorticoid activity	hypokalaemic alkalosis feminization (males); lack of normal maturation (females)

ACTH, adrenocorticotrophic hormone; AD, autosomal dominant; Aldo, aldosterone; AR, autosomal recessive; ECF, extracellular fluid; N, normal.

Table 17.6 Biochemical investigations in patients with hypertension

Investigation	Explanation
urine albumin:creatinine ratio	chronic kidney disease (see Chapter 5)
plasma creatinine	chronic kidney disease
plasma potassium	Conn syndrome, adverse effects of antihypertensive drug treatment
plasma calcium	hyperparathyroidism
plasma total and HDL-cholesterol	cardiovascular risk assessment
plasma renin and aldosterone[a]	Conn syndrome
overnight dexamethasone suppression test[a]	Cushing syndrome
urinary catecholamines/metabolites[a]	phaeochromocytoma

[a]Investigations appropriate only if indicated clinically or if simple investigations suggest a specific cause.
HDL, high-density lipoprotein.

SUMMARY

- The main lipids in the blood are **triglycerides**, an important energy substrate, and **cholesterol**, a component of the membranes of cells and their organelles. Cholesterol and triglycerides are insoluble in water and are transported in the blood in **lipoproteins**, complexes of lipids with specific proteins known as apolipoproteins.

- There are four major classes of lipoprotein: (1) **chylomicrons**, which carry exogenous, (i.e. dietary) fat (mainly triglycerides) from the gut to peripheral tissues; (2) **very-low-density lipoprotein (VLDL)**, which carries endogenous triglyceride from the liver to those tissues; (3) **low-density lipoprotein (LDL)**, which transports cholesterol from the liver to peripheral tissues, and (4) **high-density lipoprotein (HDL)**, which is involved in reverse cholesterol transport from peripheral tissues to the liver, whence it can be excreted. These particles are in a dynamic state and there is considerable exchange of lipid and proteins between them.

- **Hypercholesterolaemia**, when caused by an increase in LDL, is an important risk factor for **coronary heart disease (CHD)**; low HDL cholesterol exacerbates the risk. **Hypertriglyceridaemia** is a less important risk factor for CHD but, when very severe, can cause pancreatitis. Both hypercholesterolaemia and hypertriglyceridaemia are associated with various types of cutaneous fat deposition, or xanthomata.

- **Hyperlipidaemia may be either primary**, that is, genetically determined, **or occur secondarily to a variety of other conditions**, including diabetes mellitus, hypothyroidism, obesity, alcoholism, kidney disease and certain drugs. The diagnosis of a primary hyperlipidaemia is supported when such conditions can be excluded, especially if there is a family history; often, however, an underlying genetic tendency to hyperlipoproteinaemia is exacerbated by the presence of one of these conditions.

- The most important primary hyperlipidaemia is **familial hypercholesterolaemia (FH)**, in which a number of different molecular defects lead to decreased clearance of LDL from the blood and an increase in cholesterol synthesis. Heterozygotes for the condition occur with a frequency of ~0.4% and have a greatly increased risk of CHD. Homozygotes are rare; affected patients develop CHD in their teens. Other inherited hyperlipidaemias include familial hypertriglyceridaemia, familial combined hyperlipidaemia and remnant hyperlipoproteinaemia.

- **Screening for hypercholesterolaemia** is essential in patients with cardiovascular disease or a strong family history of this condition or of hyperlipidaemia, and in patients with other major cardiovascular disease risk factors, xanthomata or lipaemic plasma.

- The rationale for the **treatment of hyperlipidaemias** is largely related to their role in causing cardiovascular disease. The management of secondary hyperlipidaemias should be directed towards the underlying cause. Primary hyperlipidaemias that do not respond adequately to dietary and lifestyle measures require drug treatment, but (with the exception of isolated hypertriglyceridaemia, a risk factor for pancreatitis) this must always be done in the context of overall cardiovascular disease risk management including the identification and management of other risk factors.

- Biochemical tests are helpful in the diagnosis of **acute coronary syndrome (ACS)** Plasma troponin concentrations that remain within the reference range rule out ACS (but not angina), and raised concentrations in patients with chest pain indicate the need for urgent investigation even if the ECG does not show ST elevation.

- Measurements of **natriuretic peptides (BNP and NT-proBNP)** are of value in the investigation of **heart failure.** Normal results effectively rule out this condition: patients with higher plasma concentrations must be investigated further with echocardiography.

- **Hypertension** is a common clinical problem. It is usually 'essential', but investigations for treatable causes (mainly endocrine) may be appropriate. Complex investigations should be reserved for those in whom the results of simple tests are abnormal, hypertension is particularly severe or difficult to control, or in whom there are clinical features suggestive of an underlying cause.

Chapter | 18 |

Muscles, nerves and psychiatric disorders

Introduction

Disorders of muscles and the nervous system are common, although few have an obvious underlying metabolic basis. Nevertheless, biochemical tests have an important role to play in the diagnosis and management of many disorders; for example, measurement of plasma **creatine kinase (CK)** activity can be used to guide the treatment of inflammatory muscle disorders, and tests on cerebrospinal fluid (CSF) can detect abnormalities characteristic of multiple sclerosis. Normal muscle function is dependent on the integrity of the central and peripheral nervous systems, so it is not surprising that both muscle and nerve disorders frequently present with muscle weakness. Many of the conditions with a biochemical basis that affect the nervous system are rare and are beyond the scope of this book: readers are encouraged to consult other texts for a more detailed discussion.

Muscle Diseases

Skeletal muscle can be affected by several disease processes, many of which may be obvious from history and examination. Some of the terminology and more important causes of myopathy are indicated in Tables 18.1, and 18.2. Biochemical investigations in traumatic and inflammatory muscle disease are limited to the detection of muscle damage and its consequences, but investigation of suspected metabolic myopathies may involve highly specialized biochemical investigations, together with histological examination. However, muscle weakness can occur in a wide variety of conditions, including electrolyte disturbances and endocrine diseases (see Table 18.2). Simple investigations should be performed before any specialized investigations.

Investigation of muscle disease

An initial simple screen, guided by the clinical presentation of suspected muscle disease, could contain tests such as CK, thyroid function, calcium and inflammatory markers. Specialized investigations are more likely to reveal pathology if any of the following are present:
- the myalgia is exertional (normally delayed) *and* CK is >2–3 times normal
- second wind phenomenon
- muscle weakness
- muscle hypertrophy or atrophy
- a myopathic electromyogram.

Table 18.1 **Muscle disease terminology and definitions**

Terminology	Definition
myalgia	pain attributed to muscle, with or without a rise in CK
myotonia	inability of muscle to relax after contraction
myositis	inflammation of muscle, often autoimmune
rhabdomyolysis	widespread breakdown of muscle fibres with raised CK
myopathy	general term to describe any disorder of muscles

Table 18.2 **Some causes of skeletal muscle disease**	
physical damage	crush syndrome ischaemia
inflammation	polymyositis dermatomyositis viral myositis (e.g. HIV, influenza, coxsackie B) inclusion body myositis necrotising myopathy toxoplasmosis

metabolic (non-
  genetic)
	endocrine disease:
	    hypothyroidism, hyperthyroidism
	    hyperparathyroidism
	    hyperadrenalism
	vitamin D deficiency
	chronic kidney disease
	electrolyte derangement:
	    hyponatraemia
	    hypokalaemia
	    hypophosphataemia

genetic (non-
  metabolic)
	muscular dystrophies:
	    Duchenne, Becker
	    myotonic dystrophies
	periodic paralyses
	malignant hyperthermia

genetic (metabolic)	carbohydrate metabolism disorders
	    (e.g. phosphorylase deficiency)
	fatty acid oxidation disorders
	respiratory chain disorders
	    (mitochondrial disorders)

drugs	statins steroids ethanol colchicine antipsychotics beta blockers

other	myopathy associated with malignant
	    disease
	acute denervation (e.g.
	    radiculopathy)

HIV, human immunodeficiency virus.

Markers of muscle damage

The most widely used marker of muscle damage is the enzyme **CK**. Human tissues contain three forms of CK, comprising dimers of the muscle (M) and brain (B) subunits (see p. 298).

The activity of CK in the plasma varies considerably in healthy individuals and is higher in black people compared with those from other ethnic groups. Conditions that cause an increase in plasma CK activity are indicated in Box 16.8.

The highest activities are seen in association with severe muscle necrosis, for example in polymyositis and rhabdomyolysis, and in Duchenne muscular dystrophy. The elevation in CK concentration after severe exercise can be up to 10 times the upper reference limit (URL) and tends to be greater in untrained subjects. The rise begins immediately and reaches a peak after 1–2 days. Serial plasma CK measurements are of value in following the progress of myopathic disorders and their response to treatment.

Other enzymes that are released during muscle damage include aspartate aminotransferase and lactate dehydrogenase, but CK is a more sensitive and specific marker than either of these. Myoglobin is also released from damaged muscle, but its measurement provides no more information than CK. In severe muscle damage, myoglobinuria can occur and cause a brown colouration of the urine. Myoglobin can precipitate out in the kidney tubules and cause an obstructive nephropathy: the acute kidney injury associated with crush injuries is in part due to this. Other metabolic consequences of severe muscle damage include hyperkalaemia, caused by release of intracellular potassium; hypocalcaemia, caused by calcium becoming bound by damaged tissue; hyperphosphataemia; and hyperuricaemia.

Muscular dystrophies

The muscular dystrophies are inherited disorders characterized clinically by progressive muscular weakness caused by muscle degeneration. The commonest type is **Duchenne muscular dystrophy**, an X-linked condition with a prevalence of approximately 1 in 3500 live male births in the UK. It usually presents in the first decade of life; the average life expectancy is 27 years.

Duchenne muscular dystrophy is a result of a mutation in the dystrophin gene, dystrophin being an intracellular protein required to maintain the structural integrity of muscle cell membranes. Perhaps because the gene is unusually large, about a third of all cases arise from new mutations. The clinical diagnosis of the condition can be confirmed by direct analysis of a muscle biopsy for dystrophin content or by molecular genetic analysis; the latter can also be used for prenatal diagnosis. Plasma CK activity can be 50 to 100 × URL in patients with Duchenne muscular dystrophy. Female carriers are usually asymptomatic, but most have moderate elevations in CK (<3 × URL); symptoms occur in 2–3% of females depending on their pattern of X chromosome inactivation ('manifesting carriers').

Becker muscular dystrophy, a less severe condition, usually presenting later in childhood or even in adults, is about 10 times less common. It is also due to a mutation in the dystrophin gene; but whereas in Duchenne, the protein is undetectable in muscle biopsies, in Becker, it is present either in reduced amounts or is structurally altered.

Several other rare forms of muscular dystrophy have been described that typically present in early adulthood; they usually present with other patterns of muscular involvement, for example involving only proximal muscles (limb girdle muscular dystrophy) or the cranial musculature.

Metabolic myopathies

Metabolic myopathies can be divided into two main groupings (see Table 18.2): **acquired**, for example, secondarily to ethanol abuse or exposure to any of a wide variety of other drugs, and to endocrine and systemic metabolic disease; and **genetic**, caused by an inherited defect of an enzyme involved in muscle energy metabolism. There are several types of the latter; all are rare, but biochemical investigations are essential to their diagnosis. They include disorders of carbohydrate metabolism (see Case history 18.1), deficiencies of components of the electron transport chain (mitochondrial myopathies) and disorders of fatty acid oxidation.

> **!**
> Rhabdomyolysis is rare with statin use (0.1%) and ceases on statin cessation. However certain drugs increase the risk of rhabdomyolysis when co-prescribed with a statin. The commonest examples are: fibrates (e.g. gemfibrozil), amiodarone, amlodipine, diltiazem, verapamil, azole antifungals, macrolides (e.g. erythromycin and clarithromycin), ciprofloxacin and ciclosporin.

Other myopathies

Hypokalaemic and hyperkalaemic **periodic paralyses** are inherited (autosomal dominant) muscle membrane disorders that affect ion channels. Redistribution of potassium causes abnormal plasma concentrations, and patients experience episodes of generalized or localized muscle weakness. Acquired hypokalaemia (e.g. secondary to treatment with diuretics) can also cause muscle weakness. **Malignant hyperpyrexia (or hyperthermia)** is a rare, autosomal dominant condition in which certain inhalational anaesthetics or suxamethonium can trigger a rapid rise in body temperature, lactic acidosis and rhabdomyolysis with hyperkalaemia and 100-fold elevations of plasma CK activity. Lesser elevations are seen when the condition is quiescent.

Many connective tissue disorders (e.g. systemic lupus erythematosus) can cause inflammatory myopathies. Inflammation is also a feature of polymyositis, dermatomyositis and inclusion body myositis.

Myasthenia gravis, although typically presenting with muscle weakness and easy fatiguability, is a disorder of neuromuscular transmission, characterized by the presence of IgG antibodies to the acetylcholine receptor at the neuromuscular junction. The **Lambert–Eaton myasthenic syndrome** is a rare, paraneoplastic disorder (see p. 354) of the neuromuscular junction: antibodies to a specific voltage-gated calcium channel are present in the majority of patients. It is also characterized by muscle weakness, but in contrast with myasthenia gravis, this tends to improve after a few minutes of muscular activity, and previously absent tendon reflexes return.

Case history 18.1

History

An 18-year-old man was investigated for pain in his muscles associated with exercise. He said that he had experienced occasional muscle pain for years, but it had recently become more noticeable since he had started working out in a gym.

Examination

Unremarkable.

Results (see Appendix for reference ranges)

Serum:	creatine kinase	3683 U/L
	urate	672 µmol/L
Samples sent to referral laboratory	total carnitine and acyl carnitine profile	normal

Summary

Exertional myalgia with significantly raised CK and milder elevation of urate.

Discussion

The picture is suggestive of McArdle disease, glycogen storage disease type V which used to be diagnosed with an ischaemic exercise test. This has been replaced by genetic tests including, in Northern Europe, a screen for the commonest mutations and muscle biopsy to confirm low phosphorylase activity. Before muscle biopsy, electromyography can be used to exclude other muscle disorders.

Total carnitine and acyl carnitine profiles are used to screen for fatty acid oxidation defects, a group of disorders that can cause exercise-induced muscle weakness and pain. These tests are prone to false negatives and false positives.

Nervous System Disease

As with muscle diseases, there are many rare metabolic neurological disorders, but there are also many relatively common conditions with an endocrine or metabolic component that can have neurological manifestations.

Thus, although the diagnosis of some metabolic neurological disorders requires complex investigations performed only in specialist laboratories, simple investigations are frequently required. Even though most of these investigations are performed on plasma or serum, assays of CSF are also valuable in certain conditions: the examination of the CSF is discussed at the end of this section.

Coma

There are numerous causes of coma or decreased consciousness, including structural brain diseases, infection (both intracranial and systemic) and many endocrine and metabolic conditions. The history, careful physical examination and imaging will often reveal the cause. **Biochemical investigations** that may be helpful include measurement of drugs, including ethanol, and glucose (for hypoglycaemia or hyperglycaemia). The possibility of ethanol ingestion should also be considered in patients with head injuries and patients who have taken drug overdoses. Routine biochemical tests will detect hyponatraemia and kidney or liver failure. Arterial blood gases should be measured in all unconscious patients as part of the assessment of vital functions and because metabolic acidosis and respiratory failure can both lead to loss of consciousness. The clinical circumstances may indicate a need for specific tests (e.g. thyroid function tests in a comatose patient with hypothermia).

The **Wernicke–Korsakoff syndrome** is a specific disorder caused by thiamin deficiency. It is most frequently seen in alcoholics and is a risk in starved patients during refeeding if insufficient thiamin is given (see p. 140 and Case history 8.3). Although thiamin status can be assessed by direct measurement of concentrations in whole blood, in practice the diagnosis is usually made clinically and confirmed by the response to intravenous thiamin.

Dementia

Dementia is characterized by a permanent loss of intellectual function in the absence of impairment of consciousness. The most frequent causes are **Alzheimer disease** and **cerebrovascular disease**. Both are primarily diseases of the elderly, although Alzheimer disease can have its onset in middle age. Cognitive impairment can also be a feature of endocrine disorders (e.g. hypothyroidism), liver and kidney failure, chronic ethanol misuse, heavy metal poisoning, carbon monoxide poisoning and vitamin deficiencies, and can progress to dementia if severe and untreated. Simple laboratory investigations that should be performed in dementia, to identify the small number of patients with treatable causes or conditions that increase the morbidity of the condition, are shown in Table 18.3.

Most cases of Alzheimer disease occur sporadically, but familial forms occur in about 0.1% of patients, particularly

Table 18.3 Some laboratory investigations on blood, serum and cerebrospinal fluid (CSF) in patients with dementia and delirium that may be appropriate according to the clinical circumstances

Investigation	Condition
full blood count	anaemia
CRP (and/or ESR)	inflammatory or infective cause
thyroid function tests	hypothyroidism
calcium	hypocalcaemia or hypercalcaemia
kidney function	kidney failure
	electrolyte abnormality, e.g. hyponatraemia
liver function tests	liver failure, Wernicke–Korsakoff syndrome
HbA$_{1c}$	diabetes mellitus
vitamin B$_{12}$, folate	vitamin deficiency
Rare specialist and focused investigations (depending on age, presentation and risk factors)	
presentation or risk factors:	
syphilis serology	neurosyphilis
heavy metals	poisoning
autoantibodies	cerebral lupus, paraneoplastic, vasculitis
ACE	neurosarcoid
younger age:	
HIV tests	HIV dementia and brain abscess/infection
CSF MC&S, oligoclonal bands	Inflammatory or infective cause, e.g. CJD, MS
caeruloplasmin and copper	Wilson disease
Tests reserved for delirium	
glucose	hypoglycaemia
urine MC&S	infection

ACE, angiotensin-converting enzyme; CRP, C-reactive protein; CJD, Creutzfeldt–Jakob disease; ESR, erythrocyte sedimentation rate; HIV, human immunodeficiency virus; MC&S, microscopy, culture and sensitivity; MS, multiple sclerosis.

in younger people; these are usually due to mutations in one of the genes coding for the proteins amyloid precursor protein (APP), presenilin 1 and presenilin 2. At least 10 other mutations have been identified as risk factors.

Seizures

Seizures can occur in both structural and functional neurological disorders, including conditions that cause coma (see earlier discussion). The importance of monitoring plasma concentrations of certain anticonvulsants is discussed in Chapter 21.

Movement disorders

Movement disorders include conditions in which movements are either reduced (hypokinetic) or increased (hyperkinetic). Most are caused by disordered function of the basal ganglia. The most common is Parkinson disease (a hypokinetic disorder), which is caused by a degeneration of dopaminergic neurons in the substantia nigra. The best-known hyperkinetic disorder is Huntington disease, a rare, inherited (autosomal dominant) condition caused by a repeating base-triplet sequence of variable length. Of particular relevance to clinical biochemistry is Wilson disease, an inherited (autosomal recessive) disorder of copper metabolism; affected individuals are either homozygotes or compound heterozygotes for mutations in the *ATP7B* gene. Tissue damage arises from the deposition of copper in the basal ganglia and liver. Wilson disease should be considered in all patients younger than 55 years presenting with parkinsonism, tremor or dystonia, particularly if the course is progressive (see Chapter 6).

Ataxia

Ataxia is disordered control of movement. **Metabolic causes** include abetalipoproteinaemia, vitamin E deficiency, ataxia telangiectasia, cerebrotendinous xanthomatosis and various storage disorders, for example the G_{M2} gangliosidoses (hexosaminidase deficiencies, including Tay–Sachs disease). It can also be a feature of hypothyroidism, multiple sclerosis and chronic alcohol abuse. Ataxia telangiectasia typically presents in young children: the diagnosis is usually made clinically, but 90% of patients have elevated plasma concentrations of α fetoprotein, with carcinoembryonic antigen also being elevated in some. Cerebrotendinous xanthomatosis is caused by a deficiency in mitochondrial steroid 27-hydroxylase, leading to an accumulation of cholestanol in the brain and other tissues; the latter includes tendons, producing xanthomata that resemble those seen in familial hypercholesterolaemia but plasma cholesterol concentration is normal or low (see p. 313).

Multiple sclerosis is an inflammatory demyelinating condition of the central nervous system (see Case history 18.2). The most common presentation is optic neuritis followed by sensory disturbance; however, it is an important differential in those presenting with ataxia.

Case history 18.2

History

A 22-year-old woman was brought into the accident and emergency department by her flatmates having been in bed for 2 days feeling tired with a headache and now finding it difficult to stand. All of the flatmates had been suffering from a cold with headaches, but no one else had developed any neurological symptoms.

Examination

Loss of sensation and decreased muscle strength suggesting a spinal problem at the level of L4 root. No lymphadenopathy, fever or rash.

Investigation

An urgent MRI demonstrated a non-compressive myelopathy. A lumbar puncture was performed to investigate inflammatory and infective causes.

Plasma:	glucose	6.2 mmol/L
CSF:	white cell count	6×10^6/L
	protein	0.6 g/L
	glucose	5.0 mmol/L
	microbiology including PCR and serology	negative
Samples sent to referral laboratory	oligoclonal bands	detected

Interpretation

Initial investigations, normal CSF glucose and marginally raised protein and white cells, suggest inflammation but are not in keeping with bacterial meningitis. Oligoclonal bands suggest a diagnosis of multiple sclerosis.

Discussion

Multiple sclerosis is primarily a clinical diagnosis supported by neurophysiology and imaging studies. Although the CSF total protein concentration is usually only slightly raised, there is increased synthesis of IgG by a small number of B lymphocyte clones. Comparison of the electrophoretic pattern in CSF with that in a serum sample taken at the same time will demonstrate discrete 'oligoclonal' bands in the CSF which are absent from serum. Oligoclonal bands can be detected in >95% of patients with multiple sclerosis, although they may also be seen in other, less common, demyelinating diseases, such as subacute sclerosing panencephalitis, and in neurosyphilis.

Table 18.4 Some causes of peripheral neuropathy in which pathology tests may be helpful

Cause	Investigations
diabetes, metabolic syndrome	**HbA$_{1c}$ or fasting glucose** and lipid profile
kidney failure	**creatinine**
liver failure	**liver function tests**
endocrine disease (e.g. hypothyroidism, acromegaly)	**thyroid function tests**, IGF-1
paraproteinaemia (e.g. myeloma, Waldenström, MGUS, POEMS)	**serum protein electrophoresis and free light chains**
vitamin deficiency: thiamin, B$_{12}$, folate, vitamin E, pyridoxine[a]	**full blood count**, vitamins, including **vitamin B$_{12}$**
metabolic disorders (e.g. acute intermittent porphyria, amyloidosis, Fabry disease, Tangier disease, Refsum disease)	porphobilinogen, biopsy, alpha-galactosidase activity, lipid profile, phytanic acid
paraneoplastic	antineuronal antibodies
ethanol abuse	liver function tests, e.g. γGT
other systemic disease	**CRP**

[a]Pyridoxine toxicity also causes a peripheral neuropathy.
CRP, C-reactive protein; γGT, γ-glutamyltransferase; IGF-1, insulin-like growth factor-1; MGUS, monoclonal gammopathy of undetermined significance; POEMS, polyneuropathy, organomegaly, endocrinopathy, M protein and skin changes.
The commonest initial blood tests are given in bold.

Peripheral neuropathies

Peripheral neuropathies are common neurological disorders. They are diagnosed clinically and from neurophysiological studies. Many drugs and toxins can be implicated, as can metabolic and endocrine disorders (particularly diabetes mellitus). The cause is usually obvious under such circumstances. Peripheral neuropathy can be the presenting feature of lead poisoning, plasma cell dyscrasias, vitamin deficiencies, acute intermittent porphyria and other metabolic disorders (Table 18.4). Vitamin B$_{12}$ deficiency can additionally cause degeneration of the dorsal columns of the spinal cord, of which loss of vibration sensation is the most consistent early finding, with ataxia, limb weakness, spasticity and dementia developing in severe cases.

Stroke

In stroke, there is damage to brain tissue, caused by either ischaemia (80–85% of patients) or haemorrhage

(15–20%). Ischaemic stroke is usually due to cerebrovascular atherosclerosis. The diagnosis of stroke is clinical; distinction between ischaemic and haemorrhagic stroke can only be made reliably by computed tomography (CT) or magnetic resonance imaging. Most patients with cerebrovascular disease also have cardiovascular disease, and treatment with cholesterol-lowering drugs reduces the risk of both stroke and myocardial infarction. There are some rare metabolic causes of stroke, e.g. homocystinuria and Fabry disease, some metabolic conditions that mimic stroke, e.g. urea cycle defects and mitochondrial diseases, and stroke can be a rare complication of common conditions such as hyperthyroidism (atrial fibrillation leading to thromboembolic disease).

Other neurological disorders

Numerous rare inherited disorders can affect the central nervous system and cause developmental delay and poor intellectual attainment. Many are incurable and lead to death in early childhood. These conditions include lysosomal storage disorders, in which lysosomal enzyme defects lead to the accumulation of macromolecules in the brain, amino acidopathies, and others. Phenylketonuria is an example of a treatable condition, but treatment must begin very soon after birth. Neonatal screening for this condition is discussed in Chapter 19.

Examination of the Cerebrospinal Fluid

CSF is usually obtained for diagnostic purposes by lumbar puncture. Table 18.5 summarizes some of the more commonly requested CSF investigations. The protein concentration is normally 0.1–0.4 g/L and the protein is predominantly albumin; higher concentrations are found in neonates (up to 0.9 g/L) and the elderly. It is important that the CSF is not contaminated with blood because the presence of plasma proteins will completely invalidate the results of CSF protein measurement.

Examination of the CSF is most often performed in patients with suspected **meningitis**. The diagnosis of this condition is primarily the concern of the medical microbiologist, but it is usual also to request biochemical analyses for glucose and protein. The significance of the CSF glucose concentration is considered on p. 246 and in Table 18.5. In meningitis, there is secretion of IgG into the CSF, but this has little effect on the total amount of protein. However, meningeal inflammation may lead to an increase in capillary permeability and, therefore, a marked increase in CSF protein content. It is important to note that, in suspected meningitis, a normal CSF protein does not exclude the diagnosis. An

Table 18.5 Some investigations that can be performed on cerebrospinal fluid (CSF) and common causes for abnormalities

Test	Normal value	Comment
appearance	clear, colourless	turbid if high cell or protein content (including bacteria)
white cell count	$<5 \times 10^6$/L (mostly lymphocytes)	increased in meningitis, malignancy and some inflammatory disorders that affect the CNS
red cell count	none	increased with traumatic taps and subarachnoid haemorrhage
glucose[a]	60–80% of plasma glucose	decreased with bacterial meningitis and some CNS malignancies
protein[a]	0.1–0.4 g/L	increased in meningitis and some CNS malignancies
bilirubin[a] (xanthochromia)	none detectable	presence indicates subarachnoid haemorrhage
microbiology: identification of organisms, viral PCR, TB	none present	present in meningitis
lactate[a]	<2.5 mmol/L	increased in meningitis, cerebral hypoxia and some mitochondrial disorders
oligoclonal bands[a]	none detectable	present in multiple sclerosis
asialotransferrin	present	confirms presence of CSF in fluid of unknown origin

[a]CSF samples that require a paired blood sample for interpretation.
CNS, central nervous system; PCR, polymerase chain reaction; TB, tuberculosis.

increased CSF lactate concentration is characteristic of bacterial meningitis but may also be found with cerebral hypoxia and in patients with mitochondrial myopathies.

CSF protein concentration is increased in patients with tumours of the central nervous system and may exceed 5 g/L in patients with tumours that obstruct the normal circulation of the CSF (spinal block or Froin syndrome).

Examination of the CSF for xanthochromia can occasionally be useful in patients with suspected **subarachnoid haemorrhage** (SAH), which is spontaneous arterial bleeding into the subarachnoid space, usually from a berry aneurysm. There is a high mortality rate and a high risk of re-bleeding, so it is important to make the diagnosis and refer patients promptly to a neurosurgical centre for their management. However, the diagnosis is now more commonly made by a high-definition CT scan which will demonstrate blood in the subarachnoid space in almost 100% of patients if performed within 6 h of the onset of symptoms.

Rarely, CSF may leak into the nasal or aural cavities after trauma or surgery, posing a serious risk of infection ascending into the subarachnoid space. Measurement of **asialotransferrin** (also known as tau protein or β transferrin) in the fluid can distinguish normal secretions from CSF: about 25% of transferrin in the CSF is in the asialated form, but practically none is detectable in other fluids such as plasma, tears, saliva or nasal secretions.

CSF xanthochromia

If there is a high index of suspicion for SAH, or the patient has presented late (e.g. after several days), *and* the CT scan is negative, testing the CSF for bilirubin (xanthochromia) can help to confirm the diagnosis. Spectrophotometric scanning of the CSF identifies two peaks: oxyhaemoglobin, released by red cell lysis and phagocytosis, and bilirubin, produced slowly (detectable after 12 h) *in vivo* from the oxyhaemoglobin. Oxyhaemoglobin may be present as a result of either SAH or *in vitro* haemolysis of red cells introduced during a traumatic tap. A large oxyhaemoglobin peak may mask a small, but significant, amount of bilirubin. The presence of bilirubin indicates either a subarachnoid bleed *or* increased transport of bilirubin from the plasma across the meninges if there is hyperbilirubinaemia. The laboratory report should indicate whether the bilirubin is likely to be from the plasma. The least bloodstained aliquot of CSF should therefore be used for analysis (often the last one collected) obtained at least 12 h after the onset of symptoms. Bilirubin remains detectable in the CSF for at least a week after SAH, by which time <50% of patients will have an abnormality on CT scanning. Bilirubin decays rapidly when exposed to light, so samples should be covered during transport to the laboratory.

Psychiatric Disease

Although many psychiatric disorders are considered to have a biochemical basis, measurements of analytes in plasma play little part in the diagnosis of psychiatric disease, with the exception of acute confusional states (delirium), which can be caused by endocrine and metabolic disease, hypoxia and toxins (see Table 18.3). However, some organic disorders can have psychiatric manifestations (e.g. depression), psychiatric disease can affect endocrine function, and treatment with psychotropic drugs can cause metabolic and endocrine disturbances. An appreciation of these relationships is important to avoid possible misinterpretation of biochemical data. The importance of the measurement of plasma lithium concentrations in patients treated with this drug for affective disorders is discussed in Chapter 21.

Acute confusional state

Acute confusional state, or delirium, is characterized by impairment of attention, with abnormalities of perception and mood. It is a state of altered consciousness but with high arousal. It is the most common acute psychosis: >10% of older hospital inpatients develop delirium at some time during their admission. The metabolic and endocrine causes include all the conditions that can cause reduced consciousness and coma (see p. 328, see Table 18.3). Other causes include fever and structural intracranial lesions.

Other psychiatric manifestations of systemic illness

A degree of **depression** is a frequent reaction to major illness (depressive adjustment disorder), but some conditions can cause severe depression. Hypothyroid patients often appear depressed, although apathy rather than true depression is more common. It is prudent to perform thyroid function tests in patients presenting with depression. Particularly in elderly adults, hyperthyroidism can present atypically ('apathetic hyperthyroidism') and be mistaken for depression.

Depression is also a well-recognized feature of Cushing syndrome, both adrenocorticotrophic hormone (ACTH) dependent and independent. Also, patients with depression may demonstrate a failure of suppression of cortisol in response to low-dose dexamethasone (see p. 181, potentially leading to unnecessary investigation and misdiagnosis. Treatment with corticosteroids can cause euphoria. Other endocrine disorders that may have psychiatric manifestations (particularly depression) include polycystic ovary syndrome, primary hyperparathyroidism and hyperprolactinaemia.

An association between depression and diabetes has long been recognized: more recently, the association has been extended to include the metabolic syndrome. The mechanism of the association is uncertain, but insulin resistance seems likely, at least in part, to be implicated. Notably, depression is an independent risk factor for cardiovascular disease.

Endocrine and metabolic manifestations of psychiatric disorders

Abnormalities of endocrine function are a frequent finding in patients with some psychiatric diseases. Although hypercortisolaemia is found in about 50% of patients with depression (see earlier), decreased concentrations are frequent in patients with post-traumatic stress disorder; slightly low cortisol concentrations have been reported in patients with chronic fatigue syndrome. The abnormalities of thyroid function comprising the sick euthyroid syndrome (see p. 201) can be present in patients with acute psychiatric illness.

Abnormalities of the **hypothalamo–pituitary–gonadal axis** are frequent in patients with anorexia nervosa (see p. Table 8.4); women with the condition typically have amenorrhoea. Amenorrhoea is also a frequent finding in moderate or severe depression. The secretion of **prolactin** is increased by stress (which should therefore be minimized when blood is taken for its measurement); elevated concentrations are found in patients with anxiety states. Treatment of psychoses and other psychiatric disorders with dopamine antagonists also causes hyperprolactinaemia (see later).

Various other metabolic disturbances have been described in patients with psychiatric illness: hypokalaemia is frequent in anorexia nervosa and bulimia nervosa, and in the latter condition in particular may be accompanied by a hypochloraemic alkalosis secondary to self-induced vomiting (see Table 8.4). Hypophosphataemia is a feature of ethanol withdrawal and can also occur with diuretic and laxative abuse. A dilutional hyponatraemia can occur in psychogenic polydipsia.

Metabolic side effects of psychotropic drugs

Several groups of psychotropic drugs can cause metabolic derangements. Treatment with **lithium** can cause hypothyroidism, nephrogenic diabetes insipidus and, more rarely, hyperparathyroidism: regular assessment of thyroid and kidney function is essential for patients being treated with lithium, as is monitoring of serum lithium concentrations (see p. 370). Particular caution should be taken if a patient no longer has free access to water, e.g. during hospital admissions.

Dopamine antagonists such as the **phenothiazines** and **butyrophenones** stimulate prolactin secretion, sometimes resulting in plasma concentrations that may suggest a microprolactinoma. In the long term, this increases the risk of osteoporosis due to the secondary hypogonadism. Hyperprolactinaemia is less common with the newer, 'atypical' antipsychotics (e.g. **clozapine**, **olanzapine**), but these drugs can cause hyperglycaemia and hypertriglyceridaemia, as well as promoting weight gain. **Carbamazepine** and the selective serotonin reuptake inhibitors (e.g. **paroxetine**) can both cause dilutional hyponatraemia, although this is usually only mild.

The **neuroleptic malignant syndrome** occurs in up to 2% of patients being started on neuroleptic (antipsychotic) drugs. It is an idiosyncratic reaction, with fever, muscle rigidity, altered consciousness and autonomic dysfunction being the main features. Increased plasma CK activity and leucocytosis are present in most patients.

Numerous drugs can cause mild **abnormalities of liver function**, usually manifesting as a slight increase in plasma aminotransferase activity. **Chlorpromazine** can cause (usually mild) cholestasis (which may persist after withdrawal of the drug). **Sodium valproate**, a widely used anticonvulsant, occasionally causes severe hepatotoxicity, but unfortunately this is an idiosyncratic reaction and cannot be predicted from measurement of either liver function tests or plasma valproate concentrations.

SUMMARY

- Plasma **CK** activity is a valuable test for the presence of **damage to skeletal muscle**, and serial measurements can be used to monitor the progress of response to treatment of patients with muscle diseases. Many muscle diseases, such as the inherited metabolic myopathies, have a metabolic basis. Highly specialized biochemical investigations are used, together with histological investigations, in their diagnosis.
- Standard biochemical investigations are of limited value in the diagnosis and management of **neurological and psychiatric diseases.** Important applications include the investigation and management of the unconscious or de-

lirious patient and therapeutic monitoring of the plasma concentrations of certain anticonvulsant drugs used in the treatment of epilepsy, and of lithium used in the treatment of some affective disorders. Many rare neurological disorders have a metabolic origin, for which specialized investigations are required. Psychiatric disorders, and the drugs used to treat them, can cause endocrine and metabolic disturbances, and metabolic and endocrine conditions can have psychiatric manifestations.

- Examination of **CSF** can help with diagnosis in patients suspected of having meningitis, subarachnoid haemorrhage or multiple sclerosis.

Chapter | 19 |

Inherited metabolic diseases

Introduction

Many inherited diseases are known to be due to the **genetically determined absence or modification of specific proteins**. For example, in sickle cell anaemia, the protein is haemoglobin; in agammaglobulinaemia, antibody production is defective. However, in the majority of such diseases, the protein in question is an enzyme, and the effect is to cause a metabolic disorder. Other inherited metabolic diseases may be caused by defective receptor synthesis (e.g. familial hypercholesterolaemia [FH], which affects the receptor for low-density lipoprotein) or by defects involving carrier proteins (e.g. cystinuria, in which renal tubular reabsorption of cystine is impaired). Whatever the cause, the clinical features of inherited metabolic diseases stem directly from the metabolic abnormalities to which they give rise. Although individually these conditions are rare (Table 19.1), they are of considerable significance: the consequences of many of them are potentially severe, but may, in some cases, be alleviated if an early diagnosis is made and the appropriate treatment instituted.

In recent years, application of the techniques of molecular genetic analysis has massively increased our understanding of these conditions. Whereas it used to be thought that each condition was the result of a mutation in a single gene, it is now clear that many inherited metabolic diseases can arise because of one of a number of genetic defects. Furthermore, it is clear that the concept of 'one gene, one enzyme' is no longer generally applicable. Although many inherited metabolic diseases (e.g. classic phenylketonuria [PKU]) are a consequence of a mutation in a single gene affecting the synthesis of one enzyme, there are many exceptions. For example, one polypeptide chain can occur in more than one enzyme: an example is the β-subunit of hexosaminidase A (one α-, one β-chain) and B (two β-chains), deficiency of which causes Sandhoff disease, one of the gangliosidoses; inherited deficiency of the α-chain affects only hexosaminidase A and causes a related but distinct disorder, Tay–Sachs disease. The active form of an enzyme may consist of subunits coded by different genes, an example being propionyl coenzyme A (CoA) carboxylase: mutations in either gene can lead to deficiency of the enzyme, causing propionic acidaemia.

Any individual inherited disorder can be caused by many different genetic mutations, often with clustering of certain mutations in geographical areas. The phenotypic expression varies considerably depending on whether there is any residual protein function. This is exemplified by α_1-antitrypsin deficiency (see p. 288); in many affected people there is sufficient residual enzyme activity for clinical consequences to be minimal unless the individual smokes tobacco. Mutations can affect any part of the normal pathway from transcription of a protein to trafficking to the correct location: approaches to treatment may, in future, be much more specific to the type of defect. For example, in cystic fibrosis, failure to transport the transmembrane conductance regulator to the cell surface can be corrected in some patients, and in others, the function of an abnormal protein can be enhanced by specific medication (see Fig. 19.5 and p. 340).

Most inherited metabolic diseases show **autosomal recessive inheritance**; heterozygotes are usually phenotypically normal, although they are carriers of the condition. FH and most of the porphyrias are important exceptions, being inherited as **autosomal dominant** conditions. Some—disorders, for example, ornithine transcarbamylase deficiency (a urea cycle disorder) and Fabry disease (a lysosomal storage disorder)—are **X-linked**: males are more severely affected than females.

Because they are individually rare, it is important for the clinician to have a high index of suspicion and actively consider the possibility that an illness may be caused by an inherited metabolic disease. **Common clinical presentations** of

335

Table 19.1 Approximate incidences of some inherited metabolic diseases

Condition	Incidence
familial hypercholesterolaemia	1:250
non-classic steroid 21-hydroxylase deficiency	1:1000
cystic fibrosis	1:2500
α_1-antitrypsin deficiency	1:3000
phenylketonuria	1:10 000
classic steroid 21-hydroxylase deficiency	1:15000
medium chain acyl-CoA dehydrogenase deficiency	1:17 000
hereditary fructose intolerance	1:30 000
classic galactosaemia	1:48 000
glycogen storage disease (all types combined)	1:50 000
tyrosinaemia type 1	1:100 000
maple syrup urine disease	1:185 000

CoA, coenzyme A.
Note that there is considerable variation in the incidence of these conditions in different countries and in different ethnic groups.

Box 19.1 Common clinical features of inherited metabolic diseases presenting in childhood

acidosis, alkalosis
central nervous system dysfunction: irritability, coma, hypotonia, seizures
failure to thrive
frequent vomiting, other gastrointestinal abnormalities
hypoglycaemia, hyperammonaemia
unusual odour

Features may be provoked by a specific stimulus, for example, feeding or a lack of feeding.

inherited metabolic diseases are indicated in Box 19.1 and discussed in Chapter 22. Simple screening tests that should be performed when one of these conditions is suspected are shown in Table 19.3. Most inherited metabolic diseases present in infancy and childhood (sometimes in association with specific events, e.g. weaning, puberty); their diagnosis and management are the province of paediatricians, albeit usually in close collaboration with laboratory staff. With improving treatment, affected children with some conditions that were previously fatal in childhood are surviving into adulthood and being managed in dedicated adult metabolic clinics. Some inherited metabolic diseases usually present clinically only in adults, an important example being FH (see p. 313), although homozygotes for this dominantly inherited condition often develop overt atherosclerosis in childhood. The techniques of **molecular genetic analysis** are being increasingly used in the screening and diagnosis of inherited metabolic diseases (although with genetically heterogeneous diseases, phenotypic diagnosis may still be more reliable). These techniques are discussed in detail in textbooks of molecular biology and are not discussed further in this book.

In a book of this size, it is possible only to discuss a selection of the many hundreds of inherited metabolic diseases that have been described. The ones that have been chosen are either among the more common or illustrate important general principles with regard to presentation, diagnosis and management, or both. Many others are discussed elsewhere in this book.

Effects of enzyme defects

Fig. 19.1A shows a hypothetical metabolic pathway involving the synthesis of product D from substrate A by successive, enzyme-catalyzed reactions through intermediates B and C. If the formation of B from A, catalyzed by enzyme a, is rate limiting, as the first step unique to a metabolic pathway frequently is, then the concentrations of intermediates B and C will normally be low. The formation of product E from C, catalyzed by enzyme c′, is normally a minor pathway, with only a small amount of E being formed.

Three distinct sequelae of a lack of enzyme can be envisaged; these could occur alone or in combination.

Decreased formation of the product

Decreased formation of the product of a reaction is the most obvious consequence of a lack of enzyme c (see Fig. 19.1B). If enzyme c is defective, D cannot be synthesized or may be synthesized only in small amounts. Clinical features will arise if product D has an essential function and there is no alternative pathway for its synthesis.

Accumulation of the substrate

Accumulation of the substrate (C) of the missing enzyme would also be expected (see Fig. 19.1C). If this is biologically active, clinical manifestations will result. Other, earlier substrates may also accumulate if the reactions before the one blocked are reversible. This will occur particularly if there is negative feedback by the product on an early reaction in the pathway because, with decreased formation of the product, feedback will be lost, thus reversing the inhibition and stimulating the formation of the intermediate substrates.

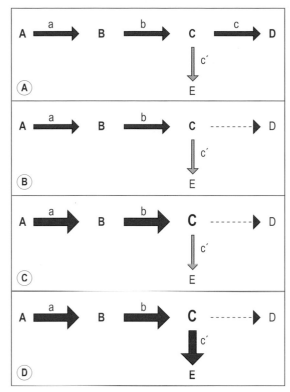

Fig. 19.1 Effects of enzyme defects. **A,** Product D is synthesized from A by a series of reactions catalyzed by enzymes a, b and c. Enzyme c′ catalyzes the formation of a small amount of product E in a minor pathway. **B,** In the absence of the enzyme c, no D is synthesized. **C,** If the conversion of C to D is blocked, the concentration of the intermediate C, and possibly other precursors, may increase. **D,** Increased formation of E may occur if the concentration of C increases and conversion of C to D is blocked.

Increased formation of other metabolites

Increased formation of E, the product of a minor pathway, may occur if the concentration of C is increased as a result of the enzyme deficiency, the reaction being promoted by a mass action effect (see Fig. 19.1D). If product E is biologically active, a clinical syndrome will result.

Inherited Metabolic Disorders

Glucose 6-phosphatase deficiency

Glucose 6-phosphatase deficiency (glycogen storage disease (GSD) type Ia) exemplifies the development of a clinical syndrome caused by lack of formation of the product of an enzyme-catalyzed reaction. Glucose synthesis from glycogen or by gluconeogenesis is blocked (Fig. 19.2) and the responses to the counterregulatory hormones (glucagon and adrenaline, which increase glucose production) are blunted. Children with this disorder are prone to **severe fasting hypoglycaemia**, because their only source of glucose is dietary carbohydrate and the small amounts of glucose that can be liberated from glycogen by the debranching enzyme.

Acute hypoglycaemia is treated with intravenous glucose infusion. Maintenance treatment is with frequent daytime feeding and overnight constant intragastric infusion with a glucose/glucose polymer feed. Older children are given uncooked corn starch, from which glucose is released only slowly in the gut.

Glucose 6-phosphatase deficiency also exemplifies the consequences of accumulation of a precursor other than the immediate substrate of the defective enzyme. **Glycogen accumulates in the liver**, causing hepatomegaly. The block in gluconeogenesis results in an accumulation of lactate, and lactic acidosis is a common finding. Hyperlipidaemia results from increased fat synthesis, and hyperuricaemia is also frequently present. Accumulation of glycogen in platelets leads to disordered platelet function and a bleeding tendency. The definitive diagnosis is made by demonstrating lack of enzyme activity in a sample of liver obtained by biopsy. In GSD types Ib and Ic, similar clinical and metabolic abnormalities occur (with an additional impairment of immune function) as a result of defects in the translocases involved in the transport of glucose 1 phosphate (type Ib) and phosphate (Ic) in the endoplasmic reticulum.

Nine other GSDs are known, each caused by the deficiency of an enzyme related to glycogen metabolism and, with one exception, leading to glycogen accumulation; glycogen synthase deficiency (GSD type 0) does not result in excessive glycogen accumulation but is included in the classification.

Galactosaemia

Three enzyme defects can cause galactosaemia and exemplify the production of a clinical syndrome caused by the accumulation of a substrate of the missing enzyme. The enzyme **galactose 1 phosphate uridyltransferase** is required for the conversion of galactose to glucose 1-phosphate (Fig. 19.3), thereby allowing galactose to be incorporated into glycogen, converted into glucose or to undergo glycolysis. Absence of the enzyme in classic galactosaemia results in the accumulation of galactose 1-phosphate. The clinical features of the condition are thought to be due directly to the toxicity of this metabolite. In addition, the plasma concentration of galactose is increased and galactose is excreted in the urine. Newborn screening programmes in some countries include testing for galactosaemia, although not in the UK.

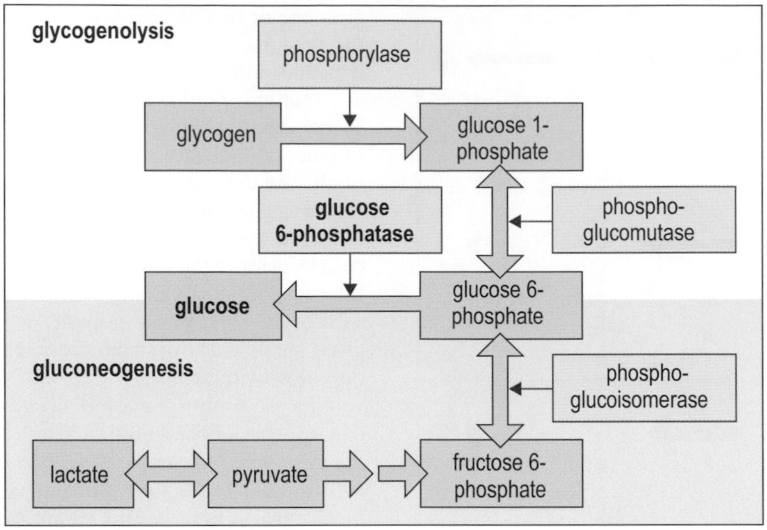

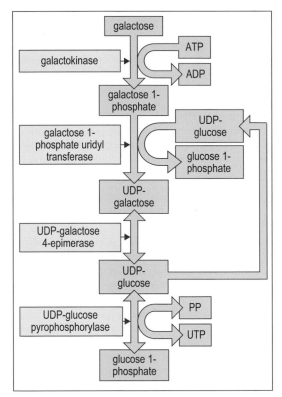

Fig. 19.2 Glucose production by glycogenolysis and gluconeogenesis. Glucose 6-phosphate is an essential intermediate in the production of glucose by either glycogenolysis or gluconeogenesis. In the absence of glucose 6-phosphatase, glucose cannot be formed from glucose 6-phosphate.

Fig. 19.3 Metabolic pathway for the conversion of galactose to glucose. ADP, adenosine diphosphate; ATP, adenosine triphosphate; PP, pyrophosphate; UDP, uridine diphosphate; UTP, uridine triphosphate.

Infants with galactosaemia **present with failure to thrive, vomiting, hepatomegaly and jaundice**. Septicaemia, particularly caused by *Escherichia coli*, is common. Cataracts may be present as a result of the conversion of excess galactose to galactitol in the lens. There may also be hypoglycaemia and impairment of renal tubular function. Galactose is a reducing sugar, and a positive test for urinary reducing substances in an infant presenting with such symptoms raises the possibility of galactosaemia. Galactose (and lactose, present in milk) should be withdrawn from the diet pending a definitive **diagnosis**, based on measurements of galactose 1-phosphate uridyltransferase in erythrocytes or genotyping. The response to **treatment** (continued exclusion of galactose from the diet) is monitored by measuring galactose 1-phosphate in erythrocytes. A case of classic galactosaemia is presented in Case history 22.2. Deficiency of the enzyme UDP-galactose 4-epimerase causes a similar clinical syndrome but is much less common. Deficiency of the enzyme galactokinase prevents the phosphorylation of galactose and leads to an increase in the plasma concentration of galactose, and thus to galactosuria. Because galactose 1-phosphate formation is blocked, this metabolite does not accumulate and, although cataracts may occur, the other clinical features of classic galactosaemia are not seen in galactokinase deficiency.

Phenylketonuria

PKU is another condition in which the accumulation of the substrate of the missing enzyme causes a clinical syndrome. The classic form of the disorder results from a mutation in

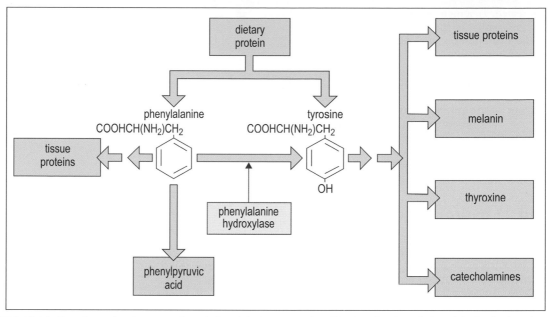

Fig. 19.4 Metabolic pathway for the conversion of phenylalanine to tyrosine. The site of action of phenylalanine hydroxylase, the enzyme deficient in phenylketonuria, is shown.

the gene for **phenylalanine hydroxylase**, which hydroxylates phenylalanine to produce tyrosine (Fig. 19.4). A rarer variant form is caused by a defect in the metabolism of its tetrahydrobiopterin cofactor.

Phenylalanine accumulates in the blood, and if the condition is untreated, it results in severe learning disability, thought to be due directly to the effect of excess phenylalanine on the developing brain. The name of the condition derives from the urinary excretion of phenylpyruvic acid, a phenylketone. This is normally a minor metabolite of phenylalanine, but is produced in excess when the major metabolic pathway is blocked. Many children with PKU have fair hair and blue eyes, because of defective melanin synthesis: tyrosine, the formation of which is blocked, is a precursor of this pigment. The diagnosis depends on the demonstration of an abnormally high concentration of phenylalanine in the blood: newborn screening for the condition is discussed later.

The **management** of PKU involves restricting the dietary intake of phenylalanine using diets based on special proteins and pure amino acids. The plasma concentration of phenylalanine should be maintained between 120 and 360 µmol/L during infancy and childhood, when there is rapid brain development. The diet is unpalatable, and adherence can be a major problem. Although there has been a tendency to allow less rigorous dietary restriction after the age of 10 years, most paediatricians now advocate a policy of 'diet for life'. Strict dietary control

is essential when a woman with PKU becomes pregnant, because maternal hyperphenylalaninaemia has been shown to affect the fetus *in utero* even if the fetus itself does not have PKU.

Because phenylalanine is an essential amino acid, a certain amount must be provided in the diet, and although tyrosine is not normally an essential amino acid, it becomes so when the intake of phenylalanine is limited: adequate quantities must therefore be provided. Dietary treatment is monitored by measuring both phenylalanine and tyrosine concentrations in finger prick blood spot samples. Some infants respond to pharmacological doses of tetrahydrobiopterin, a cofactor for the affected enzyme. Thus treated, most children in whom a diagnosis of PKU is made shortly after birth will grow and develop normally, although they rarely reach the IQ of their siblings.

Related conditions

A number of other inherited metabolic diseases are associated with abnormalities of phenylalanine and tyrosine metabolism, including tyrosinaemia and alkaptonuria.

Tyrosinaemia type 1 (caused by deficiency of fumarylacetoacetate hydrolase, a late enzyme in tyrosine degradation) causes severe progressive liver damage, leading to cirrhosis, and renal tubular damage, resulting in the renal Fanconi syndrome. It usually presents in early infancy with failure to thrive and hepatomegaly, resulting in early death if left untreated. Treatment with nitisinone, which inhibits an enzyme earlier in the tyrosine breakdown pathway, reduces the complication rate. **Alkaptonuria** (caused by deficiency of homogentisic acid oxidase) causes accumulation of homogentisic acid (a metabolite of phenylalanine and tyrosine). This polymerizes in skin and sclerae, causing brown-black discolouration (ochronosis), and in fibrous tissue and cartilage, including articular cartilage, where it can cause severe arthritis. Homogentisic acid is colourless, but it becomes oxidized in urine, causing it to become brown-black on standing. Treatment with nitisinone reduces blood concentrations of homogentisic acid but appears to have limited effect in preventing arthritis.

Steroid 21-hydroxylase deficiency

Steroid 21-hydroxylase deficiency, the commonest cause of **congenital adrenal hyperplasia**, exemplifies the effects of increased activity of a normally minor metabolic pathway, in this case the synthesis of adrenal androgens (see Fig. 10.2). As a consequence of the defective synthesis of cortisol, there is decreased negative feedback to the pituitary, and thus increased secretion of adrenocorticotrophic hormone, which stimulates the synthesis of adrenal androgens. This condition is discussed in more detail in Chapter 10.

Cystic fibrosis

Cystic fibrosis is a common inherited metabolic disease, with an incidence of 1 in ~2500 live births in the UK. The classic form is a **generalized disorder of exocrine secretion**, in which the secretions have greatly increased viscosity. The functional defect is impaired chloride transport. Affected children develop recurrent respiratory infections leading to irreversible lung disease and pancreatic insufficiency leading to malabsorption. Intestinal obstruction may occur in the neonatal period ('meconium ileus') because of the increased viscosity of faecal material. Affected men may be infertile. An increasing number of genetic mutations have been identified that cause milder variants of the disorder, such as isolated infertility.

In contrast with most inherited metabolic diseases, the basis of the functional defect in cystic fibrosis was not understood until the gene responsible had been identified, cloned and sequenced. This allowed the amino acid sequence and hence the three-dimensional structure of the gene product to be predicted. This protein, known as the **cystic fibrosis transmembrane conductance regulator (CFTR)**, is involved in the control of transmembrane chloride transport. Individual mutations affect the protein production pathway at different points. There may be almost complete failure of CFTR production or failure to transport the protein to the cell surface. Production of an abnormal

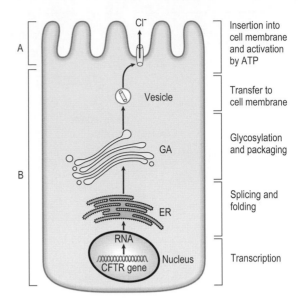

Fig. 19.5 Possible mechanisms that can disrupt protein synthesis and function caused by mutations in the gene for the cystic fibrosis transmembrane conductance regulator (CFTR). (**A**) Mutations that reduce the function of the CFTR channels at the cell surface. (**B**) Mutations that reduce the quantity of functional CFTR channels that reach the cell surface. ATP, adenosine triphosphate; ER, endoplasmic reticulum; GA, Golgi apparatus; RNA, ribonucleic acid.

protein may reduce its capacity to transport chloride ions or make it unstable, with a reduced life span (Fig. 19.5).

Sweat chloride concentration is increased in cystic fibrosis, and its measurement provides the **diagnostic test** for the condition (a concentration ≥60 mmol/L supports the diagnosis). Intervention before the condition presents clinically is beneficial, and testing for cystic fibrosis is part of the national newborn screening programme in the UK. The **screening test** is based on the detection of high neonatal plasma concentrations of immunoreactive trypsinogen, indicating pancreatic damage with blockage of the normal route of enzyme excretion. When the test is positive, sweat testing, together with molecular genetic analysis for the common mutations in the cystic fibrosis gene, can be used to confirm the diagnosis.

Management is directed towards the prevention of respiratory infections by regular physiotherapy and prophylactic antibiotic treatment, and maintenance of adequate nutrition with a good diet; pancreatic enzymes can be added to food to counter the effects of pancreatic insufficiency. CFTR-potentiating drugs are now available, although their use is limited by cost, and gene therapies are being developed.

Although the prognosis for children with cystic fibrosis has greatly improved with modern methods of treatment, this is not achieved without cost to patient and parents.

Many patients still die in early adult life. Antenatal screening for cystic fibrosis and screening of prospective parents for carrier status are discussed on p. 347.

Other inherited metabolic diseases

The disorders of phenylalanine metabolism are examples of **amino acidopathies**, a large group of disorders of amino acid metabolism encompassing a wide range of clinical severity. **Organic acid disorders**—for example, methylmalonic aciduria—are disorders of organic acid metabolism that typically present with a severe metabolic acidosis. Disorders that involve each of the enzymes of the **urea cycle** have been described, and most present with encephalopathy as a result of the accumulation of ammonia. In addition to the GSDs, numerous other **storage diseases**, involving the abnormal accumulation of, for example, lipids, glycosaminoglycans (mucopolysaccharides) and other complex molecules, have been described. Among various disorders of fatty acid transport and oxidation, **medium chain acyl-CoA dehydrogenase (MCAD) deficiency** is the most common. These conditions can present with features related to hypoglycaemia as a result of defective energy metabolism, but also can present with collapse, cardiac arrest or sudden infant death. Although many affected individuals reach adult life without any clinical evidence of the disorder, screening for MCAD deficiency is now part of the UK newborn screening programme (see p. 346).

The porphyrias

The porphyrias are a group of inherited diseases that exemplify accumulation of substrates in the metabolic pathway for **haem** (Fig. 19.6), sometimes from several steps before the deficient enzyme (Fig. 19.7). The rate-limiting step in this sequence of reactions is the first, catalyzed by δ-aminolaevulinic acid (ALA) synthase, which is susceptible to inhibition by the end product, haem. A partial deficiency of one of the enzymes of porphyrin synthesis leads to decreased formation of haem, and thus, by releasing ALA synthase from inhibition, results in the formation of excessive quantities of porphyrins or porphyrin precursors (ALA and **porphobilinogen** [PBG]). When precursors are produced in excess, the clinical manifestations are primarily **neurological** (ALA and PBG are neurotoxins). When **porphyrins** (strictly speaking, porphyrinogens: porphyrins are formed spontaneously from porphyrinogens) themselves are the major product, the predominant feature is photosensitivity: the porphyrins absorb light and become excited, inducing the formation of toxic free radicals. The porphyrias are diagnosed by their clinical features and the pattern of porphyrins and precursors present in blood and excreted in faeces and urine. This is followed by identification of the responsible mutation where possible.

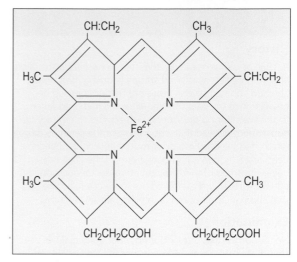

Fig. 19.6 The structure of haem, which consists of a tetrapyrrole ring, protoporphyrin IXα, linked to an iron II ion (Fe^{2+}), to which oxygen becomes reversibly bound during oxygen transport. It is found not only in haemoglobin but also in myoglobin and cytochromes, enzymes responsible for catalysing many oxidative processes in the body.

The porphyrias are classified as **acute** or **non-acute**, according to their clinical presentation, and **hepatic** or **erythropoietic**, depending on the major site of abnormal metabolism. All the porphyrias are rare. Porphyria cutanea tarda (cutaneous hepatic porphyria) is the most common, but many cases are not inherited. Of the purely genetic types, acute intermittent porphyria (AIP) is the most common (see Case history 19.1). The features of the porphyrias are summarized in Table 19.2. The genes for the enzymes involved in porphyrin synthesis have been identified and cloned, but the porphyrias are genetically heterogeneous; although genetic testing is not useful for primary diagnosis, once the mutation is known, it is used for screening other family members.

AIP is caused by deficiency of the enzyme **ALA synthase** and is characterized by a tendency towards acute attacks, separated by long periods of complete remission. **Abdominal pain and psychiatric disturbances** are nearly always present, but photosensitivity is never a feature of AIP. Peripheral neuropathy occurs in some 60% of patients. Hyponatraemia may result from stimulation of vasopressin release and inappropriate intravenous administration of hypotonic fluids. Attacks can be precipitated by various factors (Box 19.2), including many drugs; these probably act by increasing the activity of ALA synthase. Hormonal factors are also extremely important; **symptoms rarely occur before puberty** and may fluctuate in relation to menstruation or pregnancy. Women are affected more commonly than men. In some 90% of individuals who inherit the

Case history 19.1

History

A 19-year-old woman was admitted to hospital with colicky abdominal pain, which had started suddenly 12 h before. She had vomited several times but had not opened her bowels since the pain started. After she had been taken to the ward for observation, a nurse in the emergency department noticed that a specimen of the patient's urine, which had been collected for routine testing, had become a deep red although it had been normal when first passed. On being informed of this, the admitting doctor questioned the patient further and examined her more carefully. She said that she had also noticed cramping pains in her arms.

Examination

Her abdomen was tender but no other abnormalities were found. Her pulse was 140 beats per min and her blood pressure was 158/98 mmHg. She had bilateral wrist drop. A fresh sample of urine was collected, protected from light by placing it in a brown envelope and sent immediately to the laboratory.

Results

Screening test for urinary
porphobilinogen (PBG):   strongly positive
Quantitative analysis of urine:
  PBG   very high

Interpretation

The very high urinary excretion of the porphyrin precursor PBG suggests a diagnosis of acute porphyria.

Discussion

Acute porphyrias may present as an acute abdomen; systemic hypertension and sinus tachycardia are often present. They are, of course, a very uncommon cause of abdominal pain and the diagnosis is often missed, at least initially. In this case, the nurse's observation of the changed colour of the urine was crucial and led to the presumptive diagnosis of an acute porphyria being made. Colourless porphyrin precursors and porphyrinogens are unstable and will form coloured porphyrins on exposure to air and light. The diagnosis was supported clinically by the evidence of neuropathy and also by the positive screening test for PBG.

The patient's symptoms and signs resolved rapidly with appropriate treatment. It transpired that, a few days before, she had started taking an oral contraceptive pill, which probably precipitated the attacks. The diagnosis of acute intermittent porphyria (AIP) was later confirmed (in a specialist laboratory) by the demonstration that faecal coproporphyrin concentration was normal (thereby excluding hereditary coproporphyria) and that the pattern of porphyrins present in plasma was not characteristic of variegate porphyria. She was advised to use an alternative method of contraception and told which drugs she should avoid. Genetic testing was undertaken to identify other affected family members.

---

defective gene for AIP, the disease remains clinically latent throughout adult life. The **diagnosis** depends on demonstrating elevated excretion of **PBG** in the urine, usually by a screening test, followed by further investigations (see Table 19.2) to confirm the precise diagnosis.

When any form of acute porphyria has been diagnosed, blood relatives should be screened for latent disease and, if necessary, advised concerning the avoidance of precipitating factors. It is important to appreciate that the concentrations of porphyrins and their precursors in the blood, urine and faeces may be normal in latent disease, so genetic testing should be performed if the mutation is known. **Avoidance of precipitating factors** is essential in the **management** of acute porphyrias. During an attack, any such factors must be identified and treated appropriately. General supportive measures include maintenance of fluid and electrolyte balance, adequate carbohydrate intake (intravenous glucose is often beneficial) and physiotherapy. Pain can be safely relieved with narcotic analgesics. The specific treatment of choice for acute attacks is intravenous haem arginate, which decreases the activity of ALA synthase. Lists

of drugs that are considered safe to use in patients with acute porphyrias are available from expert bodies. Patients are at increased risk of developing hepatocellular carcinoma and require lifelong monitoring.

Porphyria cutanea tarda is the commonest non-acute porphyria and presents with photosensitivity resulting in erythema, vesicles and bullae, and eventually to scarring and pigmentation. This porphyria can be inherited (**familial, type II**) (15–20% of cases) or acquired (**sporadic, type I**). In both types, there is an ~50% reduction in hepatic **uroporphyrinogen decarboxylase** activity in the liver; in type II, this deficiency occurs in all tissues. Although the acquired type can develop spontaneously, it is more frequently seen in association with **excessive ethanol ingestion** (often with liver disease: 90% of patients), hepatitis C infection or as a consequence of exposure to hepatotoxins or drugs. Patients who possess the common mutation in the *HFE* gene (see p. 118) that is associated with accumulation of iron in the liver and other features of haemochromatosis are at increased risk of developing porphyria cutanea tarda. The diagnosis

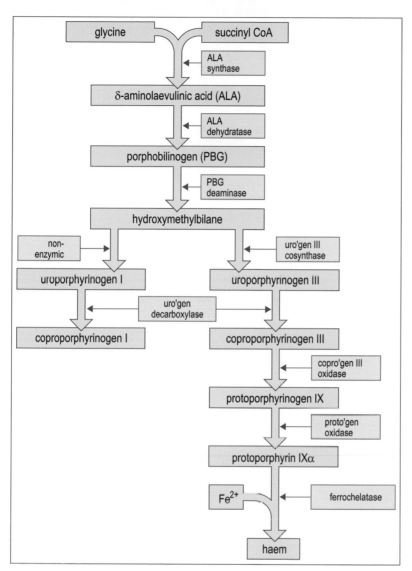

Fig. 19.7 Biosynthesis of porphyrins. PBG deaminase is also known as hydroxymethylbilane synthase and δ-aminolaevulinic acid dehydratase as PBG synthase.

depends on demonstrating the typical porphyrin patterns in urine and faeces, but the single most useful investigation is a plasma porphyrin fluorescence scan, because a normal result excludes active cutaneous porphyria. Urine PBG excretion is normal. **Management** involves the identification and **removal of precipitating factors: venesection** to remove excess iron from the liver, **avoidance of direct sunlight** and the use of **barrier creams** to protect the skin. Low-dose hydroxychloroquine can improve symptoms by enhancing excretion of porphyrinogens.

The features of all the porphyrias, including AIP and porphyria cutanea tarda, are summarised in Table 19.2.

Diagnosis

The diagnosis of an inherited metabolic disease may be suggested by clinical features and the results of simple tests (Table 19.3). However, the diagnosis will not be made if a possible metabolic origin of the symptoms is

Table 19.2 Classification and characteristics of the porphyrias

Condition	Deficient enzyme	Inheritance	Course	Erythropoietic/ hepatic	Symptomatology	Abnormal porphyrin concentrations		
						Red cells	Urine	Faeces
ALA dehydratase deficiency porphyria	ALA dehydratase	AR	acute	E	N	Zn proto-	**ALA**	
acute intermittent porphyria	PBG deaminase	AD	acute	H	N		ALA, **PBG**	
hereditary coproporphyria	copro'gen oxidase	AD	acute	H	N, P		ALA, PBG, **copro-**	copro-
variegate porphyria	proto'gen oxidase	AD	acute	H	N, P		ALA, PBG, **copro-**	copro-, **proto-**
porphyria cutanea tarda	uro'gen decarboxylase	AD[a]	chronic	H	P		**uro-**	**isocopro-**
congenital erythropoietic porphyria	uro'gen III cosynthase	AR	chronic	E	P	uro-[b] copro-[b]	**uro-**[b] **copro-**[b]	copro-[b]
erythropoietic protoporphyria	ferrochelatase	AD	chronic	E	P	**proto-**		proto-

The most important abnormalities are in bold; the changes shown for the acute porphyrias may only be present during an attack. Each porphyria also has a characteristic plasma porphyrin fluorescence profile.
[a]Eighty percent of cases are sporadic.
[b]Type I isomers.
AD, autosomal dominant; ALA, δ-aminolaevulinic acid; AR, autosomal recessive; E, erythropoietic; H, hepatic; N, neurological; P, photosensitizing; PBG, porphobilinogen.

Box 19.2 **Clinical features and factors involved in acute attacks of porphyria**

Clinical features
Gastrointestinal
abdominal pain
vomiting
constipation

Peripheral neuropathy
pain, stiffness and muscle weakness (limb and girdle
    muscles > trunk; upper limbs > lower; proximal >
    distal)
paraesthesiae, numbness

Central nervous system
seizures
depression
hysteria
psychosis

Cardiovascular
sinus tachycardia
systemic hypertension
hyponatraemia

Factors involved
anaesthesia
drugs
pregnancy
luteal phase of menstrual cycle
infection
low-calorie, low-carbohydrate diet
ethanol
stress

Table 19.3 **Diagnostic investigations for suspected inherited metabolic diseases**

Essential investigations	Examples of condition(s) that may be identified
blood gas analysis	organic acid disorders, urea cycle disorders
blood/plasma glucose	galactosaemia, fatty acid oxidation disorders, glycogen storage disorders
urinary reducing substances	galactosaemia, hereditary fructose intolerance
plasma ammonia	urea cycle disorders, organic acid disorders
liver function tests	galactosaemia, tyrosinaemia type 1, α_1-antitrypsin deficiency
plasma lactate	glycogen storage disease type I
ketones	(absence in hypoglycaemia) fatty acid oxidation disorders
Second-line investigations	
plasma/urine amino acids	amino acid disorders, urea cycle disorders
urine orotic acid	urea cycle disorders
urine organic acids	organic acid disorders
blood acylcarnitines	fatty acid oxidation disorders
urine glycosaminoglycans	mucopolysaccharidoses

not considered. Although most inherited metabolic diseases are rare, as a group they are an important cause of illness in neonates and infants. Effective treatment is now available for many of these conditions, and thus it would be tragic if treatment were not given because of a missed diagnosis.

The **definitive diagnosis** may depend on the demonstration of decreased activity of the enzyme or concentration of the protein responsible in an appropriate tissue, although genetic testing for known mutations is increasingly available for many conditions. Biopsy of an affected organ may be required, but in some cases the enzyme can be assayed in red or white blood cells. **Inherited metabolic diseases may not be diagnosed in life**. In infants with an unexplained illness who are not expected to recover, and in infants dying unexpectedly,

the collection of appropriate specimens (if necessary, *postmortem*) may allow the diagnosis to be made retrospectively. This may then be of value not only in explaining to parents the reason for their child's death but in counselling them about future pregnancy, especially if there has been a previous childhood death in the family. The identification of probable cases by newborn or prenatal **screening** merits special consideration. Contrasting examples of the clinical presentation and management of two inherited metabolic diseases are provided by Case histories 13.8 and 22.2.

Newborn Screening

Screening is designed to detect individuals affected with a condition before it is apparent clinically. This may be done prenatally, during the neonatal period or later, according to the nature of the condition. The **criteria for an effective newborn screening programme** are similar to those for screening in general (see Box 2.1). Screening is feasible for many conditions. It should, however, be appreciated that, even when a condition is relatively common and an effective test is available, screening can have adverse consequences. For every case detected, there are usually many false positive results that require further investigation (see Chapter 2) and perhaps interim treatment until the results of definitive tests become available, inducing considerable anxiety in parents. Economic considerations dictate that a screening test should be cost-effective. Even though it may be technically feasible, it is not economical to screen whole populations for rare diseases, although this is changing with the availability of new technology. Targeted screening in populations that are known to have a high incidence of a disorder, such as for galactosaemia in Eire, improves the economic balance.

The longest-established newborn screening programmes are for the detection of PKU and congenital hypothyroidism (although this is usually a developmental disorder, not an enzyme defect). The conditions included in the National Health Service Newborn Blood Spot Screening Programme in the UK (January 2020) are shown in Box 19.3. Blood samples are taken onto special filter paper from a heel prick about a week after birth, when feeding has been established. This ensures that there has been adequate substrate intake to develop the characteristic biochemical abnormalities of some of the disorders and that maternal metabolites have been cleared. If any of the screening tests are found to be positive, further definitive tests are required. In screening for metabolic disorders, the cutoff concentrations taken as positive are set such that the sensitivity of each test is virtually 100% (all cases are detected). However, because the conditions are rare, the predictive value of positive tests are low (see p. 20); thus, most positive screening tests are found not to be caused by the disorder in question.

Prenatal Diagnosis

When an inherited disease cannot be successfully treated, or the treatment imposes harsh restrictions on the patient, early prenatal diagnosis will allow parents the option of having the pregnancy terminated. The **criteria for undertaking prenatal diagnosis** are set out in Box 19.4.

Satisfactory diagnostic tests are available for many inherited metabolic diseases, but whether an attempt at prenatal diagnosis is justified depends on the risk of the procedure. Most of these conditions have a recessive mode of inheritance, and thus prenatal diagnosis should usually be considered only if there is an affected child from a previous pregnancy, if one parent is affected or if there is a strong family history of the disease. Prenatal screening of selected groups may be justified if a disease has a high incidence in a particular population, for example the lipid storage disorder Tay–Sachs disease in Ashkenazi Jews.

Maternal and fetal screening

An inherited metabolic defect may be reflected by the presence of an abnormally high concentration of a metabolite in maternal blood as, for example, in some organic acidaemias, but such metabolites, derived from the fetus, would normally be cleared by maternal enzymes. Maternal screening is not diagnostic but may point to the need to proceed to a more invasive, but definitive, test. Analysis of amniotic fluid, or cultures of amniotic cells obtained by amniocentesis, will give a more accurate reflection of fetal metabolism. Amniocentesis is usually performed in the second trimester and has an associated risk of miscarriage of <0.5%.

Fetal blood samples can be obtained by cordocentesis – transabdominal aspiration from the umbilical cord under ultrasound control.

Chorionic villus biopsy, sampling of fetal placental tissue very early in pregnancy (11–12 weeks of gestation), allows molecular genetic or chromosomal analysis for an increasingly wide range of disorders. In experienced hands, this is a safe procedure, the excess rate of fetal loss being well below 1%. As is the case with all screening procedures, the risk of fetal loss must be considered in relation to the potential benefit of early identification of a severe disorder.

Newer techniques which can isolate fetal DNA from maternal plasma offer the possibility of much less invasive testing of the fetal genome in the future.

Some of the issues relating to prenatal diagnosis are exemplified by a consideration of screening for Down syndrome and cystic fibrosis.

Down syndrome

Although Down syndrome (trisomy 21, a chromosomal disorder) is not an inherited metabolic disorder, it is convenient to discuss this important condition in the context of prenatal diagnosis. The recommended screening strategy for the detection of Down syndrome (and also Edwards and Patau syndromes) in the UK is a combination of a fetal nuchal translucency ultrasound scan and a maternal blood test for free β-human chorionic gonadotrophin (hCG) and pregnancy-associated plasma protein A (PAPP-A) at 10–14 weeks of pregnancy. Affected fetuses tend to have increased nuchal translucency and produce more hCG and less PAPP A than healthy ones. For mothers presenting later in pregnancy, a quadruple test can be performed at 14–20 weeks. This test measures α-fetoprotein and unconjugated oestriol (which tend to be low with affected fetuses) and total hCG and inhibin A (which tend to be high) in maternal blood. The age of the mother is also taken into account for the risk calculation because the incidence of Down syndrome increases with maternal age. If the calculated risk of having an affected pregnancy is high, the mother can choose to have a further, invasive test, such as chorionic villus sampling or amniocentesis for diagnostic chromosomal analysis.

Cystic fibrosis

Cystic fibrosis is an autosomal recessive disorder (see p. 340). It is a genetically heterogeneous disease, with several hundred mutations already identified in affected families. Many of these are private—that is, they occur only in one family—but ~70% of mutations causing cystic fibrosis in the UK involve the deletion of the same single codon. This mutation is designated ΔF508. It is possible to screen for this and several of the other more common mutations simultaneously. Screening can be performed on fetal tissue obtained by chorionic villus biopsy when a couple has already had one affected child, and on prospective parents from families in which the condition occurs. Screening is capable of detecting >90% of Caucasian carriers, and given the frequency of the heterozygous carrier state in the UK (~1 in 25), there has been discussion as to whether a programme for carrier screening in the population as a whole should be established. This is a complex matter, involving financial, ethical and practical issues. The availability of adequate genetic counselling is important: a positive result would indicate that an individual was a carrier, but an apparently negative result would not exclude the possibility of carriage of an unidentified mutation.

DNA Analysis

DNA analysis is now a standard technique for the investigation of an increasing number of inherited disorders. When appropriate, it can be used to genotype fetal tissue for **prenatal diagnosis** and to aid **genetic counselling** by genotyping of individuals in families in which a particular condition occurs. The index case may have been diagnosed by conventional means, but if the condition is one that is amenable to genetic analysis, other members of the family can then be studied. In some cases, notably cystic fibrosis and Duchenne muscular dystrophy, genetic analysis has led to the identification of the gene product.

It is beyond the scope of this book to discuss genetic analysis in detail. The techniques involved have many applications in medicine and science, and are explained in numerous textbooks of general biochemistry and molecular biology.

Direct detection of gene mutations is particularly suited to the diagnosis of homogeneous genetic disorders, that is, ones that are always due to the same mutation. As discussed for cystic fibrosis, when a disease can be caused by any one of several mutations in the same gene, 100% sensitivity in diagnosis would require the use of a battery of gene probes or direct gene sequencing, which between them could detect all the mutations. If these are not available, diagnosis and screening must continue to depend, at least in part, on the detection of the effects of the mutation, usually by measurement of the gene product. This technique, or, if applicable, the detection of linkage through restriction fragment length polymorphism analysis, will continue to be used for conditions where the responsible gene has not yet been identified.

It would be wrong to give the impression that the techniques of molecular genetics are applicable only to comparatively rare inherited metabolic diseases caused by single gene defects. Genetic factors play an important part in the aetiology of many common conditions, including hypertension, some cancers and coronary heart disease. For example, genetic testing for FH (see

Table 19.4 Treatment strategies for inherited metabolic diseases

Treatment	Example
restriction of substrate intake	galactose in galactosaemia
supply of missing product	cortisol in congenital adrenal hyperplasia
supply of vitamin cofactors	pyridoxal phosphate in homocystinuria
increased excretion of toxic substances	copper chelating agents in Wilson disease
replacement of missing protein	factor VIII in haemophilia
replacement of abnormal gene	organ transplantation

p. 313) can not only identify mutations known to cause FH but also give an estimate of the contribution to high cholesterol concentrations from polygenic inherited traits. It can also identify those patients who are more likely to develop statin-induced myopathy. Identification of the genes involved in many conditions will make it possible to screen for them, and thus for susceptibility to the conditions. Such knowledge would potentially be a powerful tool in preventive medicine, but its application would pose considerable ethical and economic questions. Whole genome sequencing of an individual is now technically feasible and is driving the development of 'personalized medicine'.

Treatment

Possible approaches to the treatment of inherited metabolic diseases are given in Table 19.4.

Restriction of substrate intake

Restriction of substrate intake is exemplified in the treatment of galactosaemia. If all foodstuffs containing galactose (and lactose, a dimer of glucose and galactose) are removed from the diet, clinical symptoms regress. Similarly, hereditary fructose intolerance (see p. 253) is asymptomatic if fructose (and sucrose, a dimer of glucose and fructose) is avoided. The management is less straightforward, however, if the substrate is essential for life. In PKU, the metabolism of phenylalanine to tyrosine is blocked (see p. 338), but phenylalanine is an essential amino acid, and some must therefore

be provided in the diet to allow normal growth and development.

Supply of missing product

Congenital adrenal hyperplasia is managed by giving cortisol, production of which is impaired in this condition. In salt-losing types, a mineralocorticoid must also be given. Related approaches include supplying increased quantities of a non-toxic precursor that can be converted into the missing product, providing a synthetic analogue of the product or attempting to inhibit its breakdown. The supply of the missing product will also restore negative feedback and therefore reduce synthesis of the precursor(s) and side product(s).

Addition of vitamin cofactors

If the defective enzyme has a vitamin cofactor, the supply of large amounts of the vitamin may increase cofactor binding, and thus enzyme activity, by a mass action effect. Many enzymes have separate catalytic and regulatory sites, and amino acid substitution caused by a gene mutation may affect either of such sites or alter the way in which they interact. Homocystinuria is a condition in which the conversion of homocysteine to cystathionine is blocked. The enzyme involved, cystathionine β-synthase, requires pyridoxal phosphate as a cofactor, and giving large amounts of this vitamin may be of therapeutic benefit in some patients. Some organic acidaemias may similarly respond to high-dose vitamin supplementation.

Complex formation and removal of toxic substances

Complex formation and removal of toxic substances is used in the treatment of Wilson disease (see p. 118) to remove the excess copper, which is responsible for the tissue damage in this condition. D-Penicillamine forms a soluble complex with copper, which is then readily excreted in the urine. This drug is also used in the treatment of cystinuria, an inherited disorder characterized by defective renal tubular reabsorption of cystine and the dibasic amino acids lysine, ornithine and arginine. Cystine is relatively insoluble, and there is a marked tendency to urinary stone (calculus) formation. Cystine may be kept in solution if the urine is kept sufficiently dilute and alkaline. If calculi continue to form, penicillamine (or tiopronin) can be used; the drug complexes with cysteine (from which cystine is derived) to form a more soluble compound, thus reducing the urinary excretion of free cystine. In cystinosis (see p. 97) there is a defect in the lysosomal membrane cystine transporter, resulting in accumulation of lysosomal cystine. Treatment with cysteamine slows progression by forming a cysteine–cysteamine mixed disulphide, which can be removed from the lysosome via a different (lysine) transporter.

Related techniques include strategies to block the formation of a toxic substance; in tyrosinaemia type 1, nitisinone is used to block the metabolism of tyrosine at an early step in the pathway, thus preventing the formation of fumarylacetoacetate, the toxic metabolite that is the substrate for the defective enzyme.

Replacement of missing enzyme or other protein

If the replacement of a missing protein is to be an effective method of treatment, it needs to be repeated at regular intervals, as there is a continuous turnover of proteins in the body. Replacement of gammaglobulins is the mainstay of treatment of agammaglobulinaemia, and, when necessary, factor VIII can be given in haemophilia. With the great majority of inherited metabolic diseases, the defective protein is intracellular, and thus replacement is not feasible. However, recombinant enzymes have been developed for use in type 1 Gaucher disease (glucocerebrosidase deficiency, a lipid storage disorder). The enzyme is normally active in lysosomes, and it has proved possible to modify the protein so that it is taken up by macrophages and targeted into lysosomes. Enzyme replacement therapy is also available for a small number of other storage disorders such as Fabry disease and Pompe disease.

Replacement of the defective gene

Replacement of the defective gene (or editing of the abnormal base pairs) should allow normal synthesis of the product of the gene, for example an enzyme. The technical problems are considerable, including not only the engineering of the gene but also its insertion into a sufficient number of the appropriate somatic cells in such a way that its activity is subject to normal regulation. Overexpression of a normal gene might be as harmful as the effect of the abnormal gene, and there is potential for other untoward consequences. The technique was first used to treat children with adenine deaminase deficiency, a cause of severe combined immunodeficiency, using a retrovirus to effect the transfer. Sadly, several of these children developed leukaemia as a result of unintended activation of an oncogene. Clinical trials are in progress for other disorders such as haemophilia and retinitis pigmentosa.

Organ transplantation may be appropriate in some conditions; liver transplantation has been used successfully in patients with Wilson disease and α_1-antitrypsin deficiency who have developed liver failure, and patients with kidney failure caused by cystinuria have been treated by kidney transplantation. Homozygous FH has also been treated successfully by liver transplantation. Organ transplantation effectively replaces the abnormal gene and the engrafted organ synthesizes the normal gene product.

SUMMARY

- **Inherited metabolic diseases are the result of gene mutations** that either prevent the synthesis of a protein or cause the production of an abnormal protein molecule. **In the majority of these disorders, the protein is an enzyme** and the result is a decrease in catalytic activity. In some, the defective or missing protein is a receptor (e.g. FH) or a transport protein (e.g. cystinuria).

- Hundreds of these disorders have been described: most of them are rare, some to the extent that only a handful of cases have been documented worldwide. Their effects vary in severity from the completely benign (e.g. renal glycosuria) to the invariably fatal (e.g. Tay–Sachs disease).

- Most inherited metabolic diseases have an **autosomal recessive mode of inheritance**; heterozygotes are usually phenotypically normal. Some, such as ornithine transcarbamylase deficiency, are X-linked, with boys being more severely affected than girls. Most of the porphyrias are unusual in having an autosomal dominant mode of inheritance.

- **A decrease in catalytic activity** can have a number of consequences. In the case of an enzyme involved in a synthetic pathway, there could be decreased synthesis of the product of the enzyme or pathway, accumulation of the substrate and other precursor metabolites or increased activity in a usually minor pathway which has, as its starting point, one of the intermediates that accumulates. Thus, the clinical effects may relate to decreased quantities of a product of the pathway or increased quantities of other metabolites (which may be toxic in excess), or a combination of these.

- The synthesis of the tetrapyrrole ring of **haem** involves a complex metabolic pathway from glycine and succinyl CoA through intermediates known as porphyrinogens. There are inherited metabolic disorders that affect each of the enzymes of the haem synthetic pathway, and these collectively are called **porphyrias.**

- The **definitive diagnosis** of an inherited metabolic disease requires either measurement of the activity of the relevant enzyme, a procedure that may necessitate tissue biopsy unless the enzyme is present in blood cells, or detection of the defective gene. The diagnosis can, however, often be inferred from the clinical features and

Continued

SUMMARY—cont'd

measurements of the concentrations of metabolites or precursors of the enzyme, and may then be confirmed by the response to treatment.

- **Prenatal screening** for inherited metabolic diseases may be appropriate when there is a significant risk of a fetus being affected, for instance, when a previous child is known to have had the condition or when there is a strong family history of the disorder. **Newborn screening** is technically feasible and is widely practised in the general population for many inherited metabolic disorders including PKU, cystic fibrosis, sickle cell disease and MCAD and for congenital hypothyroidism, which also satisfies the criteria for such screening. **Screening tests must be highly sensitive and specific**; the condition in question should have severe consequences that can be ameliorated by early treatment (or avoided by termination of the pregnancy in the case of prenatal screening), and the condition must occur sufficiently frequently in the population being screened for the exercise to be worthwhile.

- There is no **treatment** for many inherited metabolic diseases: others can be treated relatively simply. Congenital adrenal hyperplasia, a group of conditions in each of which one of the enzymes involved in the synthesis of cortisol is defective, can be treated by **replacing the missing product**, cortisol. Others, such as galactosaemia and PKU, can be treated by **dietary modifications**, which prevent the accumulation of toxic metabolites. A few metabolic disorders are due to decreased ability of the enzyme to bind a coenzyme; **giving large amounts of the coenzyme** may overcome this by a mass action effect and restore catalytic activity to normal.

- **The definitive treatment** for an inherited metabolic disease would be **replacement or correction of the defective protein or gene.** Some lysosomal enzyme deficiencies can be treated by enzyme replacement therapy, but this needs to be repeated frequently and is expensive. Organ transplantation for the kidney failure that can occur in cystinuria or the liver failure in Wilson disease effectively replaces the defective gene.

Chapter | 20 |

Metabolic aspects of malignant disease

Introduction

The clinical signs and symptoms in patients suffering from cancer are often directly related to the physical presence of the tumour. For example, the tumour may destroy essential normal tissue, cause obstruction of ducts or exert pressure on nerves. Systemic manifestations, including **cachexia** and **pyrexia**, are also frequently present, and indeed may be the only evidence of the presence of a tumour. In some patients, the clinical features may be those of an **endocrine syndrome**. This would be expected with a tumour of endocrine tissue such as an insulinoma (producing hypoglycaemia) or an adrenal carcinoma (causing Cushing syndrome), but often occurs with tumours not obviously of endocrine origin.

In many patients, these syndromes are caused by the secretion of a hormone by the tumour. This has been termed **ectopic hormone secretion**, because the hormone is not secreted from its normal site. Tumours can be associated with other systemic manifestations, for example a cerebellar syndrome, arthropathy, etc. The term 'paraneoplastic syndromes' encompasses all the systemic manifestations of cancer not directly related to the physical presence of the primary tumour, regardless of whether they are due to a hormone.

This chapter discusses **paraneoplastic endocrine syndromes**, certain **familial endocrine syndromes** and also **tumour markers**, that is, substances that may be present in the circulation in malignant disease and whose concentrations can be measured as an aid to the diagnosis or monitoring of tumours. The reader should refer to other textbooks for a discussion of the molecular and genetic aspects of malignancy; identification of specific mutations, including those that affect apoptosis, can be helpful for screening, diagnosis and choice of treatment in many cancers.

Paraneoplastic Endocrine Syndromes

Origins and classification

Paraneoplastic endocrine syndromes are due to the secretion of peptide hormones or other humoral factors. All somatic cells contain a full complement of genes, and aberrant hormone secretion could be explained either by novel expression of a gene that is not normally expressed in the cells from which the tumour arises, or by re-expression of a gene that is expressed during development in a stem cell from which the tumour cells are ultimately derived. The fact that these syndromes tend to be associated with certain tumours, notably small cell carcinoma of bronchus, and that some tumours cause predominantly only one syndrome favours the second explanation.

Neuroendocrine tumours

Neuroendocrine tumours (NETs, previously known as amine precursor uptake and decarboxylation [APUD] tumours) occur outside endocrine glands and are thought to arise from neuroendocrine cells that are widely distributed throughout the body. There are many different types of NET, but they share common features such as having prominent secretory granules and secreting biogenic amines and peptide hormones. They most commonly occur in the intestine (see p. 355) but can be found anywhere in the body including the bronchi. Small cell carcinoma of the bronchus is an example of a NET that is particularly associated with aberrant hormone production. Hormone secretion by tumours does not always cause an endocrine syndrome. There may not be sufficient secretion to cause a persistently raised plasma concentration (particularly because normal secretion of the hormone may be suppressed) or because the principal secretory product is an inactive precursor of the hormone.

Some tumours associated with aberrant hormone secretion are listed in Table 20.1. The most frequently encountered paraneoplastic endocrine syndromes are **Cushing syndrome, syndrome of inappropriate antidiuresis and hypercalcaemia of malignancy.** Calcitonin secretion is thought to be common but is clinically silent.

Cushing syndrome

Cushing syndrome is the condition that results when tissues are exposed to supraphysiological concentrations of glucocorticoids. It is discussed in detail in Chapter 10. Malignancy-associated causes include both adrenal and non-adrenal tumours.

Ectopic secretion of adrenocorticotrophic hormone (ACTH) by NETs is common. Evidence of it has been found in up to 50% of patients with **small cell bronchial carcinomas,** although massive secretion, causing the typical features, as shown by Case history 20.1, is uncommon. ACTH is produced by posttranslational modification of the precursor, proopiomelanocortin (POMC), and both this precursor and other products of the POMC gene (see p. 158 and Fig. 9.4) may be secreted in some patients. Alternative splicing may produce unusual forms of ACTH that are metabolically active but may not be detectable by standard biochemical assays.

The prognosis for patients who have bronchial carcinomas is usually very poor unless the tumour is suitable for surgical excision. As discussed on p. 184, medical treatment may provide symptomatic relief.

Ectopic vasopressin secretion

Ectopic vasopressin secretion is one of the causes of the syndrome of inappropriate antidiuresis (see p. 40). A patient with this syndrome is described in Case history 3.3. The secretion of vasopressin (antidiuretic hormone) by the tumour is unregulated, resulting in water retention with **dilutional hyponatraemia**. When this is mild and develops slowly, it is often asymptomatic. However, severe hyponatraemia is associated with water intoxication, which can be fatal. The clinical features (drowsiness, confusion, fits and coma) may mimic those of cerebral metastases. Ectopic vasopressin secretion is most commonly seen with small cell carcinomas of the bronchus, but other tumours may be responsible (e.g. carcinoid tumours, breast cancers and pancreatic adenocarcinomas).

Hypercalcaemia of malignancy

Hypercalcaemia is common in malignant disease. When bony metastases are present, dissolution of calcium from bone by the metastases themselves may contribute to hypercalcaemia. However, there is in general a poor correlation between the extent of metastatic bone involvement and the severity of any hypercalcaemia; also, hypercalcaemia can occur in the absence of detectable metastasis. Although hypercalcaemia can affect kidney function adversely and decrease calcium excretion, it should suppress parathyroid hormone (PTH) secretion by the parathyroid glands. This would be expected to decrease renal

Table 20.1 **Some tumours of non-endocrine origin frequently associated with aberrant hormone secretion**		
Tumour	**Hormone**	**Syndrome**
small cell carcinoma of bronchus	ACTH (and precursors)	Cushing syndrome
	vasopressin	dilutional hyponatraemia
	hCG	gynaecomastia
squamous cell carcinoma of bronchus	PTHrP	hypercalcaemia
breast carcinoma	calcitonin	none
carcinoid tumours[a]	ACTH	Cushing syndrome
	vasopressin	dilutional hyponatraemia
renal cell carcinoma	PTHrP	hypercalcaemia
mesenchymal tumours	insulin-like growth factors	hypoglycaemia

Renal cell carcinomas may also secrete erythropoietin, causing polycythaemia, but this is not ectopic secretion because this hormone is a normal product of the kidneys.
ACTH, adrenocorticotrophic hormone; hCG, human chorionic gonadotrophin; PTHrP, parathyroid hormone-related peptide.
[a]Carcinoid tumours also secrete vasoactive amines and peptides (see p. 356).

Case history 20.1

History

A retired warehouseman presented with muscle weakness and back pain. He had lost 5 kg in weight in the previous 2 months and had recently been passing more urine than usual. He had smoked 25–30 cigarettes a day for many years but had generally enjoyed good health.

Examination

His appearance was normal but he had proximal muscle weakness. His BP was 174/105 mmHg. A urine dipstick was positive for glucose.

Investigations A discrete mass was present in the left lower zone on chest radiography.

Results (see Appendix for reference ranges)

Serum:	sodium	144 mmol/L
	potassium	2.2 mmol/L
	bicarbonate	39 mmol/L
Plasma: (9:00 a.m.)	glucose	10.2 mmol/L
	cortisol	1520 nmol/L
	ACTH	460 ng/L

High-dose dexamethasone suppression test: 9:00 a.m. plasma cortisol after dexamethasone 2 mg, 4 times daily for 2 days

1500 nmol/L

Summary

Severe hypokalaemia with high bicarbonate and glucose concentrations. Markedly high cortisol and ACTH concentrations.

Interpretation

The greatly elevated plasma cortisol and ACTH concentrations are typical of ectopic ACTH secretion. Plasma ACTH concentrations are generally much higher than those seen in Cushing disease. Because ACTH secretion is not under normal feedback control, the hypercortisolaemia is not suppressed by dexamethasone. Cortisol enhances potassium loss from the kidneys which results in hypokalaemia and increased bicarbonate formation (see p. 46). It also stimulates gluconeogenesis and can increase glucose concentration above the renal threshold for reabsorption, resulting in glycosuria.

Discussion

With ectopic ACTH secretion, the clinical presentation is typically dominated by the metabolic sequelae of excessive cortisol secretion, as in this case. These include hypokalaemia with alkalosis, which exacerbates the physical weakness caused by steroid-induced myopathy, glucose intolerance, sometimes sufficient to cause frank diabetes, and hypertension. Osteoporosis predisposes to crush fractures of the vertebrae, and the presence of secondary tumour deposits may also cause back pain. The classic somatic manifestations of Cushing syndrome are often absent, a reflection of the very rapid progression of the condition in most patients. ACTH-secreting carcinoid and thymic tumours are an exception: the clinical syndrome in these patients may closely resemble Cushing disease, even to the extent that ACTH secretion, and hence that of cortisol, is suppressible by dexamethasone.

---

tubular calcium reabsorption and allow excretion of calcium mobilized from bone. However, there is often renal calcium retention caused by the involvement of humoral factors in the hypercalcaemia of malignancy. **PTH-related peptide** (PTHrP) is most frequently responsible (see p. 261 and Case history 20.2).

Hypercalcaemia is common in haematological malignancies, particularly myeloma, and is due to the release of **osteoclast-activating cytokines** (e.g. interleukin-1, tumour necrosis factor-β [TNF-β]) by the tumours. Osteoclasts may also be activated by prostaglandins produced by tumour metastases in bone, for example, metastases from breast carcinoma. Lymphomas can produce 1,25-dihydroxycholecalciferol leading to increased absorption of calcium from the gut and hypercalcaemia.

Tumour-associated hypoglycaemia

Tumour-associated hypoglycaemia is discussed in detail in Chapter 13. It is only rarely due to ectopic insulin secretion by non–β-cell tumours; it is more often associated with **large mesenchymal tumours**, such as retroperitoneal sarcoma, and is due to the secretion of **insulin-like growth factors** (somatomedins) by the tumours. Massive infiltration of the liver by solid tumours can impair gluconeogenesis resulting in hypoglycaemia.

Other paraneoplastic endocrine syndromes

Gynaecomastia may occur in patients with bronchial carcinomas, as a result of secretion of **human chorionic**

Case history 20.2

History

An elderly man presented with loin pain and increasing thirst.

Investigations

Examination of the urine showed haematuria but no glycosuria. Ultrasound examination showed an irregularly enlarged left kidney with a distorted pelvicaliceal system. Computed tomography confirmed the presence of a tumour in the left kidney. An isotopic bone scan showed no evidence of metastatic disease, and a chest radiograph was normal.

Results

Serum:	calcium (adjusted)	3.2 mmol/L
	phosphate	0.7 mmol/L
	alkaline phosphatase	80 U/L
Plasma:	PTH	<0.5 pmol/L

Summary

Hypercalcaemia with low phosphate concentration, normal alkaline phosphatase activity and suppressed PTH.

Interpretation

The combination of hypercalcaemia and hypophosphataemia is compatible with activation of PTH receptors, although the plasma phosphate may be normal or even raised if there is renal impairment. The absence of detectable PTH suggests that secretion of the hormone by the parathyroid glands is suppressed, as would be expected when hypercalcaemia is due to some agent other than PTH.

Discussion

True ectopic secretion of PTH is rare. In most patients with humoral hypercalcaemia, the cause is secretion of PTHrP by the tumour. This substance, which has some N-terminal amino acid sequence homology with PTH, binds to PTH receptors and has similar actions to PTH itself but is not detected in most assays for PTH.

At operation, a tumour was found in the upper part of the left kidney. It was later confirmed to be a renal cell carcinoma. The patient underwent nephrectomy and made an uneventful recovery. After the operation, his serum calcium concentration decreased and subsequently remained normal.

---

gonadotrophin (hCG). Precocious puberty may develop in boys with hepatic tumours secreting hCG, but this is rare. Secretion of **erythropoietin** is responsible for the **polycythaemia** that can occur in association with uterine fibromyomata and the rare tumour, cerebellar haemangioblastoma. Secretion of erythropoietin by renal cell carcinomas can cause polycythaemia, but this is not ectopic secretion because the kidneys are the normal source of this hormone. Some patients develop **acromegaly** from tumoural secretion of **growth hormone–releasing hormone** (see pp. 155 and 165). Severe phosphate wasting leading to **tumour-induced osteomalacia** is a rare feature of some mesenchymal tumours that secrete fibroblast growth factor 23 (see p. 260).

Paraneoplastic syndromes are common, but it must be remembered that an endocrine syndrome in a patient with a tumour may be caused by **coexistent endocrine disease** and not necessarily by the secretion of a hormone or other factor by the tumour. There are also several non-endocrine paraneoplastic syndromes. Many of these are immunologically mediated (e.g. the Lambert–Eaton syndrome and paraneoplastic cerebellar degeneration, see p. 327), but the cause of others is uncertain.

Other Metabolic Complications of Malignant Disease

Metabolic complications in patients with malignant disease are not always due to aberrant hormone secretion. They may be caused by some other effect of the tumour or develop as a consequence of treatment.

Acute or chronic kidney disease can occur for many possible reasons. Causes include obstruction of the urinary tract, hypercalcaemia, direct infiltration of the kidneys (e.g. by lymphoma), Bence Jones proteinuria causing light chain deposition in myeloma, antibiotics, cytotoxic drugs and the **tumour lysis syndrome**. The latter is the result of massive necrosis of tumour cells during treatment with cytotoxic drugs. Features include hyperkalaemia, hyperuricaemia, hyperphosphataemia and hypocalcaemia. It is particularly likely to occur with large, chemosensitive tumours such as some lymphomas and with leukaemias. Preventive measures include the maintenance of adequate hydration, giving allopurinol to inhibit uric acid synthesis, and careful monitoring of fluid and electrolyte status. Some drugs (e.g. rasburicase) that may be given to promote uric acid breakdown *in vivo* continue to act *in vitro* after a specimen of blood is withdrawn and may produce a spuriously low value when the concentration of uric acid is measured.

Hypomagnesaemia (often accompanied by hypokalaemia) is a particular complication of treatment with cytotoxic drugs that affect the proximal renal tubules, such as cisplatin, which is commonly used in ovarian cancer. Massive renal loss of potassium can occur in patients who require treatment with amphotericin for fungal infections, which can develop as a result of the immunosuppressive effect of some tumours and of cytotoxic drugs.

Cancer Cachexia

Cachexia, a syndrome of **weakness** and **generalized wasting**, is a common feature of malignant disease. Weight loss is attributable to loss of both fat and muscle bulk unlike in starvation where the predominant loss is from fat until a very late stage. Its causes are multifactorial and imperfectly understood. Deficient food intake, caused by either mechanical obstruction of the alimentary tract or the anorexia that is often present in malignant disease, may be partly responsible, and there may also be loss of protein from ulcerated mucosa or because of blood loss. Malabsorption may also contribute, either directly because of biliary or pancreatic duct obstruction or following treatment with drugs or radiotherapy.

Tumours require nitrogen and energy for growth, and this will be met from body stores if intake is inadequate. Associated infection or products of the tumour itself may cause pyrexia and increase energy requirements.

The metabolism of many tumours is primarily anaerobic: lactate is produced, which is converted back to glucose in the liver and kidneys. This represents a waste of energy, because glycolysis results in the net formation of only two molecules of ATP per molecule of glucose, whereas gluconeogenesis, the reverse process, consumes six.

Cachexia can be seen in patients both with large or widespread tumours and with small tumours. Indeed, it may be the presenting feature of malignancy. In many patients, production of cytokines (particularly TNF-α and transforming growth factors) may be in part responsible. TNF-α is a normal product of macrophages and may be produced by activated macrophages within tumour tissue or possibly by tumour cells themselves. Among many other effects, TNF-α increases the body's energy expenditure.

In the majority of patients, the pathogenesis of cancer cachexia is probably multifactorial. Management is difficult. Nutritional support may be beneficial, but the condition is rarely completely reversible unless the underlying tumour can be treated successfully.

Carcinoid Tumours

Gastroenteropancreatic neuroendocrine tumours (GEP-NETs) arise from neuroendocrine cells derived from the embryological gut. They commonly produce hormones and other peptides (Table 20.2), and patients may present with clinical features typical of excessive secretion. Around half of GEP-NETs are carcinoid tumours, which are most frequently found in the appendix and ileocaecal region but can also occur elsewhere in the gut, gallbladder, biliary and

Table 20.2 **Some hormones produced by gastroenteropancreatic neuroendocrine tumours**	
Hormone	**Clinical features associated with excess secretion**
serotonin (5HT)	carcinoid syndrome (see Box 20.1)
insulin	symptoms associated with hypoglycaemia (see Chapter 13)
gastrin	Zollinger–Ellison syndrome: peptic ulceration, diarrhoea (see Chapter 7)
glucagon	diabetes mellitus, necrolytic migratory erythema
somatostatin	diabetes mellitus, steatorrhoea
vasointestinal polypeptide	Verner–Morrison syndrome: watery diarrhoea
pancreatic polypeptide	none
neurotensin	none
Many gastroenteropancreatic neuroendocrine tumours also produce chromogranins, which can be useful tumour markers. 5HT, 5-hydroxytryptamine.	

pancreatic ducts, and in the bronchi. They are of **low-grade malignancy**: although they frequently invade local tissue, distant metastases are rare.

The **carcinoid syndrome** is a result of the liberation of **vasoactive amines**, such as serotonin, and **peptides**, such as ACTH, from the tumour into the circulation. It is usually seen only with **bronchial tumours**, which liberate their products directly into the systemic circulation, or when tumours in the gut have metastasized to the liver. As the greater part of the gut is drained by the portal circulation, the secreted products of tumours in the gut pass to the liver, where they are inactivated. However, the secreted products of hepatic metastases reach the systemic circulation via the hepatic veins.

Serotonin (5-hydroxytryptamine [5HT]) is synthesized from tryptophan, an essential amino acid (Fig. 20.1). In patients with carcinoid syndrome, 50% of dietary tryptophan (rather than the usual 1%) may be metabolized by this pathway, diverting tryptophan away from protein and nicotinic acid synthesis. **Pellagra-like skin lesions** caused by nicotinic acid deficiency are an occasional feature of the carcinoid syndrome. The major amine secreted by intestinal carcinoid tumours (derived from embryonic midgut) is serotonin. Bronchial carcinoids (derived from foregut) tend to produce 5-hydroxytryptophan because they often lack the decarboxylase enzyme. All carcinoid tumours may also produce histamine and kinins, which are important in the symptomatology of the carcinoid syndrome (see Case history 20.3 and Box 20.1). Furthermore, the secretion of peptide hormones (e.g. ACTH) is often demonstrable and may contribute to the clinical presentation.

The usual screening test for carcinoid syndrome is measurement of 24-h urine **5-hydroxyindoleacetic acid** (5-HIAA, a metabolite of serotonin [see Fig. 20.1]). The diagnosis is confirmed by demonstrating an increase in the excretion of 5-HIAA, which is typically more than twice the upper limit of normal and may be much greater. Foodstuffs that contain serotonin (including bananas, various other fruits and some nuts) and drugs such as reserpine, which stimulate endogenous serotonin release, must be avoided during urine collection. In patients with suspected carcinoid, but normal 5-HIAA secretion, measurement of whole blood serotonin may secure the diagnosis. Plasma **chromogranin A** is a more sensitive (but less specific) marker for carcinoid tumours and is useful to detect recurrence after treatment. It can also be produced by other NETs.

Management

Carcinoid tumours are difficult to manage, unless they can be completely excised. Symptomatic relief may be obtained with simple antidiarrhoeal agents (e.g. codeine phosphate

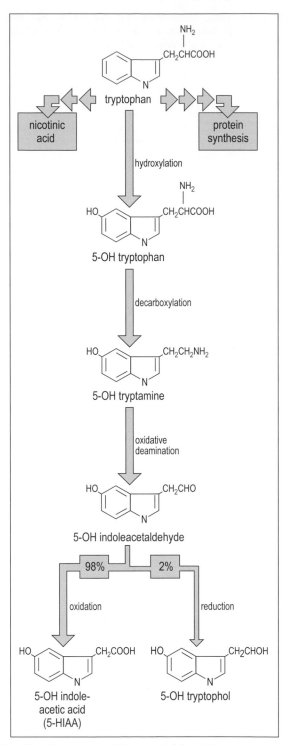

Fig. 20.1 Metabolism of 5-hydroxyindoles. 5-OH tryptamine is also known as serotonin.

Case history 20.3

History

A 50-year-old woman presented with episodic facial flushing and dizziness, sometimes accompanied by wheezing respiration. These attacks could occur at any time, but she was frequently embarrassed by them at mealtimes.

Investigations

A computed tomography (CT) scan of the liver revealed multiple nodules suggestive of tumour deposits, but the primary tumour could not be located.

Results

Urine 5-HIAA excretion: 270 µmol/24 h (10–50)

Interpretation

Very high excretion of 5-HIAA consistent with production from a carcinoid tumour. Some foodstuffs can also increase excretion but not to this degree.

Discussion

Facial flushing is the commonest clinical feature of carcinoid syndrome and may be provoked by the ingestion of food or ethanol, or by emotional stimuli. It may become continuous and spread to other parts of the body. The vasodilatation causes transient hypotension, and patients may complain of dizziness. Other clinical features are listed in Box 20.1 and include intermittent abdominal discomfort, diarrhoea and bronchospasm with wheezing. Right-sided valvular lesions of the heart, particularly pulmonary stenosis, may lead to heart failure.

Box 20.1 **Clinical features of the carcinoid syndrome**

Gastrointestinal

discomfort, hyperperistalsis and borborygmi
diarrhoea
nausea and vomiting
colicky pain

Cardiovascular

flushing
pulmonary stenosis (may lead to right heart failure and
    occasionally mitral stenosis)

Respiratory

bronchospasm
variable rate and depth of breathing

Other

pellagra
manifestations of secretion of other hormones

Box 20.2 **Glands affected in multiple endocrine neoplasia (MEN)**

MEN Type 1[a]

parathyroids
pancreatic islets
anterior pituitary

MEN Type 2a

thyroid (medullary cell carcinoma)
adrenal medulla (phaeochromocytoma)
parathyroids

MEN Type 2b

thyroid (medullary cell carcinoma)
adrenal medulla (phaeochromocytoma)
parathyroids (rarely)
various somatic abnormalities:
    Marfanoid habitus
    mucosal neuromata
    pigmentation
    café-au-lait spots

[a]Other tumours, for example, of the adrenal cortex, gut and thyroid, are sometimes present, but much less frequently than those listed.

or loperamide), but the most effective medical treatment is with a long-acting somatostatin analogue such as lanreotide or octreotide: these give symptomatic relief and may cause some tumour regression. Interferon has also been used with some success. Hepatic metastases may be destroyed by hepatic arterial embolization.

Multiple Endocrine Neoplasia

The syndromes of multiple endocrine neoplasia (MEN) are familial disorders, with an autosomal dominant inheritance, in which tumours (benign or malignant) or hyperplasia develop in two or more endocrine glands. They are uncommon, but it is important to recognize that a patient presenting with certain endocrinopathies could have one of these syndromes. The affected glands are shown in Box 20.2. Type 1 is caused by an inactivating mutation of the *MEN1*

tumour suppressor gene: genetic studies can help to identify affected family members, who require yearly screening. MEN2 is caused by an activating germline mutation in the *RET* proto-oncogene: family members should be screened for the mutation and, if affected, should be offered prophylactic thyroidectomy to prevent the development of medullary cell carcinoma. Although the syndromes are inherited, the predominant features vary in different members of the same family. Thus, one person may present with recurrent peptic ulceration caused by a gastrinoma (Zollinger–Ellison syndrome), whereas a sibling may have urinary calculi as a result of hyperparathyroidism. The individual tumours are discussed in the relevant chapters of this book.

> Although MEN is rare, it should always be considered in young people presenting with hyperparathyroidism or other associated endocrine disorders.

Tumour Markers

Tumour markers are substances that can reflect the presence or progress of a tumour. They include molecules such as enzymes, other proteins and smaller peptides, which are secreted into body fluids by tumours, and antigens expressed on cell surfaces. Clinical chemistry laboratories are usually involved only in the measurement of tumour markers falling into the first category.

An ideal secreted tumour marker could be used for:

- screening
- diagnosis
- prognosis
- treatment monitoring
- follow-up to detect recurrence.

Although some markers are reliable for some of these purposes, only one (chorionic gonadotrophin, a marker for choriocarcinoma) is widely used for all. The development of assays that use monoclonal antibodies has led to the discovery and subsequent investigation of many new tumour markers in recent years, but overall, the number of markers that are of proven clinical value remains small.

The measurement of tumour markers is not usually helpful in the diagnosis of patients with non-specific symptoms. The concentrations of many tumour markers are raised in a variety of cancers and can be raised in benign conditions. Normal plasma concentrations do not exclude cancer. The most appropriate use of most tumour markers is for serial monitoring of patients after treatment, although even this is dependent on whether further treatment is available for an individual patient.

α-Fetoprotein

α-Fetoprotein (AFP) is a glycoprotein of molecular mass 67 kDa. It is synthesized by the yolk sac and the fetal liver and gut. In the fetus it is a major plasma protein, but concentrations fall rapidly within the first few months after birth; in adults, the normal concentration is <8 kU/L. Increased plasma concentrations of AFP are seen in **normal pregnancy** because of transfer into the maternal circulation. Its use in the prenatal diagnosis of Down syndrome is discussed in Chapter 19.

AFP is a valuable marker for **hepatocellular carcinomas** (HCCs) and testicular germ cell tumours. Primary liver cancer is uncommon in the UK, and therefore population screening for the condition cannot be justified. However, some groups of patients, notably those with cirrhosis, haemochromatosis and carriers of the hepatitis B

Case history 20.4

History

A 2-year-old boy presented with progressive abdominal swelling.

Examination

He had a massively enlarged liver.

Investigations

Ultrasound and CT scans showed a large tumour in his liver, and histological examination of tissue obtained by percutaneous needle biopsy showed this to be a hepatoblastoma.

Results

Serum α-fetoprotein (AFP)   42 000 kU/L

Interpretation

Hugely raised value consistent with the histological diagnosis.

Progress

A partial hepatectomy was performed, but complete removal of the tumour was not possible because of its extent. The child was therefore started on a course of cytotoxic therapy.

Discussion

Such a massively elevated concentration of AFP in a child of this age is effectively diagnostic of hepatoblastoma (although it should be noted that infants normally have higher concentrations than adults, particularly during the first few months of life). The change in serum AFP concentration after treatment is shown in Fig. 20.2. Partial hepatectomy produced a temporary decline in AFP, but continued growth of the tumour resulted in a further increase. Cytotoxic treatment produced a sustained decline in AFP concentrations, and this corresponded to clinical remission.

virus, are at particularly high risk, and selective screening (e.g. at 6-monthly intervals) using AFP measurement may be of value. AFP concentrations are elevated in the majority of patients with cirrhosis and HCC, although in only about half of those with tumours in the absence of cirrhosis. A concentration >450 kU/L in a patient with cirrhosis makes a diagnosis of HCC highly likely. Concentrations in the range 40–450 kU/L warrant further investigation. As a tumour marker in this context, AFP lacks specificity: concentrations of up to 450 kU/L (or occasionally even higher) can occur in cirrhosis in the absence of malignancy. AFP does not appear to be of value prognostically. However, in histologically confirmed liver cancer, serial measurements of AFP are of considerable value in monitoring the response of the patient to treatment. The normal hepatic regeneration that occurs after partial hepatic resection may cause an increase in AFP concentration, but only transiently.

In patients with **non-seminomatous germ cell tumours (NSGCTs) of the testes**, AFP measurements are valuable in assessing prognosis, in staging and in monitoring therapy. A very high concentration indicates a massive tumour load and a poor prognosis (a mortality rate >50% if AFP concentration is >8300 kU/L). A rapid fall to normal after orchidectomy implies that the disease was limited to the testis. Remission is achieved in 80% of patients with metastatic NSGCT, using a combination of surgery and chemotherapy.

The efficacy of treatment can be assessed from the decline in plasma AFP concentration, which reflects the decrease in tumour mass. Once a patient is in remission, repeated measurements are essential: a rise in concentration indicates recurrence of the tumour and the need for further treatment or a change in the chemotherapeutic regimen. It should be appreciated that plasma concentrations of AFP within the 'normal' range are compatible with the presence of tumour; a rise in concentration, even if within this range, should raise the suspicion of tumour recurrence. In contrast, tumours may lose the ability to secrete AFP, so diligent clinical assessment remains an important part of the follow-up of these patients.

Around 30% of all testicular tumours are NSGCTs. More common are **seminomas** (40%): these do not secrete AFP, although some secrete hCG, another marker for NSGCTs (see p. 360).

Carcinoembryonic antigen

Carcinoembryonic antigen (CEA) is a tumour marker that is present in elevated concentrations in the plasma of 50% of patients with **colorectal cancer**, more commonly so with advanced disease (>80% if hepatic metastases are present) than with tumours confined to the colon. Concentrations may be raised in other malignancies, including pancreatic, breast and lung tumours, as well as in a variety of non-malignant conditions, including **liver disease** of various types, **pancreatitis** and **inflammatory bowel disease**, and in some people who **smoke heavily**.

CEA is neither sufficiently specific nor sensitive to be used in screening for colorectal carcinoma. CEA concentrations in plasma correlate poorly with tumour bulk, which limits the usefulness of measurements in monitoring treatment. After surgical resection of a tumour, plasma CEA concentration can be expected to fall and UK guidelines recommend monitoring for at least 3 years after apparently curative resection. However, although a subsequent rise suggests a recurrence, recurrence is not always heralded by a rise, because tumours may lose the ability to secrete CEA.

Carbohydrate antigen markers

Carbohydrate antigen (CA) markers are tumour markers that have been identified as a result of attempts to develop **monoclonal antibodies** against **tumour extracts or tumour-derived cell lines**. They are high-molecular-weight glycoproteins. Many CA markers have been identified and investigated: none has yet been identified which is specific

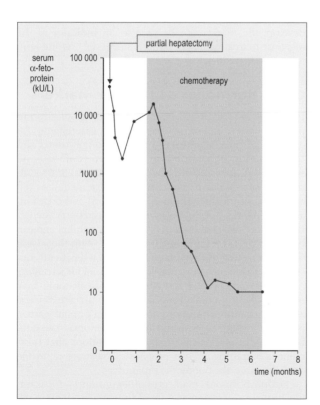

Fig. 20.2 α-Fetoprotein concentration in a patient with hepatoblastoma. (Note the logarithmic scale.)

for a particular tumour, or even tissue, and in general, those that are in use clinically are used for monitoring rather than for screening or diagnosis. An exception is **CA125**, a protein marker for **ovarian cancer** encoded by the *MUC16* gene. Women who experience persistent abdominal symptoms such as bloating or pain should be offered measurement of plasma CA125, followed by ultrasonography and gynaecological referral if the concentration is above a specified cutoff (35 kU/L). However, a normal concentration of CA125 does not exclude ovarian cancer, and increased concentrations can be found in benign conditions (e.g. endometriosis), in ascites and in non-ovarian malignancies, especially those that affect the pleura or peritoneum. There is evidence that annual monitoring of the change in CA125 concentration improves the detection of ovarian cancers compared with a single measurement, although it is not yet known whether this will translate into decreased mortality. The CA125 concentration at the time of diagnosis is of some prognostic significance, and serial measurements are valuable in monitoring patients after surgical resection of a tumour. An inadequate fall in concentration during chemotherapy suggests that the treatment is failing and needs to be reviewed and a rising concentration in a woman in remission predicts disease recurrence.

Other tumour markers of this category that are of potential value in monitoring the response of patients to treatment include **CA19-9** for **adenocarcinoma of pancreas** and possibly colorectal and gastric carcinomas, and **CA15-3** for **carcinoma of breast**. Plasma CA19-9 concentrations are elevated in >80% of patients with carcinoma of the exocrine pancreas, but only occasionally in benign disease. However, raised concentrations are also frequently found in patients with obstructive jaundice of any cause. The potential value of CA19-9 as a marker is further diminished by the fact that pancreatic cancer tends to present late and that 5–10% of the population does not express the antigen.

In carcinoma of the breast, measurement of serum CA15-3 may help to identify patients who have metastases at the time of diagnosis, and can detect recurrence before clinical signs develop.

Paraproteins

Paraproteins (see p. 292) are detectable in either serum or urine in 98–99% of patients with myeloma. Not only is their detection valuable in the diagnosis of this condition, but also paraprotein concentrations correlate well with tumour bulk, with the result that paraprotein reduction is a good indicator of the efficacy of treatment.

Human chorionic gonadotrophin

hCG is a hormone produced by the normal placenta, reaching a maximum concentration in maternal plasma by the eighth week of pregnancy. It is composed of an α- and a β-subunit: the α-subunit is identical to that of luteinizing hormone, follicle-stimulating hormone and thyroid-stimulating hormone; the β-subunit is specific to hCG. The presence of hCG in the plasma at other times indicates the presence of abnormal trophoblastic tissue or a tumour secreting the hormone ectopically. Assays for hCG as a tumour marker should measure both intact hCG and its free β-subunit (total β-hCG), because some tumours (e.g. seminomas) may produce a significant proportion of the latter. hCG is also secreted by ~50% of testicular NSGCTs and should be measured together with AFP in the follow-up of patients after treatment of the tumour.

hCG is an almost ideal tumour marker for **choriocarcinoma**, a malignant proliferation of chorionic villi that may develop from a **hydatidiform mole**, itself a potentially malignant proliferation of placental tissue, which occurs in ~1 in 2000 pregnancies in the UK. Hydatidiform mole is treated by uterine curettage, but the patient is at risk of developing choriocarcinoma if removal is incomplete. hCG is an extremely sensitive tumour marker; tumours weighing only 1 mg (corresponding to 10^5 cells) may be detectable. All patients who have had hydatidiform moles must be followed up with regular checks of plasma and urine hCG concentrations. Should a malignant tumour develop, the marker can be used as an indicator of the response to treatment and, if this is successful, in long-term follow-up thereafter.

Other hormones as tumour markers

Hormones secreted both eutopically and ectopically can provide useful tumour markers. The measurement, for example, of **catecholamines** in phaeochromocytomas and of **metabolites of serotonin** in the diagnosis of carcinoid syndrome is discussed elsewhere (pp. 190 and 356). **Calcitonin** is a valuable marker, particularly for medullary cell carcinoma of the thyroid (eutopic secretion) and occasionally in carcinoma of the breast (ectopic secretion). Medullary cell carcinoma of thyroid is frequently familial and can be part of an MEN syndrome (see p 357). With the advent of genetic testing to screen families of affected patients, calcitonin measurements are now less often used for screening. Although basal plasma concentrations of calcitonin may occasionally be normal in affected patients, an excessive rise after provocation with intravenous calcium or pentagastrin is typical in patients with medullary carcinoma. The doubling time of plasma calcitonin concentrations after treatment is helpful to predict prognosis: the more rapid the doubling time, the poorer the prognosis.

Ectopic hormonal markers of other tumours—for example, bronchial carcinomas—are of little practical use in the management of patients. They are not present sufficiently frequently to be of use in screening, and the response to treatment is, in general, so poor that their measurement provides little practical support to the clinician.

Prostate-specific antigen

Prostate cancer is the second most common cancer in men, with a higher risk in those with a family history of the disease, the elderly, African-Caribbeans and obese individuals. **Prostate-specific antigen** (PSA) is a 33-kDa glycoprotein serine protease, which is normally secreted into the prostatic duct system, although small amounts diffuse into the plasma. Plasma concentrations increase with both benign and malignant prostatic disease limiting its usefulness for diagnosis. In the UK, asymptomatic men aged >50 years can request testing following counselling. A concentration of ≥3 µg/L indicates the need for further assessment. The likelihood of cancer increases significantly at concentrations of >10 µg/L. Digital rectal examination may increase the plasma PSA concentration slightly and transiently, but significant increases can occur in both acute urinary retention and prostatitis.

Considerable effort has been expended in trying to improve the sensitivity and specificity of PSA measurement as a marker for cancer. Approaches have included the development of age-related reference ranges, determining the rate of change of concentration with time (PSA velocity) and measuring free and bound PSA. This last approach is based on the observation that, although most PSA in the plasma of normal men is protein bound, the bound proportion is higher in the presence of prostate cancer. However, prostate cancer is an unusual tumour. In many cases, it progresses relatively slowly, and many men die with prostate cancer rather than of it; in some patients, it spreads rapidly and has a poor outcome, even with treatment. Results from a major trial in the UK suggest that screening for prostate cancer in asymptomatic men using PSA has no significant effect on mortality. Widespread population screening is therefore not recommended.

Enzymes as tumour markers

Plasma enzyme activities are often increased in patients with cancer, but this is usually tumour related rather than tumour derived; that is, it is a secondary effect of the tumour rather than a result of secretion of an enzyme by the tumour. Examples include the increases in alkaline phosphatase activity seen in patients with biliary obstruction or bony metastases.

Alkaline phosphatase has several isoenzymes, and an increase in the plasma activity of the **placental type** occurs in many patients with **testicular seminomas** although measurement is no longer recommended in the UK.

Lactate dehydrogenase is used as an additional marker in the monitoring of patients with some lymphomas, leukaemias and testicular tumours and reflects tumour bulk.

Neuron-specific enolase (NSE) is an isoenzyme of enolase present in nerve and neuroendocrine cells. Small cell carcinomas of bronchus, which are neuroendocrine in origin, frequently secrete this enzyme, and when this occurs, patients' responses to treatment can be monitored by serial measurements. Raised NSE concentrations may also indicate metastatic spread of malignant melanomas of skin or ocular origin.

Other tumour markers

Thyroglobulin is a sensitive marker of disease recurrence in patients with follicular or papillary thyroid cancer who are taking suppressive doses of thyroxine (p. 206). **Faecal occult blood** analysis, using a card-based system so that samples can be sent through the post, is used in the UK national screening programme for the detection of colorectal cancer (see p. 136). **Mesothelin-related peptides** are often found in high concentration in plasma from patients with mesothelioma, a rare cancer of the pleura or peritoneal lining.

New tumour markers are continually being developed and their use investigated. Their clinical utility remains to be proved. They include S-100 for melanoma, CA50 for gastrointestinal cancers, and cytokeratin fragments (CYFRA) 21-1 and squamous cell carcinoma antigen in bronchial carcinoma.

The measurement of tumour-specific messenger RNA or DNA in plasma, urine or faeces may become a useful tool in the management of cancers in the future.

Conclusion

The clinical usefulness of secreted tumour markers for screening and diagnosis is limited to a small number of markers (Table 20.3) and relatively uncommon tumours. Other markers are of use in monitoring the response of patients to treatment, and there is considerable research in progress in this field. Antibodies developed against tumour cell-surface antigens are of considerable value in the differential diagnosis of lymphomas and leukaemias, although their measurement is not usually the responsibility of the clinical biochemist.

It should be appreciated that the existence of a marker for a cancer, however sensitive and specific (and most are not), does not on its own imply clinical utility. The aim of using markers, whether for screening, diagnosis or monitoring the response to treatment, should be to improve outcome. This depends not only on the properties of the marker but on the availability of safe and effective treatment. It can be argued that tumour markers, like drugs, should only be introduced into routine use when they have been shown to be of proven benefit. In practice, markers are often measured when there is little evidence that this can benefit the patient and without a full understanding of their limitations.

Table 20.3 **Some clinically useful tumour markers**

Marker	Tumour	Uses
α-fetoprotein	hepatocellular carcinoma germ cell	SDMF DPMF
human chorionic gonadotrophin	germ cell choriocarcinoma	DPMF SDPMF
carcinoembryonic antigen	colorectal carcinoma	MF
paraproteins	myeloma	DMF
calcitonin	medullary thyroid carcinoma	SDMF
prostate-specific antigen	prostate carcinoma	MF
CA125	ovarian carcinoma	SPM
CA19-9	pancreatic carcinoma	DPM
CA15-3	breast cancer	MF

D, diagnosis; F, follow-up; M, monitoring treatment; P, prognosis; S, screening (only in individuals at high risk).

SUMMARY

- Patients with malignant disease frequently suffer from disorders not directly attributable to the physical presence of the tumour. These **'paraneoplastic' syndromes** include metabolic disorders, notably those in which **ectopic hormone secretion** occurs. This term refers to the secretion of a hormone (or a substance with hormone-like activity) by a tumour of non-endocrine origin. The clinical features produced can closely resemble those seen when a hormone is secreted in excess by its normal tissue of origin (eutopic secretion). Examples include **Cushing syndrome** and the **syndrome of inappropriate antidiuresis** caused by the production of adrenocorticotrophin and vasopressin, respectively, by small cell carcinomas of bronchus and various other tumours; **hypercalcaemia**, particularly in some patients with squamous cell carcinomas of bronchus and renal cell carcinomas; and **hypoglycaemia**, which may occur in patients with large mesenchymal tumours, caused by secretion of insulin-like growth factors. Other hormones that are secreted by non-endocrine tumours include chorionic gonadotrophin, growth hormone-releasing hormone, calcitonin and erythropoietin. The mechanism of ectopic hormone secretion is unclear, but it is presumed that selective de-repression of the appropriate genes occurs in the tumour cells.
- **Cancer cachexia**, a non-specific syndrome of weight loss, anorexia and weakness, is common in patients with cancer. It is probably multifactorial, but the secretion of a humoural substance by the tumour may be partly responsible.

- **Carcinoid tumours** are part of the family of NETs. They are mainly found in the gut, are of low-grade malignancy and may go unnoticed unless metastasis occurs. They tend to secrete serotonin; when hepatic metastases are present, serotonin reaches the systemic circulation and may produce the **carcinoid syndrome.** The diagnosis is made by demonstrating an increased urinary excretion of the serotonin metabolite, 5-HIAA.
- Some tumours occur in association and this tendency is often inherited. There are several syndromes of **MEN.** Tumours that may be present in these syndromes include parathyroid adenomas, medullary cell carcinomas, phaeochromocytomas and pancreatic endocrine tumours.
- **Tumour markers** are substances that can be measured in body fluids in patients with cancer. They include hormones secreted by tumours, such as **calcitonin** from medullary cell carcinoma of the thyroid and **catecholamines** from phaeochromocytomas. Some tumours regularly secrete substances that are normally found only in low concentrations in the plasma, and these may be useful markers both for diagnosis and for following the progress of a malignancy. The best established examples of such tumour markers are **AFP** (testicular tumours and HCC), **hCG** (choriocarcinoma and testicular tumours), **PSA** (carcinoma of prostate), **CEA** (colorectal carcinoma), **CA125** (ovarian cancer), **CA19-9** (pancreatic cancer), **CA15-3** (breast cancer) and **paraproteins** (myeloma).
- New tumour markers are constantly being sought, but most fail to provide the benefits expected.

Chapter | 21 |

Therapeutic drug monitoring and chemical aspects of toxicology

Introduction

Clinical chemistry laboratories are called on to measure drugs in body fluids for three main purposes:

- to provide information relevant to the diagnosis and management of patients taking drugs therapeutically
- to provide such information in patients suspected to have taken drug overdoses
- to screen for the presence of drugs of abuse.

This chapter covers these topics and discusses the metabolic sequelae of some common poisonings.

Therapeutic Drug Monitoring

The questions that should be addressed when prescribing a drug are summarized in Box 21.1. All patients treated with drugs should be **monitored clinically** to assess the efficacy of treatment and to detect any adverse effects; **laboratory assessment** may also be helpful for these purposes. Thus, it may be possible to measure a particular index of therapeutic response, for example the blood glucose concentration in a patient with diabetes treated with insulin, or thyroid function tests in a patient with thyrotoxicosis treated with carbimazole. In addition, the laboratory may be asked to monitor for possible toxic effects; for example, elevated aminotransferase activity in patients treated with statins, or abnormalities of thyroid function in patients treated with the iodine-containing antiarrhythmic drug amiodarone.

An individual's response to a particular drug is dependent on many factors. These can be divided into two categories: **pharmacokinetic**, relating to the effect of the body on the drug (e.g. transport and distribution, metabolism and excretion); and **pharmacodynamic**, relating to the action of the drug on the body (e.g. interaction with receptors, and the presence of agonists and antagonists). Age, sex, kidney function and the concurrent administration of other drugs are of particular importance. These factors should be borne in mind when deciding what dose of drug to prescribe, but in many cases the optimum dosage can be achieved by commencing treatment with a standard dose and modifying this as necessary in light of the observed response.

This approach is suitable for the many drugs whose effects can be assessed reliably, such as antihypertensive agents, anticoagulants, insulin and antidiabetic drugs, but it is not universally applicable. Obviously, optimization of drug dosage in this way is impossible when the effect of treatment is not easily ascertainable. An example is the use of immunosuppressants following kidney transplantation. The clinical features of organ rejection appear late and can be difficult to distinguish from drug toxicity. It is also difficult to adjust dosage on the basis of the therapeutic effect when a drug has a **low therapeutic ratio** (i.e. the dose required to produce a therapeutic effect is close to that at which features of toxicity are seen, as is the case, for example, with lithium), especially if the adverse effects are difficult to recognize. In such cases, measurement of the concentration of the drug in the plasma may provide valuable objective information.

It is outside the scope of this chapter to discuss in detail the many factors that can influence the relationship between the dose of a drug and the intensity of its effects. Some of these are listed in Fig. 21.1. It is reasonable to assume that there will be a greater correlation between the intensity of a drug's effect and its plasma concentration than with the dose of the drug that the patient takes. Despite this, plasma concentrations and tissue effects may

What effect is it hoped to achieve?
Is the drug chosen capable of producing the desired effect?
What are the side effects of the drug and, if they are predictable, do the likely benefits of using the drug outweigh the disadvantages?
Are there any special factors in the patient that increase the likelihood of an abnormal response to the drug?
How should the effect of the drug be monitored?
If the drug is not effective, or produces undesirable effects, why does this happen?

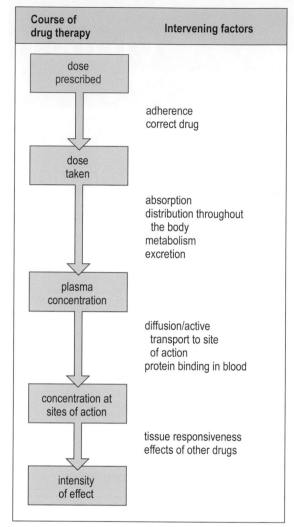

Fig. 21.1 Factors that influence the relationship between drug usage and the intensity of its effect; the latter is not necessarily directly related to the plasma concentration but may be more closely related to it than the dose prescribed.

correlate poorly, because the drug must first be transferred from the plasma to its site of action and, once there, the responsiveness of the tissues may not be constant or predictable. In addition, there may be no correlation at all when a drug is itself inactive but is metabolized to an active substance in the body, or when it acts irreversibly.

Nevertheless, the correlation between the plasma concentration and pharmacological effect is surprisingly strong for many drugs and provides the rationale for the use of concentration measurement in **therapeutic drug monitoring** (TDM). It is important that any experimentally determined relationship between plasma drug concentration and the effect of a drug is confirmed in a clinical setting, and that plasma drug concentrations are interpreted in the particular clinical context. The **time of sampling** in relation to the **time of dosage** may be critical and the sensitivity of the target organ may vary, being influenced by individual pharmacokinetic and pharmacodynamic factors.

Even if there is good evidence that measuring the plasma concentration of a particular drug can provide useful information, in individual cases there should always be a rational reason for the request (i.e. a specific question should be asked, the answer to which will influence management); the right specimen (particularly with regard to timing) must be provided, and the analysis must be accurate and its result interpreted correctly. Finally, appropriate action should ensue.

In addition to individualizing drug therapy, measurements of plasma concentrations of drugs can be useful in the diagnosis of suspected toxicity and in the assessment of adherence to treatment (compliance or concordance). Failure to take a prescribed medication (non-adherence or non-concordance) is a common cause of failure to achieve a therapeutic response. Non-concordance is costly for health services, resulting in wasted dispensed drugs and potentially invasive investigations or changes in medication for patients wrongly thought to be resistant to treatment.

Although TDM is based mainly on serum or plasma measurements, there has been some interest in developing assays using saliva. Ideally, these should reflect the plasma concentration of the non-protein-bound drug (i.e. free drug) that is directly available to the tissues; the advantage of this technique is that venipuncture is not required, but the assays are technically challenging. Salivary assays are unsuitable for drugs that are actively secreted into saliva (e.g. lithium) or are strongly ionized at physiological hydrogen ion concentration (pH) (e.g. sodium valproate).

Measuring plasma concentration

The most frequently used assays measure the total plasma concentration of a drug (see Lightbulb on p. 22 for an explanation of the use of the terms serum and plasma). With drugs that are protein bound, changes in plasma protein concentration may have a disproportionate effect on the total drug concentration relative to the amount free in the plasma and thus available to tissues. The assay chosen must be specific for the drug itself (or its active metabolite where appropriate) and should not measure inactive metabolites or be affected by other drugs that the patient may be taking.

As with other biochemical measurements, plasma concentrations of drugs are compared with standard data. The term 'reference range' is inappropriate in this context, because healthy people will not be taking the drug. The term 'therapeutic' or 'target' range is used instead. This is the range between the minimum effective concentration of the drug and the maximum safe concentration. In some cases, notably with some antiepileptic medications, only the upper limit is stated, because a drug may be efficacious in certain individuals at concentrations below the generally accepted minimum effective concentration. In contrast, optimum management may sometimes require that the concentration of a drug is maintained above the upper limit of the therapeutic range. Such ranges are not absolute: for example, hypokalaemia increases sensitivity to digoxin and effectively lowers the upper limit. **The plasma concentrations of therapeutic drugs must always be considered in context with clinical information: decisions should not be based on concentrations alone, unless these are in an unequivocally toxic range.**

Readers should be aware that the concentrations of drugs (and toxins) in body fluids may be reported in either **mass units** (e.g. mg/L) or **molar units** (e.g. mmol/L). In the UK, the consensus view is that mass units should be used, except for a few substances that have always been reported in molar units (including iron, lithium, methotrexate and thyroxine).

When a drug is first taken, the plasma concentration rises relatively rapidly as it is absorbed, and then falls, more slowly, as it is taken up into tissues, metabolized and excreted. Many drugs are taken in doses and at intervals such that a **steady-state plasma concentration** is achieved. This occurs after a period equivalent to **five half-lives** and is often the most relevant concentration to measure. For some drugs with short half-lives, significant fluctuations in plasma concentration occur and it is the **peak** or **trough concentrations**, achieved shortly after and immediately before the drug is taken, respectively, that are measured.

In the following section, the use of plasma measurements of a few representative and commonly used drugs is discussed to illustrate the general principles of TDM.

Monitoring of Specific Drugs

Immune system modulating drugs

Immunosuppressive drugs have been used for many years to prevent rejection of transplanted organs and TDM is essential to maintain adequate but safe drug concentrations at various stages postoperatively. Examples include ciclosporin, tacrolimus, mycophenolate mofetil and sirolimus. Newer classes of immune modulators are increasingly being used to treat systemic disorders in which immune system regulation is disrupted, such as rheumatoid arthritis and ulcerative colitis. Many of these are monoclonal antibodies, e.g. infliximab and adalimumab, and measurement of plasma concentrations can help to guide treatment.

Ciclosporin, a calcineurin inhibitor, is widely used in high doses after transplant surgery but is nephrotoxic. The dose and target trough whole blood concentration decrease with time after transplant and patients require close monitoring. Measurements of blood ciclosporin concentration may also help to distinguish between drug toxicity and incipient rejection of a transplanted kidney, both of which can cause an increase in plasma creatinine concentration. Lower doses of ciclosporin can be used to control disorders such as psoriasis and alopecia, in which case TDM is not usually required, although regular monitoring of kidney function and blood pressure is recommended.

Tacrolimus is chemically dissimilar from ciclosporin but has a similar mode of action and is also nephrotoxic; it is also neurotoxic and can cause hyperglycaemia. Different branded formulations have varying pharmacokinetic properties and switching a patient from one to another without careful monitoring of trough whole blood concentrations risks toxicity or graft rejection. **Sirolimus** is also used following kidney transplantation and its concentration is measured in whole blood. The target concentration depends on the type of assay used for its measurement so patients should always be monitored by the same laboratory. It is cleared by the liver and patients with liver disease may require smaller doses and more frequent monitoring. **Mycophenolate** is used following solid organ transplants and has a range of toxic effects, including myelosuppression. There is considerable debate about the usefulness of routine monitoring of blood concentrations and there is little consensus about target therapeutic concentrations.

Azathioprine and mercaptopurine are thiopurine drugs widely used to suppress the immune system following organ transplantation and in inflammatory and autoimmune disorders such as rheumatoid arthritis and Crohn disease. Azathioprine is metabolized to mercaptopurine, which in turn is metabolized predominantly by the enzyme **thiopurine methyltransferase** (TPMT) to form an inactive metabolite, **6-methylmercaptopurine nucleotide**

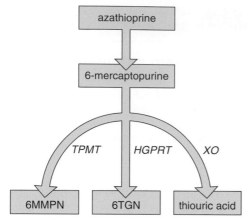

Fig. 21.2 Metabolism of azathioprine. 6TGN is the active cytotoxic metabolite which can also cause myelosuppression. 6MMPN is an inactive metabolite that can cause hepatotoxicity in high concentration. TPMT, thiopurine methyl transferase; HGPRT, hypoxanthine–guanine phosphoribosyl transferase; XO, xanthine oxidase; 6MMPN, 6-methylmercaptopurine nucleotide; 6TGN, 6-thioguanine nucleotide.

(6MMPN) (Fig. 21.2). Azathioprine is also metabolized to an active but myelotoxic metabolite, **6-thioguanine nucleotide** (6TGN), by hypoxanthine–guanine phosphoribosyl transferase (HGPRT, see pp. 279 and 281). In patients with a genetically determined low TPMT activity, the HGPRT pathway assumes more importance, and there is a greater risk of toxicity when azathioprine is used. Such patients should be identified before starting treatment by measurement of red cell TPMT activity. One in 10 of the general population is heterozygous for deficiency, with intermediate enzyme activity, and ~1 in 300 is completely deficient. Genotyping can be used to confirm TPMT status if enzyme deficiency is found. Patients with complete deficiency are not treated with thiopurine drugs, as they are at high risk of severe toxicity. Those with partial deficiency may respond to lower than usual doses, without developing myelosuppression. Occasionally patients have higher than normal TPMT activity and require higher than usual doses of azathioprine to achieve a clinical response; however, the resulting increased concentration of 6MMPN may lead to hepatotoxicity.

If patients develop symptoms of azathioprine toxicity, measurement of the concentration of metabolites (6MMPN and 6TGN) can be helpful for dose adjustment (see Case history 21.1), especially in those with partial TPMT deficiency. Measurement of 6MMPN is helpful to distinguish those who are non-compliant with medication or taking too low a dose from those who have resistance to azathioprine because of increased TPMT activity. The former have appropriately low concentrations, whilst the latter have

disproportionately high concentrations of 6MMPN compared with 6TGN.

Antitumour necrosis factor-α (TNF-α) drugs (e.g. infliximab, adalimumab) are used for the treatment of refractory inflammatory diseases such as rheumatoid arthritis, ankylosing spondylitis and Crohn disease. They are humanized or chimeric monoclonal antibodies (biologics) that bind plasma and membrane TNF-α, thus preventing activation of intracellular TNF-α receptors. They are given by intravenous infusion at 2- to 8-week intervals. However, the response to standard doses of these drugs is highly variable, partly because the plasma drug concentration achieved is unpredictable and partly because patients can develop antibodies to them. Measurement of trough drug and antibody concentrations in patients who are responding poorly to treatment can help to identify those who have not reached adequate therapeutic concentrations and could benefit from an increased dosage. Spuriously low drug concentrations are also found in patients who have developed antibodies against the drugs, in which case patients are unlikely to benefit from further doses and are at increased risk of infusion hypersensitivity reactions (see Case history 21.2).

Anticonvulsants

Phenytoin is no longer recommended for use as a first-line drug for epilepsy in the UK, although it is still used as adjunctive therapy in patients with complex disorders or with status epilepticus. However, its therapeutic effectiveness is difficult to assess without monitoring. It has a **low therapeutic ratio**, and the signs of toxicity may mimic the neurological diseases that can be associated with epilepsy. It is extensively protein bound, and changes in plasma albumin concentration can affect the availability of the drug in the free (active) form. Furthermore, phenytoin has unusual pharmacokinetic properties: the enzyme responsible for the elimination of the drug (hepatic CYP2C9) becomes **saturated within the therapeutic range of plasma concentrations**, giving rise to zero-order kinetics. This phenomenon has several important implications. In particular, the relationship between plasma concentration and dose is **non-linear;** thus, small increments in dose may lead to disproportionate increases in steady-state plasma concentrations. In contrast, even if the dose is unchanged, a small decrease in drug-metabolizing enzyme activity, or the presence of other drugs that inhibit phenytoin metabolism, can increase the plasma concentration to within the toxic range.

The measurement of plasma phenytoin concentration is also useful if adverse effects occur, if there is an unexplained deterioration in the patient's control, during intravenous therapy in status epilepticus and if a drug known to interact with phenytoin has to be prescribed. As emphasized earlier, measurements should be interpreted in light of clinical

Case history 21.1

History

A 60-year-old woman with a history of ulcerative colitis became acutely unwell with severe bloody diarrhoea. She was admitted to hospital where she was diagnosed with pancolitis. She was started on azathioprine 150 mg daily. Several weeks later, her large bowel symptoms had reduced in severity but she felt nauseated. Her dose of azathioprine was halved, after which her nausea resolved without further exacerbation of her colitis.

Results

Blood:		
	red cell thiopurine methyltransferase (TPMT) (pretreatment)	121 mU/L (68–150)
	6MMPN (on treatment)	16 770 pmol/8 $\times 10^8$ cells (<5700)
	6TGN (on treatment)	430 pmol/8 $\times 10^8$ cells (235–450)
	6MMPN (after dose reduction)	1190 pmol/8 $\times 10^8$ cells (<5700)
	6TGN (after dose reduction)	325 pmol/8 $\times 10^8$ cells (235–450)

Summary

Normal pretreatment TPMT activity but very high posttreatment 6MMPN concentration which decreased after dose reduction.

Interpretation

Although this patient had normal TPMT activity, she was started on a relatively high dose of azathioprine and developed toxic concentrations of the non-active metabolite, 6MMPN. The concentration of the active metabolite, 6TGN, remained within the therapeutic range even after dose reduction.

Discussion

Azathioprine is metabolized to 6-methylmercaptopurine nucleotide (6MMPN) and 6-thioguanine nucleotide (6TGN) (see Fig. 21.2). Its therapeutic cytotoxic effect is mediated by 6TGN, which is incorporated into DNA as false bases. The alternative metabolite, 6MMPN, is potentially hepatotoxic and is produced by the action of TPMT. It can accumulate in patients on high-dose azathioprine or in those with a genetic variant resulting in high enzyme activity. Azathioprine itself can induce the activity of TPMT. Measurement of red cell TPMT activity is therefore recommended in all patients before treatment is started. Measurement of red cell metabolite concentrations can be helpful in patients who develop side effects during treatment or in those who fail to respond to treatment. In this case, dose reduction was sufficient to reduce the toxic metabolite to acceptable concentrations while still retaining adequate control of her ulcerative colitis. If symptoms of inflammatory bowel disease persist despite adequate concentrations of 6TGN, additional or alternative treatments are required.

---

circumstances: some patients achieve effective control of seizures only at plasma concentrations greater than the upper limit of the therapeutic range, yet do not experience toxicity, whereas others, particularly older patients, may achieve good control at concentrations below the range.

The value of measuring the plasma concentrations of some other anticonvulsant drugs is shown in Table 21.1. Carbamazepine induces its own metabolism and interactions occur with other anticonvulsants. Monitoring (of trough concentrations) is valuable when carbamazepine is first prescribed, if seizure control is difficult to achieve and if other anticonvulsants are being used, but it is complicated by the fact that the drug has active metabolites, which are not measured in standard assays. The dosage of ethosuximide can often be adjusted on clinical grounds, because toxicity is easily recognizable when the drug is being used alone. The plasma concentration of lamotrigine reflects its effect, and TDM is usually recommended when the drug is used with phenytoin or carbamazepine (which reduce its plasma half-life) or valproate (which prolongs it). With sodium valproate/valproic acid there is no clear safe maximum concentration, there is a poor correlation between plasma concentration and efficacy, and hepatotoxicity, which is rare, cannot be predicted from plasma concentration. There is a poor correlation between plasma concentrations of phenobarbital and either clinical or toxic effects, so that routine monitoring is of little value. TDM of vigabatrin is unnecessary; plasma concentrations show little relationship with clinical effect, probably because the drug binds irreversibly to its target enzyme (γ-aminobutyric acid transferase) in the brain. TDM for clonazepam, clobazam, gabapentin, topiramate, levetiracetam or oxcarbazepine is of doubtful value.

Digoxin

Digoxin is used in the management of atrial fibrillation, although less frequently than previously. It is no longer recommended as first-line treatment for uncomplicated heart failure. It is cleared mainly via the kidneys, and if patients have coexisting chronic kidney disease, monitoring of plasma concentration

---

Case history 21.2

History

A 30-year-old woman was admitted to hospital with fistulating Crohn disease. She had been treated with corticosteroids and azathioprine but still had active disease. She was started on regular infusions of infliximab.

Her symptoms improved, with healing of her fistula over the first 6 months, but the frequency of her diarrhoea began to increase again after this.

Examination

She was underweight with a body mass index of 18.3 kg/m^2.

Results (see Appendix for reference ranges)

Blood:	haemoglobin (preinfliximab)	110 g/L
Faeces:	calprotectin (preinfliximab)	>1000 µg/g (<50)
Serum:	infliximab (6 months after first infusion, trough sample)	<0.3 µg/mL
	anti-infliximab antibody	30 AU/mL (<10)

Summary

Markedly increased calprotectin excretion pretreatment. Undetectable infliximab with significantly raised anti-infliximab antibody after 6 months of infusions. Mild anaemia.

Interpretation

The high faecal calprotectin excretion is in keeping with her symptoms of active inflammatory bowel disease (see p. 131). Anaemia is common in chronic inflammatory disorders and is a result of decreased red cell production or survival. The development of neutralizing anti-infliximab antibodies results in loss of therapeutic effect and spuriously low measured drug concentrations because of assay interference.

Discussion

Infliximab (an anti-tumour necrosis factor α drug) can be an effective treatment for patients with refractory inflammatory disorders. However, because of its structure (a chimeric antibody), there is a significant risk that patients will develop neutralizing antibodies. If a patient on regular infliximab infusions fails to improve (primary failure) or loses their initial response (secondary failure, as in this case), a preinfusion blood sample should be collected to measure trough drug and antibody concentrations. If both drug and antibody concentrations are low, an increase in dosage should be considered to achieve therapeutic drug concentrations. If the antibody concentration is high, an increased dosage is unlikely to be effective and alternative treatments should be sought.

---

is recommended. If kidney function is normal, monitoring of plasma creatinine and electrolytes (see later) is usually sufficient unless toxicity or non-concordance is suspected.

The therapeutic range for plasma digoxin concentration is generally taken as 0.5–2.0 µg/L, although for the few people still treated with digoxin for heart failure, a lower range is more appropriate (0.5–1.0 µg/L). There is a significant increase in plasma concentration following a dose of the drug, and a **minimum period of 6 h** should elapse before blood is drawn for assessment of the mean steady-state concentration. In practice, a blood sample taken shortly before a dose is due is satisfactory for clinical purposes.

The therapeutic effect is minimal when the plasma concentration is <0.5 µg/L, and there is in general a rather poor correlation between plasma concentration of digoxin and therapeutic effect. Toxicity becomes more common at concentrations >1.0 µg/L and is almost invariable if concentrations exceed 3.0 µg/L. Box 21.2 summarizes various factors that alter either the therapeutic response to a given plasma concentration of digoxin or the plasma concentration achieved on a particular dosage. The clinical setting is thus very important when assessing the significance of plasma digoxin concentrations. **Hypokalaemia** is a particular

problem because many patients treated with digoxin are also receiving diuretics, which may cause this (see Case history 21.3). It is good practice always to measure the plasma potassium concentration when digoxin is measured.

Some of the features of **digoxin toxicity** are relatively non-specific (e.g. nausea and vomiting), whereas others include dysrhythmias that could also be a complication of the underlying heart disease. Patients with severe toxicity can be treated with antidigoxin antibody fragments, but it should be noted that these interfere with assays for digoxin, so further measurements of plasma concentration are not possible for several days, until the fragments have cleared. If a patient taking digoxin is symptom free yet has a plasma concentration <0.5 µg/L, it is likely that the drug is not required and can be withdrawn under supervision.

The occurrence of endogenous substances that bind to the antibodies used in digoxin immunoassays (digoxin-like immunoreactive substances) can occasionally cause spurious apparent elevations in digoxin concentrations, especially in neonates. Some herbal remedies contain naturally occurring cardiac glycosides that are also detected in immunoassays for digoxin. Such interferences should be suspected if unexpectedly high concentrations are found.

Table 21.1 Therapeutic monitoring of anticonvulsant drugs

Drug	Therapeutic range	Monitoring
phenytoin	10–20 mg/L	essential
carbamazepine	4–12 mg/L	useful if on combination therapy
ethosuximide	40–100 mg/L	useful if on combination therapy
phenobarbital	10–40 mg/L	tolerance makes upper limit imprecise
valproic acid	50–100 mg/L	not proven to be useful, range not well defined
lamotrigine	3–15 mg/L	useful if on combination therapy

Therapeutic limits are for guidance only. Some patients benefit from concentrations outside the quoted range.

> **!** Digoxin toxicity occurs most frequently in patients who develop hypokalaemia or have deteriorating kidney function. Plasma potassium and creatinine concentrations should be monitored regularly in patients taking digoxin.

Box 21.2 Sensitivity to digoxin

Increased sensitivity

hypokalaemia
hypercalcaemia
hypomagnesaemia
hypoxia
hypothyroidism

Decreased sensitivity

hypocalcaemia
hyperthyroidism

Acute or chronic kidney disease and hypothyroidism may increase the plasma concentration of digoxin in relation to the dose taken; hyperthyroidism may decrease it.

Case history 21.3

History

An elderly woman with a history of congestive cardiac failure and atrial fibrillation presented with increased confusion and falls. She was being treated with digoxin, a thiazide diuretic, an angiotensin-converting enzyme (ACE) inhibitor and warfarin. Her estimated glomerular filtration rate determined 3 months previously was 41 mL/min/1.73 m².

Results

Serum:		
	digoxin (12 h after previous dose)	2.9 µg/L
	potassium	3.0 mmol/L
	urea	11.2 mmol/L
	creatinine	160 µmol/L
	eGFR	26 mL/min/1.73 m²

Summary

High digoxin concentration with hypokalaemia and low eGFR.

Interpretation

The digoxin concentration is well above the therapeutic range of 0.5–2 µg/L and hypokalaemia increases the risk of toxicity. Her kidney function has deteriorated over the last 3 months, resulting in decreased clearance of digoxin.

Discussion

Drug interactions are an important cause of ill health at all ages, but particularly in elderly adults. Confusion in a patient treated with digoxin should raise the suspicion of digoxin toxicity. Digoxin toxicity is enhanced by hypokalaemia: thiazide diuretics are an important cause of this (see p. 369). The elevated serum creatinine concentration with a history of a low eGFR indicates chronic kidney disease with a more recent acute deterioration; this can impair the excretion of digoxin and lead to its accumulation in plasma. Both diuretics and ACE inhibitors can cause a deterioration in kidney function. The risk of toxicity outweighs the benefit of digoxin in many patients, especially elderly people. Digoxin is therefore no longer recommended as a first-line treatment for uncomplicated heart failure and its use in other conditions is also diminishing.

Other antidysrhythmics

Methods are available for the measurement of many other drugs used in patients with heart disease, in particular antidysrhythmics. The arguments relating to the value of plasma concentrations in monitoring treatment are complex, and the place of TDM is debatable. It may be useful under some circumstances in patients treated with amiodarone.

Lithium

Lithium is used in the **treatment** of **acute hypomania** and **mania** and for **prophylaxis** in **bipolar affective disorder**. The optimum therapeutic serum concentration varies from patient to patient: in acute treatment, concentrations of up to 1.2 mmol/L may be required, but for long-term maintenance, concentrations of 0.4–0.8 mmol/L are usually sufficient. Lithium has a low therapeutic ratio and there are wide interindividual differences in dose requirements; monitoring of serum concentration is vital to the management of patients on lithium therapy. Blood samples for monitoring should be taken 12 h after the previous dose; up to a week may be needed after the dosage is changed before a new steady state is attained.

Lithium is nephrotoxic (it can cause nephrogenic diabetes insipidus) and is excreted by the kidneys, and consequently toxicity may be self-perpetuating. Renal handling of lithium is also related to sodium balance, and diuretics may cause lithium retention. Lithium can cause hypothyroidism and hyperparathyroidism and patients should be monitored for these conditions.

Serum concentrations >1.5 mmol/L should be avoided. Toxicity is treated with measures to increase urinary excretion (a high fluid and sodium intake, but not diuretics), but severe toxicity (features include hyperthermia, fits, oliguria and coma) is a medical emergency and dialysis may be required to remove the drug.

Antipsychotic drugs

Therapeutic ranges have been determined for numerous antipsychotic drugs, but TDM is readily available for relatively few. Plasma concentrations reflect binding to brain receptors reasonably well. Patients taking clozapine require close clinical monitoring, particularly to detect agranulocytosis, a recognized adverse effect of the drug. Several antipsychotic drugs affect lipid, and patients should be assessed for cardiovascular risk, especially since patients with mental health problems are often already at increased risk of atherosclerosis.

Antidepressants

A case can be made for TDM of the tricyclic antidepressant amitriptyline when used as an antidepressant, although since the introduction of selective serotonin reuptake inhibitors (e.g. fluoxetine), which are as effective, have fewer side effects and are safer in overdose, amitriptyline is now mainly used for the treatment of neuropathic pain and in the prophylaxis of migraine, for which monitoring is not required.

Theophylline and caffeine

Theophylline is a **bronchodilator** used in the treatment of **asthma** and, rarely, **neonatal apnoea**. Response to theophylline in different patients varies considerably in relation to dosage but correlates well with plasma concentration. The therapeutic range is 10–20 mg/L (5–15 mg/L in infants); toxicity (principally cardiac dysrhythmias) may occur at higher concentrations. Patients who require intravenous theophylline for severe asthma may already be treated with an oral preparation. In such circumstances, measurement of drug concentration is required urgently before an infusion is started, to avoid toxicity. In infants in whom the drug is sometimes used as a respiratory stimulant, significant metabolism to caffeine occurs; this metabolite is also pharmacologically active. It is, however, more common to administer caffeine directly to infants, unless the bronchodilatory effect of theophylline is also required. Routine monitoring of caffeine concentrations is no longer recommended as it is much less toxic than theophylline.

Aminoglycoside antibiotics

Aminoglycoside antibiotics (e.g. gentamicin) are nephrotoxic and ototoxic, but relatively high concentrations are needed for bactericidal effects. They have a short plasma half-life. Toxicity appears to relate to the **trough concentration** (i.e. that found immediately before a dose); bactericidal action requires a sufficient **peak concentration** (achieved shortly after a dose has been given). The peak and trough concentrations can be manipulated independently by altering the dose and the frequency of dosage. With once-daily dosing in patients with normal kidney function, the monitoring of trough concentrations is adequate. In patients with a reduced glomerular filtration rate, further doses are given only when trough drug concentration has fallen below a predetermined value. An alternative approach is to give a standard dose of drug and to use a nomogram to determine dosing interval based on drug concentration at 6–14 h.

Methotrexate

Methotrexate (a cytotoxic drug) inhibits dihydrofolate reductase and depletes intracellular stores of reduced folate. At high concentrations, this depletion may become potentially harmful to the host, as well as the tumour, by causing bone marrow suppression. Marrow damage becomes maximal later than the effect on tumour cells, and can be prevented by the use of folinic acid 'rescue' treatment if methotrexate is not cleared rapidly enough from the plasma. Such treatment is usually required only with high-dose methotrexate regimens. The risk of harmful effects varies between individuals; factors that suggest high risk of bone marrow suppression include plasma methotrexate concentrations >5.0 at 24 h or >0.5 μmol/L at 48 h after the infusion, or an initial plasma half-life of >3.5 h. Monitoring of weekly, low-dose methotrexate treatment is discussed on p. 111; it does not require measurements of drug concentration.

Toxicology

Poisoning is a common reason for hospital admission. In most cases, the patient has taken a deliberate overdose of a prescribed or over-the-counter drug, but poisoning may also be the result of accident (particularly in children), environmental or occupational exposure to toxins, or attempted homicide; the range of toxic substances is vast, including industrial and domestic chemicals, plants and fungi, as well as drugs.

Metabolic abnormalities (particularly **acid–base disturbances, hypokalaemia** and **hypoglycaemia**) are common in poisoned patients. They may be caused by direct toxic effects of the poison or by non-specific effects on vital functions. Poisoning with some agents causes relatively specific metabolic disorders, for example hypocalcaemia with ethylene glycol. **Rhabdomyolysis**, which may lead to acute kidney injury, can occur as a direct toxic effect of some drugs (particularly amphetamines and related drugs such as 3,4-methylenedioxymethamfetamine [MDMA, 'ecstasy']) or secondary to pressure-induced muscle damage in comatose patients.

The **drugs most frequently taken in overdose** include **ethanol, paracetamol** and **salicylates** (each of which causes significant, specific metabolic derangements), and **opioids, benzodiazepines** and **antidepressants** (which do not). Other relatively frequent causes of poisoning include carbon monoxide, ethylene glycol, methanol and heavy metals. In some parts of the world, venomous bites (e.g. by snakes) are a hazard, as is poisoning by herbicides and pesticides (particularly in developing countries).

Management

Specific antidotes (Table 21.2) or other forms of treatment are available for some poisons (although they may

Table 21.2 Examples of specific antidotes for poisons and their mechanisms of action

Poison	Antidote	Mechanism of action
carbon monoxide	oxygen	competes with poison at site of action
iron	desferrioxamine	formation of inert complex
methanol and ethylene glycol	fomepizole	inhibits rate of formation of more toxic metabolite
benzodiazepines	flumazenil	competitive antagonist at receptor
opioids	naloxone	competitive antagonist at receptor
organophosphorus insecticides	atropine	blocks cholinergic receptors responsible for mediating toxicity
paracetamol	N-acetylcysteine	promotes detoxification (see p. 372)

themselves not be without risk). Other potential therapeutic measures include prevention of further absorption (e.g. by giving oral activated charcoal, for most organic poisons) or enhancement of elimination of the drug from the body. Measurement of the plasma concentration of the poison may indicate the need to institute such forms of treatment and monitor their efficacy. Support of vital functions is an important aspect of the management of any poisoned patient, and the clinical biochemistry service has a role in monitoring such treatment, for example by measuring plasma creatinine concentration.

Few poisons produce specific physical signs: the patient's history, if available, may not be reliable and mixed drug overdoses are common. There is, therefore, a need for an analytical service to identify what poisons may have been ingested, particularly if a patient does not respond to conventional management. This presents an entirely different problem for the laboratory, because what is required is a screening service capable of identifying any of a large number of toxins, rather than providing quantitative data on a small number.

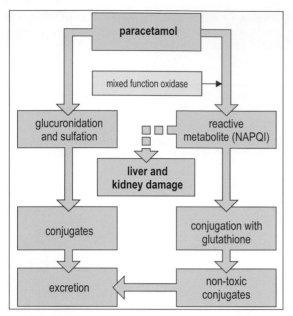

Fig. 21.3 Metabolism of paracetamol. When the drug is taken in therapeutic doses, the toxic metabolite formed, *N*-acetyl-*p*-benzoquinoneimine (NAPQI), is detoxified by conjugation with glutathione; when taken in overdose, glutathione supplies are rapidly exhausted and NAPQI accumulates, causing cell damage.

Poisoning With Specific Agents

Paracetamol (acetaminophen)

A specific antidote is available for paracetamol, the metabolism of which is summarized in Fig. 21.3. The major products of its metabolism are harmless glucuronide and sulphate conjugates, which are excreted in the urine together with a small amount of the unchanged drug. Small quantities of a highly hepatotoxic metabolite (*N*-acetyl-*p*-benzoquinoneimine [NAPQI]) are also formed through the action of the mixed function oxidase (cytochrome P450) enzyme system: this is normally detoxified by conjugation with glutathione. However, the glucuronidation and sulfation pathways are saturable so that when an overdose of the drug is taken, a greater proportion is converted to NAPQI. Glutathione supplies are limited, and if they are insufficient to detoxify this metabolite, liver damage will result. In addition, depletion of glutathione reduces the liver's defence mechanisms against oxidizing damage. NAPQI is also nephrotoxic, and its generation in the kidneys can cause acute kidney injury in paracetamol poisoning.

Box 21.3 Signs and symptoms of paracetamol poisoning

<24 h

anorexia, nausea and vomiting

24–48 h

abdominal pain, hepatic tenderness, prolonged prothrombin time (INR), elevated plasma aminotransferases and bilirubin

>48 h

jaundice, encephalopathy, liver failure, acute kidney injury

INR, international normalized ratio.

Clinical features

Paracetamol is an insidious poison because there may be no clinical disturbance during the first 24 h after taking an overdose, except anorexia, nausea and vomiting (Box 21.3). Patients remain conscious unless a sedative drug has been taken concurrently. If liver damage occurs, abdominal pain with hepatic tenderness will develop and liver function tests become abnormal (increased international normalized ratio (INR) or prothrombin time, plasma aminotransferase activity and bilirubin concentration). The INR is the best marker of severity. With massive overdoses, patients may develop liver failure (see p. 110). If kidney injury occurs, the plasma creatinine concentration is a better indicator of renal function than that of urea, because hepatic urea synthesis may be decreased. An increase in plasma creatinine concentration and the development of systemic acidosis are both indicators of a poor prognosis.

It is possible to predict the likelihood of liver damage from the plasma concentration of paracetamol. The blood sample must be taken **at least 4 h after ingestion** of the drug. The plasma concentration, interpreted in relation to the time of ingestion, can be used as a guide to decide whether to treat the patient with an antidote (Fig. 21.4). Unfortunately, the time at which the drug was taken may not be known, and it is then wisest to treat the patient actively if the concentration falls anywhere within the treatment zone. Treatment should also be given to patients who have taken staggered doses, because plasma concentrations do not predict toxicity in these circumstances. Even if a patient presents >15 h after ingestion of paracetamol, its measurement is valuable to confirm the diagnosis and, together with the INR, plasma aminotransferase activities and acid–base status, to assess the need for treatment.

Management

The antidote of choice is **N-acetylcysteine**, which is given by intravenous infusion. Plasma creatinine concentration,

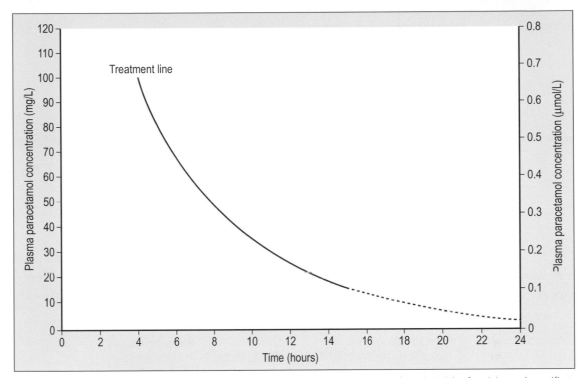

Fig. 21.4 Plasma paracetamol concentrations and prognosis in paracetamol poisoning. There is a risk of toxicity and specific treatment is indicated if the concentration is on or above the curve joining concentrations of 100 mg/L at 4 h and 15 mg/L at 15 h.

aminotransferase activity and the INR should be checked before starting and at the end of treatment. *N*-acetylcysteine acts by promoting hepatic glutathione synthesis, thereby increasing the capacity of the liver to detoxify the active metabolite. It may also repair oxidative damage, and there is evidence of benefit from its continued use even once liver damage has occurred. Oral **methionine** (which also promotes glutathione synthesis) is no longer recommended.

In treating paracetamol poisoning, general emergency measures must not be forgotten. Administration of activated charcoal is only of proven value if given in the first hour after an overdose. The patient must be kept hydrated, preferably using 5% dextrose because there may be a tendency towards hypoglycaemia with liver damage. Vitamin K can be given prophylactically. If liver failure develops, the patient should be referred to a specialist unit to determine whether liver transplantation is required.

> In a patient who has taken a paracetamol overdose, the development of systemic acidosis or acute kidney injury indicates a poor prognosis requiring immediate transfer to a specialist unit if possible.

Salicylates

Salicylate poisoning, usually with **aspirin** (acetylsalicylic acid), is less common than in the past. It can produce profound metabolic disturbances, and although there is no specific antidote, measures can be taken to increase the excretion of the drug. These are effective but not without hazard in themselves.

The effects of salicylates that lead to metabolic disturbances are summarized in Fig. 21.5, and include **stimulation of the respiratory centre** (causing a respiratory alkalosis), a **metabolic acidosis, uncoupling of oxidative phosphorylation** and a **central emetic effect** (see Case history 21.4). Tinnitus is an early symptom of toxicity.

Management

There is no specific antidote to aspirin. It is metabolized by hydrolysis to salicylic acid, the active form of the drug, which is excreted unchanged in the urine; other metabolites include various inactive conjugates. The conjugation pathways are saturable, and once they are saturated, urinary excretion becomes the major route for elimination of the drug. If the urine is acidic, salicylic acid is not ionized and, although filtered by the glomeruli, is reabsorbed by the tubules. If the

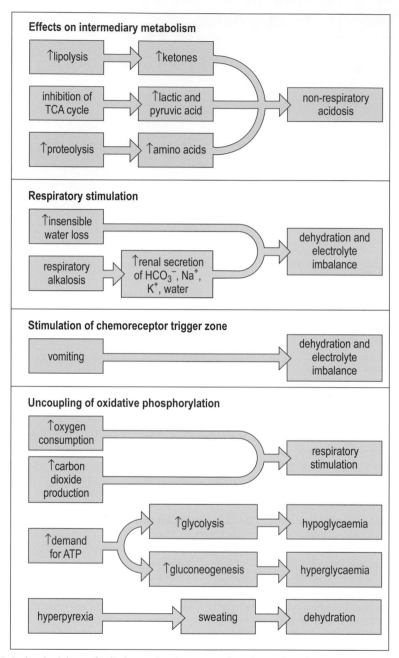

Fig. 21.5 Pathophysiology of salicylate poisoning. ATP, adenosine triphosphate; TCA, tricarboxylic acid.

urine is alkaline, salicylic acid ionizes: its tubular reabsorption is decreased and urinary excretion is enhanced. This is the rationale for alkalinization using sodium bicarbonate infusions in the treatment of salicylate poisoning. However, this process is in itself potentially dangerous and requires careful monitoring. It should not be attempted if the patient already has a systemic alkalosis or if the urine pH exceeds 8, the aim being to maintain a urine pH of 7.5–8 during treatment. An additional benefit of giving bicarbonate is that it reduces blood hydrogen ion concentration, thereby increasing the ionization of salicylate and reducing its ability to enter cells, particularly in the brain. Potassium supplements

History

A 20-year-old male student was brought into hospital in a confused state, having been found at home by his flatmate with an empty bottle of aspirin tablets on his desk.

Examination

He was hyperventilating and sweating profusely. He was pale but not anaemic. He was not grossly dehydrated, but the inside of his mouth was dry and there was a smell of ketones on his breath. His pulse was 112/min, blood pressure 110/60 mmHg and temperature 39.5°C.

Results

Serum:	sodium	131 mmol/L
	potassium	3.2 mmol/L
	bicarbonate	10 mmol/L
	urea	10 mmol/L
	salicylate	520 mg/L
	paracetamol	<10 mg/L
Arterial blood:	hydrogen ion	62 nmol/L (pH 7.20)
	P_{CO_2}	3.5 kPa
Plasma:	INR	1.3
	glucose	3.2 mmol/l

Summary

Partially compensated metabolic acidosis with hyponatraemia, hypokalaemia and raised urea concentration. High salicylate with glucose concentration at the low end of the reference range.

Interpretation

The salicylate concentration is above 500 mg/L, indicating severe toxicity. The high urea is consistent with dehydration. Hyponatraemia and hypokalaemia reflect renal losses. The low bicarbonate concentration is consistent with metabolic acidosis and is exacerbated by renal losses in the early stage of poisoning. The low P_{CO_2} indicates respiratory compensation by hyperventilation. Although within the reference range for a healthy individual, the glucose concentration is low for someone in a stressed state. The INR is slightly raised but unlikely to result in bleeding.

Discussion

The results are consistent with the metabolic effects of salicylates described in the text. There is an acidosis, compensated to some extent by hyperventilation (see Chapter 4). The initial acid–base disturbance (in adults, but usually not in children) is a respiratory alkalosis due to direct stimulation of the respiratory centre. This is often overwhelmed by the developing acidosis, but during the alkalotic phase any compensatory renal excretion of bicarbonate will deplete the capacity of the body to buffer excess hydrogen ions, thus making the acidosis more dangerous.

Patients who have taken overdoses of salicylates are rarely comatose; irritability is an early feature, and later hallucination and delirium may occur. Tinnitus may be a prominent feature. Hyperpyrexia is thought to reflect the uncoupling of oxidative phosphorylation that occurs with toxic doses. Blood coagulation, as determined by the INR, may be prolonged because of decreased hepatic activation of clotting factors, but the effect is usually minor and intervention is seldom required. Salicylates also inhibit platelet aggregation. However, although gastric erosions may occur, owing to the direct action of salicylate on the gastric mucosa, severe bleeding is uncommon in aspirin overdosage.

are required (administration of bicarbonate can cause hypokalaemia, which may hinder effective alkalinization of the urine); dehydration and hypoglycaemia must be corrected, and fluid balance, plasma glucose, arterial blood hydrogen ion concentration and urine pH must be monitored. A high intravenous fluid input is no longer recommended because of the risk of fluid overload.

Aspirin is absorbed only slowly from the gut: activated charcoal can be used to reduce absorption of the drug. The decision whether to embark on active treatment should be based on clinical grounds but be guided by laboratory data. Maintenance of adequate hydration and general supportive measures are important for all patients. Alkalinization should be considered if plasma salicylate concentration exceeds 500 mg/L in adults and 300 mg/L in children, particularly if there is acidosis. If the initial concentration exceeds 700 mg/L and if there is renal impairment or if other therapeutic measures fail, haemoperfusion or haemodialysis will usually be necessary.

Plasma salicylate concentrations may continue to rise for several hours after ingestion because of delayed absorption. Measurements should therefore be repeated every 3 h after a confirmed overdose until the concentration begins to fall.

Iron

Iron poisoning, although much less common now than in the past, still occurs and can cause severe illness, especially in young children. Iron causes necrosis of the gastrointestinal mucosa, with resultant bleeding and fluid and electrolyte loss. Patients may develop encephalopathy and acute kidney injury with circulatory collapse, and acute liver necrosis may develop in those who survive these complications.

Severe poisoning is indicated by plasma iron concentrations >90 µmol/L. Management involves the use of **desferrioxamine**, an iron-chelating agent, to promote iron excretion, together with appropriate supportive measures.

Lead

The toxic effects of lead are a result of its propensity to bind to functional chemical groups (e.g. amino groups) and to substitute for calcium and thus affect, for example, nerve and muscle function. Acute lead poisoning is very uncommon, but chronic poisoning occurs more frequently. In **children**, the source may be old paint or toys, and imported cosmetics or medicines. In **adults**, most cases are associated with **occupational exposure** (e.g. battery manufacture, smelting, ship-breaking). Lead poisoning is a notifiable industrial disease. Lead is concentrated in erythrocytes, and in adults who are not occupationally exposed to the metal, a blood concentration >10 µg/dL (0.48 µmol/L) requires follow-up. In male lead workers, the action limit for blood lead is 50 µg/dL (2.4 µmol/L). Symptomatic lead poisoning is usually associated with concentrations >80 µg/dL (3.8 µmol/L), but in children symptoms may be present at lower concentrations. In the UK, lead concentrations are reported as µmol/L for clinical purposes but as µg/dL when monitoring occupational exposure.

Although blood lead measurement is the screening method of choice for excessive exposure, other biochemical abnormalities may be observed. Lead interferes with several steps in porphyrin synthesis (see p. 343), and porphyrinuria (mainly caused by coproporphyrin III) may be present in lead poisoning, although this is not a very sensitive test. An excess of δ-aminolaevulinic acid in the urine is also characteristic but is not specific. An excess of protoporphyrin in erythrocytes is a more sensitive indicator of excessive exposure to lead, but again is not specific, also occurring in iron deficiency.

Clinical features and management

Lead poisoning causes nausea, vomiting and severe abdominal colic. In the nervous system, encephalopathy with convulsions and impairment of consciousness may lead to coma and death. In severe cases, usually caused by acute lead poisoning, treatment is with a chelating agent, for example oral dimercaptosuccinic acid, to promote lead excretion. For an asymptomatic patient whose blood concentration indicates excessive exposure to lead, the source

of lead should be identified and removed or the exposed person removed from the source.

Other metals

Chemical pathology laboratories are involved in screening for other industrial toxins, especially heavy metals such as cadmium and mercury. Also, people with some types of metal-on-metal joint replacements are at risk of absorbing trace metals from particulate matter within the joint space, and in the UK it is now obligatory to check blood concentrations of **chromium** and **cobalt** in such patients.

Ethanol

Although there is no specific antidote to ethanol, drug overdose is often complicated by the simultaneous ingestion of ethanol. It potentiates the action of many drugs, and measurement of blood ethanol concentration may provide the explanation for an unexpected delay in a patient's recovery.

Blood ethanol measurements may also be of value in the management of patients with head injuries. The effects of ethanol may make it difficult to assess the clinical effect of the injury, but a low ethanol concentration should suggest that the head injury, rather than the alcohol, is the cause of any neurological deficit.

Clinical features and effects

Acutely, ethanol is a central nervous system (CNS) depressant; its metabolism increases the lactate/pyruvate ratio, causes hyperlactataemia and inhibits gluconeogenesis, which can cause hypoglycaemia, especially in children and malnourished individuals (see p. 250). Excessive intake, particularly on a background of chronic ingestion, can cause ketoacidosis. Chronic alcoholism is a major health problem in many areas of the world. In addition to its well-known harmful effects on the liver, chronic ethanol ingestion can damage many organs and tissues in the body. Metabolic sequelae include hypertriglyceridaemia, hypoglycaemia, hypogonadism, hyperuricaemia, a form of Cushing syndrome, thiamin deficiency and porphyria cutanea tarda (cutaneous hepatic porphyria, see p. 342).

The combination of a raised plasma γ-glutamyltransferase and increased mean red cell volume is a characteristic index of excessive ethanol intake in recent weeks, although not a specific one. The values may be normal in some individuals with a high ethanol intake, and increases in each can be caused by many other possible disorders. Measurement of carbohydrate-deficient transferrin (plasma concentration tending to increase with a high ethanol intake) has been promoted as a useful test in this context, but as with other tests, significant numbers of false negative results occur.

Case history 21.5

History

A garage mechanic was admitted to the emergency department unconscious, having been found in this state at home by his flatmate. He had been acutely depressed since the death of his girlfriend in a road traffic accident 2 weeks before.

Examination

He was unrousable. Temperature, blood pressure and pulse were normal, but he was hyperventilating.

Results

Serum:		
	sodium	138 mmol/L
	potassium	5.2 mmol/L
	bicarbonate	4 mmol/L
	urea	7.0 mmol/L
	creatinine	110 µmol/L
	eGFR	69 mL/min/1.73 m^2
	adjusted calcium	1.5 mmol/L
	osmolality	326 mmol/kg
	phosphate, protein and 'liver function' tests were within reference limits	
	paracetamol, salicylate	not detected
Plasma:	glucose	4.5 mmol/L
Blood:	hydrogen ion	104 nmol/L (pH 6.98)
	$P\text{CO}_2$	2.0 kPa
	ketones	0.4 mmol/L (<0.6)

Summary

Profound metabolic acidosis with severe hypocalcaemia and high osmolality.

Interpretation

There is a severe acidosis with a low $P\text{CO}_2$ indicating a degree of respiratory compensation. Diabetic ketoacidosis is excluded by the normal glucose and ketones. The calculated osmolarity is ~288 mmol/L, giving an osmolar gap of 38 mmol/L (see p. 38).

Discussion

The osmolar gap indicates the presence of some other osmotically active substance(s) in the blood. A lactate concentration high enough to account for the osmolar gap of 38 mmol/L would be exceptional even in severe lactic acidosis. The substance could be ethanol (although the acidosis of ethanol poisoning is usually a ketoacidosis) or some other alcohol. The clue to the diagnosis is provided by the low calcium concentration. The combination of severe acidosis and hypocalcaemia is characteristic of ethylene glycol poisoning. This substance (a component of antifreeze) is metabolized to various organic acids, including oxalic acid, which combines with calcium to form insoluble calcium oxalate. This can precipitate in tissues and in the renal tubules and urine. Acute kidney injury may occur. Ethylene glycol assays are available for confirmation and monitoring but results are rarely available in time to institute treatment.

Ethylene glycol poisoning is treated by giving a competitive inhibitor of alcohol dehydrogenase to block the metabolism of ethylene glycol to toxic organic acids. Ethanol has been used for this purpose, but 4-methylpyrazole (fomepizole) is now preferred. Hypocalcaemia and acidosis may require correction. Haemodialysis may be required in severe cases.

The detection of ethanol in urine or blood is the most reliable indicator of very recent ingestion of ethanol. Measurement of ethanol in breath or blood is required to establish acute toxicity. Poisoning with other alcohols is discussed in Case history 21.5.

Poisons causing formation of abnormal haemoglobin derivatives

Methaemoglobin is oxidized haemoglobin, with iron in the Fe^{3+} form. It is incapable of carrying oxygen. A small amount is normally produced spontaneously in red blood cells but is reduced back to haemoglobin enzymatically. Excessive methaemoglobin (**methaemoglobinaemia**) can be **congenital** or **acquired**. It can occur as a result of the ingestion of large amounts of certain drugs, such as sulphonamides, and also in some haemoglobinopathies, with an inherited deficiency of the reductase enzyme. In toxic methaemoglobinaemia, the presence of free methaemoglobin in the urine may give it a brown colour.

Acute toxic methaemoglobinaemia causes symptoms of anaemia and may lead to vascular collapse and death. The major clinical manifestation of congenital methaemoglobinaemia is **cyanosis**. Methaemoglobinaemia can be treated with **methylthioninium chloride** (methylene blue) or **ascorbic acid**, agents that reduce the abnormal derivative back to haemoglobin.

Carboxyhaemoglobin (COHb) is formed from haemoglobin in the presence of **carbon monoxide**, the affinity of the pigment for this gas being some **200× greater than for oxygen**. Because of this, even small quantities of carbon monoxide in the inspired air can result in the formation of large amounts of COHb, and hence greatly reduce the oxygen-carrying capacity of the blood. The binding of carbon monoxide to haemoglobin causes a left shift in the oxyhaemoglobin dissociation curve (see p. 378), further decreasing the availability of oxygen to tissues.

Carbon monoxide is produced by the incomplete combustion of fuels. Small amounts of COHb (<2%) are commonly present in the blood of urban dwellers, and greater amounts (up to 10%) may be found in the blood of tobacco smokers. Chronic carbon monoxide poisoning is usually the result of poorly fitted or maintained gas appliances in the home. Exposure to motor car exhaust in a confined space (e.g. a closed garage) is a well-recognized means of suicide and, occasionally, homicide.

Measurement of COHb is critical to the diagnosis of carbon monoxide poisoning. Treatment is to provide a high inspired concentration of oxygen, sometimes at greater than atmospheric pressure in a hyperbaric oxygen chamber, to increase the rate of dissociation of carbon monoxide from the haemoglobin molecule.

These derivatives of haemoglobin can be identified by their spectral characteristics. Most blood gas analyzers incorporate a **co-oximeter** to measure the concentrations of haemoglobin, methaemoglobin and COHb in this way.

Other poisons

The amfetamine derivative MDMA (ecstasy) is widely used as a recreational drug. Although significant toxicity is uncommon, it can cause hyperpyrexia, leading to increased fluid intake, and this, coupled with stimulation of vasopressin secretion, can cause severe hyponatraemia.

The possibility of poisoning should always be investigated in a comatose patient when no cause is obvious. Poisoning can usually be diagnosed from the history (obtained from a witness if necessary), clinical examination and simple laboratory investigations. In addition, measurement of plasma osmolality and comparison with the calculated value may sometimes reveal the presence of a foreign substance in the blood, as demonstrated in Case history 21.5. Expert advice is always available in the UK through the National Poisons Information Service.

Screening for Drugs

When a toxin does not have a specific antidote, precise knowledge of its plasma concentration contributes little to patient management. Nevertheless, qualitative rather than quantitative measurement of a toxic agent may be desirable. If a patient is admitted to hospital **unconscious for no readily discernible reason**, identification of a drug may help to eliminate other possible causes. It may also draw attention to possible specific complications or suggest treatment (e.g. haemofiltration or dialysis) to remove the drug from the body.

Screening for drugs is also necessary in cases of **suspected brain death**. Symptoms of apparent brain death may be caused by the presence of CNS-depressant drugs, and it is vital that this possibility is eliminated before true brain death is diagnosed. When drug measurements are made for medicolegal reasons, it is essential that secure evidence of a chain of custody is maintained, so that there is no doubt about the identity of the specimens subjected to analysis.

In cases of **suspected homicide**, the identification of any poisons present is critical and must be carried out by suitably qualified personnel whose testimony would be accepted in court as witnesses.

It is not practical for all laboratories to provide facilities for screening for all possible toxins. In the UK, there is a network of poisons reference laboratories that provide advice and an analytical service for such purposes.

Drug and substance abuse

Many drugs and chemicals are widely abused, and laboratories play an important role in screening for some of these. This may be required for medicolegal reasons (e.g. for monitoring drivers of some heavy goods vehicles) but is also important to confirm what drugs are being taken and to monitor adherence to treatment in drug dependent patients (e.g. for those on methadone maintenance programmes for opiate addiction). Increasingly, screening tests are performed within substance misuse clinics by point-of-care technology, although all positive results should be confirmed by more specific analytical methods that allow identification of individual substances, because some prescribed or over-the-counter medications can cross-react in the screening tests. Some point-of-care tests are optimized for use with saliva.

Samples for drugs-of-abuse testing should be collected after consultation with the local laboratory. Urine is, in general, more useful for screening or confirmation than blood, because many drugs and their metabolites are cleared rapidly from the blood but will be present in higher concentration in the urine. Patterns of misuse of therapeutic drugs, 'recreational' drugs and drugs of abuse are always changing. As a result, laboratories must keep their repertoire of drug tests under constant review, so that they are able to offer an appropriate analytical service. Considerable expertise is required in both the analyses and the interpretation of the results, so this service is generally provided by a small number of specialist laboratories.

Sample collection in patients with suspected poisoning

If a patient is admitted to hospital acutely unwell or comatose, it can be difficult to tell whether poisoning is the cause or even a contributory factor. Although assays for some commonly used poisons such as salicylate and paracetamol are rapidly accessible, most toxicology investigations are not available in a time frame suitable for immediate patient management. If poisoning is suspected, it is good practice to ask the laboratory to save samples of blood and urine in case subsequent testing is required. Stomach contents may also be worth storing, as are any tablets or materials thought to be involved with the poisoning. Although it is rarely helpful to perform a wide toxicology screen, targeted analysis (based on the clinical presentation of the patient and advice from a toxicology centre) can be informative. The laboratory should also be alerted if there is involvement by the coroner or the police so that samples can be handled and stored appropriately.

Pharmacogenomics

The body's reaction to drugs is determined by many factors, including genetics. Polymorphisms in enzymes involved in drug metabolism may affect the rate at which a drug is metabolized, whether to an inactive or an active metabolite. It is likely that, in the future, genetic analysis of individuals may allow a more bespoke usage of drugs (both in relation to choice of drug and dosage). Such an approach might be of particular value when the use of an especially expensive drug, or a drug known to have a significant risk of causing toxicity, is being considered. The genetic influences on azathioprine metabolism have already been discussed and pretreatment screening for deficiency of TPMT is routine in many countries. More recently, the gene responsible for the enzyme that metabolises 5-fluorouracil (5FU, an anticancer drug), has been sequenced. Almost 10% of the population have genetic variants that reduce or abolish the activity of the enzyme and are at risk of severe toxicity from 5FU. Although not yet widely available, genetic testing can identify those patients in whom treatment with 5FU should be avoided.

SUMMARY

- **TDM** is the measurement of the concentration of drugs, usually in blood, to provide a guide to the dose to prescribe. It is valuable for drugs that have a low therapeutic ratio (i.e. the dose required for a therapeutic effect is only slightly lower than that which causes toxicity) and when it is difficult to assess their effects clinically.
- Drugs for which TDM is useful include **phenytoin, lithium, digoxin, aminoglycoside antibiotics, theophylline, ciclosporin, tacrolimus and sirolimus.**
- TDM is **not required** for drugs whose effects can readily be assessed clinically or by other clinical or laboratory measurements, or when a drug of low toxicity has a virtually guaranteed effect when given in a standard dose. It is of no value when the effect of a drug is due to a metabolite, unless the concentration of the metabolite can be measured.
- Measurements of antidrug antibodies in patients being treated with some of the newer 'biologics' (e.g. infliximab) can differentiate inadequate dosing from acquired resistance to treatment.
- Measurements of drug concentrations in body fluids are valuable in the investigation and management of patients who have taken **overdoses of drugs** or been **poisoned.** While the management of many forms of poisoning and drug overdosage is essentially conservative, so that identification of the substance is of little direct use in management, for those drugs for which specific antidotes exist,

or for which it is possible to take measures to promote their excretion, measurement of plasma concentrations may be very helpful. Examples include **paracetamol**, for which the value of treatment with N-acetylcysteine to prevent hepatic damage can be predicted from the plasma paracetamol concentration, and **aspirin**, for which the plasma salicylate concentration provides a guide to the use of urinary alkalinization to accelerate excretion of the drug.
- Other toxins for which measurement of plasma concentrations can be valuable in management include **iron** and **lead.**
- Some poisons reduce the oxygen-carrying capacity of haemoglobin, for example, by forming **COHb** or **methaemoglobin.**
- Many drugs and poisons cause metabolic disturbances, particularly in acid–base, glucose and sodium, water and potassium homoeostasis, and clinical chemistry laboratories have an important role in the management of patients who develop such disturbances.
- A further role is in relation to the detection of **drugs of abuse**, and the monitoring of patients on treatment programmes for drug dependency.
- Increasingly, genetic or enzyme tests are being used to predict how a patient will metabolise a drug, e.g. measurement of thiopurine methyltransferase in patients being considered for treatment with **azathioprine.**

Chapter | 22 |

Clinical chemistry in children

Introduction

The investigation and management of illness in children is affected by a number of specific special issues. These include:

- different patterns of disease
- different presentation of disease
- different reference ranges.

Chronic disease and polypharmacy are fortunately less common in this age group, and generally healing processes are faster and there is good functional organ reserve. Caution should still be taken, as during development children may be very sensitive to pathological and pharmacological insult with long-term sequelae, and the functional reserve can mask early pathology until the child presents *in extremis.*

For children, a particular problem for the clinical biochemist relates to the size of the blood sample. For the very young, it is essential to apply analytical methods that will use the smallest possible amount of plasma, and this may mean using special equipment. Small quantities of capillary blood can be conveniently collected by pricking the baby's heel, but this should be done by experienced personnel, as the results obtained may be affected by haemolysis or by contamination with tissue fluid. If the sample obtained is particularly small, it is advisable to prioritize the tests that are the most important for that infant.

Complete, accurately timed collections of urine are difficult to obtain in children. It is usually more reliable to relate the concentrations of urinary constituents to urinary creatinine concentration.

In the immediate neonatal period, the concentrations of metabolites in infants may still reflect maternal metabolism and may be affected by the function of organs that are relatively immature. Pharmacokinetics can also be different in neonates compared with older children or adults. Many conditions present exclusively, or predominantly, in the neonatal period; examples include many congenital diseases and inherited metabolic disorders (see Chapter 19). Other disorders may become apparent at any time during childhood; in particular, disorders of growth and of sexual differentiation and development. The occurrence of some tumours is confined to, or significantly greater in, childhood. Examples include neuroblastoma, hepatoblastoma and acute lymphoblastic leukaemia. Biochemical investigations are of value in the diagnosis of the first two of these (catecholamines and α-fetoprotein) and are discussed on pp. 190 and 358, respectively.

Paediatric medicine no longer begins with the birth of the child. It is now becoming possible to treat some fetal disorders *in utero,* and clinical biochemistry laboratories will be required to provide an appropriate service to support this.

In a book of this size, it is possible only to outline some of the more important areas where paediatric medicine and clinical biochemistry interact. The reader seeking more detailed information should consult more specialized textbooks.

Reference ranges

The reference ranges for certain analytes are different in the newborn from the adult (Table 22.1) and may vary through childhood; some even continue to change throughout adulthood, such as plasma low-density lipoprotein (LDL) cholesterol which continues to rise from birth and uric acid which, after a rapid reduction in the first year, continues to rise gradually with age. A result should always be interpreted in light of the reference range appropriate to the child's age. The age-related changes in plasma alkaline phosphatase and immunoglobulins are discussed in Chapter 16 and Case history 22.1. The glomerular

Case history 22.1

History

A 26-month-old boy was brought to hospital with a history of diarrhoea for a week. His older sibling had caught gastroenteritis at school, but his parents were concerned about the longer duration of his symptoms and the fact that he had been eating things in the garden.

Examination

Normal, and no significant weight loss as, except for the first 2 days, he had been eating well and the loose stools were infrequent.

Results (see Appendix for reference ranges)

Serum:		
calcium (adjusted)	2.32 mmol/L	
total bilirubin	12 µmol/L	
alanine aminotransferase	22 U/L	
alkaline phosphatase	868 U/L (156–369)	

Summary

Isolated hyperphosphatasaemia.

Interpretation

Alkaline phosphatase activities are higher in children than adults and peaks occur during growth spurts (see p. 296 and Fig. 16.5). However, the result is higher than expected (reference range given is for males aged 1–10 years old) and therefore, in the absence of any other concerning features, this could represent transient hyperphosphatasaemia.

Discussion

Transient hyperphosphatasaemia is a diagnosis of exclusion in children under 5 years of age with an isolated increase in alkaline phosphatase and no clinical or biochemical evidence of liver or bone disease (or bone fractures). Liver and bone isoforms, if measured, are both elevated, and the condition resolves within 6 months with no adverse sequelae. Measurement of alkaline phosphatase should be repeated within 3–4 months and further investigations for other causes undertaken if the increased enzyme activity has not resolved.

Table 22.1 Common analytes with different reference ranges in children

Analyte	Difference
potassium	mean and upper limit higher in newborn
calcium	higher at birth; normal adult concentrations by 72 h
phosphate	higher at birth, then falls but remains higher than adult concentrations throughout childhood; rises at puberty, then falls to adult concentration
alkaline phosphatase	as phosphate but more marked rise and fall at puberty
creatinine	rapid decrease after birth; gradual increase to adult values, particularly after puberty
thyroid-stimulating hormone	rapid increase for a few days immediately after birth; slightly higher than adult values maintained throughout childhood
free thyroxine	higher for first month, slowly falling to reach values similar to adulthood by 1 year

Screening

The well-established programmes for neonatal screening for phenylketonuria, congenital hypothyroidism, cystic fibrosis, sickle cell disease and medium-chain acyl-CoA dehydrogenase deficiency, as well as other rarer disorders, are discussed in Chapter 19. Screening programmes for other conditions are being introduced or piloted: although the number of conditions for which screening is theoretically possible is considerable, it is important to assess both the benefits and the potential pitfalls of doing so before introducing nationwide programmes (see Box 2.1).

The rapid increase in the identification of mutations responsible for many inherited metabolic diseases, together with the development of techniques for obtaining and analyzing fetal DNA, is increasing the availability of reliable antenatal screening, particularly in high-risk pregnancies (i.e. where there is a strong family history of a particular disorder). The increasing use of molecular techniques to define disease conditions in both adults and children has allowed more definitive disease classification and presymptomatic detection in children of all ages. The myriad benefits of this approach must be balanced by the problems associated with medicalising what might otherwise have been a normal childhood.

filtration rate (GFR) increases throughout childhood as the kidneys grow, but if scaled for surface area, which is a marker of kidney size, it reaches adult values by the age of 2 years. The formulae used to calculate estimated GFR in adults are not valid in children, in whom it can be estimated using a formula that includes the child's age, sex and height.

Changes in disease prevalence in childhood may also influence future screening programmes. For example, HbA_{1c}, which is used in targeted screening for type 2 diabetes mellitus in adults, is not currently recommended routinely for diagnosis in children as, until recently, they have suffered almost exclusively from type 1 diabetes mellitus. With the increasing prevalence of childhood obesity, type 2 diabetes now accounts for ~2% of the paediatric population with diabetes in the UK. If this trend continues, future targeted screening with HbA_{1c} measurement in the highest risk groups could allow early intervention and prevention of diabetes.

Childhood disorders

Neonatal hypoglycaemia

Neonatal hypoglycaemia is an important condition that is discussed in Chapter 13. It is particularly likely to occur in low birthweight infants, both premature and 'small-for-dates' infants born to diabetic mothers, and infants who are ill or who have feeding problems. In such infants, blood glucose measurements should be made every 4 h for the first 48 h and at appropriate intervals thereafter to monitor treatment if hypoglycaemia has occurred. Persistent hypoglycaemia or requirement for a high-rate glucose infusion to prevent hypoglycaemia should prompt a search for metabolic and endocrine causes (see Fig. 13.8).

Neonatal hypocalcaemia and hypomagnesaemia

The clinical signs of hypoglycaemia include irritability, twitching and convulsions. If the baby's plasma glucose concentration is not low, hypocalcaemia or hypomagnesaemia, which present with similar signs, should be suspected.

Plasma calcium concentration, which at birth is higher (up to 3.00 mmol/L) than in healthy adults, falls rapidly and then rises to reach adult values by the third or fourth day of life. This transient, physiological hypocalcaemia is rarely symptomatic but tends to be exaggerated, and may be symptomatic, in preterm infants, infants born to mothers with diabetes and following birth asphyxia. It can be prevented by giving adequate calcium; if the baby is not feeding normally, intravenous calcium may be required.

Hypocalcaemia occurring after the first 2–3 days of life is uncommon. Causes are shown in Box 22.1. Most of these conditions are discussed in Chapter 14. Hypocalcaemia is a potential complication of exchange blood transfusion (clotting of donor blood is prevented by chelation of calcium ions) and can be prevented by giving calcium during transfusion.

Hypocalcaemia is often accompanied by hypomagnesaemia, and magnesium supplements should be given together with calcium in treating hypocalcaemia. If magnesium is not given, hypocalcaemia is often resistant to

> **Box 22.1 Causes of hypocalcaemia in infancy**
>
> high phosphate intake (unmodified cows' milk)
> vitamin D deficiency
> hypoparathyroidism including DiGeorge syndrome
> pseudohypoparathyroidism
> blood transfusion (exchange transfusion)
> hypomagnesaemia
> transient neonatal hypocalcaemia

treatment. Isolated hypomagnesaemia is rare: it most frequently occurs in the infants of mothers with diabetes.

Jaundice

Most newborns become mildly jaundiced shortly after birth. This **'physiological' jaundice** is due to immaturity of the hepatic conjugating enzymes, normal postnatal haemolysis and enterohepatic circulation of bilirubin (conversion of bilirubin to urobilinogen in the gut cannot occur until the gut becomes colonized with bacteria). In physiological jaundice, the bilirubin is primarily unconjugated and its plasma concentration rarely exceeds 100 μmol/L; the jaundice is never present at birth and does not persist beyond 14 days of life. Physiological jaundice can be exacerbated by various factors, including dehydration, hypoxia, prematurity, breast-feeding and birth trauma leading to bruising or a cephalohaematoma.

At high concentrations of unconjugated bilirubin (>340 μmol/L in a full-term newborn) there is a **risk of brain damage** (kernicterus) developing. The risk is higher in premature infants. As unconjugated bilirubin is bound to albumin, the risk is greater if the plasma albumin concentration is decreased or bilirubin is displaced from albumin, for example by hydrogen ions in acidosis, by certain drugs or by high concentrations of free fatty acids. Unconjugated hyperbilirubinaemia can be treated by increasing water intake, phototherapy or exchange transfusion as appropriate, and of course by treatment of the underlying cause if this can be ascertained and treatment is feasible. National treatment thresholds in the UK for phototherapy, followed by exchange transfusion, are based on gestational age and time since birth in hours. Circumstances that should prompt investigation of neonatal jaundice are given in Box 22.2.

Other causes of unconjugated hyperbilirubinaemia in the newborn are given in Box 22.3. There are also many causes of **conjugated hyperbilirubinaemia** (i.e. >25% of total bilirubin is conjugated, or conjugated bilirubin

> Jaundice before 24 hours of life is never physiological and must be investigated urgently. Plasma bilirubin concentration must be measured within 2 h and the necessary management instigated without delay.

concentration is >25 µmol/L): this is **always pathological**. Some of the more important causes are listed in Box 22.4.

Inherited metabolic disorders

Although inherited metabolic diseases are **individually rare**, they are collectively an important cause of illness in

the neonatal period. Conditions that may present at this time include disorders of amino acid, organic acid and carbohydrate metabolism, and urea cycle disorders (see Case histories 22.2 and 22.3). If an inherited metabolic disease is suspected, accurate diagnosis is essential. It is important to collect and preserve appropriate samples (usually blood and urine) at presentation, because treatment may reverse the typical (often diagnostic) biochemical abnormalities.

The **clinical features** of metabolic disorders are rarely specific to any one condition; the salt loss and virilization of female infants with steroid 21-hydroxylase deficiency (see p. 188) are exceptional in this respect. Some clinical features, such as severe acidosis and coma (see p. 336), suggest that a metabolic disorder may be present, but in many cases they are non-specific, with babies affected by such disorders presenting, for example, with vomiting or 'failure to thrive'.

The determination of the precise **diagnosis** of a metabolic disorder may require complex and lengthy investigation, so it is important to be able to carry out some simple screening tests to indicate whether a metabolic disorder may be the cause of a baby's illness. An appropriate selection is shown in Table 19.3. If the results of these are all normal, a metabolic disorder is unlikely; if there are abnormalities, the pattern of these may suggest a possible diagnosis or indicate what further investigations would be appropriate. It is important that the child should, if at all possible, be on a normal diet when these tests are done: potential abnormalities may otherwise be masked. Thus, disorders associated with an abnormal pattern of amino acid excretion may be missed if the infant does not have a normal protein intake.

If a baby suspected of having an inherited metabolic disease appears likely to die before a diagnosis has been established, it is essential that samples of blood, urine and skin (for fibroblast culture) are taken during life or immediately *postmortem*. Making a diagnosis after death will be valuable in counselling and management should another pregnancy be contemplated. Samples of liver and muscle may also be helpful for this purpose. Guidelines for investigating sudden unexpected deaths in infants and children are produced by various societies and professional bodies.

Failure to thrive

Failure to thrive is a term used to describe a failure of infants to grow and develop normally. It is a common paediatric problem, and can be a consequence of any acute illness in neonates and more chronic conditions at any time in infancy: some of the more important examples of the latter are listed in Box 22.6. Most are discussed elsewhere in this book. Accurate clinical and anthropometric (e.g. measurement of growth velocity) assessment is essential, but when there are no clinical features, either in the history or on examination, to suggest a specific diagnosis, the results of tests listed in Table 19.3, together with simple haematological tests and

Case history 22.2

History

A female infant, born at 38 weeks by spontaneous vaginal delivery to a primigravid woman, presented at day three with slow feeding and frequent vomiting after feeds. The parents had noticed she looked yellow.

Examination

Jaundiced with an enlarged liver and bilateral cataracts.

Results

Serum:		
	total bilirubin	168 µmol/L
	conjugated bilirubin	45 µmol/L
	alanine aminotransferase	122 U/L
	alkaline phosphatase	244 U/L
		(90–273)

Summary

Significant conjugated hyperbilirubinaemia in a neonate with elevated aminotransferase but normal for age (reference range given for females <14 days old) alkaline phosphatase activity.

Interpretation

This pattern is typical of 'neonatal hepatitis'—a term used to denote hepatic inflammation with patent bile ducts—the causes of which include infection (congenital and acquired) and various metabolic disorders. Conjugated hyperbilirubinaemia in neonates is always pathological. The presence of cataracts suggests a diagnosis of galactosaemia (see p. 337).

Discussion

The child was started on a galactose-free feed and improved clinically. The diagnosis was confirmed by the finding of a low erythrocyte galactose 1-phosphate uridyltransferase activity. False negatives can occur if samples are taken within 3 months of a blood transfusion, in which case carrier status can be confirmed in the parents whilst awaiting the appropriate opportunity to sample the child. Testing for urine-reducing substances is neither a sensitive nor a specific test for galactosaemia, but their presence in a symptomatic infant may trigger further investigation for this disorder.

Case history 22.3

History

Thirty-six hours after birth, born at term after a normal pregnancy, a male infant was brought to hospital with vomiting. He then developed grunting respiration and rapidly became lethargic and unresponsive. The parents were first cousins; it was the woman's first pregnancy.

Examination

He appeared physically normal.

Results

A metabolic screen revealed a very high plasma ammonia concentration (>1000 µmol/L), but the infant was not acidotic. The plasma urea was at the lower end of the reference range. Subsequently, plasma amino acid analysis showed an excess of glutamine and alanine.

Summary

Hyperammonaemia, with a presentation and clinical signs typical of toxic encephalopathy.

Interpretation

Although there are many causes of hyperammonaemia (Box 22.5), a case as severe as this, without any suggestion of liver disease, and in a child born of a first-cousin marriage should raise the suspicion of an inherited metabolic disorder. The excess plasma amino acids, low–normal urea and lack of acidosis are consistent with a urea cycle disorder. Patients with organic acidaemias and hyperammonaemia are usually acidotic: patients with urea cycle disorders are usually not. This child's urine was found to contain a high concentration of orotic acid. This pattern of abnormalities suggests ornithine transcarbamylase (OTC) deficiency, and this was confirmed by enzyme analysis of a *postmortem* biopsy of the liver as despite intensive treatment, including peritoneal dialysis, the baby died 72 h after birth.

Discussion

Hyperammonaemia is an important cause of both morbidity and mortality in infants: urgent analysis must be performed in acute paediatric presentations. Consanguineous parents, or a history of a previous neonatal death, should increase suspicion that an inherited metabolic disease may be responsible for a child's illness. In this patient, however, parental consanguinity was coincidental, because OTC deficiency is an X-linked disorder.

Deficiencies of all five enzymes of the urea cycle occur. The plasma amino acid profile is specific in citrullinaemia (arginosuccinic acid synthetase deficiency), arginosuccinic aciduria (argininosuccinase deficiency) and arginase deficiency, but may be normal or non-specifically abnormal in OTC deficiency and carbamyl phosphate synthetase deficiency; of these two, orotic aciduria occurs only with OTC deficiency. All five disorders can be diagnosed by measurement of enzyme activity in a liver biopsy.

a screen for infectious disease, will in many cases provide a starting point for definitive investigation.

A significant increase in growth rate occurs during puberty, and delayed puberty may be diagnosed (particularly in boys) because of short stature. Notably, growth hormone deficiency is a rare but important cause of growth failure, as it can be effectively treated by hormone replacement, with the best results obtained if this is started early in childhood. It is considered in more detail

---

Box 22.5 Some causes of hyperammonaemia in infancy

transient neonatal hyperammonaemia[a]
inherited disorders of the urea cycle[a]
other inherited metabolic disorders[a] such as organic
   acidaemias
liver disease (including Reye syndrome[b])
severe systemic illness[a] (asphyxia, infection, sepsis)
parenteral nutrition (excessive amino acid input)
sodium valproate therapy

---

[a]Important causes in the newborn.
[b]Reye syndrome is a cause of encephalopathy in children, associated with fatty infiltration of the liver and hyperammonaemia; the cause is not known, but there is an association with aspirin treatment.

Box 22.7 Some causes of precocious puberty

Gonadotrophin dependent

idiopathic (particularly females)
pineal tumours, hypothalamic hamartomas
raised intracranial pressure (trauma, hydrocephalus)
cerebral palsy
cranial irradiation

Gonadotrophin independent[a]

congenital adrenal hyperplasia
adrenal tumours
ovarian and testicular tumours

---

[a]Also known as pseudoprecocious puberty.

Box 22.6 Some causes of failure to thrive

malnutrition
malabsorption
inherited metabolic diseases
infection
chronic diseases
   renal
   hepatic
   pulmonary
   cardiac
psychosocial deprivation
hypothyroidism
hypopituitarism

Box 22.8 Disorders of sexual development (DSD)

Male DSD

(46, XY: genotypic males with incomplete masculinization)
decreased androgen production:
   various inherited enzyme abnormalities
impaired androgen metabolism:
   5α-reductase deficiency
   androgen insensitivity syndromes
complete and partial gonadal dysgenesis

Female DSD

(46, XX: genotypic females with virilization)
androgen excess
   congenital adrenal hyperplasia
   Cushing syndrome
   premature adrenarche
   androgen-secreting ovarian tumours
gonadal dysgenesis (ovotesticular and testicular DSD)

Sex chromosome DSD

Turner syndrome (45, XO and variants)
Klinefelter syndrome (47, XXY and variants)
45, XO / 46, XY (mixed gonadal dysgenesis)
46, XX / 46, XY (chimeric)

---

in Chapter 9, as are the effects and diagnosis of growth hormone excess.

Disorders of sex development and abnormal puberty

Precocious sex development, which may become apparent shortly after birth, is rare: some causes are given in Box 22.7. True precocious puberty (also known as gonadotrophin-dependent precocious puberty), in which the gonads are fully developed and contain gametes, should be distinguished from pseudoprecocious puberty (which is gonadotrophin independent), in which they are not. Pseudoprecocious puberty is often amenable to treatment, whereas true precocity is often not. Delayed puberty is much more common: it is discussed in detail in Chapter 12.

Virilization of females is also discussed in Chapter 12. It is rare in children: causes include congenital adrenal hyperplasia (CAH), Cushing syndrome, adrenal tumours and premature adrenarche (in all of which the adrenals are the source of the excess androgens), and ovarian tumours. Some disorders of sex development present with ambiguous genitalia at birth. It is worth noting, however, that although this may be obvious

in genetically female (XX) patients, it may be less obvious in genotypic males (XY). This can result in delayed diagnosis, for example of some of the rarer types of adrenal hormone deficiency, until they present later with severe salt-losing crises (see p. 189).

These conditions can be very complex: some examples, classified on the basis of the karyotype, are listed in Box 22.8. Although rare, all these conditions are of immense importance to the patients and their parents, and laboratory investigations are vital in their diagnosis and management.

SUMMARY

- **Many biochemical and physiological functions change with age**; some of these are related to specific events, in particular puberty, but for others the change is more gradual. This must be borne in mind when interpreting biochemical results, and ideally, such results should, where appropriate, be compared with age-related reference ranges. Examples include plasma phosphate concentration and alkaline phosphatase activity (both higher) and cholesterol and urate (both lower in childhood).

- **Screening programmes** prevent avoidable morbidity and mortality, and many are well established. Progress in test and treatment development and changes in disease patterns will influence the future repertoire of screening tests and programmes.

- **Metabolic problems** that occur particularly frequently in the newborn include **hypoglycaemia, hypocalcaemia and hypomagnesaemia.**

- **Jaundice** occurs frequently in the first few days of life, but in most cases this is benign. This 'physiological' jaundice is due to an increase in unconjugated bilirubin. Conjugated hyperbilirubinaemia is always pathological.

- The clinical features of **inherited metabolic disorders** presenting in infancy and childhood are often non-specific. For children who, for example, fail to thrive or show unusual irritability or lethargy, simple screening tests on urine and plasma should be performed to identify any abnormality that might be caused by an inherited metabolic disease. Samples should be collected and preserved as quickly as possible after presentation, because treatment may reverse the typical biochemical abnormalities.

- There are many causes of **growth failure**, including systemic disease, social deprivation and malabsorption; relatively few cases are due to growth hormone deficiency. Again, the results of accurate clinical assessment, combined with simple laboratory tests, will often indicate the diagnosis, and thus the appropriate mode of treatment.

- **Disorders of sex development** are uncommon but, after clinical assessment, the results of laboratory tests (e.g. measurement of the concentrations of adrenal and gonadal hormones, and gonadotrophins) are often of vital importance in formulating a differential diagnosis and indicating the course of further investigations. This is also true of delayed puberty, a much more common complaint.

Appendix

Adult Reference Ranges

These adult reference ranges are provided for the interpretation of data presented in the case histories. Readers should note that reference ranges may differ between laboratories; this applies particularly to hormones and enzymes. All values are for concentrations (activities in the case of enzymes) in serum or plasma, except where indicated otherwise. Uniform reference ranges have been introduced across the UK for many common analytes, but this has not yet been achieved where, for example, there are significant differences between the analytical methods used or in their standardization. Reference ranges for some other, less frequently measured analytes are given within the relevant case history.

adrenocorticotrophic hormone (ACTH) at 09.00 h	<50 ng/L
alanine aminotransferase (ALT)	10–50 U/L
albumin	35–50 g/L
alkaline phosphatase	30–130 U/L
ammonia	10–50 µmol/L
amylase	<120 U/L
bicarbonate (total CO_2)	22–29 mmol/L
bilirubin (total)	3–20 µmol/L
calcium (adjusted)	2.2–2.6 mmol/L
carbon dioxide (P_{CO_2}) (arterial blood)	4.5–6.0 kPa (35–46 mmHg)
cholesterol:	
total	<4.0 mmol/L[a]
high-density lipoprotein (HDL)	>1.2 mmol/L[a]
low-density lipoprotein (LDL)	<1.8 mmol/L[a]
non-HDL-cholesterol	<2.5 mmol/L[a]
copper	12–19 µmol/L
cortisol at:	
09.00 h	140–690 nmol/L
24.00 h	<100 nmol/L
C-reactive protein	<10 mg/L
creatine kinase (total):	
males	40–320 U/L
females	25–200 U/L

creatinine:	
males	60–110 µmol/L
females	50–95 µmol/L
α-fetoprotein (AFP)	<8 kU/L
follicle-stimulating hormone (FSH):	
males	1.5–12.4 IU/L
females	
follicular phase	3.5–12.5 IU/L
postmenopausal	>25 IU/L
glucose (fasting)	2.8–6.0 mmol/L
γ-glutamyltransferase (γGT):	
males	<70 U/L
females	<37 U/L
growth hormone:	
after glucose load	<0.3 µg/L
after stress	>5.0 µg/L
haemoglobin (whole blood):	
males	130–180 g/L
females	120–160 g/L
HbA_{1c} (glycated haemoglobin): see Fig. 13.4	
hydrogen ion (arterial blood)	35–46 nmol/L (pH 7.36–7.44)
insulin (in hypoglycaemia)	<18 pmol/L

luteinizing hormone (LH):		sodium	133–146 mmol/L
males	1.7–8.6 IU/L	testosterone:	
females		males at 09.00 h	9–30 nmol/L
follicular phase	2.4–12.6 IU/L	females	0.5–2.2 nmol/L
postmenopausal	7.7–58.5 IU/L	thyroid-stimulating hormone (TSH, thyrotrophin)	0.3–4.0 mIU/L
magnesium	0.7–1.0 mmol/L		
osmolality	275–295 mmol/kg	thyroxine (T4): free	12–22 pmol/L
oxygen (P_{O_2}) (arterial blood)	11–15 kPa (85–105 mmHg)	triglyceride (fasting)	0.4–1.7 mmol/L
		triiodothyronine (T3): free	3.9–6.7 pmol/L
parathyroid hormone	2–7 pmol/L	troponin T (cardiac, high sensitivity)	<14 ng/L
phosphate	0.8–1.5 mmol/L		
potassium	3.5–5.3 mmol/L	urea	2.5–7.8 mmol/L
prolactin:		uric acid:	
males	<300 mIU/L[b]	males	200–430 µmol/L
females	<500 mIU/L[b]	females	140–360 µmol/L
progesterone (females):		vitamin D	<25 nmol/L deficient
follicular phase	<4 nmol/L		25–50 nmol/L insufficient
luteal phase (ovulatory)	>30 nmol/L		>50 nmol/L sufficient
protein: total	60–80 g/L		
sex hormone binding globulin:			
males	20–75 nmol/L		
females	30–130 nmol/L	zinc	12–20 µmol/L

[a]Indicates ideal values in patients with established cardiovascular disease, see p. 317.
[b]Plasma prolactin concentrations <700 mIU/L are unlikely to be of clinical significance.

Index

Page numbers followed by '*f*' indicate figures, '*b*' indicate boxes, and '*t*' indicate tables.

Index